Stronger Than Infertility

The
Essential Guide
to Navigating Every Step
of Your Journey

Heather R. Huhman

WORKMAN PUBLISHING · NEW YORK

The tools and information presented herein are not intended to replace the services of a doctor or other health professionals, or be a substitute for medical or mental health advice. You are advised to consult with your health care professional with regard to matters relating to your physical or mental health, and in particular regarding matters that may require diagnosis or medical attention.

Any links or references to third-party resources are provided as a convenience and for informational purposes only; they do not constitute an endorsement or an approval by the author or publisher of any products, services, or opinions of a third party. While the information provided in this book is based upon sources that the author believes to be reliable, neither the author nor the publisher can control the accuracy, legality, accessibility, or content of any external site or resource referenced here. Please address any questions regarding third-party content to the owners of the external resource.

Library of Congress Cataloging-in-Publication Data is available.

ISBN 978-1-5235-0432-9

Design by Janet Vicario
Illustrations by Rachel Krohn
Alamy: Constantin: Cover and Back Cover background. **Shutterstock:** Crystal Eye Studio: p. 8; VerisStudio: Cover, Title Openers. **CanStock Photo:** sdCrea: Image repeated throughout.

Workman books are available at special discounts when purchased in bulk for premiums and sales promotions as well as for fundraising or educational use. Special editions or book excerpts can also be created to specification. For details, please contact special.markets@hbgusa.com.

Workman Publishing Co., Inc.,
a subsidiary of Hachette Book Group, Inc.
1290 Avenue of the Americas
New York, NY 10104

workman.com

WORKMAN is a registered trademark of Workman Publishing Co., Inc., a subsidiary of Hachette Book Group, Inc.

Printed in the United States of America on responsibly sourced paper.
First printing June 2023

10 9 8 7 6 5 4 3 2 1

Stronger Than Infertility

Contents

Foreword

I have always been a champion of educating people about their bodies so they can take control of their health. We spend most of our young lives learning how to avoid unwanted pregnancies. When we are ready for a family, we can be undereducated about how our bodies work, the unwavering countdown to ovarian shutdown, and our options when we need help.

As a board-certified reproductive endocrinologist, I have been trained in the ultra-specialized and high-tech field of infertility. I have also personally experienced the full range of infertility care and pregnancy loss.

I was sure that becoming pregnant with my second child would come easy after conceiving my first child easily and quickly as an ob-gyn resident. But this was very far from reality. It took years—along with multiple rounds of fertility treatment, inseminations, IVF, and embryo transfers, and multiple losses—to get pregnant with my second child, all while studying to be a fertility specialist. It seemed inconceivable that I was a fertility doctor who couldn't get pregnant! During my journey, I experienced grief, isolation, and sadness. I was so embarrassed that I didn't talk to others about what I was experiencing until long after my last child was delivered. That's when I finally had the courage to use my voice to help others realize they aren't alone.

Heather Huhman and I started working together in 2015 on the *Beat Infertility* podcast with a shared mission of educating and empowering people experiencing infertility. She found my infertility blog and reached out to see if I would be willing to be a medical contributor for her podcast. Like me, Heather has been a patient who has experienced infertility care and pregnancy loss and, like me, feels driven to help infertility patients understand their diagnosis, prognosis, and treatment options so they can advocate for themselves.

Infertility patients have to navigate so much misinformation (from well-intentioned family and friends, TikTok trends, and celebrities sharing "news" about the dangers of fertility treatment or sharing about their "natural" pregnancy at age 48 with twins without disclosing the fact they needed donor eggs). Unfortunately, there are even many educated medical providers who just don't have an expertise in infertility and do their patients the disservice of treating them too long with minimally invasive but minimally successful treatment.

As a TikTok and Instagram creator with more than 1.3 million followers combined, the author of my own book, *We Need to Talk About Vaginas*, as well as the medical contributor on the *Beat Infertility* podcast, using my voice has shown me how much people crave to understand and advocate for themselves!

Rapid technological advances in the laboratory and procedures such as in vitro fertilization, egg freezing, and genetic testing are among some of the amazing and powerful tools we have to help people build the healthy families of their dreams.

But you don't know what you don't know. And Heather wants to make sure you *know* what you need to know! In this book, she goes beyond the typical broad overview of fertility treatments and goes into the important details so you can truly understand your options for treatment, know what questions to ask your medical provider, and feel empowered to get a second opinion. Her comprehensive approach is evidence-based and easy to digest.

Infertility journeys can be overwhelming, but with Heather as your coach, you can start advocating for yourself. *Stronger Than Infertility* is the new infertility bible for all those trying to build their family.

—Allison K. Rodgers, MD

Board-certified in Reproductive Endocrinology and Infertility at Fertility Centers of Illinois in Chicago

Medical contributor for the *Beat Infertility* podcast

Author of *We Need to Talk About Vaginas*

Introduction: Stronger Than Infertility

For years, infertility robbed me of control over my life. I suffered in silence, and not because I'm meek or afraid to stand up for myself. It was because, in our society, we *whisper* about infertility. We hide our struggle. We wear masks over our emotions. We feel shame because we can't perform a basic biological function of our species: having children.

But the truth is infertility is not uncommon. One in eight couples in the United States struggles to build a family. Worldwide, it's one in four couples. Yet we are all so scared to talk about it, which impedes the exchange of information about the issues and what they really entail. Without knowledge, we face infertility unarmed and, in turn, lose any sense of power over our present situation or our hope for the future.

What if, instead of keeping everything pushed down, the infertility community felt empowered to speak up?

We could ask the tough questions. We could trade war stories. We could get real about what it's like to struggle to build a family. We could find strength together.

This idea of becoming stronger than infertility is what led me start my online community and podcast, *Beat Infertility*. My mission was to bring to light all the aspects of infertility we have been conditioned not to talk about. It was an instinctual pursuit of answers that I had been unable to find up to that point in my journey.

Yet, as I heard the stories of other people facing infertility and as I looked back at my own difficulties, I noticed a common need: self-advocacy.

As a community, we infertility warriors have to find our voice. We need to learn how to be persistent in our pursuit of knowledge, treatment options, and a fair chance to build our families.

This realization is where the book idea began. I wanted to compile stories, information, and expert advice in one place with the goal of not only educating, but also empowering. To that end, I've tried to cover all aspects of infertility from scientific, emotional, and practical perspectives. The purpose isn't to show you that there is one correct route to build your family; it's to give you the information and skills to determine *the right route for you*.

Since I started writing this book, I've become a full-time infertility coach, helping people from all over the world navigate their own journeys. This includes single parents, couples (hetero and queer), trans people, people pursuing surrogacy or adoption, people who are experiencing secondary infertility, and more. No two infertility warriors have the same story—but there is so much we do share on this journey.

I will tell you here what I tell my clients. I cannot promise that you will end up with a child. No one can make that promise. But I *can* promise you that when you are armed with information, when you take the time to understand and weigh your options, and when you can give yourself the grace (and find the support) to weather the emotional highs and lows, *you will feel stronger than infertility*—braver, better equipped to tackle the journey, and come out a survivor on the other side.

Every Journey Starts with a Single Step

Whether you're just beginning down your path toward parenthood, have been trying and struggling for years, or have reached a happy conclusion at least once already but are having trouble now, you are an infertility warrior. That's a badge you should wear with pride. While no one *wants* to be an infertility warrior, those who are fight with unparalleled strength.

Throughout this book, I'll give the details of my own infertility story. I consider this book a safe place to share my pain, mistakes, and struggles. And I'm so grateful that hundreds of infertility warriors have shared their stories with me on *Beat Infertility* and now in these pages. While some are my clients, the vast majority aren't. They are members of our worldwide community. You'll hear their stories and hard-won wisdom throughout this book. We share our journeys to heal, educate, and show that *you are NOT alone.*

As an infertility coach, a big part of my job is to translate all the best information, latest research, and evidenced-based medical advice for my clients—and to help them decode the information they receive from their doctors. I do not have formal medical training and this is not a medical textbook, but I interviewed dozens of experts—ranging from reproductive endocrinologists to mental health professionals to insurance agents—and their wisdom is quoted throughout. Readers should be aware that doctors often have differing opinions and, for example, what one RE recommends may

not be what your RE recommends. My hope is that you can use the information in this book to help you communicate with your medical team so that they can help you make the right choices for *you.*

Hopefully by the time you reach the end of the book, you will have the courage and sense of support to also speak up. You'll quickly see this as you read, but the more we—infertility warriors, fertile individuals, health-care providers, and our society as a whole—talk about infertility, the less power it has.

This book is chock-full of data: statistics, dosages, graphs, illustrations . . . you name it, it's here. Science, fortunately for us, is constantly evolving. There are always new treatments, changes to the accepted orthodoxy, even new ways too look at old tests. The data and recommendations in this book will most certainly date—and in the case of infertility, that's probably a good thing! Your doctor will (read: should) have the most up-to-date information so be sure to consult with them each step along your journey. I also refer you to many incredible online resources throughout the book that will likely stay on top of the latest developments.

Wherever possible, I've used inclusive language to account for the shape and experience of many types of infertility warriors. The reality is that much of the science and language of infertility is still very much rooted in the binary and relies on gendered studies and medical trials. However, my hope is that you will still be able to glean the information that best suits you and your family.

I don't expect this book to be read in a linear fashion, because infertility is not a straight road with set on- and off-ramps. While I've done my best to organize the chapters in an order that makes sense, not every chapter or situation will be applicable to your journey.

However, there are a few overarching themes to this book—and to how I approach my work as a coach—that I'd like to call out here:

- **Infertility is not your fault.** I know it's hard to convince yourself of this sometimes, but you did not cause your infertility. Don't believe me? I have a book full of quotes from experts to back me up.

- **Every infertility journey is different.** We've hinted at this a bit already, but know that there is likely no one else facing the *exact* same situation as you. There are others who will understand and empathize, but no one else is in your specific shoes—not even your partner, if you have one. This is why it's important to learn about all the available options and advocate for *your* best path to parenthood.

- **Honor your emotions, and practice healthy coping mechanisms.** Infertility will dredge up countless emotions, and not all of them will be pretty. In fact, some common feelings downright suck. But don't try to shove those feelings down—they'll just build up and get worse. Throughout the book, we'll go through different ways to cope with the negative emotions you might experience. Practice them, and discover which methods work best for you.

- **Lean on your support system.** Infertility is isolating. You're going to feel like there's no one you can turn to, but there are people— some currently in your life and some you've yet to meet—who can help ease your burden. In most cases, having a mental health professional as part of your system is key. Know now that the sooner you begin working through challenges with a therapist, the better. *Don't try to face infertility alone.* We're striving to become stronger than infertility, and your support system will be a big source of your strength.

- **There are no "wrong" choices.** You can only make decisions based on the available information about your current situation. While you should always ask questions and educate yourself on your options, you are not omnipotent. Some of your choices might not work out for the best, but don't blame yourself for not choosing differently. Process your pain, learn from the outcome, and focus on the present and future.

One of the main purposes of this book is to empower you during your infertility journey, no matter what stage you are at. Often, the biggest obstacle keeping you down is uncertainty. But knowledge is power. Right now, you may lack the information to make educated decisions or you may fear exploring your greatest concerns. This book is meant to guide you through the reality of infertility so you can take ownership of your journey. It's meant to give you room to safely work through your emotions, doubts, and choices not only without judgment, but with a sense of community.

With *complete* confidence I can tell you:
You are not alone.
You are not defined by infertility.
You are not powerless.
You are stronger than infertility.
I believe in you,

Heather

PART ONE

The Basics

Infertility 101

I REMEMBER MY PRECONCEPTION appointment like it was yesterday. After 6 years of marriage, building our careers, and developing some semblance of financial security, my husband and I were *finally* ready to expand our family.

"Be careful," my doctor warned me. "You're only just starting prenatal vitamins, and they won't have had time to build up in your system if you get pregnant quickly."

Oh, the irony!

The months flew by, but my period continued to show up.

I was traveling with my husband when I noticed I hadn't used the pads I had packed. I looked at my calendar. I was late. Definitely late.

I took a pregnancy test. The three minutes I spent waiting for the results were among the longest of my entire life. The incredibly faint line that appeared—most would call it a "squinter"—indicated a positive.

The next day, Mother's Day, I began bleeding. I was devastated.

Five months later, I still wasn't pregnant. It was time to get serious. I started meticulously tracking my cycles. I bought ovulation prediction kits (OPKs) and began taking my basal body temperature (BBT) every morning.

It was September and we were on another trip, this time to Germany. I brought an enormous stash of pads. When I hit day 35 of my cycle without breaking into them, I sent my husband out for a pregnancy test. The instructions were,

of course, in German. I had no clue how to read the results, but according to the pictures on the back of the box, the first test appeared invalid.

Before using the second test in the box, I sent my husband back to the pharmacy for further instruction. He returned triumphant, and back to the bathroom I went. This time, we waited together—only to have another squinter. We took it as a win. Here we were, on this amazing trip, and I was pregnant! It was time to sit back, relax, and let the embryo settle in.

I woke up one morning near the end of our trip in agonizing pain. I was weak, dizzy, and confused. It was all I could do to make it onto our flight home.

Back in the United States, after catching a few hours of much-needed sleep, we headed to the ER. I was seen quickly and instructed to pee in a cup. Despite the pain and dizziness, I'd not had any bleeding. Imagine my surprise when the urine in the cup was black.

But the ER doctor took one look at the cup, rolled his eyes, and told me all of my symptoms were PMS and I should go home. He discharged me with no evaluation. He didn't even test the urine. I left in a haze of red-hot anger, confusion, and overwhelming sadness—not to mention pain.

I'd had enough of trying to conceive on our own. It was time to get help. Probably way past time. I made an appointment with the reproductive endocrinologist that Google Maps told me was closest to our house. (Seriously, I did no other research.) We met her exactly 1 year after our preconception appointment. It was the first time someone told me I had infertility.

That was the day I became one of 48.5 million people who experience infertility. At the time, I felt isolated and alone. But now I know that a lot of people hoping to get pregnant—15 percent, according to the CDC—were right there with me.

Every infertility journey is different. And learning that you have or will have trouble conceiving happens in different ways. For some, it comes after an unexpected medical event. Lindsey from Wyoming had been trying to conceive for 6 months until she blacked out in the shower. She and her husband, Grant, went to the ER.

"They found seven cysts on my ovaries, and I was encouraged to follow up with my ob-gyn," says Lindsey. "I truly believe that if I hadn't blacked out, we probably would've tried on our own for years not knowing any better."

Her ob-gyn suggested laparoscopic surgery, which confirmed that Lindsey had endometriosis—a common, painful, chronic disease where the uterine lining grows in areas other than the uterus, such as the ovaries, where it can cause cysts to form. Her cysts were drained and her endometriosis lesions were removed. But, as Lindsey found out, the disease carries long-term fertility risks. "My ob-gyn told me there is a chance I could have issues conceiving on my own," she says.

Three months later and still not pregnant, she went back to her ob-gyn, who ordered blood work for a fertility workup. "As soon as the results came in, she called me to explain that I had signs of diminished ovarian reserve. She suggested I go to a reproductive endocrinologist."

For others, it's a miscarriage—and especially recurrent pregnancy loss—that leads to a diagnosis. Rachel of North Carolina experienced two miscarriages in a year.

"After the second miscarriage, we started taking more active steps to discover the problem," she explains. "We found a fertility clinic and started with basic blood work and genetic tests, as well as testing hormone levels at various stages of my cycle."

Age is another factor that drives many people to seek help with their fertility. We live in a time when celebrities such as Alanis Morissette, Gwen Stefani, Marcia Cross, and many more have announced pregnancies in their mid- to late-40s (Janet Jackson gave birth at 50!), it can sometimes come as a surprise to people that age is still very much a factor in fertility.

Melinda from New York began trying to conceive with her partner when she was 34 but didn't visit a fertility clinic until she was 38.

"We tried for about 4 years on our own," she says. "I had always heard about women my age getting pregnant, so I did not think too hard about it—except that it was always so heartbreaking and frustrating to get my period each month."

Eventually she felt it was time to consult a reproductive endocrinologist. "She warned me to not wait too long because the likelihood of getting pregnant on my own—seeing as how I was not successful to that point—was getting lower with each passing day."

However you found your way to dealing with infertility, I believe that knowledge is power and a firm understanding of the science of fertility will give you a strong foundation to navigate your journey with confidence. You are your own best self-advocate!

What Is Infertility?

Simply put, infertility is defined as the inability to get pregnant after 12 months of regular unprotected sexual intercourse. But what about infertility is ever simple?

Many official definitions of infertility don't take into account what infertility may look like for the LGBTQ+ couples or single people who are struggling to conceive through methods other than sexual intercourse, or folks like me who can get pregnant but not stay pregnant. In 2017, an international group of medical organizations hammered out a more expansive and inclusive definition of infertility:

Failure to establish a clinical pregnancy after 12 months of regular, unprotected sexual intercourse or due to an impairment of a person's capacity to reproduce either as an individual or with a partner. Fertility interventions may be initiated in less than 1 year based on medical, sexual, and reproductive history, age, physical findings, and diagnostic testing. Infertility is a disease, which generates disability as an impairment of function.

Infertility can also be broken down into two different categories (though these definitions aren't as inclusive as the one above):

Primary infertility. A condition in which pregnancy has not been achieved after at least 1 year (6 months for females 35 or older) of having sex without any form of birth control.

Secondary infertility. A condition in which pregnancy has been achieved in the past but can no longer be achieved after at least 1 year (6 months for females 35 or older) of having sex without any form of birth control.

Understanding Female Fertility

Let's take a trip down memory lane to junior-high health class. If you want to understand your infertility, you need to understand how the female reproductive system is *supposed* to work. This information will help you ask good questions and better understand your doctor. You may want to return to it as a glossary once you read future chapters.

The Female Reproductive System

The female reproductive organs are exclusively internal and are made up of the following organs:

• **Vagina.** A muscular tube located between the external genitals and the cervix.

• **Cervix.** The lowest region of the uterus that attaches to and provides a passageway between the uterus and vagina.

• **Uterus.** A pear-shaped, hollow, expandable organ located in the lower abdomen between the rectum and bladder. This is where fertilized eggs implant and gestate before birth. Also known as a womb.

• **Oocytes.** Female sex cells, also known as eggs. (Sex cells—whether female or male—are sometimes also called gametes.) A person is born with one to two million eggs but starts losing them immediately. By puberty, only 300,000 to 500,000 remain.

• **Ovaries.** The small, internal glands located on both sides of the uterus that produce eggs.

• **Follicle.** A small, fluid-filled sac in the ovary that contains one immature egg.

• **Ovum.** A mature egg ready for ovulation. Once the menstruation cycle begins, eggs grow slowly—approximately 1 to 2 mm per day—until one takes the lead and matures, eventually reaching 17 to 20 mm.

• **Ovulation.** Release of an ovum. But before the ovum releases, the body has a lot of work to do. It needs to produce and increase levels of luteinizing hormone (LH). Then, just a few hours before ovulation, the lead egg is divided in a process called *meiosis*, which gives it twenty-three chromosomes.

• **Corpus luteum.** A temporary cyst that develops after ovulation from the follicle that releases an egg. It quickly degenerates unless

Female Reproductive Organs

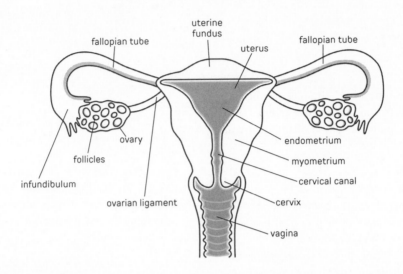

pregnancy has begun. Follicles that do not release an egg are absorbed back into the ovary until every egg is gone and menopause occurs.

• **Cumulus.** A circular, mucous-based barrier created by the egg-releasing follicle to protect and support the egg.

• **Zona pellucida.** The membrane just beneath the cumulus. A sperm must fight its way through the cumulus *and* the zona pellucida to fertilize an egg—usually 12 to 24 hours after ovulation—in the fallopian tube.

• **Fallopian tubes.** A pair of tubes attached to the upper part of the uterus. Fertilized eggs journey through them from the ovaries to the uterus.

• **Endometrium.** The mucous membrane that thickens during the first half of the menstrual cycle to prepare for possible implantation. Also known as the uterine lining.

Female Reproductive Hormones

A healthy female reproductive system must continuously produce five important hormones to maintain that system: estrogens (E1, E2, E3), progesterone (P4), gonadotropin-releasing hormone (GnRH), follicle-stimulating hormone (FSH), and luteinizing hormone (LH).

• **Estradiol (E2).** The most important of the three estrogens during the reproductive years. It's secreted from follicles on the ovaries and impacts the growth of reproductive organs, such as the vagina, fallopian tubes, uterine lining, and cervical glands.

• **Estrone (E1).** Produced by both the ovaries and fat cells. When estrone levels are high, they promote weight gain, which then causes more estrone production, and so on.

• **Estriol (E3).** The weakest of the three estrogens. It's released by the placenta—the organ that develops around a fetus—and thus is present only during pregnancy.

• **Progesterone (P4).** Produced by the ovaries. During the menstrual cycle, levels of this hormone fluctuate. When the corpus luteum forms after ovulation, it produces progesterone to enable implantation and support pregnancy until the placenta can take over production.

• **Gonadotropin-releasing hormone (GnRH).** Secreted by the brain. The release of GnRH stimulates the production of FSH and LH.

• **Follicle-stimulating hormone (FSH).** Produced in the pituitary gland at the base of the brain. Together with LH, it regulates follicular function in the ovary. FSH stimulates follicles to increase estrogen and progesterone levels during the follicular phase of the menstrual cycle. Follicles grow until one takes the lead, secreting the most estrogen. Rising estrogen levels eventually signal to the brain that it's time for ovulation and to stop producing FSH.

• **Luteinizing hormone (LH).** Produced in the pituitary gland at the base of the brain. Together with FSH, it regulates follicular function in the ovary. Rising estrogen levels signal to the pituitary gland when it's time to release LH, which initiates ovulation.

The Menstrual Cycle

The menstrual cycle is, on average, 28 days, although cycles can be longer or shorter. Many people turn their attention to their cycle only when their period arrives—or doesn't. However, understanding the significance of each day in your cycle is important when it comes to understanding your body and recognizing when there's an issue.

Menstrual Phase

Days 1–5. Enter the period—also known as "Aunt Flo" (AF) within the infertility community—when your uterine lining breaks down and leaves your body. You must have a full flow, as opposed to spotting, to be considered on cycle day 1 (CD1). Normal bleeding can last anywhere from 4 to 7 days. Both estrogen and progesterone levels are low. Follicles, each containing one egg, begin to develop in the ovaries during this time.

Early Follicular Phase

Days 6–7. One—or sometimes two and very rarely three—lead or dominant follicle continues growing to maturity. The others stop and are absorbed back into the ovary as estrogen rises.

Late Follicular Phase

Days 8–13. By the time day 8 arrives, that dominant follicle has grown much larger, period bleeding has subsided, and the increased estrogen levels cause your uterine lining to thicken in preparation for implantation.

Ovulatory Phase

Day 14. Estrogen levels peak, causing LH levels to rise. LH then causes the mature follicle to burst open and release an egg. Women who have intercourse in the 3 days before, the day of, and/or the day after ovulation are most likely to get pregnant because sperm can live for 3 to 5 days in a woman's reproductive organs when estrogen levels are at their highest.

Luteal Phase

Days 15–24. The newly released egg travels away from the ovary, through the fallopian tube, and toward the uterus. The corpus luteum produces progesterone, further supporting uterine lining development. If the egg is fertilized by a sperm in the fallopian tube, its cells begin dividing and it eventually becomes a blastocyst—a ball of hundreds of cells. Meanwhile, it continues its journey through the fallopian tube and attempts to attach to the uterus; this process is also known as implantation. If an egg remains unfertilized, it breaks apart.

Days 24–28. If implantation doesn't take place, the blastocyst doesn't remain attached, or the blastocyst doesn't continue to develop, and estrogen and progesterone levels drop. This change can impact your mood, causing irritability, anxiety, or feelings of depression. The menstrual cycle comes to an end when the

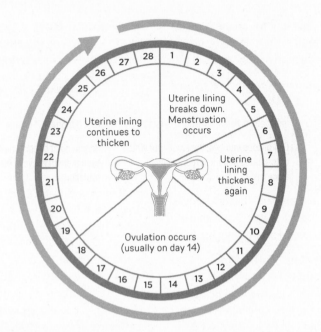

unfertilized egg exits the body with the uterine lining, which takes us back to day 1, and a new period begins.

Remember that everyone is different—and so is each cycle. Your cycle is still considered "regular" if your period comes every 25 to 35 days (counting from the first day of your last period to the start of your next).

Some people's periods function like clock-work, making it easy to predict the day it'll arrive. Others are still regular but know only a general range of days when they might expect their period to begin. Many people battling infertility, however, have erratic or even non-existent periods.

What You Need to Know About Egg Health

Typically, between 300 and 400 eggs—approximately one per menstrual cycle, though that number declines with age—will reach ovulation during a person's reproductive lifetime. But what's going on with those eggs

prior to ovulation? It all starts before you're even born.

Approximately 95 percent of embryo health is derived from the egg, according to Dr. Allison K. Rodgers, a board-certified reproductive endo-crinologist with Fertility Centers of Illinois in Chicago. There are a number of factors that can lead to poor egg health.

Age
As much as we hate to admit it, a biological clock *does* exist. As Dr. Rodgers explains, when we talk about age and fertility, "we're talking about the percentage of eggs that have the ability to do their job of making a baby."

When a woman is in her 20s, between 50 and 75 percent of her eggs should be of good quality. That percentage goes down to between 25 and 50 percent by her mid-30s and 15 per-cent by the time she's 40 years old. (For more information, see the advanced reproductive age "diagnosis" in the appendix.)

Perhaps not surprisingly, research con-ducted by RESOLVE: The National Infertility Association and Shady Grove Fertility found

THE EGG DEVELOPMENT PROCESS		
STAGE	DESCRIPTION	TIMELINE
Primordial	Most immature stage; dormant and small	First 5 months of gestational development within the womb
Primary (or preantral)	Initial cell division, leading to growth	Last 3 months of gestational development
Secondary	Cell divides into two, the smaller of which deteriorates and the larger of which advances to the next stage	Beginning at puberty, new follicles grow each menstrual cycle; 90 days before ovulation
Early tertiary	Basic structure of the mature follicle has formed and no novel cells are detectable	10 days before ovulation
Late tertiary	Majority of the follicles that started growth have died; eventually, only one will be viable (dominant follicle)	5 days before ovulation

that 87 percent of respondents younger than 35 and 81 percent older than 35 wish they had better understood the link between age and fertility earlier.

Dr. Shruti Malik, a board-certified reproductive endocrinologist with Shady Grove Fertility in Fair Oaks, Virginia, explains, "As [people] age, hormonal changes begin to take

BUSTED

Myth: I've got time.

Dr. Lynn Westphal, a reproductive endocrinologist and chief medical officer at Kindbody in New York, says it's not uncommon to see stories of people giving birth in their late 40s or early 50s and think, "If they can get pregnant, I've got plenty of time." But the truth is these people are the exception, not the rule. And most likely, they did not get pregnant easily.

"Many people are not aware of the decline in fertility with aging," says Dr. Westphal. "Also, many lose track of time and don't realize that there is a big difference even between ages 35 and 40."

place. There is a lot going on, but of particular interest are the two main hormones controlling the development and release of the egg each month. These are follicle-stimulating hormone (FSH) and luteinizing hormone (LH)."

If age has begun to impact your egg health, one of the first symptoms you might notice is your cycles shortening. Dr. Rodgers says, "If they were always 28 days and now they're 24 days, that's something that can happen when quality declines. Additionally, you might have true menopausal symptoms, such as hot flashes and vaginal dryness. But that's not until things get really severe."

Dr. Rodgers adds, "There's so much variability, and that's why it's really important to meet with a doctor if you're having trouble conceiving." In other words, if you are older than 35 and are having trouble conceiving, the sooner you visit your doctor, the better.

Poor Blood Flow

Healthy eggs require oxygen-rich blood flowing to your ovaries. Low oxygen levels may result in immature eggs that don't fertilize, implant, or develop properly. Lack of exercise, dehydration, and thick blood can all reduce blood flow.

Hormonal Imbalance

An imbalance of any of the five crucial hormones—estrogens (E1, E2, E3), progesterone (P4), gonadotropin-releasing hormone (GnRH), follicle-stimulating hormone (FSH), and luteinizing hormone (LH)—can result in poor-quality eggs or no ovulation at all.

Although some over-the-counter supplements purport to help regulate these hormones to normal levels, be wary—and *never* take supplements or adjust dosages without your doctor's knowledge and ongoing monitoring. Sometimes they can do more harm than good.

Instead, it's good practice to receive a full fertility workup (as described on page 34), once a year—and more often if diagnostics come back showing something abnormal. Work with your doctor to develop a plan to regulate abnormal hormone levels through a combination of prescription medication and approved supplements.

Lifestyle Factors

A variety of lifestyle factors may impact your egg quality:

- Smoking and using recreational drugs

- Exposure to environmental chemicals (parabens, phthalates, bisphenol A, bisphenol S, flame retardants, and pesticides)

- High caffeine and/or alcohol intake

- Being underweight or overweight (BMI of less than 18.5 or more than 25)

- An unbalanced diet, especially one low in fertility-fueling foods (see chapter 8)

- Not getting enough sleep on a regular basis

Just remember: Your actions are one aspect over which you have control throughout this journey. Feel empowered by that!

Certain Health Conditions

Certain health conditions can impact your fertility. In fact, you may already have been diagnosed with a condition—such as polycystic ovary syndrome (PCOS) or endometriosis—earlier in life and weren't told at the time how it would impact your future fertility.

Not all people who have PCOS produce unhealthy eggs. However, if you have elevated male hormone (predominantly testosterone) levels, you are likely to have poor egg quality.

Endometriosis is often associated with higher levels of inflammation from macrophages (a type of white blood cell) and cytokines (secreted by cells in the immune system). Some believe the presence of this inflammation is toxic to eggs, impacting their quality and ability to develop into healthy embryos.

Those of us with endometriosis, myself included, often develop ovarian cysts called endometriomas. These cysts are filled with a combination of menstrual debris, endometrial tissue, blood, and more. Their dark brown pigment has earned them the nickname "chocolate cysts." Endometriomas cause hormonal imbalances that impact egg development, quality, and even overall count.

Endometriosis can also leave scar tissue throughout your reproductive system, blocking blood flow to or within your ovaries. And remember, your ovaries need plenty of blood flow to produce healthy eggs.

> ### WARRIOR WISDOM
> #### Don't Wait If You Have a Known Condition
> ....
> *Sarah, Ontario, Canada*
>
> Sarah knew she had an autoimmune disease. What she *didn't* know, however, is how this disorder needlessly extended her journey to pregnancy. "I wish I had known then that you don't have to wait a year if you have an existing medical condition that impairs fertility."

There are many other medical conditions that can cause infertility. In the appendix, you'll find the nitty-gritty on each.

Signs and Symptoms of Female Infertility

Let's look at some general signs that might indicate a fertility issue.

• Irregular cycles

• Rarely or never menstruating

• Periods lasting longer than 7 days

• Short luteal phase

• Hormonal imbalance

• Pain during sex

• Recurrent miscarriages

• Chronic health issues and past illnesses

• Certain medications

Irregular Cycles

If your menstrual cycle is less than 25 days or longer than 35 days, it's considered irregular.

Cycles lasting less than 25 days indicate you likely are not ovulating. (You can still bleed even if you don't ovulate.) A short cycle could also be a sign of low egg quality and/or quantity (diminished ovarian reserve). As the number of available eggs decreases throughout your reproductive years, the brain releases higher amounts of FSH, which results in earlier follicle development and ovulation—and thus shorter menstrual cycles.

Cycles lasting longer than 35 days indicate you likely are not ovulating or are ovulating much later than expected. If you don't ovulate, progesterone is never released by the corpus luteum. Instead, your uterine lining continues to thicken in response to estrogen levels.

Eventually, your lining thickens to the point of instability and your period begins, often consisting of heavy, prolonged bleeding.

Rarely or Never Menstruating

Dr. Rodgers explains, "If you're not having a monthly cycle, you're probably not ovulating—or not ovulating strongly or regularly."

If your body mass index (BMI) is less than 18.5, this could explain your lack of a period. Remember, fat cells produce estrogen. So, if you don't have enough body fat, you also won't have enough estrogen for your cycle to function properly. Sometimes this is easily resolved by gaining weight to return to a normal BMI range (18.5 to 25).

If you've never had a period, there may be a development problem with your uterus or vagina. If your once-regular period has stopped, it could indicate a uterine abnormality, like scar tissue or the premature onset of menopause.

Periods Lasting Longer Than 7 Days

Dr. Rodgers says, "If your periods are very heavy or very long, this may be a sign of a hormone imbalance or an anatomic issue with the uterus." Polyps, fibroids, an infection within the uterus or cervix, endometriosis, and even cancer can result in a long period, prevent implantation, and possibly increase your chance of a miscarriage should implantation occur. More rarely, it can indicate a blood clotting condition, which should be evaluated and treated by a hematologist.

Short Luteal Phase

The average luteal phase lasts for 12 to 16 days. When your luteal phase is less than 12 days, it's a sign that your body doesn't produce enough progesterone—perhaps because the corpus luteum has failed—and your uterine lining is not thick enough for healthy implantation. In this case, if you do become pregnant, the result might be an early miscarriage.

Laura and her husband from Michigan had been trying to conceive for only a few months after she stopped taking birth control—which regulates your hormones and might mask any natural hormonal imbalances—when she suspected there might be an issue. "I was tracking my cycle and realized there was not enough time between when I ovulated and when I started spotting. I also spotted several days before my period started, and I no longer had any breast tenderness leading up to my period and always had before. They seemed like small things, but I could tell something was off."

A short luteal phase is a red flag, and if you find yourself in the same position as Laura, it's time to consult a doctor.

Hormonal Imbalance

Other signs of a hormonal imbalance include:

- Excessive hair growth in unwanted places, such as the lips, breasts, or lower abdomen

- Thinning hair

- Weight gain or loss

- Milky white discharge from your nipples (unrelated to breastfeeding)

BUSTED

Myth: If there's no family history of infertility, I can't possibly have it.

"Every woman's fertility is different, and even very fertile families may have someone with a fertility problem," explains Dr. Westphal.

People might also feel shame around their infertility. There's good chance that if someone in your family went through it, they might have kept it to themselves.

When Elisa from Missouri stopped birth control to try to conceive, she observed changes in her body. "My period started disappearing—4 days turned into 30 light hours. I also noticed many symptoms that pointed toward a hormonal imbalance—long cycles, weight gain, dark hair growth on my face (and thighs and stomach and toes!), night sweats, migraines, and so much spotting." Turns out she had PCOS.

Other Signs

Your body has many other ways of telling you that something may be off, including:

- **Pain during sex.** Pain during sex can be a warning sign for endometriosis or scar tissue in the pelvis.

- **Recurrent miscarriages.** Experiencing multiple miscarriages typically points to issues with sustaining a pregnancy rather than getting pregnant. (But remember, recurrent loss is a type of primary infertility.)

- **Chronic health issues and past illnesses, including cancer and sexually transmitted infections (STIs).** Chronic health issues from diabetes to thyroid disorders to endocrine-related conditions can impact fertility. Cancer-related issues, such as surgery or chemotherapy and radiation, can damage eggs or sperm. STIs can cause scarring or blockage in reproductive organs, including the fallopian tubes, where damage to the tissue can prevent fertilization or the transport of the embryo into the uterus.

- **Certain medications.** Many psychiatric and epilepsy medications can increase prolactin levels, which can inhibit FSH and GnRH and thereby interfere with cycles. Be up-front with your doctor about what medications you're taking and ask how they might impact your fertility.

Myth: Infertility is a female-only problem.

Male-factor infertility is just as common as female-factor infertility, accounting for one-third of all cases. Another one-third of cases can be attributed to female infertility, and the rest are due to a combination of issues between male and female partners or unknown causes.

Understanding Male Fertility

Male partners are often overlooked during the initial fertility workup and early diagnostic exploration. Many don't even have a semen analysis until pretty deep into the process—they either don't want one or the doctor doesn't suggest it. Yet male fertility is on the decline and has been for a while. Four decades ago, the average sperm count was approximately 50 percent higher than today. However, sperm count is only one possible cause of male infertility. So let's go back to health class for a refresher on the male reproductive system.

The Male Reproductive System

The male reproductive system is both external and internal.

External reproductive parts:

• **Sperm.** These are the male sex cells—and they're 10,000 times smaller than eggs. The sperm development cycle is known as spermatogenesis. Every second, the average person produces approximately 1,500 sperm. If you do the math, that's more than 500 *billion* sperm over the course of a lifetime. These little packets of DNA have one goal: to fertilize an egg by swimming from the bottom of the cervix up into the fallopian tube.

• **Penis.** The penis has three parts: the root (attached to the wall of the abdomen); the body, or shaft; and the glans, or head (the dome-shaped end of the penis). The glans is covered with a loose layer of foreskin (if the penis has not been circumcised). At the tip of the glans is the opening of the urethra, which transports semen and urine. Semen, which contains sperm, is ejaculated through the end of the penis when it is erect and reaches sexual climax.

• **Scrotum.** A loose sac of skin that hangs directly behind the penis. Inside are the testicles, many nerves, and blood vessels. Even though the scrotum *seems* tender, it actually provides protection for the testicles. The testicles must be slightly cooler than body temperature for normal sperm development, so the scrotum acts as their climate control. When testicles are cold, the scrotum contracts to bring them closer to the body for warmth. When they're too warm, it relaxes, allowing them to cool down away from the body.

• **Testicles (testes).** Each oval teste is secured at both ends by a structure called the spermatic cord. The testes are in charge of making testosterone (the primary male sex hormone). But this isn't their only—or most important—job. Within the testes are tubes, called seminiferous tubules, that are responsible for producing sperm cells.

• **Sertoli cells (nurse cells).** These cells are located within the seminiferous tubules and aid the early sperm development process.

• **Epididymis.** A long, coiled tube resting on the back of each testicle. It acts like a parental figure to young sperm by carrying and storing them, then bringing them to maturity.

Internal reproductive parts:

• **Vas deferens.** A long, muscular tube travels from the epididymis into the pelvic cavity and behind the bladder. Once the epididymis has finished helping the sperm mature, the vas deferens transports it to the urethra in preparation for ejaculation.

• **Ejaculatory ducts.** These are formed by the fusion of the vas deferens and the seminal vesicles. The ejaculatory ducts empty into the urethra.

• **Urethra.** The urethra serves a dual purpose. This tube runs through the center of the prostate gland and carries urine from the bladder. Additionally, it's in charge of ejaculating semen full of sperm when the man reaches sexual climax. When the penis is erect, the flow of urine is blocked from the urethra, allowing only semen to be ejaculated.

• **Seminal vesicles.** Sperm need a sugar rush to get moving. The seminal vesicles—sac-like pouches attached to the vas deferens near the base of the bladder—produce a sugar-rich fluid that provides sperm with a source of energy and helps them move. In fact, this fluid makes up the majority of a man's ejaculate.

• **Prostate gland.** Those tiny sperm need all the nourishment they can get, and that's exactly what the prostate gland provides. This walnut-sized structure is located below the bladder and in front of the rectum. Just like the seminal vesicles, the prostate gland contributes fluid to the ejaculate.

• **Bulbourethral glands.** Just below the prostate gland, on the sides of the urethra, you'll find the bulbourethral glands, or Cowper's glands. They're small, pea-sized structures that produce a clear fluid that empties directly into the urethra. The fluid lubricates the urethra and neutralizes any acidity caused by residual drops of urine.

• **Leydig cells.** These cells, found adjacent to the seminiferous tubules, produce testosterone in the presence of luteinizing hormone (LH).

Male Reproductive Hormones

The entire male reproductive system is dependent on five primary hormones that regulate the activity of cells and organs.

• **Gonadotropin-releasing hormone (GnRH).** Secreted by the brain. The release of GnRH stimulates the production of FSH and LH.

• **Follicle-stimulating hormone (FSH).** Produced in the pituitary gland at the base of the brain. FSH stimulates the Sertoli cells to produce an androgen-binding protein. (Androgen is a male sex hormone.) This protein initiates testosterone production and kicks off spermatogenesis.

• **Luteinizing hormone (LH).** Produced in the pituitary gland at the base of the brain. LH plays a smaller role by stimulating more testosterone production in the testes to continue the process of spermatogenesis.

• **Testosterone.** Produced by the Leydig cells located next to the seminiferous tubules inside the testicle. It's stimulated by LH and required for normal spermatogenesis.

• **Inhibin.** Produced in the testes and released by the Sertoli cells. As testosterone levels increase, inhibin slows spermatogenesis by inhibiting GnRH, FSH, and LH production. Once the sperm count drops to 20 million/ml, the Sertoli cells cease producing inhibin, allowing spermatogenesis to continue.

What You Need to Know About Sperm Health

Most male infertility occurs as a result of issues with sperm production or delivery. The sperm cell is the smallest in the body, whereas the egg cell is the largest. Although

THE SPERM DEVELOPMENT (SPERMATOGENESIS) PROCESS		
PHASE	DESCRIPTION	TIMELINE
Mitosis of the spermatogonia	Undeveloped germ cells (type A spermatogonia) in the seminiferous tubules undergo mitosis, splitting into type B spermatogonia and new type A spermatogonia. The type B spermatogonia divide into primary spermatocytes.	First 16 days of spermatogenesis
First meiosis	Primary spermatocytes develop in their complexity and double their internal DNA. Each primary spermatocyte becomes two secondary spermatocytes.	Next 24 days of spermatogenesis
Second meiosis	Each secondary spermatocyte divides to become two spermatids, each with only half of the original DNA material.	Next several hours of spermatogenesis
Spermiogenesis	Spermatids transform into sperm cells	Final 24 days of spermatogenesis

sperm is about 10,000 times smaller, it contains the same amount of DNA as the egg. Sperm take approximately 64 days to develop and an additional 5.5 days to travel the length of the epididymis. Their development can be broken down into four phases.

Sperm production begins in the brain with the hypothalamus. The hypothalamus is constantly monitoring blood testosterone levels, which communicate the level of testicular activity. When blood testosterone starts slipping, the hypothalamus starts its engine and secretes GnRH. GnRH flows to the pituitary gland, stimulating the production of LH and FSH.

LH travels away from the pituitary gland and into the testicles, where it stimulates cells in the connective tissue surrounding the seminiferous tubules to secrete testosterone. Once testosterone is secreted, FSH concentrates it into the seminiferous tubules, where sperm are finally made.

Sperm starts as a germ cell that divides and becomes a baby sperm, or spermatid. A spermatid is then nourished by nurse cells in the testicle, where it slowly grows a tail—which is crucial for the swimming process in the race for fertilization. Once it's developed, the sperm

is released from the testicle's nurse cells and sent into the epididymis. This is where it finishes maturing, prepares to swim, and is stored until it is ejaculated out of the body.

Fertilization and Conception

The great migration for those warrior sperm cells has just begun—and most won't survive to become the king of fertilization. But the sperm aren't going down without a fight.

After ejaculation, the liquid portion of semen continues to protect the sperm and prevent them from getting turned around and going in the wrong direction.

The capable sperm go into the cervical canal—a much more sperm-friendly environment full of cervical mucus. During ovulation, that mucus is stretchy, clear, and thin and will carry the sperm to the egg.

The sperm cells aren't finished—or safe—yet. Newly ejaculated sperm cells spend close to an hour undergoing biochemical changes, picking up a tail-thrashing pace just to make it into the uterus and fallopian tubes.

The key to any rendezvous is timing. If you're in the right place at the wrong time, you will miss meeting your soulmate. The same goes for sperm cells as they're racing to reach an egg. That egg isn't just sitting around waiting for a sperm to come find it, though. The egg is on its own journey through a fallopian tube from the ovary.

Sperm that reach the fallopian tube too quickly could die before the egg even shows up. Those that are late will miss their chance with the now-departed egg.

The sperm that reach the egg win a chance for a date. But they still have some wooing to do before an egg gives in to fertilization. The sperm now needs to tunnel through the hard outer layer of an egg—alongside hundreds of other sperm fighting the same battle.

Once a clear sperm winner has successfully penetrated the outer layer, the egg experiences an immediate chemical reaction, preventing other sperm cells from also penetrating (in most cases, anyway). The chromosomes carried by both the sperm and egg join together, officially fertilizing the egg.

Within just a few hours, the newly fertilized couple divides multiple times. After a week, a ball of about one hundred cells (a blastocyst) finds the uterus, settles in, and gets comfy-cozy in the uterine lining. The sperm and egg have officially gone beyond fertilization and reached implantation.

Possible Causes of Poor Sperm Health

Although only 5 percent of embryo health is derived from sperm, it obviously still plays an important role. Like with eggs, sperm development and delivery can run into issues.

Age

Yes, age impacts sperm, too. The older you are, the more likely you are to have more chronic health issues, like diabetes and high blood pressure, that impact your fertility. Additionally, as you age, you may produce more sperm with DNA abnormalities, which can lead to miscarriages or birth defects. You are also more likely to experience erectile dysfunction and weight gain.

Advanced paternal age is generally considered older than 40 or 45 years old. However, you never stop producing sperm, except in cases of disease or structural damage.

Most studies show that age negatively impacts sperm health, although some have mixed results.

Although age is not a barrier you can change, the action you *can* take is getting a semen analysis—and potentially a physical examination and blood work by a reproductive urologist—as soon as possible.

Hormonal Imbalance

An imbalance of any of the five crucial hormones—GnRH, FSH, LH, testosterone, and inhibin—can result in abnormal semen parameters.

SEMEN PARAMETER	DESCRIPTION	REDUCTION OVER 20 YEARS, FROM AGES 26–46
Concentration	Total sperm count	66% fewer sperm
Motility	What percentage of the sperm moves	15% less movement
Morphology	The shape and appearance of the sperm	4%–18% fewer normally shaped sperm
Volume	How much semen is ejaculated at once	3%–4% less seminal volume

Source: Harris, Isiah D., Carolyn Franczak, Lauren Roth, and Randall E. Meacham. "Fertility and the Aging Male." *Reviews in Urology* 13, no. 4 (2011): e184–e190. https://doi.org/10.3909/riu0538.

Lifestyle Factors

Lifestyle factors may contribute to poor sperm health:

- Smoking and using recreational drugs

- Exposure to toxins and testicular heat

- High caffeine and/or alcohol intake

- Being underweight or overweight (BMI of less than 18.5 or more than 25)

- An unbalanced diet, especially one low in antioxidant-rich foods

- Not getting enough sleep on a regular basis

- Overexercising

Chronic Health Conditions

Chronic conditions such as diabetes and liver cirrhosis can cause abnormal ejaculation. Again, it's best to consult a reproductive urologist if you have any ongoing health concerns that might impact your fertility.

Signs and Symptoms of Male Infertility

- Changes in hair growth or sexual desire
- Pain, lump, or swelling in testicle(s)
- Problems with erection or ejaculation
- Small, firm testicles
- Being underweight or overweight (BMI of less than 18.5 or more than 25)
- Past cancer treatments
- Exposure to toxins or heat

Changes in hair growth or sexual desire. Either of these could indicate a hormonal imbalance.

Pain, lump, or swelling in testicle(s). Swelling could be a varicocele—a swollen varicose vein in the testicle. This dramatically decreases sperm count and, in turn, decreases your chances of successfully conceiving. Pain or a lump could be a sign of testicular cancer.

Problems with erection or ejaculation. Either of these could be due to a hormonal imbalance.

Small, firm testicles. This is another sign of a possible hormonal imbalance. In more serious instances, small, firm testicles are a symptom of premature testicular failure.

Being overweight. Being overweight can produce an excessive amount of estrogen and decrease sperm production.

Past cancer treatments. Chemotherapy can damage a testicle's ability to produce sperm.

Exposure to toxins or heat. Sperm are very sensitive to toxins and heat. People who are often exposed to chemicals can have a lower sperm count and difficulty conceiving. A low sperm count can also be caused by heat from hot tub use, hot baths, and excessive bike riding.

When to See an Ob-Gyn vs. a Reproductive Endocrinologist

Many warriors were initially reluctant to seek medical advice. Melinda waited 4 years—until she was 38—before seeing a reproductive endocrinologist (RE).

Lilly from Indiana had previously given birth, so she never thought conceiving again would be an issue.

"I was very naive and didn't think anything was wrong with me," she admits. "I kept assuming it wasn't happening because my husband was a long-haul truck driver and gone for 10 to 12 days at a time."

After about a year, Lilly saw her ob-gyn but didn't find the appointment helpful. A year later, she consulted another general practitioner, who sent her for blood work and an ultrasound, but the results were never shared with

---

BUSTED

Myth: Infertility is something shameful.

Many people feel that infertility makes them "less than"—less valuable to their partner or a disappointment to their family. If there's anything I want you to take away from this book, it is that your infertility is not your fault. It's important to feel all your feelings surrounding infertility, rather than trying to shove them down. But struggling with infertility isn't shameful. It does *not* define you or affect your worth as a human being.

---

her. Finally, after more than 4 years of trying for another child, she and her husband, Paul, went to a fertility clinic for help.

Brad from Illinois was not ready to consult an RE until he and his wife, Lisa, had been trying unsuccessfully for more than 2 years.

"We started trying when I was just a month shy of 27," Lisa explains. "I had regular periods prior to going on the pill when we got married and had no worries about being able to become pregnant. The month after going off the pill, my cycle returned and came every month on the dot. A year passed, with no positive test. My husband was not ready to see a doctor. Another year and a half went by before we called the RE my PCP recommended."

Unfortunately, they had to wait 2 additional months for the initial fertility clinic consultation, which is not uncommon.

Greg from Vermont also wanted to wait before seeking medical help. Although his wife, Suzanne, knew they should see a doctor after only 6 months due to their ages, he wasn't on board until they had been trying for 10 months—at least partially due to stress in other areas of his life.

"It was very stressful after the first 3 to 4 months," says Suzanne. "We started trying to time things better, but it felt like sexual coercion and I hated it. We also were going through some difficult times with his father dying and his mother falling ill and needing intensive care. So, there were a lot of stressors."

If you are still on the fence, consider this: If you are 35 or older and have been trying for 6 months, or if you are younger than 35 and have been trying for a year, and you have not achieved pregnancy or have experienced more than one loss, it's time to get evaluated.

Dr. Rodgers says, "It really breaks my heart to hear stories of people trying for years without success when, sometimes, easy minimal treatment could have helped them have a child years sooner."

Once you decide to schedule a preconception appointment at a minimum, there's another determination to make: whom to ask for help. Advocating for yourself and your future family isn't an easy job. You need the best team of doctors supporting you along the way, and you have a few options about where to start.

It's *extremely* likely that your ob-gyn has expertise in general women's health and pre- and postnatal care—not helping people become pregnant. Unless there's an obvious cause, most ob-gyns won't be looking for signs of infertility.

"Most ob-gyn offices are focused on health maintenance and addressing current issues," points out Dr. Westphal. "They may not have time or may not feel comfortable bringing up the topic of fertility."

Dr. Rodgers points out that many ob-gyns do great low-invasive infertility work. However, those who are interested in it usually stick to prescribing Clomid (an ovulation-stimulating drug—more on this in chapter 5) and timed intercourse (see chapter 6). And sometimes this just isn't enough.

"If you've done three courses of treatment and you're not successful, it's time to move on," she advises. Some patients, such as those of advanced reproductive age, would benefit from seeing an RE even sooner.

An RE starts out as an ob-gyn and then receives 3 years of *additional* training that focuses specifically on reproductive endocrinology and infertility.

Sarah, the woman with an autoimmune condition, had no choice but to start with her ob-gyn because, in Canada, "they are the gatekeepers to the fertility world." However, she regrets not seeing a specialist sooner. "In retrospect, I spent a lot longer with the ob-gyn than I should have before going to an RE."

Emily from Oregon also started with her ob-gyn because "the cost of an RE made me scared to go that route." Looking back, she too has second thoughts about that decision. "I wish I had just started with an RE. It would have saved me precious time."

If you're particularly attached to your ob-gyn, perhaps start by having an open and honest discussion. Find out how they'll assess you, what treatments they're willing and able to administer, and if they feel your situation requires the immediate attention of an RE. Divyagiri from Germany says, "My ob did an exploratory laparoscopy with hysterosalpingogram, which came back normal. Then we were referred to the RE, who did a full workup for both my husband and myself."

But you don't have to wait. "If you are even thinking about it, you shouldn't hesitate to make an appointment [with an RE]," says Dr. Rodgers. "A reproductive endocrinologist will be able to identify whether there is something preventing your success. Remember that you are the captain of your fertility journey and have the power to make decisions about what you want and don't want. It's important to find a doctor who is a good fit and can work as a teammate with you to empower and involve you in clinical decisions."

OB-GYNS VS. REPRODUCTIVE ENDOCRINOLOGISTS		
	OB-GYNS	**REPRODUCTIVE ENDOCRINOLOGISTS**
Specialization	Focused on women's health and pre- and postnatal care. Most are not trained extensively in fertility.	Ob-gyns with years of *additional* medical training who specialize in both female and male aspects of fertility.
Cost	A visit is typically inexpensive and, in most cases, covered by insurance.	Appointments and treatments are more expensive and may not be covered by insurance.
Fertility treatments offered	Many, but not all, can help with timed intercourse or intrauterine insemination.	Trained in a wide variety of fertility treatments, from timed intercourse to in vitro fertilization (IVF).
When to make an appointment	You should be seeing your ob-gyn annually. When you've decided to start building your family, you can schedule a preconception visit to request an initial female and male workup.	When you're younger than 35 and haven't conceived after a year of trying, or when you're older than 35 and haven't conceived after 6 months of trying. Also consider making an appointment if you have known health conditions that can impact fertility.

It's essential to set up a supportive foundation at the beginning of your journey.

WARRIOR ACTION STEPS
Discuss Possible Infertility with Your Partner

When you start to suspect that you and your partner are facing a fertility issue, find a time—when both you and your partner are calm and unemotional—to have a conversation. Without placing blame or being judgmental, discuss the following topics:

• **How important it is to build your family.** Most couples have this conversation more than once throughout the course of their relationship. But as situations change, so do people's feelings. Infertility journeys are marathons, and it's important to discuss early and often how important it is—for you as a couple and as individuals within the relationship—to build your family.

• **Your worries about possible infertility.** Are you scared your partner will leave you? Or vice versa? Does infertility threaten your identity?

Is it painful to think that your path to a family won't look like what you had hoped? Get your fears out in the open so you can both be sensitive to each other's needs.

• **Why you love each other.** You didn't pick your partner based on their ability to have children. It was their personality, your shared values, and a million other factors that brought you two together. Reassure each other as you begin on this journey—and throughout.

WARRIOR ACTION STEPS
Single Parents: Gather Your People

I've worked with and interviewed many single infertility warriors over the years and all agree that building a support system is vital. No one should walk this journey alone.

• **Find a support group.** There are a lot of options. Motherhood Reimagined, led by single mom Sarah Kowalski, is my favorite. RESOLVE: The National Infertility Association also has local support groups all over the country, so check out the map on its website. There are also Facebook groups, such as Surviving Single Parenthood.

• **Don't forget friends and family.** Unless someone you know has told you they struggled with infertility or is pursuing single parenthood, you might feel like you're living alone on an island. But if you already have any close relationships, consider inviting them into your world.

• **Narrow down your circle.** The exact number of people is up to you, but most people cast a wide net and select only a handful for regular, ongoing updates and support.

• **Check your gut.** Sometimes sources of support—online, in-person, friend, family— can get overwhelming, especially for people who are already stressed out by the infertility journey. As always, do what feels best for *you*.

WARRIOR WISDOM
Know When to Ask for Help

"I have never been someone to ask others for help. My mother died when I was young, and I have been fiercely resourceful. Learning to ask for help and seeing people rise to the call and go above and beyond was gratifying and a life lesson beyond infertility."— Allison, New York

WARRIOR CHECKLIST
Understanding Infertility

❑ Learn the definition of infertility and the difference between primary and secondary infertility.

❑ Get familiar with both the female and male reproductive systems and how they should function.

❑ Understand the factors that impact egg and sperm health and how they can cause infertility.

❑ Know the signs and symptoms of both female and male infertility.

❑ Consider whether it's time for you to see a reproductive endocrinologist.

❑ Begin practicing coping mechanisms and leaning on your support system to make it through the tough times.

Add more items to your Warrior Checklist or jot down any notes here:

_____

_____

_____

_____

_____

_____

_____

_____

_____

_____

_____

_____

_____

_____

How to Select the Right Doctor and Prepare for Your First Visit

I MET MY FUTURE HUSBAND IN MY second week of college. I had just started a job as a staff writer at one of the university's student newspapers. The paper's photo editor, Brett, offered to lend me a camera for my first story. Because we'd only communicated via email, he suggested that we meet at the dumpster next to the main administration building on campus. Why the dumpster? His rationale was that no one else would be standing there, so it would be easy to identify each other. I later learned that he'd fallen in love with me that fateful day by that stinky dumpster. "She's beautiful," he told one of his best friends at the time, "and I'm going to marry her one day."

And marry we did, three years later.

I've always been a focused, driven person, but that doesn't mean I was uptight. Pre-infertility, one might have even called me easygoing. Things, especially with me and my husband, just had a way of working out. For example, our destination wedding was a disaster from start to finish: our wedding bands didn't fit, our train to the airport caught fire, the flight to Jamaica was canceled, my mom lost her dress, the men's suits hadn't been

properly hemmed and had to be held together with pins, and my husband forgot the music for our first dance. Oh, and it was June and the heat index in beautiful Montego Bay was about 100 degrees. Nearly all of our wedding photos are of people fanning themselves—you can practically chart the time of day based on the makeup-to-sweat ratio.

Even the earthquake that hit the island 2 days later, while we honeymooned, didn't (pardon the pun) shake us. We rolled with all of it.

If I planned a big event *today* and everything went wrong, I honestly would not be as relaxed and accepting. Infertility has changed me. I used to go with the flow—whatever happened, it wasn't the end of the world. Earthquakes, train fires, dancing our first dance as a married couple in absolute silence—I could handle it. We both could. We loved each other and that was all that mattered.

When my husband wasn't ready to start trying to conceive like I was a year after we were married, I didn't press the issue. After all, we weren't financially ready to support another human being, and I was more than

Myth: I can choose my reproductive endocrinologist the same way I pick other doctors.

It's not only okay to have high standards when you're looking for a reproductive endocrinologist, it's encouraged. You *deserve* this! It's important to consider the level of specialty care you're seeking. Jody Madeira, a law professor at Indiana University, sifted through hundreds of interviews with infertility patients and doctors to write the book *Taking Baby Steps*. She points out that you wouldn't use the same criteria to find a doctor to treat a sinus infection as you would to perform open-heart surgery. That same principle applies to picking a reproductive endocrinologist.

"They're actually helping you and your partner to create life," she says.

---

happy to focus on building my career in public relations—for a while, at least.

Five years later, when he gave the green light, I was excited—but I still wasn't overly anxious or impatient.

Even after my second miscarriage, I didn't feel particularly hurried or concerned. We were sad about our two losses, of course, and desired answers, but we were certain that ultimately everything would just *work itself out*. We were so laid back that we selected our first fertility clinic based on how close it was to our house—because, you know, traffic.

And it was that sense that *things will work out* that kept me at that clinic for 8 months without a treatment plan, much less a pregnancy.

Finally, we were to start a timed intercourse cycle (see chapter 6), but the clinic lost my baseline blood work. In that moment, it

hit me: *I didn't have to stay and shouldn't just roll with the punches.* If I wanted things to work out, I had to play an active part—a role I hadn't assumed up until then. So, I did what I should have done originally and identified the *best* fertility clinic—not the closest—to help us achieve our goal.

How to Choose the Best Fertility Clinic

Deciding to seek help from a reproductive endocrinologist is a *huge* step. It's a scary, internal admission that something might be "wrong" with your (and/or or your partner's) body, and as a result, the path that possibly lies ahead feels daunting.

Making an educated decision about your fertility clinic and reproductive endocrinologist is a complicated process that involves weighing several factors, from location to reputation to success rates.

In this chapter, I'll help you figure out *your* priorities and provide a framework to help you walk through this big decision.

I cannot say this enough: *Not all fertility clinics are created equal.* I've come up with nine criteria for selecting a clinic—a list I wish I had when I was starting my own journey.

1. Your insurance coverage

2. The clinic's location

3. The size of the clinic and the services it offers

4. Recommendations and reviews

5. The perfect-fit fertility treatment team

6. The quality of the clinic's lab

7. Your experience at the initial consultation

8. The doctor's sense of urgency and ability to empathize

9. Your gut feeling

Your Insurance Coverage

Don't become a patient at a clinic *just* because it's covered (in part or in full) by your insurance. Free or discounted infertility treatments will be of little comfort when you've been unsuccessful over and over again because you are at a subpar clinic.

⚡ As someone who spent tens of thousands of dollars to have my daughter, I know that expenses throughout this journey are not taken lightly. However, I encourage you to consider cost as only one of many factors when making your decision. (See chapter 20 for creative funding options.)

The Clinic's Location

Treating infertility means a lot of appointments. A lot. If there are excellent clinics around you, then by all means pick the one that is most convenient. But if you have to travel an hour (or two) or across state lines to see the top specialist versus 15 minutes to see your third or fourth choice, to me, the answer is obvious: Go the distance. Yes, it's a pain. And yes, you will have to do some explaining at work (see chapter 21). But it will be worth it in the long run.

Most clinics can accommodate you even if you're hundreds (or thousands) of miles away. Kara lives in North Dakota, a state where there is only one fertility clinic—200 miles away from Kara's home. Luckily, the staff worked to limit how much she needed to travel.

"In the first few treatments that we did, a lot of it was remote where I would—here in my own town—get the ultrasounds done so that they could look at my follicles. Then I would Skype with the doctors. They would get my blood work, and we would decide where to go from there," she says.

The Size of the Clinic and the Services It Offers

There are several types of fertility clinics, from solo practitioners to sprawling fertility networks. Weigh the pros and cons of a clinic's size and services, and choose the one that best aligns with *your* needs.

WARRIOR TIPS
Discovering What Your Insurance Covers

Hopefully you're one of the lucky ones who lives in a state with mandated infertility coverage. As of this writing, those states include Arkansas, California, Colorado, Connecticut, Delaware, Hawaii, Illinois, Louisiana, Maine, Maryland, Massachusetts, Montana, New Hampshire, New Jersey, New York, Ohio, Rhode Island, Texas, Utah, and West Virginia (see chapter 19). If you don't live in one of those states, call your insurance company to see what, if anything, they cover. (Mine, for example, covers all diagnostic procedures, including ultrasounds.)

When researching how your insurance coverage will impact your fertility clinic options, find out the following:

- What types of medications, diagnostics, and treatments are covered

- If there's a limit on the number of cycles or overall dollar amount they cover

- If they cover only certain doctors or clinics

- If there's supplemental coverage you can purchase

- How you can appeal a denied claim

Solo Practitioners and Small Practices

These specialty doctors offer treatment on a smaller scale. Some will offer only the treatments they're familiar with and thus may have to refer you to other specialists as needs arise.

Pros:

- Most offer a personable experience.

- Direct access to your doctor rather than a fertility nurse

Cons:

- Accept fewer patients and might be more selective about whom they choose to treat

- May not offer as many services

- Limited resources when compared to large-scale practices

- Limited discounts and financing options

- May have you take birth control pills to time treatment cycles around their limited availability rather than your unique body

- May not be open on weekends

Large, Full-Service Practices

This collection of multiple specialists and doctors works together to provide mostly in-house treatment to patients.

Pros:

- Typically have in-house, state-of-the-art labs, equipment, and other resources

- More financing options than small practices

Cons:

- May be impersonal; you are one of hundreds of patients

- You may not see the same doctor every visit, and your doctor might not be the one to perform procedures like IUI and IVF.

- You are more likely to communicate with a fertility nurse and other staff than with your doctor.

Fertility Networks

A fertility network is a group of clinics—typically large practices—that operate under the same parent company.

Pros:

- Often have even more resources than large practices

- More financing options than large practices

Cons:

- May be impersonal; you are one of thousands of patients

- You may not see the same doctor every visit, and your doctor might not be the one to perform procedures like IUI and IVF.

IUI and IVF: What do they stand for?

- IUI, or intrauterine insemination, is a procedure where the doctor bypasses the vagina and cervix and puts sperm directly into the uterus using a small tube (catheter).

- IVF, or in vitro fertilization, is a procedure where eggs are retrieved from the ovaries, fertilized by sperm in a lab, developed into embryos, and transferred back into the uterus using a catheter.

- You may have to travel to other office locations for certain procedures.

- You are more likely to communicate with a fertility nurse and other staff than with your doctor.

University- or Hospital-Based Clinic

These treatment centers are affiliated with academic institutions or larger health-care organizations, often with a focus on research or teaching.

Pros:

- Particularly when tied to a university, the doctors tend to take a research- and teaching-based approach, which could mean access to experimental techniques and steep discounts.

- Access to resources similar to that of large clinics

Cons:

- Medical students may observe appointments.

- You likely have to navigate a lot of red tape and bureaucracy.

WARRIOR WISDOM

You Don't Have to Jump on the IVF Train

Beware of clinics that offer only IVF—or at least push it much, much harder over other less expensive and less invasive treatment options. Many infertility cases don't require even IUI—just some Clomid and timed intercourse (see chapter 6). It's worth going to the initial consultation appointment and hearing them out, but if the reproductive endocrinologist jumps straight to IVF without a really good reason—*and* you're just not ready to take that step—that's a major red flag that this clinic might not be a great fit.

Recommendations and Reviews

Infertility warriors understand the difficulty of choosing a clinic and doctor, so many will leave *detailed* reviews of the clinics and doctors they've used. Seriously, we write pages and pages about our experiences on review sites like FertilityIQ to make sure others have the best information at their disposal. Take advantage of these reviews. (FertilityIQ is a great resource, offering the latest research and a searchable database of doctors and clinics.)

But don't just look at the overall score. Remember, everyone has different priorities in choosing a doctor, so actually read the reviews so you can give more weight to reviewers who went through situations similar to yours.

For Brianna from Pennsylvania patient-doctor relationship and communication were important, so she wanted "someone with 'raving' reviews." To achieve that goal, after much research, she chose an out-of-state clinic about an hour away from her home.

Also, don't be afraid to ask other infertility warriors—even people you've met online—for their recommendations. They can provide insights about how the clinic as a whole treats patients.

If you start with your ob-gyn, the doctor might refer you to an RE. (Your insurance may even require this step.) However, proceed with caution, advises Katie from Wyoming. "I found my first RE through the recommendation of my ob-gyn. I later learned that this clinic aggressively recruited referrals from area ob-gyns through frequently taking them out to very fancy dinners. So, referrals may have substance, or they may mean nothing."

The Perfect-Fit Fertility Treatment Team

A team-based approach to treating fertility is becoming more and more common. There are always outliers, especially in remote areas and at solo practitioner clinics, but chances are your fertility clinic team will consist of at least some of the following professionals: a reproductive endocrinologist, a fertility nurse, a reproductive urologist, and an embryologist.

Reproductive Endocrinologist

As noted earlier, reproductive endocrinologists are ob-gyns who specialize in infertility. Their focus isn't on pregnancy itself but rather achieving it.

I can't stress enough how important it is that your RE is board-certified. This holds them to a higher standard. In order to renew their board certification, for example, they must complete a certain number of continuing education credit hours, which means staying up-to-date on the latest research and techniques.

Katie and her husband, Michael, from Kansas initially went to the clinic where Katie's sister had been successful. "I regret not meeting with any other clinics," Katie says. "My husband didn't like the RE, but I ignored that because I tended to do what my sister always did, especially in this realm of unknown medical territory."

Looking back, Katie wishes she and Michael had advocated for themselves. "I think it's necessary to get more than one opinion to see if your RE is a good fit for you, personality-wise, and if you are comfortable with them. I wish I would've slowed down a little bit, talked to my husband more about his opinions, and met with at least two or three different clinics before making a decision."

Once you choose an RE, they will direct your diagnostic testing and treatment plan. In many cases, they will also perform your fertility treatments. However, know that this isn't *always* the case. At some clinics, especially the large practices and fertility networks, a different doctor might perform your IUI or IVF cycles.

WARRIOR TIPS
Understanding SART Data

The Society for Assisted Reproductive Technology (SART) collects the results of cycles performed at every fertility clinic and offers it on their website, so you can make an educated decision about your chances of success with a particular clinic. However, this information isn't completely cut-and-dried. Remember the following factors when reviewing a clinic's SART numbers:

• **Live births vs. pregnancies.** Unfortunately, getting pregnant does not guarantee a baby. You're looking for a clinic that has a high rate of live births.

• **Clinics don't have to accept all patients.** There are some clinics that refuse to take on difficult cases because high-risk patients can hurt their success rates.

Supplement SART scores by asking clinics how many cases they turn away and why.

• **eSET vs. 2BET.** eSETs are single embryo transfers, and 2BETs are double embryo transfers. Clinics more confident in their results will trend toward eSET. However, SART does not include the number of embryos transferred during a reported cycle. So, the "success" listed could be as a result of an eSET or 2BET—you'll never know. But don't make the mistake of thinking more embryos means a higher chance of success. Transferring two embryos just increases the odds of multiples and the associated complications of those pregnancies (see chapter 9).

Fertility Nurse

Nurses are the linchpin of the fertility treatment team cogwheel. As Amber Kiddie, a fertility nurse with Fertility Centers of Illinois in Chicago, explains, although the RE leads your care and finalizes medical decisions, a nurse will likely be your main point of contact.

"The doctor will put together a treatment plan," she says, "and the nurse really helps orchestrate it. We're the ones who communicate with the patient. We order the medications. We do the training about how to give the medications. We really help facilitate this process. Of course, the doctor's the head of the team and they help us know which way we're going, but we're bridging that gap between the doctor and the patient to help them to get to where they need to be."

Your nurse will also monitor treatment cycles, assist with ultrasounds, and perform some in-office procedures, like IUI. And they are an invaluable guide, helping patients understand the procedures, their test results, and medical terminology.

WARRIOR WISDOM
Asking for a Different Nurse
● ●

Just as you don't have to stick with a doctor you don't mesh with, you also have the right to ask for a nurse who better meets your needs.

"Sometimes there's a nurse who you just don't agree with or seems to not return calls," says Jody Madeira, author of *Taking Baby Steps.* "If you are part of a clinic that has a nurse pool, you can often just ask for another nurse or work around that individual."

It might be awkward, but over the course of your journey, the person you're going to spend the most time with is your nurse. They offer you emotional support and take your calls. It's vital that you and your nurse are a good fit.

"We also really help advocate for the patient," says Kiddie. "If the doctor wasn't aware of something going on, we can say, 'Hey, this is what's going on in their life. Can we adjust this in this sort of way?' We have to help them think outside of the box. It's a really nice and unique position to be in."

Urologist (or Andrologist)

"Male reproductive problems are often complicated because there are multiple systems involved," explains Dr. Craig Niederberger, a professor at the University of Illinois at Chicago and board-certified urologist specializing in male infertility. "A urologist who specializes in male reproductive medicine and male reproductive surgery is a really good resource."

Most fertility clinics will run a semen analysis and blood work at your initial consultation appointment, although some may request it in advance. A laboratory technician analyzes the semen sample and blood for abnormalities. If the results are normal, it's unlikely you'll ever even meet a reproductive urologist. If the results are *abnormal*, a separate appointment is scheduled—and I recommend both partners attend.

Embryologist

If you decide to pursue IVF, a final member joins your fertility clinic treatment team: an embryologist. The embryologist "builds" embryos by placing the egg and sperm together—or in the case of intracytoplasmic sperm injection (ICSI), injecting the sperm directly into the egg. They also monitor the progression and status of embryos while they are in the clinic's lab and ensure proper cryopreservation (this goes for eggs and sperm, too, not just embryos). Jody Madeira says she once met an embryologist who described her job as "the first babysitter that couples will ever have."

The importance of an embryologist's role cannot be overstated. Sometimes embryologists discover *additional* diagnoses while analyzing eggs, sperm, and embryos. After my second retrieval cycle yielded only one poor-quality embryo and nothing left to freeze, the embryologist determined that I produce poor-quality eggs, likely due to my endometriosis and frequent ovarian cysts. It turned out we'd been extremely lucky with embryo quality during my first fresh transfer that had resulted in our twins. Had I known that further study of the embryos could be useful, I could have asked the embryologist for feedback at that time instead of 18 months later.

Finally, embryologists assist with preimplantation genetic testing (see chapter 4). For these tests, the embryologist removes a single cell from the embryo and sends it on for further testing to determine whether or not chromosomal abnormalities exist within that specific embryo.

WARRIOR WISDOM
Be Aware of the Medical Review Board
....

While your fertility treatment team hopefully lives and breathes your case, there's a good chance that a medical review board composed of people who've never met you is pulling the strings behind the scenes. Never forget that fertility clinics are *businesses*. If your reproductive endocrinologist finds something in your initial testing that makes you a less-than-optimal candidate for IVF, the most invasive (and expensive) procedure, you might be turned away.

If this does happen, I consider it a good thing. Why? Because if that's how the clinic makes its decisions, you didn't want to be a patient there anyway. A fertility clinic that turns down a patient just because that patient might impact their success rate is one you want to run away from as far as possible. Fertility clinics *should* work to be successful on the first try, but it should be for the right reasons.

The Quality of the Clinic's Lab

If you end up needing IVF, the quality of the lab at your fertility clinic is a vital factor. The clinic is responsible for fertilization (successfully inseminating eggs with sperm); growing embryos (developing healthy embryos into blastocysts); biopsying embryos (removing cells for genetic testing); and storing eggs, sperm, and embryos (ensuring cryosurvival).

According to Jake Anderson-Bialis of FertilityIQ in San Francisco, which he co-founded with his wife, Deborah, after struggling to find the best fertility doctor, we should evaluate the following in a lab:

• **Laboratory volume.** High volume means that the lab is experienced. Look for the total cycle volume to be *at least* 200 cycles per year—but the more the better. Anderson-Bialis reports that clinics with fewer than 200 cycles per year have lower success rates per IVF patient (63 percent versus 69 percent).

• **Embryologist experience.** Remember when I said the importance of an embryologist cannot be overstated? Anderson-Bialis recommends seeking out clinics with embryologists who perform at least one procedure per day and have a minimum of 2 to 5 years of training.

• **Intracytoplasmic sperm injection (ICSI) fertilization rate.** Even without a male factor playing a role in the fertility issues, there is a more than 60 percent chance that ICSI (see chapter 7) will be utilized during an IVF cycle. This chance increases to 95 percent when a male factor is present. The clinic should have an ICSI fertilization rate of at least 70 percent—meaning if you provide ten eggs, at least seven of them fertilize.

• **Incubator type and oxygen.** Ideally, your lab would use "desktop incubators," which have separate chambers for each sample, and 5 percent oxygen—not 20 percent, like nearly one-third of labs in the United States. The air we breathe contains around 20 percent oxygen, but the oxygen level *within our bodies*—where embryos grow and develop—is about 5 percent. If the lab uses "big-box incubators," ask how many other patients share the same incubator. Incubators with more samples inside will be opened more frequently, which can increase oxygen levels and decrease temperature. If the incubator is shared, Anderson-Bialis suggests

asking if your samples can get their own shelf, preferably the middle shelf.

• **Blastocyst conversion rate.** By day 5, at least 30 to 40 percent of embryos should become blastocysts—embryos with two distinct cell types, cells that have started to differentiate, and a central cavity filled with fluid (see chapter 7). By day 6, the number of embryos that become blastocysts should increase to 40 to 50 percent. Although there are individual cases in which transferring embryos prior to day 5 make sense, defaulting to earlier transfers should be a red flag.

• **Staffing and availability.** Labs should have at least two embryologists and should be operational 7 days a week. Each embryologist should oversee no less than 100 cycles but no more than 150 cycles per year.

• **Natural disaster plan.** From hurricanes to earthquakes and everything in between, natural disasters—and the subsequent power outages—are unavoidable. So, it's important the clinic have real-time incubator monitoring and a plan in place should systems fail.

• **Number of embryos transferred per cycle.** Guidelines from the American Society for Reproductive Medicine (ASRM) currently read as follows: "In patients of any age, transfer of a euploid embryo has the most favorable prognosis and should be limited to one. Even in patients of advanced maternal age where euploid embryos are available, a single blastocyst transfer should be the norm." Clinics that perform an overwhelming number of eSETs are following ASRM's best practices and likely have the most cutting-edge lab equipment.

• **Success rate of fresh donor egg cycles.** Fresh donor eggs (versus frozen) should, in theory, be of similar quality across clinics. Patients most often refer to success rates provided by SART and the CDC. However, as we already discussed, this data is often skewed, as clinics can selectively treat low-risk patients or report only select data to the organization.

⚡ Most clinics will be willing to share this information with you if you simply ask. Some will even grant a tour of their lab. If they won't answer your questions, consider another clinic.

Your Experience at the Initial Consultation

Once you've found a fertility clinic that looks good on paper, schedule an initial consultation—and prepare to self-advocate. Think of it as a job interview where *you* are the employer. Your main duty is to yourself, your partner (if you have one), and your future child(ren)—*not* the clinic or doctor. I'm looking at you, people-pleasers!

WARRIOR TIPS
Do Your Homework and Come Prepared to Ask Questions

Research the questions you want to ask. This is important! Write down your questions in advance so you don't forget to ask them. Some examples include:

- Why haven't we/I been able to conceive?

- How does our/my age affect our/my fertility and chances for a healthy pregnancy?

- What type of testing will we/I need to determine the cause of our/my infertility?

- How long do you think it will take to get the initial fertility workup completed and potentially start some form of treatment? How can we/I best get these tests scheduled?

- If we/I already know what's causing our/my infertility, is this condition likely to get worse over time, stay the same, or maybe improve?

- If our/my infertility diagnosis remains unexplained after the initial fertility workup, what additional tests will you run to narrow down the possible causes?

- What do you think about lifestyle modifications? Is there anything we/I can do to increase our/my chance of becoming pregnant?

- What type of treatment should we/I try first, and why?

- What does this treatment involve? Walk us/me through it step-by-step.

- What are your success rates with this treatment for patients like us/me? How do you define success?

- Are there any risks or side effects of your recommended treatment?

- How many cycles do you recommend before we/I try something else?

- What does this treatment cost? What if our/my insurance doesn't cover certain aspects of this treatment? Do you offer financing plans?

- Do you see patients every day of the week? What are your monitoring hours?

- Do you have an after-hours line for emergencies?

- Who is the best person to contact if we/I have any questions? How do we/I contact this person?

- Do you truly believe you can help us/me build our/my family?

- Are there any other questions you think we/I should be asking?

Finally, inquire whether or not you need to follow any special instructions. Should you be fasting for certain blood tests? Should a male partner get a semen analysis in advance? How long does he need to refrain from ejaculating before his semen analysis? (Typically, it's no less than 1 and no more than 11 days.) Is there anything else you need to do to prepare for the tests?

"I personally have met doctors who are rushed. And I've met doctors who could talk with you all day to the point the patient would want to leave before the doctor would want to conclude the appointment," says Madeira.

Before the Consultation

Gather your medical records from your primary care physician, ob-gyn, and other specialists—anything and everything that might be relevant and useful to your reproductive endocrinologist. If you have a partner, bring their medical records as well.

If possible, fill out the clinic's required paperwork in advance so you don't have to rush through it before your appointment. Additionally, consider preparing an overview

BUSTED

Myth: I have to be an "ideal" patient.

I understand this instinct. (My husband and I actually dressed up for our initial consultation, as though we would be judged on our potential as parents based on our appearance!) Your fertility team is working to make your dream of being a parent come true, so you feel like you have to make their lives as easy as possible. Jody Madeira's research found that most infertility warriors feel a pressure to seem calm, educated, and unemotional in front of their doctor.

However, this couldn't be further from your medical professionals' expectations.

"In fact," says Madeira, "[doctors are] kind of alarmed when they expect patients to be emotional—like after a negative pregnancy test—and the patient is completely, 'OK, so what?'"

Your journey will be a lot easier and possibly faster if you are open and honest. After all, they've agreed to treat you, not a robot.

of your journey thus far—how long you've been trying, whether or not you've been temping and charting, and so on—to turn in with the rest of the forms. Don't forget to bring a copy for yourself for reference!

During the Consultation

If you have a partner and they cannot attend for some reason—although I always recommend partners make every effort to be there—or if you are embarking on this journey by yourself, bring a friend who can help you take notes so you can actively listen and participate in the conversation. You'll need to absorb and process a lot of new information to make an informed decision about next steps. Ask questions, but prepare a list of topics to research when you get home.

In general, during the initial consultation, you're grading the clinic and its team in two ways: (1) whether their operations meet your needs and expectations and (2) whether they mesh with you and your personality.

Let's start with operational considerations.

• **Whether or not they see patients 7 days a week.** To me, this is nonnegotiable, but you might feel differently. Just remember, the ideal time to perform an IUI, IVF egg retrieval, or embryo transfer—or the first day of your period—doesn't always happen during non-holiday weekdays.

• **How they communicate with patients.** At the first clinic I went to, if I had any questions, I had to leave messages with the front desk and wait for the doctor to call me back. My second clinic was a large practice in a fertility network, so I was assigned a nurse whom I could reach during normal business hours via both phone and email. And she heard from me a lot! That arrangement worked for me, but if you prefer direct communication with your doctor, seek out a clinic that offers that relationship. They do exist!

• **How accessible they are after-hours.** While I didn't expect my nurse to take care of my needs at all hours of the day, it was nice to know my clinic had an answering service for evenings and weekends.

• **Their hospital affiliation.** If you experience a complication that requires hospitalization, you want to make sure they plan to send you to a hospital covered by your insurance. These kind of complications don't happen often, but they *can* happen. And anyway, I'm a big believer in being prepared for all possibilities.

• **Their financial options.** Most clinics require you to pay for procedures 100 percent up front, but if you're paying out of pocket, they should have programs to help you with the burden (see chapter 20).

• **What diagnostic tests they plan to perform.** Educate yourself on the many tests that should be performed (on both you and your partner; see the next section). If the clinic didn't plan on testing a specific hormone you feel might be relevant to your case, this shouldn't be a deal-breaker. Remember, you can always self-advocate!

⚡ Some infertility warriors don't understand why personality should play into their decision when they're choosing a clinic. If the doctor gets you pregnant, what else matters? But as Madeira points out, how your experience *feels* is important.

"Patients really love when their physicians are personable and empathic. Cold and clinical providers can be alienating, and leave patients wondering if they can ask questions or discuss the more emotional or relational impacts of going through treatment," she says. "Patients really like when their physicians know their names, listen to them, and converse with them, making them feel as if they are the physician's immediate priority, and that the physician responds to them as individuals."

WARRIOR WISDOM
Use Only Reliable Resources
• •
Dr. Google is not your friend. Instead, search for information on these sites:

• American Society for Reproductive Medicine (asrm.org)

• Fertility Answers by MedAnswers (fertility.medanswers.com)

• FertilityIQ.com

• Healthline.com

• ReproductiveFacts.org

• RESOLVE: The National Infertility Association (resolve.org)

Look for the following:

• **How you're greeted.** Does the staff seem warm and welcoming? Do you feel like a number—just another patient—or like you've finally found "your people"?

• **How they define success.** Again, live births should be the only statistic that matters—to both you *and* your clinic. If you've never seen those two pink lines, you might think being pregnant even for a short time is better than never being pregnant at all, but *you deserve better.*

• **What wellness and mental health services they provide.** Do they offer support groups or counseling? What about acupuncture? Even if they don't offer these resources in-house, they should have a list of pre-vetted providers.

• **Whether they seem hopeful for you—and make you feel hopeful for yourself.** You should walk away from this appointment feeling *energized*—a little overwhelmed, perhaps, but definitely energized.

That last point is huge. Although they can never offer guarantees, you want a team who strongly believes they can help you complete your family. Beth from Utah says her doctor filled her and her husband, Wesley, with optimism from the very first day and throughout their journey.

"He made us feel like there was definite hope, and he was for sure going to get us pregnant. I never let go of that hope. I always felt like there was a next step in the right direction," she says.

Regardless of what kind of clinic you choose, the initial consult and fertility workup should look pretty much the same.

Fertility Workups for Women

Ideally, you should schedule it for day 2 or 3—or day 4 at the *latest*—of your menstrual cycle. Again, ask for any special instructions, like whether you need to fast before the test, in advance.

The appointment typically starts with a conversation about your medical, surgical, gynecological, and obstetric history, as well as your lifestyle (whether you smoke, drink, regularly exercise, and so on). Although the doctor might not be able to answer many of your questions until you've completed an initial fertility workup, this is a great opportunity to go through your list—especially the questions about doctor-patient communication and overall clinic operations. Just keep in mind that you might need to circle back to your treatment plan questions after your results are available.

If you are on cycle day 2, 3, or 4, you should receive a transvaginal ultrasound (see chapter 3) to visually assess your uterine lining and ovaries, including an antral follicle count (AFC). The number of antral follicles—or "resting" follicles containing immature eggs—along with blood work and your age allow the doctor to estimate your ovarian reserve and anticipated response to ovarian stimulation medications.

Again, assuming you are on cycle day 2, 3, or 4, here's the blood work the doctor should order (we'll talk more about normal ranges and what abnormal results might mean in chapter 3):

- **Anti-Müllerian hormone (AMH).** Secreted by the antral follicles found in the ovaries at the start of the menstrual cycle. Can help indicate the size of your ovarian reserve.

- **Dehydroepiandrosterone sulfate (DHEA-S).** A hormone produced by the adrenal glands. High levels can interfere with ovulation.

- **Estradiol (E2).** Stimulates the growth of follicles and the production of fertile cervical mucus. Thickens and prepares the uterine lining for the implantation of a fertilized egg.

- **Follicle-stimulating hormone (FSH).** Stimulates egg development.

- **Luteinizing hormone (LH).** Stimulates ovulation.

- **Progesterone (P4).** Maintains the health of the uterine lining in preparation for the implantation of a fertilized egg. Supports early pregnancy.

- **Prolactin.** Inhibits FSH, which stimulates egg development, and gonadotropin-releasing hormone (GnRH), the hormones that trigger ovulation and allow eggs to develop and mature. *This test requires fasting, so inquire in advance of your appointment. You likely will also be asked to avoid exercise, intercourse, and hot showers in the 24 hours beforehand.*

- **Testosterone.** High levels in women can interfere with ovulation.

- **Thyroid-stimulating hormone (TSH).** Produced by the pituitary and controls thyroid gland activity. Low levels indicate hyperthyroidism. High levels result in high prolactin levels and indicate hypothyroidism.

- **Thyroxin (T4) and triiodothyronine (T3).** Produced by the thyroid, T3 is the more active form of thyroid hormone that tells cells what to do, and T4 is converted into T3 inside the target cells. Low levels can result in high levels of prolactin and indicate hypothyroidism. High levels indicate hyperthyroidism.

- **Vitamin D.** Low levels of this fat-soluble vitamin have been linked with infertility.

- **Infectious diseases.** Hepatitis B, hepatitis C, HIV, and other infectious diseases may impact fertility.

⚡ If you've experienced two or more pregnancy losses, advocate for a recurrent pregnancy loss (RPL) panel. The tests included in a RPL panel are extensive and look for autoimmune, genetic, and thrombophilic (blood clotting) abnormalities—all of which have been most strongly associated with recurrent miscarriage.

Workups for Men

For male patients, you will have to give the doctor information about your medical and surgical history. You'll also answer questions about your lifestyle and factors that might put you at higher risk for infertility issues.

With regard to your semen analysis (we'll talk more about normal ranges and what abnormal results might mean in chapter 3), the doctor is looking at:

- **Abnormal cells.** The presence or absence of white or red blood cells or immature sperm.

- **Concentration.** Your total sperm count.

- **Liquefaction time.** How long it takes your fresh sample to break down into seminal fluid.

- **Morphology.** The shape and appearance of your sperm.

- **Motility.** What percentage of your sperm moves.

- **pH.** The level of acidity in your semen.

- **Total motile count.** The amount of sperm typically left following a sperm wash (determined by multiplying the volume by the concentration, then multiplying that number by the motility percentage, then multiplying that number by the percentage of sperm with normal morphology, and finally dividing the resulting number by half).

- **Viscosity.** The thickness and consistency of the sample.

- **Vitality.** The percentage of dead cells in the sample.

- **Volume.** How much semen you ejaculate at once.

If you provided a semen analysis in advance and it revealed any abnormalities, your doctor may also run blood tests checking your hormone levels—estrogen, LH, FSH, and testosterone. They may also perform blood tests for hepatitis B and C, HIV, and other infectious diseases.

If the appointment is early in the morning, you might receive most of the blood work results later that afternoon, although some may take up to a week. However, the testing doesn't end there—especially if you fall under the dreaded "unexplained infertility" category. You'll learn more about additional diagnostics in chapter 3.

After the Consultation

You should have a follow-up with your reproductive endocrinologist when all of the initial fertility workup results are available. Some of the questions listed earlier—especially the ones about specific treatment paths—might not be answerable until this follow-up. Bring that list and any other questions you have to this appointment.

Remember, evaluating your doctor and clinic is an ongoing process. Your initial consultation could be fantastic, but subsequent appointments might reveal issues. Continue paying attention to:

• **How your doctor explains results, plans, outcomes, and next steps.** Unless you have a medical degree, the information you discuss may be confusing. Ask your doctor to break everything down and explain what it means for you moving forward. If you do this and continue to leave appointments confused, that's not a good sign.

• **The ease of scheduling follow-up appointments.** Even if you had to wait for your initial appointment, all subsequent appointments should be easy to schedule.

• **The proactiveness and creativity of your doctor.** You should always have a treatment plan, even if you cannot execute it right away for one reason or another. And it shouldn't be a cookie-cutter approach. All treatments should be tailored to you as an individual or couple—and tweaked when needed. When a doctor continues trying the same unsuccessful approach over and over, that's a red flag.

• **Staff turnover.** Over the course of your infertility journey, it's likely that some of your nurses or other friendly faces will change jobs. However, if you notice that the office seems to have a revolving door, it could be a bad sign.

The Doctor's Sense of Urgency and Ability to Empathize

Let's say you found a clinic that you felt comfortable with after the initial consultation and you've just completed the diagnostic phase.

At this point, the only person more excited and ready to get started with a treatment plan than you should be your doctor. If they have no sense of urgency and don't prompt you with a clear plan of action immediately after testing is complete, you may want to take your results and transfer to another clinic.

"It hurts me when a patient doesn't get pregnant or loses a pregnancy, and it elates me when everything goes well," says Jill Mathews, an embryologist at Fertility Centers of Illinois. "Some of my proudest moments are when former patients seek me out to share their stories and show off their beautiful, healthy babies. It is really gratifying when we see that we have helped to positively change [someone's] life in that way."

Doesn't that sound like someone you'd want managing your care?

BUSTED

Myth: I have to stick with my doctor.

I'm living proof that sometimes firing your doctor is the right choice.

While I'd like to tell you my situation is unique, many infertility warriors find it necessary to make a change. Some people know right away, like Stephani from Kansas. "I saw a reproductive endocrinologist for one appointment, and he really rubbed me the wrong way. He didn't read my history. He went straight to recommending IVF and didn't ask me very many questions. It all felt very impersonal and didn't really fit for us."

Even if you've spent months or years with a doctor or clinic, you don't have to stick it out if you have doubts.

Your Gut Feeling

Time for some more self-advocacy talk. While you're not a medical expert, trust your intuition when something tells you that you're not getting the care you deserve. "You know your case better than any RE ever will," encourages Katie, whom we heard from earlier in this chapter. "You have your own ideas about what is wrong that are likely being continually brushed off by doctor after doctor. Stick with those ideas, and find a clinic that will take them seriously."

And don't be afraid to get a second opinion, whether you've been with your current clinic for a day or a year. It took Katie *four* clinics before she found the right fit, and she expresses doubt that she would ever have been successful had she stuck with her first clinic.

She says, "Despite all ostensibly doing the same things, each of these experiences has been so completely different. I tell [anyone] going through this to seek out multiple opinions—even if you like the first clinic. For most of us, this is such a huge investment that it is worth knowing what different options are out there. Maybe something will feel like a better fit than the first clinic that you set foot in."

Carley from Illinois said that listening to her gut and speaking up put her on a path with which she was more comfortable.

"I sought out a second opinion after my second miscarriage and have never been happier," she shares. "My new RE tested me using

WARRIOR TIPS
When to Seek a Second Opinion

A second opinion may come from another doctor within the same practice—especially if it's a large one or part of a network—or from another clinic altogether. If you find yourself in any of the following scenarios, it's time to seek one:

• You feel you cannot trust your doctor or are questioning their advice after you've raised valid concerns. Expect nothing less than to be taken seriously at every turn.

• Your doctor isn't changing your treatment plans despite repeated failed cycles.

• The clinic staff is rude, insensitive, or incompetent.

• Your doctor is *too* optimistic given your medical history. In other words, there is realistically little hope of conceiving or carrying a child with a particular fertility treatment (such as IUI), yet your doctor encourages you to continue. This might be an indication that they just want your money.

the recurrent loss panel and found out that I have a blood clotting disorder that was interfering with pregnancy. I'm now happily pregnant because of the medical interventions I was able to get thanks to my new RE."

Never feel like you don't have options when it comes to your fertility clinic. You don't owe your doctor or the clinic a long-term relationship. If you have doubts, trust your instincts and move on.

Every reproductive endocrinologist and fertility clinic is different. Identifying your needs and expectations is the first step to making your decision less overwhelming.

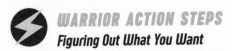

WARRIOR ACTION STEPS
Figuring Out What You Want

Think about the following topics to find the medical support that is right for you:

- **The size of your team.** Some people prefer a lot of one-on-one time with just a few health-care providers. Others want access to as many specialists as possible. Think through the pros and cons of each option and determine how to move forward—at least at first. Keep in mind that your needs might change.

- **The type of alternative support you want.** If you have a predisposition for certain mental illnesses, having access to a therapist might be a must-have (see chapter 14). Other infertility warriors may want to balance Western medicine with Eastern practices.

- **Your deal-breakers.** Identifying your deal-breakers before choosing a doctor and clinic ensures you're on the lookout for red flags from the beginning. You can have a clear idea about when you absolutely need to walk away from a medical care provider.

- **If you have a partner, make sure you're on the same page.** You're going to be on this journey together—it's important you both start on the same foot.

WARRIOR WISDOM
Finding the Empathy You Deserve

"I decided to go with the RE mostly because of the empathy he displayed. Although I am pretty independent and okay with people being straightforward with me, [when things are] incredibly stressful, I want somebody who's going be able to show me empathy."— Lindsay, Missouri

WARRIOR CHECKLIST
Selecting a Fertility Clinic

- ❏ Know the nine criteria to consider when researching doctors and fertility clinics.
- ❏ Remember that not all fertility clinics are created equal, and know your priorities.
- ❏ Become familiar with the different people who might be on your fertility team.
- ❏ Understand what you should expect during your first appointment at a fertility clinic and how to prepare.
- ❏ Don't be afraid to change doctors if your first choice turns out to be a bad fit.

Getting—and Understanding— Your Diagnoses

MY FIRST PERIOD ARRIVED on my 12th birthday. I was at a sleepover and the rush of blood woke me. Of course, I was not prepared. I was particularly upset about the timing—having to sneak away from my friends in the middle of the night—but there was so much blood, and I was in a tremendous amount of pain. It was nothing like my mom had described.

Once the floodgates opened, they didn't really stop. I would have a couple of days of relief, then my period would return. I could hardly change pads quickly enough. Because my school system did not allow students to use the bathroom during class, my thick pads often overflowed. To prepare for the inevitable, I began carrying a cleaning spray, paper towels, and a coat to tie around my waist. I passed frequent, large clots. And the pain, oh the pain. I doubled over—and at times, completely blacked out.

My parents didn't know what to do with me. My dad had no interest in discussing "women's troubles," and my mom had always had light, painless periods, so this was foreign to her.

Over the years, I saw many gynecologists, all of whom told me to "suck it up" and "this is just how periods are." Eventually, I believed them.

In the summer of 2007, then 23 years old, I had been in such constant, excruciating pain—particularly on my right side—that my husband and I actually switched sides of the bed because I could no longer comfortably lie on the right. I couldn't take it anymore and reached out to a doctor at Johns Hopkins University, begging him to see me. I was in his office 3 days later.

A transvaginal ultrasound identified the problem—or at least one: an ovarian cyst the size of a baseball on my right ovary. I had been on various forms of hormonal birth control pills since I turned 18 to reduce my period symptoms. The doctor told me the cyst was likely *from* the birth control pills and to stop them immediately.

A few weeks later, I felt the cyst burst. I honestly thought I was going to bleed out and die. I contacted my doctor and headed into laparoscopic surgery. When I woke up, he told me and my husband that he'd found endometriosis in multiple places, including my bladder. He showed us lots of pictures and said he'd removed it all. But, he warned, the surgery wasn't a cure—it would return.

Still, I felt satisfied that he'd removed it for the moment. My periods became shorter—sometimes I had a whole week in between bleeds—and slightly less painful.

But honestly, I mostly pushed the diagnosis out of my mind.

My first reproductive endocrinologist performed another laparoscopy in January 2013 to clear out my endometriosis again, but for the most part, endometriosis was treated as a non-factor in my fertility. The same was true when I switched clinics and underwent my first IVF retrieval cycle. It hardly even came up.

All of that changed following my second retrieval, in April 2015.

Despite our success the first time around, this time we ended up with only one barely viable embryo, whereas in the first cycle we had had six.

BUSTED

Myth: Everyone gets a diagnosis.

If only. Many infertility warriors never receive concrete answers about why they're struggling to conceive. And as Elizabeth from California puts it: "Unexplained infertility is kind of a funny diagnosis because a lot of us are problem-solvers, and so it's frustrating to not have a problem to solve."

However, you don't need a diagnosis to start fertility treatments. Your reproductive endocrinologist (RE) will most likely recommend that you start with the least invasive treatment options—which might provide some answers—while you continue to undergo additional testing. You also might work your way up to IVF or get pregnant and never identify the underlying issue. Sue from Michigan went through seven IVF cycles and transferred forty embryos before one finally implanted.

"My doctors told me that my cycles were 'picture perfect.' But if everything was so perfect, then why couldn't we get pregnant?" she says. "Infertility was the toughest battle we fought!"

Turns out, I had poor-quality eggs—because of the endometriosis. Finally, it was time to discuss it.

Introduction to Diagnostic Tests

In this chapter, we'll go through the *diagnostic process*—the possible diagnostic tests you'll get, how to navigate the ups and downs of the process, how to learn more about a diagnosis, and how to process and accept the results of all that testing.

⚡ Once your initial fertility workup results are in, it's time to review them with your doctor at a follow-up consultation. I recommend asking for a copy of your results in advance of this appointment so that you can come armed with questions.

There are a few things to keep in mind:

• It's possible that the test you need is not described here because it is rare or was developed after this writing.

• I've noted which tests you'll likely receive first. The majority of these tests are conducted once a problem has been identified or once you've been lumped in the "unexplained infertility" category.

• Use this section as a reference guide when reading about the various diagnoses described later in this chapter and in the appendix.

• Note that what is considered a "normal range" may change overtime. Be sure to consult with your doctor for the latest wisdom.

Female Diagnostic Tests

The initial diagnostic phase of your journey might feel long—especially depending on what's found—but it's a crucial step in the overall process. After all, it's hard to make sound decisions without data.

Initial Fertility Workup

It's important to understand not only what tests should be included in the fertility workup, but also the normal ranges for each and what abnormal results might mean.

For a woman, the workup usually begins with a transvaginal ultrasound, which visually assesses your uterine lining for thickness and appearance and your ovaries for an antral follicle count (AFC). The number of antral follicles, your blood work results, and your age allow the doctor to estimate your ovarian reserve and anticipated response to ovarian stimulation medications.

Your doctor or the sonographer will insert the ultrasound wand several inches into your vagina. Using high-frequency sound waves, it creates an image of your reproductive organs. This process is routine and painless, although you may be asked to place the wand yourself to ensure your comfort.

UTERINE LINING THICKNESS RESULTS

MENSTRUAL CYCLE PHASE	NORMAL RANGE	WHAT ABNORMAL RESULTS COULD MEAN
Menstrual phase	2–4 mm	Too thick: Endometrial hyperplasia, a noncancerous condition caused by too much estrogen and not enough progesterone
		Too thin: Amenorrhea (the absence of menstrual periods) or another condition that results in low estrogen production
Early follicular phase	4–6 mm	Too thick: Endometrial hyperplasia or irregular ovulation, especially with long cycles
		Too thin: Amenorrhea (the absence of menstrual periods) or another condition that results in low estrogen production
Late follicular phase	6–8 mm	Too thin: Poor ovarian response, use of certain ovarian stimulation medications (such as Clomid; see chapter 5), or amenorrhea (the absence of menstrual periods) or another condition that results in low estrogen production
Luteal phase	≤ 12 mm	Too thick (15+ mm) or too thin (< 6 mm): Reduced likelihood of embryo implantation or increased likelihood of early miscarriage
		Too thin (< 6 mm): Poor ovarian response or luteal phase defect, caused by low levels of progesterone after ovulation

UTERINE LINING PATTERN RESULTS

GRADE	NAME	DESCRIPTION
A	Homogeneous and hyperechogenic	Lacks a central line
B	Isoechogenic	Poorly defined or absent central line
C	Trilaminar	Triple layered, with a clearly defined outer layer, central line, and inner layer

ANTRAL FOLLICLE COUNT

ANTRAL FOLLICLE COUNT (AFC)	COUNT CONSIDERED	EXPECTED RESPONSE TO OVARIAN STIMULATION MEDICATION	CHANCES FOR IVF SUCCESS
Less than 4	Extremely low	Very poor or none	Cycle cancellation likely
4–9	Low	Possible poor response	Lower than average
10–19	Average	Usually good	Good
20–29	High	Excellent, although at greater risk for ovarian hyperstimulation syndrome (OHSS)	Excellent
More than 30	Polycystic	Excellent, although at high risk for OHSS; cycle cancellation possible due to high estrogen levels	Cycle cancellation possible due to high estrogen levels

Antral Follicle Count (AFC)

As you learned in chapter 1, follicles are the small cavities that surround developing eggs. Antral follicles (or "resting" follicles) contain immature eggs, each with the potential to mature. Using a transvaginal ultrasound administered on cycle day 2, 3, or 4, a sonographer will count and measure the number of follicles on each ovary. No matter your results, remember that quality is more important than quantity!

Endometrial Stripe

Your uterine lining, or endometrium, appears as a dark line during a transvaginal ultrasound. This dark line is your endometrial stripe. Your doctor will measure the thickness and grade the pattern of your endometrial stripe to evaluate how receptive your uterus is to embryo implantation. If the stripe is too thick or too thin or the pattern is not grade C immediately before ovulation, insemination, or an embryo transfer, your doctor might recommend canceling your cycle (see box on page 41).

Blood Tests

The rest of your initial female fertility workup consists of blood tests. Again, assuming you are on cycle day 2, 3, or 4, here's the blood work the doctor should order, the normal ranges, and what abnormal results might indicate.

Anti-Müllerian Hormone (AMH)

AMH is secreted by the antral follicles found in the ovaries at the start of the menstrual cycle. Together with other tests—specifically those for AFC and follicle-stimulating hormone (FSH)—it helps indicate your ovarian reserve.

AMH RESULTS	
AGE	NORMAL RANGE
< 33	≥ 2.1 ng/mL
33–37	≥ 1.7 ng/mL
38–40	≥ 1.1 ng/mL
41+	≥ 0.5 ng/mL

Dehydroepiandrosterone Sulfate (DHEA-S)
DHEA-S is a hormone produced by the adrenal glands. High levels can interfere with ovulation.

DHEA-S RESULTS	
AGE	NORMAL RANGE
20–29	65–380 µg/dL 1.75–10.26 µmol/L
30–39	45–270 µg/dL 1.22–7.29 µmol/L
40–49	32–240 µg/dL 0.86–6.48 µmol/L

Estradiol (E2)
E2 stimulates the growth of follicles and the production of fertile cervical mucus. It thickens and prepares your uterine lining for the implantation of a fertilized egg. At the start of your cycle, E2 should be 25 to 75 pg/mL. While low levels are preferred, too low can potentially cause a slow response to ovarian stimulation medication and/or a uterine lining that does not properly thicken. High levels, on the other hand, may indicate the presence of an active or functional (estrogen-producing) ovarian cyst or diminished ovarian reserve (DOR).

E2 RESULTS		
CYCLE DAY TESTED	NORMAL RANGE	WHAT ABNORMAL RESULTS COULD MEAN
3	25–75 pg/mL	May indicate the existence of a functional cyst or diminished ovarian reserve
LH surge day	200+ pg/mL per mature (18+ mm) follicle	Poor ovarian response

Follicle-Stimulating Hormone (FSH)
FSH stimulates egg development. A high FSH level may reduce the likelihood of pregnancy and mean primary ovarian insufficiency (also known as premature ovarian failure) or impending age-related menopause.

FSH RESULTS	
AGE	NORMAL RANGE
< 33 years	< 7.0 mIU/mL
33–37 years	< 7.9 mIU/mL
38–40 years	< 8.4 mIU/mL
41+ years	< 8.5 mIU/mL

Luteinizing Hormone (LH)
LH stimulates ovulation and should be less than 7 mIU/mL. If your LH level is higher than your FSH level on cycle day 3, it could indicate polycystic ovary syndrome (PCOS).

LH RESULTS	
CYCLE DAY TESTED	NORMAL RANGE
3	< 7 mIU/mL
LH surge day	> 20 mIU/mL

Progesterone (P4)
P4 maintains the health of your uterine lining in preparation for the implantation of a fertilized egg and supports early pregnancy.

P4 RESULTS	
CYCLE DAY TESTED	NORMAL RANGE
3	< 1.5 ng/mL
Post-ovulation	> 3 ng/mL
21	≥ 20 ng/mL

Prolactin

Prolactin inhibits the production of hormones that trigger ovulation and allow eggs to develop and mature. *This test requires fasting, so inquire in advance of your appointment.* You likely will also be asked to avoid exercise, intercourse, and hot showers in the 24 hours beforehand.

PROLACTIN RESULTS	
CYCLE DAY TESTED	NORMAL RANGE
3	< 24 ng/mL

Free Thyroxin (T4) and Free Triiodothyronine (T3)

Produced by the thyroid, T3 is the more active form of thyroid hormone that tells cells what to do, and T4 is converted into T3 inside the target cells.

FREE T4 AND FREE T3 RESULTS		
THYROXIN (T4)		
CYCLE DAY TESTED	NORMAL RANGE	WHAT ABNORMAL RESULTS COULD MEAN
Any time	0.8–2.0 ng/dL	Low levels can result in high levels of prolactin and indicate hypothyroidism, and high levels indicate hyperthyroidism.
TRIIODOTHYRONINE (T3)		
CYCLE DAY TESTED	NORMAL RANGE	WHAT ABNORMAL RESULTS COULD MEAN
Any time	1.4–4.4 pg/mL	Low levels can result in high levels of prolactin and indicate hypothyroidism, and high levels indicate hyperthyroidism.

Testosterone

High levels in women can interfere with ovulation. Total testosterone measures testosterone concentration in the blood. Free testosterone measures the "bioavailable"—free rather than attached to a protein—testosterone. Total testosterone will always be greater than free testosterone.

TESTOSTERONE RESULTS		
TYPE	CYCLE DAY TESTED	NORMAL RANGE
Total testosterone	3	6–50 ng/dL
Free testosterone	3	0.7–3.6 pg/mL

Thyroid-Stimulating Hormone (TSH)

TSH is produced by the pituitary and controls thyroid gland activity. Abnormal TSH levels disrupt both ovulation and the luteal phase—potentially preventing pregnancy or resulting in poor implantation and an early miscarriage.

TSH RESULTS		
CYCLE DAY TESTED	NORMAL RANGE	WHAT ABNORMAL RESULTS COULD MEAN
Any time	Normal TSH levels range from 0.5–4.0 uIU/mL. For conception, you want your range to be between 1.0 and 2.0 uIU/mL—although it can be as high as 2.5 uIU/mL.	Low levels indicate hyperthyroidism, and high levels result in high prolactin levels and indicate hypothyroidism.

Vitamin D

Vitamin D is a fat-soluble vitamin needed for overall health, maintaining strong bones, and optimal fertility.

VITAMIN D RESULTS	
CYCLE DAY TESTED	NORMAL RANGE
Any time	Good: 30+ ng/mL Better: 40+ ng/mL Best: 50+ ng/mL

Additional Tests for the Initial Fertility Workup

Like assessing your AFC and evaluating your hormones, there are some additional tests you should undergo at a specific time in your menstrual cycle. However, these take place during the mid-to-late follicular phase.

Hysterosalpingogram (HSG)

It's important to note that although the HSG might be included in your initial fertility workup, many reproductive endocrinologists are moving away from it in favor of the saline infusion sonogram.

With this test, your doctor uses an X-ray and contrast dye to evaluate your uterus for abnormalities and your fallopian tubes for any blockages. The HSG is conducted after your period ends but prior to ovulation to avoid the chance of disrupting a pregnancy and reduce the risk of infection.

You will be asked to change into a gown, lie on your back, and put your feet into stirrups, just like you would for a gynecological exam. A radiologist will place a speculum in your vagina, clean your cervix, and possibly inject a local anesthetic into your cervix to reduce potential pain. A long tube (cannula) will be inserted into your cervix, at which point the speculum is removed. Contrast dye is injected into your uterus and fallopian tubes through the cannula. An X-ray machine takes pictures, and you may be asked to change positions to get all the angles the radiologist requires.

Many women, including me, find this test painful, especially if a blockage is discovered. Jahsmyn from Queensland, Australia, had a very difficult experience with this test: "My doctor tried pushing the dye through six times with no success. Everyone heard my screams from the waiting room. Afterward he said cheerfully, 'Well, IVF is your only option.' I was destroyed and still in so much pain that I couldn't breathe. My husband carried me out of the hospital."

Katie from Kansas says she's happy she didn't know what she was getting into prior to her HSG and describes it as "probably the most painful [experience] I've ever had." However, she says it didn't last long. She went alone and advises other warriors to bring someone to drive them home.

"But even through the pain," she adds, "it felt good to be actively doing something to help me get answers."

For Katie from Wyoming, on the other hand, the pain was manageable. "For me, the HSG was not bad. The technicians were very kind and went slowly, and the pain was not bad with some ibuprofen taken a couple of hours before the procedure. It was uncomfortable, but not for very long."

Because of the risk of pain, your doctor may suggest premedicating with over-the-counter or prescription pain medication.

Saline Infusion Sonography

Saline infusion sonography (SIS), sometimes called sonohysterography (SGH), is an ultrasound that evaluates your uterine structure and lining. If your doctor wants to check your fallopian tubes for blockages, this procedure—performed at the same time—is called a sonosalpingogram.

As previously mentioned, the SIS/SHG is often now the initial female reproductive system diagnostic test of choice over the HSG. If you've never been pregnant or have had miscarriages, this test can help doctors understand why. In addition to getting a good look at your fallopian tubes, it allows doctors to identify scar tissue, abnormal growths (fibroids or polyps), and irregularities in the uterine lining and to visualize the shape of your uterus.

A SIS/SHG is conducted after your period ends but prior to ovulation to avoid the chance of disrupting a pregnancy and reduce the risk of infection. You will be asked to empty your bladder, lie on your back, and put your feet into stirrups. The first step is a transvaginal ultrasound (explained on page 41) to obtain an image of the uterine lining. Your doctor will then place a speculum in your vagina, clean your cervix, insert a tube, and send liquid through the tube to widen your uterus and make the uterine lining easier to see. Finally, your doctor will reinsert the transvaginal ultrasound probe, send more liquid through the tube, examine your uterine lining, and observe how the liquid flows from your uterus into your fallopian tubes.

At this point, you may feel pain from the liquid entering your uterus. Some doctors will use the ultrasound's Doppler feature to identify blood flow blockages, blood clots, and blood supplies to polyps and other abnormalities. The SIS/SHG is a common, safe test with a very low risk of infection, although you may experience spotting or cramping afterward.

Further Diagnostic Testing

If your doctor discovers an issue during your initial fertility workup, or if your fertility issues have been categorized as "unexplained," or if you've had recurrent implantation failure or pregnancy losses, your doctor might recommend that you undergo additional diagnostic testing.

Abdominal Ultrasound

This procedure allows your doctor to see organs and structures inside your abdomen. Abdominal ultrasounds are common, safe, and pain-free. You may be asked to remove your clothes and change into a gown or simply to lift your shirt. You'll lie on a table with your abdomen exposed, and a sonographer will use lubricating jelly and an ultrasound wand to send high-frequency sound waves that echo as they hit dense objects, like your organs.

Endometrial Biopsy

This test may be used in several possible ways to evaluate the lining of your uterus:

- **Hormone ranges.** Recall from chapter 1 that your uterine lining requires both progesterone and estrogen to grow and stabilize to allow implantation and support a pregnancy. An endometrial biopsy may be taken by your doctor around cycle day 21 and sent to a pathologist for hormonal evaluation.

- **Abnormal bleeding.** If you are bleeding too much, not at all, or at the wrong time of your cycle, your doctor may take an endometrial biopsy and send it to a pathologist for hormonal evaluation and/or the presence of fibroids or polyps.

- **Chronic endometritis.** An endometrial biopsy, in this case called an analysis of infectious chronic endometritis (ALICE), may be used to test for chronic endometritis—inflammation of the uterine lining caused by an infection. It is often asymptomatic and either hinders implantation or causes early miscarriages. Thankfully, this condition is easily addressed with antibiotics.

- **Endometriosis.** Not to be confused with endometritis, endometriosis is when your uterine lining grows outside the uterus. A test called ReceptivaDx can detect the type of inflammation of the uterine lining that is most commonly caused by endometriosis, and an endometrial biopsy is conducted during your implantation window in order to collect a sample for that test.

• **Uterine receptivity.** A biopsy to assess uterine receptivity—also known as an endometrial receptivity analysis (ERA)—is often recommended when you've had two or more failed frozen transfers—either no implantation or biochemical pregnancies—with genetically normal embryos. It must be taken during your implantation window. It determines whether your lining is prereceptive (not ready to receive an embryo), receptive (optimal time for implantation), or postreceptive (past the optimal time for implantation). The biopsy sample is sent to a genetics company for gene expression evaluation.

• **Endometrial microbiome.** The endometrial microbiome metagenomic analysis (EMMA) test helps identify potential reasons for recurrent implantation failure. It looks for the presence of bacteria associated with higher pregnancy rates and determines if the uterine environment is friendly at a microbial level.

To conduct the biopsy, your doctor will place a speculum in your vagina, insert a small catheter into your uterus through your cervix, and remove a small sample of your uterine lining. You might have light spotting afterward—it could even last until your next period. A word of caution: Do not try to conceive during the same cycle as an endometrial biopsy, as the test could disrupt the chance of pregnancy.

The procedure is short, but I personally found it very painful. However, most doctors will tell you that you'll feel "a pinch and some cramping," so it's quite possible you'll have a better experience, like Rachel from North Carolina. "It was much like a Pap smear, only more uncomfortable," she says. "They had to take a few samples and it was not terribly pleasant, but it was over fairly quickly and well worth the knowledge we gained from the results."

Rachel had a ReceptivaDx biopsy to test for endometriosis after exhausting all other possible reasons for her recurrent miscarriages. "After the biopsy came back positive, I had laparoscopic surgery to confirm and remove the endometriosis. They found and removed stage two endometriosis, mostly on one of my ovaries and some on my uterus."

Laura from California had unexplained infertility for 3 years before the ReceptivaDx test provided some answers. "It wasn't until after our first failed frozen embryo transfer that I pushed to have a ReceptivaDx biopsy, which revealed probable endometriosis. I felt relieved that there was finally something I could direct my research energies toward, but also nervous that I might develop more pain with each cycle that did not result in pregnancy."

Three years after my daughter was born, I did an ERA at the recommendation of my doctor in preparation for a frozen embryo transfer. With my daughter, I had taken 123 hours of progesterone prior to the embryo transfer. However, my uterine receptivity seemed to have changed because the test came back showing me to be prereceptive—and suggesting 149 hours of progesterone instead. That's an extra 26 hours of progesterone! Had we followed the same plan we'd used for my previous transfer, we would have been unsuccessful.

Hysteroscopy

In this procedure, a device with a light and small camera is inserted into your uterus to look for abnormalities. A hysteroscopy is conducted after your period ends but prior to ovulation to avoid the chance of disrupting a pregnancy and reduce the risk of infection.

Depending on the complexity and length of the procedure, a hysteroscopy might take place at your fertility clinic, a surgical center, or a hospital. Also depending on the scenario, you might be fully awake, under light anesthesia, or completely asleep under general anesthesia.

You will be asked to change into a gown, lie on your back, and put your feet into stirrups. Your doctor will dilate your cervix and insert the device through your cervix and into your uterus. Because there is normally no open area in your uterus, a gas or liquid will be sent through the device into your uterus to help widen it. The light and camera help your doctor see your uterus and the openings of your fallopian tubes.

If an abnormality is discovered and you are already under anesthesia, your doctor may correct it without the need for another procedure. Afterward, you may experience cramping, spotting, and/or shoulder pain (if carbon dioxide was used).

Possible complications include infection, uterine scarring, heavy bleeding, or side effects related to anesthesia.

Contact your doctor if you develop a fever, experience heavy bleeding, or are in pain post-procedure.

Laparoscopy

A laparoscopy is a surgical procedure that allows your doctor to examine your abdominal organs and potentially correct any issues discovered. Most often, a laparoscopy is performed when endometriosis, pelvic inflammatory disease, pelvic adhesions, or ectopic pregnancy are suspected. Other situations in which a laparoscopy might be suggested include when:

- Hydrosalpinx (explained in the appendix) is suspected.

- At least one fallopian tube is blocked or in need of repair.

- A large ovarian cyst is blocking a tube or causing severe pain.

- A fibroid is blocking a fallopian tube or distorting your uterus.

BUSTED

Myth: I always knew I would have trouble conceiving due to preexisting health conditions, so the diagnosis won't sting now.

Some diseases and disorders that impact fertility are diagnosed as early as in utero. That means these infertility warriors have known, at some level, for years that they might struggle to build a family. But even all that time may not temper the pain when you finally decide to try to conceive.

"I was told I would likely struggle with fertility when I was 18, but at that age, you don't really comprehend the gravity of what is being said," says Sarah from Ontario, Canada.

Give yourself time to grieve your diagnosis all over again, if necessary. And be prepared to feel new emotions this time.

- You are a good candidate for ovarian drilling due to a polycystic ovary syndrome diagnosis (explained in the appendix).

Laparoscopy for diagnostic purposes, such as looking for suspected endometriosis, is controversial and definitely not for everyone. A laparoscopy is performed in a hospital under general anesthesia. Your doctor will make a small incision near your belly button, which will be used to fill your abdomen with gas so your doctor can maneuver around, see your pelvic and abdominal organs with a laparoscope, and potentially take a biopsy for testing. Sometimes two or three more incisions are needed to get a better view or make surgical corrections.

As with the HSG, your doctor may decide to inject a contrast dye through your cervix to see if your fallopian tubes are open. If no surgical repairs were made, you may feel pain or soreness around the incision(s) and your shoulders for a couple of days. If repairs were made, recovery may take 1 to 2 weeks. Common complications include postsurgery bladder infection and irritation around the incision(s). Less common complications include uterine adhesions and infection. Contact your doctor if you develop a fever or experience severe pain, or if your incision site(s) ooze or bleed.

Male Diagnostic Tests

Male patients require diagnostic testing, too! Don't let any reproductive endocrinologist convince you otherwise. After all, remember that male-factor infertility accounts for one-third of all cases and another one-third are due to a combination of issues between male and female partners (or unknown causes). However, like much of this process, they have it a bit easier than female patients.

Initial Fertility Workup

The initial fertility workup begins with semen analysis. Semen is typically collected at your doctor's office, but it can be done at home as long as the semen is kept at body temperature and arrives at the office within 45 minutes of ejaculation.

⚡ If you think it might make the process easier and less stressful, ask for a special collection condom so that you can collect the sample during intercourse. Most fertility clinics will have them.

What is considered a "normal range" may change overtime. Be sure to consult with your doctor for the latest wisdom.

Abnormal Cells Analysis

An abnormal cell analysis looks for the presence or absence of white or red blood cells or immature sperm in the semen sample.

CELLS ANALYSIS	
NORMAL RANGE	WHAT ABNORMAL RESULTS COULD MEAN
≤ 1 million/mL	Possible infection

Sperm Concentration

The concentration is the total sperm count in your semen sample.

SPERM CONCENTRATION	
NORMAL RANGE	WHAT ABNORMAL RESULTS COULD MEAN
≥ 20 million	Something is blocking sperm release or the testicles are not properly producing sperm

Liquefaction Time

Liquefaction time is a measure of how long it takes your fresh semen sample to break down into seminal fluid.

LIQUEFACTION TIME	
NORMAL RANGE	WHAT ABNORMAL RESULTS COULD MEAN
15–25 minutes	Issues with viscosity

Morphology

This is the shape and appearance of your sperm. Normal sperm has:

- A smooth, oval-shaped head that is 5 to 6 micrometers long and 2.5 to 3.5 micrometers wide (less than the size of a needle point)

- A well-defined cap (acrosome) that covers 40 to 70 percent of the sperm head

- No visible abnormality of the head, neck, midpiece, or tail

- No fluid droplets in the sperm head that are bigger than one half of the sperm head size

MORPHOLOGY	
NORMAL RANGE OF ABNORMAL SPERM	WHAT ABNORMAL RESULTS COULD MEAN
≥ 4–5%	Abnormal sperm decrease the chances of pregnancy due to their inability to properly penetrate the egg

After 6 months of trying to conceive, Brianna and Chad from Pennsylvania visited Brianna's ob-gyn. The doctor ordered a semen analysis, which revealed that Chad's morphology was less than 1 percent—in other words, 99 percent of his sperm were abnormal. "As soon as this test came in, our ob-gyn advised us to see a urologist regarding the male factor infertility. The urologist was very blunt and told us 'based on the semen analysis, your best chance is IVF.'"

However, it's important to point out that semen analysis results can vary each time, which was the case for Chad. "During each IUI cycle, his semen analysis report was provided, showing slight variations with his results."

Sperm Motility

How your sperm move. Your sperm will be graded—yes, graded!—as follows:

- **Grade 0:** No movement

- **Grade 1:** Sluggish movement

- **Grade 2:** Slow movement in a poorly defined direction

- **Grade 3:** Slow or curved forward movement

- **Grade 4:** Fast movement straight forward

SPERM MOTILITY	
NORMAL RANGE	WHAT ABNORMAL RESULTS COULD MEAN
≥ 40% of sperm graded 3 or 4	Pyospermia (high number of white blood cells in the semen), antisperm antibodies (immune system attacks a man's semen as a mistaken invader), varicocele, sperm ultrastructural abnormalities, partial ductal obstruction, lifestyle issue (smoking, alcohol, chemicals from a job or hobby, or caffeine intake), or hormonal problems

Six months after stopping the birth control pill, Ana from Belgium still had not regained her period. So she and her boyfriend, Tom, went to a fertility clinic. She was surprised to learn that they had dual—both female and male—infertility. "He had poor motility, but the doctor never explained really what that meant. I was puzzled because my boyfriend had had two accidental pregnancies with two ex-girlfriends, although neither resulted in a live birth."

She adds, "Tom thought the semen analysis was quite embarrassing, but he could laugh about it."

Like Brianna's husband, whose morphology changed from cycle to cycle, Katie's husband, Michael, also received varied results. "The first time his motility came back low. He got retested three months later, and his numbers came back normal. He mentioned to the doctor that he had smoked pot a couple weeks before the first analysis, and the doctor said that it could affect his motility. He didn't smoke at all prior to the second test."

pH Level

A simple pH test assesses the acidity of your semen sample.

PH LEVEL	
NORMAL RANGE	WHAT ABNORMAL RESULTS COULD MEAN
7.2–8.0	Low pH (acidic): Blockage in the seminal vesicles
	High pH (basic): Possible infection

Total Motile Count

This is a calculation of the total number of motile sperm in the semen sample. It is determined by multiplying the volume by the concentration, then multiplying that number by the motility percentage, then multiplying that number by the percentage of sperm with normal morphology, and finally dividing the resulting number by half to account for the number of sperm typically lost in the vagina, in the cervix, or following a sperm wash.

MOTILE COUNT	
NORMAL RANGE	WHAT ABNORMAL RESULTS COULD MEAN
≥ 20 million moving sperm	10–20 million: IUI may be suggested
	< 10 million: IVF may be recommended

Viscosity

Viscosity is a measure of the thickness and consistency of the semen sample.

VISCOSITY	
NORMAL RANGE	WHAT ABNORMAL RESULTS COULD MEAN
Low to moderate thickness	Thick (highly viscous) semen may inhibit sperm motility

Vitality

Vitality is a measurement of the percentage of dead cells in the semen sample.

VITALITY	
NORMAL RANGE	WHAT ABNORMAL RESULTS COULD MEAN
≤ 58% dead cells	Lower chance of pregnancy

Volume

How much semen you ejaculate at once.

VOLUME	
NORMAL RANGE	WHAT ABNORMAL RESULTS COULD MEAN
1.5–5 mL	A volume less than the normal range indicates a blockage or dysfunction in the seminal vesicles or prostate

Blood Tests: FSH and Testosterone

The rest of the initial male fertility workup consists of blood tests, specifically for FSH and testosterone. Additional hormone levels are typically evaluated only if FSH and testosterone levels are abnormal.

Recall from chapter 1 that FSH is produced in the pituitary gland at the base of the brain. It stimulates the Sertoli cells to produce an androgen-binding protein. This protein initiates testosterone production and kicks off spermatogenesis. We also learned that testosterone is produced by the Leydig cells located next to the seminiferous tubules inside the testicles. It's stimulated by LH and required for normal spermatogenesis.

Abnormal FSH and/or testosterone levels could indicate low sperm concentration, gonad failure (hypogonadism), and diminished testicular function.

FSH AND TESTOSTERONE RESULTS	
HORMONE	NORMAL RANGE
FSH	1–18 mIU/mL
Total testosterone	270–1,100 ng/dL
Free testosterone	0.95–4.3 pg/mL or 0.3–5%

Further Diagnostic Testing

If your doctor discovers an issue during your initial fertility workup, which also includes a physical examination, you might undergo additional diagnostic testing.

Chromotubation

This procedure is used to diagnose an ejaculatory duct obstruction. During a transrectal ultrasound (see page 53), your doctor will inject a colored dye into the seminal vesicles. The doctor will then place a small scope through the penis. If no dye emerges from the ejaculatory ducts into the urethra, then an ejaculatory duct obstruction is likely.

Ejaculatory Duct Manometry

An ejaculatory duct manometry determines whether an ejaculatory duct obstruction is partial or complete and physical or functional by measuring the pressure at which fluid enters the urethra.

A transrectal ultrasound (see page 53) measures the pressures inside the seminal vesicles with pressure-sensitive probes. The backup of fluid will increase pressure if an obstruction is present and remain normal if it is not. This procedure is relatively new and not widely available.

Post-Ejaculate Urine Test

This one tests for retrograde ejaculation—when semen travels to the bladder rather than exiting through the penis during ejaculation. After abstaining from ejaculation for 2 to 7 days, you will be asked to urinate to empty your bladder, wait 30 to 40 minutes, ejaculate into a collection cup for analysis, and then urinate into another collection cup until your bladder is empty.

This is most often done at the doctor's office, but it can be done at home as long as the semen is kept at body temperature and arrives at the office within 45 minutes of ejaculation. The lab will divide the number of sperm found in the urine by the total number of sperm found in the ejaculate and urine combined to produce the overall percentage of retrograde ejaculated sperm.

Seminal Vesicle Aspiration

During a transrectal ultrasound (see page 53), a long, narrow needle is placed into the seminal vesicles to aspirate fluid and diagnose an ejaculatory duct obstruction. The fluid is examined for sperm, which should not be present in the seminal vesicles.

This test has several limitations. First, it does not definitively determine whether the problem is an ejaculatory duct obstruction or seminal vesicles that accept abnormally large amounts of fluid. Additionally, it's possible for sperm to enter the seminal vesicles after extended periods of abstinence. Finally, because the doctor is inserting a needle through your rectal wall, there's a risk of infection. To reduce this risk, you will be provided pre-procedure bowel preparation instructions and prescribed antibiotics.

Sperm Chromatin Structure Analysis (SCSA) or DNA Fragmentation Test

This detects sperm that have a high percentage of DNA fragmentation—small breaks in the chromosomes. After treating sperm with a special dye, sperm with fragmented DNA turn red and normal sperm turn green. The entire sample is then run through software that determines the DNA fragmentation index (DFI)—that is, the green-to-red sperm cell ratio.

To conduct this test, you must ejaculate into a collection cup. Semen is typically collected at the doctor's office, but it can be done at home as long as the semen is kept at body temperature and arrives at the office within 45 minutes of ejaculation.

Testicular Biopsy

This biopsy analyzes a tissue sample taken from a testicle. It can diagnose the cause of sperm production problems, identify the condition and location of a testicular lump, and even obtain sperm for use during IVF.

There are three types:

• Percutaneous biopsy

• Core needle biopsy

• Open biopsy

You will be asked to lie on your back, and your scrotum will be cleaned. If general anesthesia is not being used, local anesthesia will numb the area. During a percutaneous biopsy, a thin needle collects testicular tissue for analysis. It does not require an incision. A core needle biopsy is a variation of a percutaneous biopsy in which a hollow, spring-loaded needle collects a larger specimen of cells—also known as a core sample—without an incision. An open biopsy, on the other hand, is a surgical procedure where the doctor makes an incision in both the skin and testicle. A small sample is removed for analysis, and stitches close the incision.

Although it is a helpful procedure, testicular biopsies are not performed until blood work and a semen analysis indicate a need for further information. Testicular biopsies may be performed at the doctor's office or a hospital, depending on whether anesthesia is used. The procedure is short—typically only 15 to 20 minutes—but because you have to remain perfectly still, some doctors prefer to do it under general anesthesia. Post-procedure instructions will vary depending on the type of biopsy. However, in general, you will likely be directed to abstain from sexual activity and ejaculation for 1 to 2 weeks, keep the biopsy site dry, wear an athletic supporter for several days, and avoid aspirin for 1 week. Swelling, discomfort, discoloration, and even a small amount of bleeding for a few days are all normal. However, contact the doctor if a fever develops or you experience severe bleeding, pain, or swelling.

Testicular Ultrasound, Testicular Sonogram, or Scrotal Ultrasound

In this procedure, the doctor evaluates your testicles and surrounding tissues in the scrotum with an ultrasound machine. Using high-frequency sound waves, the test can determine whether a lump in the scrotum is solid or filled with fluid, identify the cause of pain or swelling in the testicles, and evaluate possible testicular torsion or varicoceles.

You will be instructed to undress from the waist down, lie on a table with your legs spread, and move your penis to the side not being examined. Tape might be used to position the scrotum. The doctor may raise the sac slightly. After applying gel, the doctor will move the ultrasound wand over the scrotum to capture images. The procedure is routine and painless.

Transrectal Ultrasound (TRUS)

For this ultrasound, you will be asked to change into a gown, lie on your back or side, and bend your knees. The doctor inserts a small wand into the rectum to evaluate the prostate and look for blockages in the ejaculatory ducts and seminal vesicles. Using high-frequency sound waves, it measures seminal vesicle diameter and length and ejaculatory duct width.

Because a TRUS offers an excellent view of the entire reproductive tract, it sometimes can identify the source of an obstruction. However, like all tests, it has limitations. Not all patients with an ejaculatory duct obstruction have dilated ejaculatory ducts and seminal vesicles. Additionally, it does not definitively determine whether the problem is an ejaculatory duct obstruction or seminal vesicles that accept abnormally large amounts of fluid.

This is a safe, common procedure. Although your rectum might feel sore for a couple of days afterward, other than potentially prescribing an antibiotic to prevent infection, the doctor likely will not provide any additional care instructions.

Transrectal Ultrasound–Guided Seminal Vesiculography

During a transrectal ultrasound, a long, narrow needle is placed into the seminal vesicles to inject contrast dye. Using X-ray, the doctor examines whether or not the contrast travels into the urethra and bladder. This test will determine if there is an ejaculatory duct blockage but does not rule out the possibility that the seminal vesicles accept abnormally large amounts of fluid. To reduce the risk of infection, you will be provided pre-procedure bowel preparation instructions and prescribed antibiotics.

Vasogram

A vasogram diagnoses an ejaculatory duct obstruction (explained in more detail in the appendix). The doctor makes a small opening in the vas deferens to check for sperm. If sperm are found, the doctor will inject a contrast dye into the vas deferens and take X-rays. As with a seminal vesiculography, if the contrast flows into the seminal vesicle but not the urethra or bladder, an ejaculatory duct obstruction is likely. Vasal scar tissue is a risk of this procedure.

Other Diagnostic Tests

Sometimes infertility is caused by genetic conditions (see chapter 4) and other medical issues. If your doctor suspects any of these are the issue, or if your infertility is still undiagnosed, you may undergo some of these tests.

Genetic Factors

You may have genetic conditions that could affect your fertility. Although most people's results come back normal, I've met more than a few who were surprised by what these tests revealed.

Carrier Test

After a simple blood draw, your doctor can check whether you are a carrier of one of the hundeds of genetic conditions that impact fertility.

Chromosome Karyotyping

This genetic blood test looks for structural problems or other abnormalities in your chromosomes. Abnormalities include:

- Extra chromosomes

- Missing chromosomes

- Missing portions of a chromosome

- Extra portions of a chromosome

- Portions that have broken off one chromosome and reattached to another

Chromosome Microarray

This genetic blood test looks at your chromosomes in more detail than karyotyping. It can identify *extremely* small pieces of missing or added DNA.

Single Gene Test

A single gene test looks only at the gene associated with a known genetic condition. It is conducted via a simple blood draw.

Physical Factors

If female patients have unexplained abdominal or pelvic pain or suspected adenomyosis or a müllerian duct anomaly (see appendix) or male patients have a suspected varicocele (see appendix), a doctor may run some of these tests."

Computerized Tomography (CT or CAT)

Using computers and X-ray, a CT or CAT creates images of your body that are more detailed than those of a normal X-ray. In addition to bones, it shows your doctor soft tissues and blood vessels.

You will be asked to change into a gown, remove any metal like glasses and jewelry, and lie faceup on a sliding table. Depending on the area of your body your doctor wishes to examine, you may be given a contrast dye via injection, a drinkable liquid, or an enema in your rectum. You must remain perfectly still on the table while the X-ray machine rotates around you. You may hear soft noises during the scan. Although a CT scan exposes you to more radiation than a typical X-ray, it is considered very safe. However, if you are allergic to iodine and contrast is planned, alert your doctor beforehand.

MRI (Magnetic Resonance Imaging)

With magnets and radio waves, MRIs produce detailed images of your organs and tissues, allowing your doctor to check for abnormalities.

You will be asked to change into a gown, remove any metal like glasses and jewelry, and lie faceup on a sliding table. You must remain perfectly still on the table while the machine rotates around you. It is very loud, so you may be offered earplugs. Take them. The scan is longer than a CT and may take 30 to 90 minutes, depending on the area of your body your doctor wishes to examine. Unlike a CT scan, no radiation is used, and thus the MRI is considered safer.

Getting Your Results

Your initial test results often indicate at least one obvious diagnosis. You'll likely feel a wave of emotions—relief at having an answer and fear about the future. Dr. Rodgers assures us this is completely normal. "Getting a new diagnosis can be overwhelming and scary. But knowledge is power, and the more information a patient is given on their diagnosis and prognosis, the better."

In an ideal world, your reproductive endocrinologist will:

- Tell you the diagnosis

- Explain the diagnosis and what it means for your fertility

- Answer any immediate questions you have

- Provide a treatment plan and overall next steps

- Hand you a stack of resources catered to your diagnosis

- Suggest that you schedule a follow-up appointment so you can ask additional questions once you've processed the information

Unfortunately, many doctors gloss over most of these details, as was the case for me. As always, come to this appointment with prepared questions, including:

- How common is this diagnosis?

- What are the causes and symptoms?

- How often do you treat this diagnosis?

- Can you recommend any resources to help us/me better understand this diagnosis?

- Do you recommend any additional diagnostic testing?

- What do you think about lifestyle modifications? Is there anything we/I can do to increase our chance of becoming pregnant?

- What are our/my chances of conceiving without treatment?

- What type of treatment should we/I try first, and why?

- What does this treatment involve? Walk us/me through it step-by-step.

- What are your success rates with this treatment for patients like us/me? How do you define success?

- Are there any risks or side effects of your recommended treatment?

- How many cycles should we/I go through with this treatment before trying something else?

- What does this treatment cost? What if our/my insurance doesn't cover certain aspects of this treatment? Do you offer financing plans?

- Do you truly believe you can help us/me build our family?

- Are there any other questions you think we/I should be asking?

Keep in mind that while your doctor will have treatment plan recommendations, solidifying the next steps should be a *collaborative* process—and you should feel comfortable with the direction.

Dr. Samuel Ohlander, assistant professor of urology and director of andrology at the University of Illinois at Chicago, adds, "Fertility is tricky because treatment options come in the context of a couple, so considerations for both partners must come into play. There isn't a clear-cut answer to most scenarios. It's important to understand what options exist and how different options may impact their overall reproductive treatment plan. Then the couple can make the decision that they are most comfortable with."

Sometimes, a diagnosis—or the specific cause of a diagnosis, which is also important—isn't obvious and more investigation is required.

Although hope is complicated, Dr. Rodgers leaves us one final reminder: "Often, patients—even with the most serious diagnosis—still have

BUSTED

Myth: My doctor will give me all the information I need.

Unfortunately, many doctors don't realize all the support you need in that moment.

"The medication explanation from our doctor was very vague, and to this day, I am still unsure and confused at her reasoning," Brianna says. "This is why I believe it is so important to be armed with as much information as possible—you should feel empowered to ask questions and push for clarification."

Practice your self-advocacy skills. After you're diagnosed, keep a running list of questions that pop into your mind. As you continue to process and research, you'll discover the additional information you need.

an excellent prognosis. I believe it's incredibly important to convey that there is hope and that we can achieve parenthood through a variety of options. While a diagnosis is a roadblock, it is also a sign of progress because it can help tailor a treatment plan to precise needs."

Possible Diagnoses

You'll find a comprehensive list of diagnoses in the appendix. Each one includes a brief description, possible causes and symptoms, how it's diagnosed (refer back to the list of diagnostic tests in this chapter starting on page 40), and how it might be treated and approached by your doctor. I suggest reading through each one, even if your doctor hasn't mentioned them as a possible cause of your fertility issues.

If the symptoms of a particular diagnosis are a potential fit with your experience, feel empowered to initiate a conversation with your doctor.

Receiving a diagnosis can be liberating. Finally having an answer allows you to start moving forward in a more direct way. But the relief is often short-lived.

"It was a really intense day emotionally—to realize this diagnosis isn't something I'm making up. This isn't me being melodramatic. This is an actual medical condition. Now we can work together as a team to solve this specific problem," says Elyse from Minnesota. "It also made it all feel so much more real. And the weight of that took a few months to really sink in."

Coping with your diagnosis is going to be a process. As time passes, you'll learn more about what the condition means and how it impacts your chances of building a family. Be patient with yourself and allow yourself time to come to terms with your diagnosis. Practicing self-care will be essential.

Another big part of accepting your diagnosis will be gathering information and learning more about the condition. But whatever you do, do not go to Dr. Google. You'll just end up going down a rabbit hole that will pile on the emotional distress. Think of Dr. Google as your ex—you left that relationship for a reason, so stop going back to it! Stick to reputable sources of information like medical journals and studies or resources written by actual experts.

Also, try to limit how much research you do at a time. Staying up late every night reading articles on your phone will just be overwhelming. You won't have time to properly digest all the information.

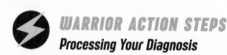

WARRIOR ACTION STEPS
Processing Your Diagnosis

It takes time to work through the emotions surrounding your diagnosis—or lack thereof. But there are strategies to help you reach acceptance. When you're trying to understand your diagnosis, be sure to:

• **Ask your doctor to repeat information three times.** Don't assume that just because you understand the literal definition of your doctor's words, you're truly absorbing their meaning. By having your doctor repeat information three times in different ways, you'll process it better.

• **Bring someone else to your diagnosis appointment.** It never hurts to have a second set of ears. Your partner or a friend can take notes

and ensure there's a record of what the doctor says so you can review it later when you're less overwhelmed and doing additional research.

• **Find others with your diagnosis.** Ideally, your doctor will give you the best information and make the best recommendations. But as we've seen throughout this book, that doesn't always happen. Meeting other infertility warriors with your condition will allow you to compare notes so you can be confident you're well informed.

WARRIOR WISDOM
Getting Answers

"When I got that diagnosis, I actually felt very relieved because I knew something was wrong. In fact, I was the one who requested this particular blood test after doing lots of research. I knew it was something that was treatable, and we could go from there."— Mindi, Ohio

→

WARRIOR CHECKLIST
Understanding Your Diagnosis

❑ Prepare for the fact that you may not get a full diagnosis or that your doctor may not give you all the information you need.

❑ Learn about infertility diagnostic tests and see if any might be right for your situation.

❑ Know normal test result ranges and what abnormal results could mean.

❑ Get familiar with possible infertility diagnoses, their causes, and the treatments that are available. (See the appendix.)

❑ Write a list of questions to ask your doctor so you get all the information you need to make the right choice for you.

❑ Accept that coping with your diagnosis will take time, and give yourself room to feel and process.

Add more items to your Warrior Checklist or jot down any notes here:

_____

_____

_____

_____

_____

_____

_____

_____

_____

_____

_____

_____

_____

_____

_____

_____

_____

The Role of Genetics in Infertility

ENETICS IMPACT INFERTILITY in different ways. Your genetic makeup, or your partner's, can lower your odds of conceiving. Or a mutation in your gamete cells (eggs and sperm) can lead to miscarriage or genetic disorders. In some cases, a mutation can occur as the embryo cells divide, which can lead to lower chances of viability.

For people who have had trouble getting pregnant or staying pregnant, genetic testing can offer insight into the possible causes.

Genetics 101

A discussion of the relationship between genetics and infertility could fill its own book, and as you might imagine, it's incredibly complicated.

Let's start with the basics and a refresher on some terms you probably haven't heard since high school. All human cells contain **chromosomes**. The chromosomes house **DNA**, the chain of "links" that determines how the different cells in your body will function. **Genes** are sections of DNA that define fundamental inherited traits. Each human cell has approximately 30,000 genes.

Our genes determine how we look and how our body functions, all of which is dictated by **gene expression**. A **mutation** is some aspect of your genetics that is different from the norm. You can inherit mutations from your parents, or mutations can develop as your cells divide and grow during gestation. Certain environmental factors can also lead to mutations, even after you are born. You can be a **carrier** of a gene mutation, which means you may not exhibit any of the traits but can still pass it on to your biological children.

Every cell contains twenty-three pairs of chromosomes, or forty-six chromosomes in total. These include the **allosomes**—chromosomes X and Y, or sex chromosomes—and twenty-two pairs of **autosomes**, or non-sex chromosomes. Eggs and sperm each contain twenty-three single chromosomes. During fertilization, the egg and sperm come together to contribute one chromosome for each pair to the resulting embryo, yielding forty-six chromosomes.

However, mistakes can happen during the egg and sperm pairing and cell division process. Chromosomally abnormal embryos have a low rate of implantation. If an abnormal embryo *does* implant, the pregnancy may

Genetics 101

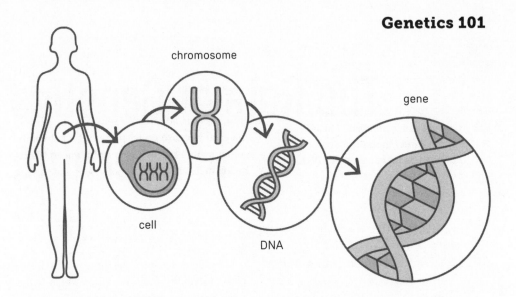

result in miscarriage or the birth of a baby with physical, developmental, or mental delays or disabilities.

Dr. Kimberly Martin, senior global medical director of the Women's Health franchise at genetics testing company Natera in San Carlos, California, says, "If we look at pregnancies that are unsuccessful, about half of those miscarriages are actually caused because of too much or too little genetic information. [The errors are] not inherited from the parents—it was just a random mistake that happened around the time of conception."

Chromosomal Abnormalities

Chromosomal abnormalities can be numerical or structural. **Numerical abnormalities** are those in which an embryo or person has less than or more than the standard forty-six chromosomes. They are more likely to occur in people of advanced maternal age because, over time, the chromosomes within eggs are less likely to divide properly. **Structural abnormalities** in chromosomes, on the other hand, are not associated with maternal age. They can be passed from parent to child in many complex ways and can be the cause of recurrent implantation failure, miscarriages, or birth defects.

Aneuploidy. An embryo has too many or too few chromosomes.

The most common type of chromosome abnormality, an aneuploidy is more likely to occur in embryos from women of advanced reproductive age. If the extra or missing chromosome is an autosome (chromosomes 1 to 22), the embryo may not implant or may stop normal development soon after attaching and result in a miscarriage. In the event that the embryo does implant and carry to term, the child may have physical or mental developmental delays.

Deletion. A chromosome has a missing piece.

Unlike an aneuploidy, which involves a whole extra chromosome or an entirely missing one, a deletion is when only a piece of a chromosome is missing. One example is Y chromosome infertility, a result of deletions of genetic material in the regions that provide instructions for making sperm.

Myth: You can't defeat genetics.

When your genetic tests reveal you have DNA abnormalities, it seems like game over. After her husband's karyotyping (see page 63) revealed an abnormality, Laurie from Florida panicked. "I heard chromosomes and I thought, 'Oh my God, they can't fix that because it's DNA. And you can't mess with DNA.'"

While that is true, it doesn't leave you without options. Preimplantation genetic testing (see page 63) can help your doctor identify embryos with the best chance of success. It becomes a bit of a numbers game because the chances of a normal embryo are lower, but success *is* possible. It took Laurie and her husband, Wayne, two egg retrievals, but they produced a normal embryo and now have a son.

Duplication. A chromosome has an extra, duplicated piece.

Duplication is when a piece of a chromosome is duplicated (there are two copies). Although the total number of chromosomes is typically normal, extra genetic material is present. This extra genetic material may cause dysfunction in that particular gene—and result in abnormal fetal development. One example is Pallister-Killian syndrome, a rare developmental disorder where part of chromosome 12 is duplicated.

Inversion. A chromosome has an upside-down segment.

When there are two breaks in a chromosome and the segment between the breaks is reinserted, but in reverse orientation, it's known as an inversion. Genetic material may or may not be lost during this process. Pregnant people with an inversion may experience recurrent losses.

Translocation. Chromosome pieces are attached to the wrong chromosome.

A translocation is when pieces of different chromosomes have been interchanged or when chromosomes attach to each other. There are two main types: In a **balanced translocation,** there is no additional or missing genetic material because equal parts of two chromosomes switch places. In an **unbalanced translocation,** there *is* additional or missing genetic material because unequal parts of two chromosomes switch places. People with a translocation may experience recurrent pregnancy loss or have a child affected with potentially fatal physical and neurological problems.

Single-Gene Diseases

A single genetic mutation in either the egg or sperm might result in an embryo that carries a genetic disorder. Single-gene diseases are usually inherited in one of several patterns, depending on the chromosome where the gene is located and whether one or two normal copies of the gene are needed for normal function.

Autosomal dominant. One mutated copy of a gene.

Remember, we get two copies of our genes: one from the egg and one from the sperm. If one of our copies has an autosomal dominant mutation, the mutated genetic trait is expressed. If either biological parent has the disease, then each child has a 50 percent chance of inheriting it. These diseases can also occur spontaneously when a random mutation occurs in one gene at conception. They tend to happen in every generation of an affected family.

Autosomal recessive. Two mutated copies of a gene.

Both biological parents of affected children are usually carriers—unaffected individuals each with a single copy of the mutated gene. When both biological parents are carriers, there is a 25 percent chance the child will have the disease, a 50 percent chance the child will also be a carrier, and a 25 percent chance the child won't have the disease or be a carrier. These do not typically occur in every generation.

X-linked dominant. One mutated gene on the X chromosome.

Because females have two X chromosomes, a mutation in one of the two copies of the gene causes the disorder. Males, on the other hand, have only one X chromosome, so a mutation in the only copy of the gene causes the disorder. In most cases, males experience more severe symptoms of the disease than females. Biological fathers cannot pass X-linked traits to their male children.

X-linked recessive. No normal copies of the X chromosome.

Because males have only one X chromosome, one altered copy of the gene causes the condition in males. Females, on the other hand, have two X chromosomes, so a mutation would have to occur in both copies of the gene to cause the disease. Because this is unlikely, males are affected much more frequently than females. Again, biological fathers cannot pass X-linked traits to their male children.

Y-linked. A mutated gene on the Y chromosome.

Because only males have a Y chromosome, this disease can only be passed from biological fathers to their male children.

Mitochondrial. Mutations in either mitochondrial DNA or nuclear DNA.

Because only egg cells contribute mitochondria to the developing embryo, only females can pass on mitochondrial mutations to their children. However, both males and females can be affected. These diseases can appear in every generation of an affected family.

BUSTED

Myth: Preimplantation genetic testing is cut-and-dried.

In most cases, genetic testing companies give PGT results in a simple manner: normal, abnormal, or mosaic (contains both normal and abnormal chromosomes—more on that in a bit). But in reality, there's a gray area. Testing is not perfect, unfortunately, and it is possible for an embryo deemed abnormal to be perfectly fine—and vice versa.

Chrissy from British Columbia, Canada, had two mosaic embryos after her first retrieval. Her clinic told her that they would not transfer them. So she went through two additional unsuccessful IVF cycles.

"But there is so much that they do not know about the DNA makeup of an embryo," she explains. "We were told mosaic embryos were not able to be transferred as they were abnormal. Later [we found] out that they could be, with risks, and my healthy son was born from that 'abnormal' embryo."

Testing for Genetic Issues

There are two categories of genetic testing: patients and embryos.

Dr. Martin says, "People who are thinking about utilizing some type of technology to become pregnant understandably might wonder if the chromosomes [in a particular embryo] have undergone the normal division, or if something's gone astray and the embryo has an extra or missing piece of genetic information."

You're probably already aware that you can perform several genetic tests—such as amniocentesis and chorionic villus sampling (CVS)—during pregnancy to determine the health of a baby. But if you're having trouble getting pregnant or staying pregnant, or if you would simply like to prevent passing on a genetic defect, those tests are likely of little comfort. Luckily, there are other options.

Tests for Patients

Karyotyping

A karyotype is performed on the patient via a simple blood draw *before pregnancy* to test for **chromosome abnormalities**. Cells from the blood are cultured, studied in a lab, and evaluated for size and shape. Specialized photographs are taken that allow the analysis of chromosome number and structure.

Some clinics say you should undergo genetic testing only if you've had recurrent miscarriages or don't produce any sperm. However, I recommend both the sperm and egg contributors be tested as soon as they seek medical help no matter what—you never know what you might find.

BUSTED

Myth: If my partner and I have no genetic issues, neither will our child.

Mutations arise in a variety of—often unpredictable—ways. Take Jackie and her husband, Tim, from Texas. They are both healthy, and genetic screening cleared them both of 160 different abnormalities. Still, after Jackie's first egg retrieval, they ended up with three embryos: one abnormal, one mosaic (see page 64), and only one normal embryo.

This happens all the time with couples who *aren't* facing infertility. They rarely know, however, because the embryo never implants or the woman miscarries before she knows she's pregnant. Infertility warriors, who need all the information they can get, are often forced to dig deeper into the "why" behind every aspect of each cycle.

Carrier Testing

Like karyotyping, carrier testing is performed on the patient via a simple blood draw *before pregnancy* to test for **gene mutations** and the likelihood of passing on a **genetic disease or disorder** to a biological child. Your doctor may recommend testing only the female patient—or at least testing her first—but as we've learned, there are some conditions that are passed on only by the male parent.

My karyotyping revealed I had one abnormal copy of the MTHFR gene. This is the least severe form of the mutation, and it's highly debated whether or not *any* form impacts fertility. My doctor chose to "treat" me anyway by prescribing a specially formulated folate supplement because the mutation may be associated with miscarriages, birth defects (spina bifida and anencephaly), and pregnancy complications (pre-eclampsia).

Other than that, the carrier testing came back normal, but I was glad we did it because it ruled out an important question on our minds—whether we had a genetic issue we didn't know about.

Tests for Embryos

Preimplantation Genetic Testing for Aneuploidy (PGT-A)

This test looks for aneuploidy (see page 60) in an embryo. Melissa Maisenbacher, a board-certified genetic counselor at Natera in San Carlos, California, explains the process:

• **Egg retrieval and fertilization.** During an IVF cycle, the egg retrieval takes place on what is considered day 0. The following day, or day 1, you should receive a fertilization report— how many eggs were successfully penetrated by sperm to become embryos.

• **Embryo biopsy.** To perform PGT-A, any embryos developing as expected are biopsied— a few cells are removed from the part of the embryos that will form the placenta—on day 5, 6, or 7. At this stage, embryos are likely blastocysts, which contain hundreds of two distinct types of cells. Embryos on day 3 or 4, called morulas, only contain between 10 and 30 cells. Biopsying a blastocyst increases the accuracy because several cells can be tested, versus just one with a morula. Your embryos remain at your fertility clinic, while the cells are shipped off for testing.

• **Analysis.** The genetic testing company analyzes each sample for chromosome abnormalities, identifying each one as euploid (normal), aneuploid (abnormal), or mosaic.

• **Results.** Typically, results are received by your clinic about 2 weeks later. Some labs can deliver results faster, though.

• **Embryo transfer.** One benefit of testing a morula is the possibility of a day 5 or 6 fresh embryo transfer if the genetic testing results come quickly enough. Unfortunately, testing blastocysts means a fresh transfer is not possible. Biopsied blastocysts are always frozen on day 5, 6, or 7 for future use. The best embryos are chosen for transfer.

As maternal age increases, so does the risk of having chromosomally abnormal embryos, says Maisenbacher. "With day 5 testing, for women who are less than 30 years of age, the risk for each embryo sample that's tested to be abnormal is about 30 percent. For women in their early 30s, the risk goes up to about 35 percent. For women in their late 30s, the risk goes up to about 50 percent. And then for women who are 40 years and older, the risk is about 75 percent. You can see it drastically raises as maternal age goes up."

When my embryos went through the PGT-A process in 2015, there were only two designations: normal or abnormal. Now, **mosaicism** has become a hot—and complicated—topic.

In the simplest terms, a mosaic embryo is one that contains both normal and abnormal chromosomes.

"We can think of it as a traffic light," says Michael Large, senior director of research and development at CooperGenomics and a sought-after expert on mosaicism. "Normal embryos are the green light, abnormal embryos are the red light, and mosaic embryos are the yellow light. They're somewhere in between."

What's more, mosaicism is incredibly common.

"Seven out of eight embryos either have no indication of abnormality or have a full chromosome change that we know is incompatible with life. PGT-A is very reliable—black and white—for those embryos. But about one in eight embryos has mosaic-only chromosomes," he explains.

"PGT-A really is more of a prioritization tool. It helps us identify a completely abnormal embryo—we know that we don't want to use that one. We can eliminate the abnormal ones, and then we're left with just embryos that appear to be healthy or appear to be mosaic."

Sarah and her husband, Kyle, from Massachusetts decided to move forward with PGT-A because of her history with recurrent early pregnancy loss. "With PGT-A testing, we knew that if an embryo came back as abnormal, it would not survive and would likely end in a failed transfer or another miscarriage. We are happy we did the testing to learn *why* we were experiencing miscarriages. And for us, if we can avoid that heartbreak again, we'd like to."

As is the case with so many other areas of your infertility journey, the cost of PGT-A is not simple and straightforward. In fact, the bills will likely be from multiple sources:

• Embryo biopsies
  (charged by your fertility clinic)

- Shipping of the embryo biopsies (charged by your fertility clinic)

- PGT-A processing and results (charged by the genetic testing lab)

Altogether, you're looking at a total of between $2,500 and $5,000, and few insurance plans cover it. (For more about figuring out what your insurance does and doesn't cover, see chapter 19.)

One potential cost-saver is to "batch" your embryos—biopsying embryos from back-to-back retrieval cycles and saving the samples for a single shipment. The cost of PGT-A typically includes up to a certain number of embryos—I believe my genetic testing company's cutoff was eight. So, whether we biopsied and shipped samples of one embryo or eight, the cost was the same. If genetic testing is important to you, look into batching to minimize your costs.

Jackie and Tim underwent karyotyping and carrier testing, which all came back normal. However, she reminds warriors that it's possible for their genetics to be normal, but once

egg and sperm are combined, the results may be abnormal. "Out of three frozen embryos, we had one normal, one abnormal, and one high-level mosaic. We were expecting all to come back normal."

Had Tracey and her husband, Matthew from Georgia not used PGT-A, her story could have had a heartbreaking ending. "We decided

PROS AND CONS OF PGT-A	
PROS	**CONS**
• Especially for people of advanced reproductive age, those who have had repeated implantation failure, or patients who have experienced recurrent pregnancy loss, PGT-A can decrease the time it takes to have a live birth.	• For people who are young and healthy, with a good chance of getting pregnant, PGT-A does not increase pregnancy rates.
• Potentially saves time and money overall by making it possible to transfer only genetically normal embryos	• Because embryos go through the biopsy and freezing process, there is a *potential* for damage—even to embryos that testing determines are normal.
• Potentially reduces the chance of a miscarriage	• Results may not be 100 percent reliable.
• Could potentially provide information useful to future treatment decisions	• The cost ranges between $2,500 and $5,000.
• Could potentially reduce or eliminate the need for invasive testing during pregnancy	• You must pay for subsequent frozen embryo transfers when you choose to freeze all your embryos.
• Increases the confidence in transferring a single embryo, reducing the likelihood of multiples	• Does not guarantee embryo implantation will not result in a miscarriage

that, with our ages, this was the route we wanted to take. I am happy we did it, especially [because one] embryo . . . had Edwards syndrome."

Babies born with Edwards syndrome typically don't survive their first year—and as few as 60 percent make it through their first week. "I don't know what I would have done with losing a child [so soon] after being born."

Preimplantation Genetic Testing for Monogenic Disorders (PGT-M) and Preimplantation Genetic Testing for Structural Rearrangement (PGT-SR)

PGT-M looks for single-gene (monogenic) abnormalities. PGT-SR looks for translocation (structural rearrangement) abnormalities. The process is similar to that of PGT-A, but there are some key differences. Again, Maisenbacher explains:

• **Genetic counseling.** The PGT-M and PGT-SR process is highly customized to the specific genetic issues of the patients involved, so the first step is to meet with a genetic counselor and get an idea of the situation. Some patients will have known about potential problems in their medical history for a long time, while others might have only recently learned about them through karyotyping.

• **DNA samples.** DNA samples are collected from both biological parents, as well as additional family members as needed.

NOTE: When testing for structural rearrangements, as opposed to single-gene diseases, the two steps above may be skipped.

• **Test design.** Because of the customized nature of PGT-M and PGT-SR, the genetics testing company must design a test specific to the genetic issues involved.

• **Egg retrieval and fertilization.** The rest of the steps from here are very similar to those of PGT-A. During an IVF cycle, the female patient stimulates her ovaries to produce as many eggs as is safely possible, followed by an egg retrieval and hopefully fertilization by sperm.

• **Embryo biopsy.** In PGT-M and PGT-SR, a few cells from any embryos that are developing as expected are biopsied. The embryos remain at the fertility clinic, while the cells are shipped off for testing.

• **Analysis.** The genetic screening company analyzes each sample, focusing specifically on the gene that carries the mutation under scrutiny. The results confirm whether each embryo is affected or unaffected.

• **Results.** Due to the complex nature of PGT-M and PGT-SR, results tend to take a bit longer than with PGT-A. When they're ready, the results are sent directly to your clinic.

• **Embryo transfer.** The unaffected embryos are chosen for transfer.

"Most couples are not at risk for single-gene disorders," says Maisenbacher. "Most individuals are actually carriers of four to six different genetic diseases, but their partner is usually not a carrier for the same genetic disease. For most of these single-gene conditions that we do PGT-M and PGT-SR for, *both* parents need to be carriers in order to have a risk of having an affected child.

"There are some other rare cases where parents are known to be carriers of a genetic disease because they've had an affected child, but the mutations that caused that genetic disease cannot be identified because technology just hasn't caught up yet. And so, unfortunately for those families, if a mutation has not been found, we can't design a PGT-M or PGT-SR test."

Maisenbacher says to start with the PGT-A percentages as the base, then multiply by the chance that the embryo will inherit a single-gene disease.

"For recessive conditions, which are most of the conditions that are tested for because they are more common, like cystic fibrosis and sickle cell anemia, each embryo [of biological parents who are both carriers] has a 25 percent risk of being affected with those types of diseases. But there are some diseases that are inherited in an autosomal dominant fashion. Those would be conditions like Marfan syndrome, which is one of the more commonly heard of conditions. And those carry a 50 percent risk of passing on."

Due to the complex nature and added steps of PGT-M and PGT-SR, the total cost ranges between $5,000 and $7,000, which again includes fees charged by both your fertility clinic and the genetic testing company. Depending on the lab, PGT-A might also be conducted at no extra cost. As is the case for PGT-A, your insurance likely will not cover PGT-M or PGT-SR, but you should always ask just to be sure.

WARRIOR TIPS
When to Consider PGT-M and PGT-SR
• •

Unlike PGT-A, which might be beneficial in most situations, PGT-M and PGT-SR were designed with very specific circumstances in mind:

- Both parents are carriers of the same autosomal recessive disease.

- The female patient is a carrier of an X-linked disease.

- Either patient has an autosomal dominant disease.

- Either patient has a mutation associated with a hereditary cancer syndrome, such as BRCA1 and 2.

- Either patient is a carrier of a chromosome rearrangement (translocation or inversion).

- Either patient had a child or previous pregnancy with a single-gene disease or chromosome rearrangement (translocation or inversion).

Consulting a Genetic Counselor

Genetic counselors are specially trained health-care professionals who have expertise in genetics *and* counseling. They can:

• Explain how personal and family medical histories might impact the likelihood of inherited conditions and diseases.

• Discuss with individuals and couples how chromosome abnormalities and single-gene diseases might impact them and their future biological children.

• Help patients decide which genetic tests might be the right choice for them and what to expect from those tests.

• Interpret genetic test results (for both patients and embryos).

• Provide information and support and present available next-step options.

Especially if you're on the fence about PGT-A, PGT-M, or PGT-SR, they can also explain the processes in more detail.

Dr. Martin says, "I'm a big fan of genetic counseling for anyone who feels that they would like the opportunity to really explore their history and to review their options so that they can make the best choice for them. One of the things about genetic counselors and geneticists is that we never answer the question, 'What would you do?' We believe that everyone should have the opportunity to make their own decisions about how much information they want. We're one of the few health-care professionals that never recommend you have a test. We're really supportive no matter what you decide."

As you would for other specialists, consider choosing a genetic counselor who is board-certified. Visit the American Board of Genetic Counseling (ABGC) website to find a certified provider in your area.

Finding out information about your genetics can be stressful because the outcomes feel unchangeable. Take a deep breath and remember that discovering new information—even if it's hard to hear—means filling in one more piece of the puzzle.

Identifying Your Needs

Before your test results come in—or even before you elect to have genetic testing—think about how good or bad news might trigger you. If you have a partner, make sure to share your feelings with each other. Then weigh how having the information stacks up against the potential emotional stress you'll feel. If the information will calm your anxiety about having a miscarriage, testing could give you peace of mind.

- **Your religious and ethical beliefs.** Consider the ethical and religious arguments against genetic testing. Make sure your belief system aligns with making decisions based on the results of these tests. (For more on this, see chapter 18.)

- **What you're comfortable telling family and friends.** People can have strong opinions about genetic testing, so you might not want to share information with everyone in your life. Right now, you need support, not judgment.

- **How much information you want.** Some clinics will tell you more than the genetic status of an embryo. They can also tell you the specific anomalies and the sex of the embryos. You may not want all of this information, especially for embryos that won't be transferred.

Communicating Your Needs

Be clear when you're discussing this topic with others in your life. And most important, know when to walk away from the conversation. "So many people have their own opinion about things, and the ones that have not been through it always seem to have the most opinions," says Tracey.

- **Practice your responses to negativity.** If you decide to talk with others about genetic testing, there's a chance they'll respond poorly. Have responses ready so you can enforce your boundaries despite feeling a sense of shock.

- Be clear with your treatment team. If you're comfortable transferring mosaic embryos, but your clinic is not, it's better to find out sooner rather than later. Make sure everyone is on the same page so there aren't any surprises if there's bad news.

WARRIOR TIPS
When to Consider Genetic Counseling

- You are older than 35.

- You have experienced recurrent pregnancy loss.

- You are doing IVF.

- You and/or your partner (if you have one) receive abnormal results from a karyotype test.

- You and/or your partner have a known family history of a single-gene disease.

- You and/or your partner are carriers of chromosome rearrangement (translocation or inversion) or single-gene disease.

- You and/or your partner have had a child with a single-gene disease or chromosome rearrangement.

- You and/or your partner are a member of a certain ethnic group at risk for specific genetic diseases (for example: Black and African Americans for sickle cell anemia; central or eastern European Jews for Tay-Sachs disease; and Italians, Greeks, and those of Middle Eastern descent for thalassemia).

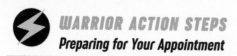

WARRIOR ACTION STEPS
Preparing for Your Appointment

• **Get your family history.** Collect information about your family medical history, including the age of living family members, the age of family members when they died, major diseases or diagnoses in the family and the age at diagnosis, and the results of previous genetic tests.

• **Collect your own medical records.** Some aspects of your past health might not seem relevant to you, but the information can help fill in gaps for your genetic counselor. Also, be sure to bring a printed version of your genetic results.

• **Write down a list of questions and concerns.** You're going to be sifting through *a lot* of overwhelming information. As you would for any other appointment, organize your thoughts beforehand so you can make sure all of your questions are answered.

WARRIOR WISDOM
Making the Right Choice for You

"Do I wish I hadn't done PGT? Sometimes. I would be more hopeful, but knowledge is power, so by knowing, I perhaps am setting myself up for less heartache of actually miscarrying. I've never been pregnant. But which is worse . . . taking hundreds of tests over the years with only one pink line [a negative test] or miscarrying?" — Jackie, Texas

WARRIOR CHECKLIST
Diving into Genetics

❑ Dispel all the misunderstandings you had about genetics and how they impact your ability to have a biological child.

❑ Understand chromosomes and their possible abnormalities.

❑ Learn about the different single-gene disorders and how they can be passed on from parent to child.

❑ Know the different types of genetic testing available and decide whether they might be beneficial in your situation.

❑ Come up with a plan for coping should you get bad news after genetic testing.

Add more items to your Warrior Checklist or jot down any notes here:

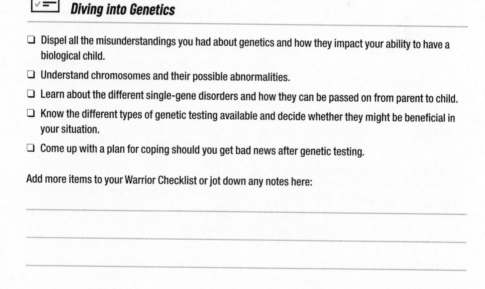

An Introduction to Fertility Medications

CHAPTER 5

AT THE START OF MY INFERTILITY journey, I was really, really afraid of needles.

Before my first hormone injection, my husband mixed and drew up the Menopur (a medication designed to stimulate follicle development and maturation) and cleaned the injection site. Fearing I might faint, I sat on the edge of our bed, closed my eyes, and turned my head away. He pinched some skin on my stomach as instructed and injected the medication.

The physical reaction was immediate. A large swath of my stomach turned a reddish purple, and the sensation was overwhelming. I felt as if I was being burned from the inside out.

Eyes wide with surprise and fear, my husband yelled, "Is it supposed to do that?!"

"How the hell would I know?!" I screamed back. "I've done this just as many times as you!"

He looked startled. I paused and took a breath. "We should call the emergency line," I suggested, referring to the after-hours line at my fertility clinic.

"This doesn't feel like an *emergency* . . ." he trailed off, reading the now-angry look on my face.

Instead, he consulted Dr. Google and found the reaction was indeed common. And more importantly, it would—eventually—go away on its own. We finished the injections for the evening, and I shot off an email to my nurse. She responded the next day reassuring me that this happens all the time, and she had a trick to minimize my body's reaction. (I love her—but wouldn't it have been nice to know her trick *beforehand*?)

That was my first series of injections, but it certainly wasn't my last. For 4 years, I cycled through rounds of Menopur, Clomid (an estrogen modulator), and Lovenox (an anticoagulant). Needless to say, I stopped being afraid of needles.

Who Needs Fertility Medication

The truth is, although some people diagnosed with infertility may benefit from fertility medication, not everyone does. If, for example, you ovulate on your own but have hostile cervical mucus, unmedicated IUI might be the best first step.

To determine whether you need fertility medication—and if so, what type—your doctor will take into consideration:

WARRIOR ACTION STEPS
Deciding to Move Forward with Fertility Medication

Many fertility medicines have uncomfortable or slightly painful side effects. (I'm looking at you, Lovenox!) So, you need to seriously consider whether to take—or continue taking—these medications. Make an informed decision with the following steps.

Step 1: Listen. Your doctor will have a specific plan in mind for helping you get pregnant. *You* have to decide whether you are ready for that plan, but start by listening and taking notes.

Step 2: Research. Consider this book your go-to reference guide. We've got answers galore here for your questions about fertility medications and point you toward reliable online resources for even more information. Reflect on which medications you are comfortable—and not comfortable—taking.

Step 3: Have a conversation. Take your research back to your doctor and have a conversation. Apply the lessons you learned about self-advocacy in the introduction. Don't be afraid to speak your mind, especially if a

certain medication makes you truly uncomfortable! However, because your doctor must prescribe all medications, understand that they do have the final say and will not prescribe you a medication that makes *them* uncomfortable.

Step 4: Solidify the plan. Walk away from this conversation with a solid understanding of which medications you'll use and how and when to take them.

Step 5: Take action. If you and your doctor decide to move forward with fertility medication, call around for the best prices—and ask your clinic if they have any donated medicine you can have. Order your new prescriptions, pick them up or arrange for them to be delivered, and take them as instructed.

- Your medical history
- How long you've been trying to become pregnant
- Whether you've had any pregnancy losses
- Your signs and symptoms of fertility issues
- Any known conditions or diagnoses that arise following initial diagnostic testing

As the patient, it's best to familiarize yourself with the various fertility medications your doctor might prescribe. But, in the face of fear or questions, Dr. Allison K. Rodgers, a board-certified reproductive endocrinologist with Fertility Centers of Illinois in Chicago, reminds us that all final decisions rest with the patient.

"You have control," she says. "In this situation where it feels like you have no control, remember that your treatment choices are

yours. What you do and when you do it or when you stop is completely under your control."

Dr. Edward Marut, a board-certified reproductive endocrinologist with Fertility Centers of Illinois, agrees and adds, "There is generally flexibility in putting together a treatment plan, including specific drug protocols. The patient may have legitimate reasons for opposing certain approaches, but there should be room for altering the strict course."

Common Medications

Over the course of fertility treatments, many people end up taking one or more medications. And any time you introduce new chemicals into your body, it's essential to be educated about their effects.

Whether or not you have a hormonal imbalance, REs—and even some ob-gyns—might use fertility medications to develop the most ideal conditions possible within your reproductive system.

Although your particular protocol—the combination of fertility medications and the timeline on which you take them—might include a medication not listed on the following pages, this broad overview includes **medication categories** (in alphabetical order), **popular brand names** you might recognize, **how it works**, **why your doctor might recommend it**, **how it's typically administered**, and **possible side effects**. As always, speak to your doctor to discuss whether these medications are right for you. Note this overview is for reference only, be sure to follow the protocol as described by your doctor.

You'll find more information about specific protocols as they apply to timed intercourse and IUI in chapter 6 and to IVF and frozen embryo transfers in chapter 7.

ANTICOAGULANT

Brand names (generic names):

- Heparin Sodium ADD-Vantage (heparin)
- Lovenox (enoxaparin)

How it works:

- Stops blood clots from forming to reduce the chance of having a stroke or a blood clot traveling to your lungs
- Helps blood flow through your blood vessels (rather than actually "thinning" your blood)

Why your doctor might recommend it:

- To prevent blood clots
- To improve blood flow in the uterus and improve chances of implantation

How it's typically administered:

- Injected subcutaneously
- Will require frequent blood tests to make sure the medicine is working well

Possible side effects:

- Stinging pain during the injection
- Redness, warmth, or skin changes where the medicine is injected
- Mild itching of your feet
- Bruising around the injection site

AROMATASE INHIBITOR

Brand name (generic name):

- Femara (letrozole)

How it works:

- Lowers your estrogen levels so your pituitary gland will produce FSH to help you make more eggs

Why your doctor might recommend it:

- **Timed intercourse or IUI cycle:** Aromatase inhibitors result in higher birth rates (27.5 percent) than selective estrogen receptor modulators such as Clomid (19.1 percent) and also higher ovulation rates—especially in women with polycystic ovary syndrome (PCOS).
- **IVF cycle:** For women with poor ovarian response, using aromatase inhibitors during an antagonist protocol (see chapter 7) improves the number of mature eggs retrieved.

How it's typically administered:

- Take orally as a pill for 5 days, starting on cycle day 3, 4, or 5.

Possible side effects:

- Mood swings
- Hot flashes
- Vaginal dryness

ASPIRIN

How it works:

- Decreases the stickiness of blood platelets

Why your doctor might recommend it:

- To increase uterine blood flow, reduce inflammation, and aid implantation

How it's typically administered:

- Taken orally as a pill
- Some doctors recommend taking it daily when you start trying to actively conceive and continuing to take it until 34 weeks of pregnancy.

Possible side effects:

- Could increase your risk of bleeding; let your doctor know if you have a known blood clotting disorder.
- Can interact poorly with heparin, corticosteroids, some antidepressants, and other medications

BIRTH CONTROL PILL (BCP)

Brand names (generic names):

- Comes in many names

How it works:

- Releases man-made estrogen and/or progesterone
- Prohibits the production of naturally occurring estrogen and progesterone
- Prevents ovulation and makes your uterus more hostile to sperm

Why your doctor might recommend it:

- Allows coordination of your cycle with your clinic's availability to perform your egg retrieval or embryo transfer
- "Quiets" or suppresses your ovaries prior to ovarian stimulation to increase the likelihood that your follicles will develop at an even rate

How it's typically administered:

- Taken orally as a pill, once a day, starting on cycle day 3 and continuing for at least 2 weeks

Possible side effects:

- Change in sexual desire
- Bleeding between periods (most often with progestin-only pills)
- Sore breasts
- Headaches
- Nausea

DOPAMINE AGONIST

Brand name (generic name):

- Parlodel (bromocriptine)

How it works:

- Blocks the release of prolactin from the pituitary gland

Why your doctor might recommend it:

- To treat elevated levels of prolactin, a condition called hyperprolactinemia, which interferes with ovulation

How it's typically administered:

- Taken orally as a pill
- 2 to 3 weeks after taking the full dose, check prolactin levels again.
- If you're pregnant, you'll likely continue taking it until 8 weeks.

Possible side effects:

- Dizziness
- Upset stomach
- Mild headache

ESTRADIOL

Brand names (generic names):

- Delestrogen (estradiol valerate)
- Estrace (estradiol)
- Minivelle (estradiol transdermal system)
- Vivelle (estradiol transdermal patch)

Why your doctor might recommend it:

- To help develop and thicken your uterine lining in preparation for implantation during an embryo transfer cycle

How it's typically administered:

- **Delestrogen:** An intramuscular injection
- **Estrace:** A pill taken orally or vaginally
- **Minivelle and Vivelle:** Administered via an abdominal skin patch
- If you become pregnant, your doctor will begin weaning you off estradiol sometime after pregnancy is confirmed, and you will discontinue it completely by 10 weeks at the latest.

Possible side effects:

- Gastrointestinal issues (nausea, vomiting, etc.)
- Vaginal discharge
- Bloating
- Breast tenderness
- Weight gain
- Headaches

GLUCOCORTICOID

Generic names:

- Dexamethasone
- Prednisolone
- Prednisone

How it works:

- **Dexamethasone:** Decreases male hormones (androgens) and progesterone produced by the adrenal gland, which interfere with egg development and growth
- **Prednisone and prednisolone:** Suppresses your immune system

Why your doctor might recommend it:

- **Dexamethasone:** To improve the results of ovarian stimulation that is hindered by the excessive production of androgens or progesterone; used in conjunction with an estrogen modulator like Clomid or follicle-stimulating hormones like Gonal-F, Follistim, and Menopur
- **Prednisone and prednisolone:** To address an autoimmune disease—such as the presence of antithyroid antibodies or high levels of natural killer cells—after several failed embryo transfers

How it's typically administered:

- **Prednisone:** An oral medication that comes as a tablet, syrup, or liquid solution and should be taken with food or milk. If you are prescribed the tablet form, do not crush, break, or chew it.
- **Prednisolone:** An oral medication that comes as a tablet, liquid, or concentrated liquid and should be taken with food. If you are prescribed the tablet form, do not crush, break, or chew it.
- **Dexamethasone:** A low-dose oral pill taken starting on day 2 or 3 and ending at ovulation

Possible side effects:

- Dizziness
- Fatigue
- Headache
- Mood changes
- Weight gain

GONADOTROPIN-RELEASING HORMONE (GNRH) AGONIST

Brand name (generic name):

- Lupron Depot (Leuprolide acetate)

How it works:

- Lowers estrogen levels by triggering the release of FSH and LH from your pituitary gland
- Inhibits the pituitary gland's ability to control the ovary

Why your doctor might recommend it:

- **Endometriosis management:** To provide pain relief and reduce the size of endometriosis lesions

During any cycle using ovarian stimulation injections, such as Gonal-F and Menopur, you run the risk of developing ovarian hyperstimulation syndrome (OHSS). It's caused by the development of too many follicles—and thus high estrogen levels. This is a serious condition that requires immediate treatment. If you experience any of the following symptoms, notify your doctor:

- Mild to moderate abdominal discomfort and bloating

- Severe abdominal pain

- Persistent nausea and vomiting

- Swelling or discoloration in your legs

- Rapid weight gain

- Shortness of breath

Brianna from Pennsylvania was never formally diagnosed with OHSS, but she believes she had it—and has some advice for other warriors: "During my first cycle with supplemental hCG (Pregnyl), I had almost every symptom of OHSS for an entire day, but it eventually subsided. I experienced nonstop vomiting, shakes, and abdominal pain and cramping. It was very scary, and looking back, I wish I would have called my doctor."

- **Antagonist (or short) IVF protocol:** As a "trigger shot" to stimulate final follicle maturation and ovulation approximately 36 hours later and decrease the risk of ovarian hyperstimulation syndrome (OHSS). It may be used with or without human chorionic gonadotropin (hCG).

- **Long Lupron (or Lupron downregulation) IVF protocol:** To allow injectable FSH and LH to control your ovarian stimulation and prevent unintended ovulation

- **Flare (or microdose Lupron) IVF protocol:** To improve ovarian stimulation results if you have had a poor response to other protocols

Note: See chapter 7 for a discussion of these IVF protocols.

How it's typically administered:

- Injected subcutaneously

Possible side effects:

- Hot flashes

- Headaches

- Mood swings

- Insomnia

- Vaginal dryness

GONADOTROPIN-RELEASING HORMONE (GnRH) ANTAGONIST

Brand names:

- Cetrotide

- Ganirelix

How it works:

- Suppresses your LH surge by immediately downregulating your pituitary gland

Why your doctor might recommend it:

- To prevent unintended ovulation

How it's typically administered:

- Injected subcutaneously

- Used during any IUI or IVF cycle that uses injectable medication (not all do), this medication is typically started when the majority of follicles have reached 12 to 13 mm in size (around ovarian stimulation day 6 or 7) and continued until the "trigger shot" (a medication given to stimulate final follicle maturation and ovulation approximately 36 hours later).

Possible side effects:

- Hot flashes

- Headaches

- Nausea

- Weight gain

HUMAN CHORIONIC GONADOTROPIN (hCG)

Brand names (generic names):

- Ovidrel (currently no generic brand)
- Pregnyl (chorionic gonadotropin) and Novarel (chorionic gonadotropin)

How it works:

- Releases man-made hCG, a hormone that occurs naturally during pregnancy, to trigger an LH surge

Why your doctor might recommend it:

- As a "trigger shot" to stimulate final follicle maturation and ovulation approximately 36 hours later
- May be used with or without Lupron
- May be used in low doses with Gonal-F or Follistim in place of Menopur to slowly increase LH during ovulation stimulation

How it's typically administered:

- **Ovidrel:** Injected subcutaneously. Typically started when the majority of follicles are 18 to 20 mm in size (around ovarian stimulation day 9, 10, 11, or 12).
- **Pregnyl and Novarel:** Injected intramuscularly into the upper outer quadrant of your buttocks. Although it's possible to do this yourself, due to the injection's particular location, it's advisable to ask a partner or friend for help.

Possible side effects:

- Breast tenderness
- Nausea
- Mild abdominal swelling
- Irritability

Note: These medications stay in your system for 7 to 12 days, depending on the dosage and other factors.

HUMAN MENOPAUSAL GONADOTROPIN (HMG)

Brand name:

- Menopur

How it works:

- Releases a combination of man-made FSH and LH

Why your doctor might recommend it:

- Stimulates follicle development and maturation
- Mostly used during IVF but may be part of your IUI protocol in lower doses—with a goal of developing one to three mature follicles—if you do not respond well to letrozole or Clomid

How it's typically administered:

- Injected subcutaneously
- Typically started in the evening of cycle day 3 and continued until your doctor advises you to stop—usually when the majority of your follicles reach maturity

Possible side effects:

- Mood swings
- Headache
- Generalized weakness or achiness
- Enlargement or tenderness in the breasts
- OHSS

INSULIN-SENSITIZING DRUG

Brand names (generic names):

- Glucophage, Riomet, Glumetza (Metformin)

How it works:

- Lowers blood glucose and insulin levels by suppressing your liver's glucose production, increasing the sensitivity of your body to the insulin it makes

Why your doctor might recommend it:

- To improve ovulation, regulate menstrual cycles, reduce hirsutism symptoms, and assist with weight loss

- Most often prescribed to patients with type 2 diabetes and PCOS, particularly those with insulin resistance

How it's typically administered:

- Taken orally as a pill, with food

Possible side effects:

- Gastrointestinal issues like diarrhea, nausea, and gas. Avoiding sugary and processed foods will minimize these side effects.

- Long-term use can increase the likelihood of developing a vitamin B_{12} deficiency.

Medroxyprogesterone

Brand name:

- Provera

How it works:

- Releases man-made progesterone

Why your doctor might recommend it:

- To treat abnormal uterine bleeding or restore absent periods

How it's typically administered:

- Taken orally as a pill, typically once a day for 5 to 10 days during your luteal phase—the post-ovulation phase of your menstrual cycle

- If it works as expected, your period will begin 3 to 7 days after discontinuing the medication.

Possible side effects:

- Mood swings
- Lethargy
- Vaginal discharge
- Breast soreness
- Bloating

Progesterone

Brand names (generic names):

- Crinone (progesterone gel)
- No brand name (Endometrin)
- No brand name (Progesterone in oil [PIO])
- No brand name (Prometrium)

How it works:

- Releases man-made progesterone to prepare your uterine lining for implantation and support a pregnancy until the placenta takes over

Why your doctor might recommend it:

- Prescribed as standard practice for an IUI or IVF cycle during the luteal phase

- May also be prescribed during a timed intercourse cycle if your body's natural progesterone production isn't sufficient

How it's typically administered:

- Typically started 2 or 3 days after ovulation or insemination and 5 days before a day 5 embryo transfer

- **Crinone:** A vaginal gel inserted using an applicator

- **Endometrin:** A vaginal suppository inserted using an applicator

- **Progesterone in oil (PIO):** Injected intramuscularly into the upper outer quadrant of your buttocks; although it's possible to do this yourself, due to the injection's particular location, it's advisable to ask a partner or friend for help

- **Prometrium:** Micronized capsule taken orally (and considered significantly less effective than other delivery methods)

- If you become pregnant, your doctor will begin weaning you off progesterone sometime after your pregnancy is confirmed, and you will discontinue it completely by 10 weeks at the latest.

Possible side effects:

- Mood swings
- Lethargy
- Depression
- Breast soreness
- Possible delay in the onset of your period
- Nodules, or small hard bumps, in the skin when using the injectable form
- Allergic reactions to the progesterone (but more often to the oil used)

- Possible irritation of the vagina when taken intravaginally

RECOMBINANT FOLLICLE-STIMULATING HORMONE (RFSH)

Brand names:

- Gonal-F
- Follistim

How it works:

- Releases man-made FSH

Why your doctor might recommend it:

- Stimulates follicle development and maturation

- Mostly used during IVF but may be part of your IUI protocol in lower doses—with a goal of developing one to three mature follicles—if you do not respond well to letrozole or Clomid

How it's typically administered:

- Injected subcutaneously

- Typically started in the evening of cycle day 3 and continued until your doctor advises you to stop—usually when the majority of your follicles reach maturity

Possible side effects:

- Headache
- Pelvic pain or tenderness
- Bloating
- Injection-site reactions (redness, pain, bruising, irritation)
- Breast tenderness
- Acne

SELECTIVE ESTROGEN RECEPTOR MODULATOR (SERM)

Brand name:

- Clomid

How it works:

- Tricks your body into thinking it has either too little or too much estrogen

- Causes the hypothalamus and pituitary gland—located in your brain—to release the hormones GnRH, FSH, and LH to help you make more eggs

Why your doctor might recommend it:

- Stimulates follicle development and maturation

- Effective in about half of women who take it

How it's typically administered:

- Taken orally as a pill for 4 days, starting on cycle day 3, 4, or 5

Possible side effects:

- Feeling emotionally down, like you do when your estrogen is low, such as right before your period

- Vaginal dryness

- Hot flashes

- For women prone to ovarian cysts, can increase the likelihood of producing one or more

What You Need to Know About Injections

Although many fertility medications are taken orally or vaginally, some are injected. If possible, I strongly recommend delegating injections to a partner, friend, or family member.

Amy from Victoria, Australia, is a nurse, so she gave herself the subcutaneous injections and convinced colleagues to give her the intramuscular injections. "It's a very weird feeling injecting yourself. Even after years of giving injections to other people, I hesitate every time. But the actual injection isn't as bad as the anticipation."

She joked, "My husband is not qualified to be coming at me with needles!"

Brianna on the other hand, turned to her husband. "I personally did not give myself any injections. My amazing husband administered them all. I winced at the thought of sticking myself with a needle, and my husband stepped up to the plate and did a great job. He even learned how to premix and fill the syringes for me!"

BUSTED

Myth: I'll never be able to handle all the injections.

Injections can be particularly intimidating if you have to administer them to yourself. But know that most infertility warriors get used to them.

Carley from Illinois admits that injections of progesterone in oil were her biggest fear early in her journey.

"It is a huge needle and has to be injected slowly," she shares. "After the initial shock of the first shot, I realized that although it wasn't fun to have to do, it wasn't so bad." Brianna offers warriors some words of encouragement: "Other than the emotional side effects and occasional physical side effects, I feel as though the injections were very manageable. The pain was minimal, and we learned quickly how to properly mix and administer."

Building a routine around your injections can help. Put on some soothing music. Have a cup of tea waiting. Practice meditation before it's time for the shot to ease your mind. Eat a cookie or a piece of chocolate after each injection. You've earned it!

Types of Injections *

Intramuscular Injection

What it means:

- An injection into the muscle under your skin

Where you can give it:

- **Dorsogluteal buttocks muscle:** On the right or left upper outer quadrant of your buttocks
- **Ventrogluteal hip muscle:** On your right or left side, in the area between your pointer and middle finger if you place your hand on your hip bone and rest the tips of your fingers on your pelvis

How to do it:

- Thoroughly wash your hands for at least 20 seconds—or approximately the time it takes to sing the "Happy Birthday" song twice.
- Choose an injection area.
- Using an alcohol wipe, clean the planned injection area. Let it dry and do not touch it again before the injection.
- Hold the syringe with your dominant hand, between your thumb and pointer finger, with the barrel resting on your middle finger. Pull off the needle's protective cover with your other hand.
- Insert the needle at a 90-degree angle.
- Once the needle is completely in, inject the medication by pushing the plunger down.
- Remove the needle, and put pressure on the injection area with a gauze pad for approximately 60 seconds.
- Discard the syringe and needle into the hard plastic container you were provided.
- Use a new injection site each day to reduce pain and bruising.

Subcutaneous Injection

What it means:

- An injection into the fatty tissue under your skin

Where you can give it:

- **Abdomen:** On the right or left side of your abdomen, at least 2 inches from your belly button, into the fattiest part
- **Thigh:** On the front or outer right or left thigh, about halfway between your hip and knee, into the fattiest part
- **Upper arm:** About halfway between your shoulder and elbow, into the fattiest part

How to do it:

- Thoroughly wash your hands for at least 20 seconds—or approximately the time it takes to sing the "Happy Birthday" song twice.
- Choose an injection area.
- Using an alcohol wipe, clean the planned injection area. Let it dry and do not touch it again before the injection.
- Hold the syringe with your dominant hand, between your thumb and pointer finger, with the barrel resting on your middle finger. Pull off the needle's protective cover with your other hand.
- With your nondominant hand, pinch an inch or two of skin in your chosen injection area.
- Insert the needle at a 45-degree (for those without a lot of fatty tissue to grab) or 90-degree (for everyone else) angle into the skin you've pinched.
- Once the needle is completely in, inject the medication by pushing the plunger down.
- Remove the needle, pulling it out at the same angle you inserted it, and wipe the injection area with a gauze pad.
- Discard the syringe and needle into the hard plastic container you were provided.
- Use a new injection site each day to reduce pain and bruising.

*Your doctor will go through these steps with you, but use this box as a refresher.

Here are some definitions and general step-by-step instructions, which may vary slightly depending on the person doing the injecting and the specific medication being injected. You can find instructional videos on the Freedom MedTEACH website. And as Brianna advises, "Fully read and review the instructions for your specific medication injection. If you have *any* questions at all— even if they seem silly—ask your nurse or pharmacist for a full explanation."

SYRINGE

The parts:

- **Needle:** What actually goes into your skin
- **Cap:** The protective plastic around the needle
- **Barrel:** Holds the medicine and has measurement markings
- **Plunger:** Used to pull up and push out medicine

How to use it:

- Attach the needle—with the cap still on— to the syringe.
- Remove the cap and clean the rubber stopper on the vial of medicine with an alcohol wipe.
- Fill the syringe with air by drawing back the plunger to the prescribed medication dosage.
- Without touching the needle, remove the cap, insert the needle through the vial's rubber stopper, and inject the air into the vial.
- With the syringe still inserted, turn the vial upside down and draw out the prescribed medication dosage by pulling back the plunger.
- *Gently* tap the syringe and push the plunger just enough to remove any air bubbles.

Affording Fertility Medications

Depending on the medicine and your insurance coverage, the cost of fertility drugs can range from a couple of bucks to thousands of dollars.

"It's like any of the costs involved in IVF. It's expensive and a struggle at times. But you do what you can to manage," says Amy. "If you need to take a break because the finances don't allow you to continue at that stage, then do it."

Here are a few methods that can help reduce the cost of your medications.

Understand Your Insurance Coverage

Insurance is a complicated topic (see chapter 19), but it's important to know the ins and outs so that you can maximize your benefits. My insurance, for example, covered fertility medications during timed intercourse and IUI cycles, but not for IVF—even if the medication itself was exactly the same.

"It is important to understand your insurance coverage," advises Maria Patswald, who works in financial services at Shady Grove Fertility in Rockville, Maryland. "If you have combined medical and prescription coverage, pulling from one lifetime financial cap, many patients find that using their coverage on their medical treatment, and paying out-of-pocket for their medications, leads to the best coverage and out-of-pocket spending."

Brianna had to take an extra step with her insurance company—*applying* for a discount. But doing so dramatically lowered her costs. "Any remaining balance was paid out-of-pocket, which was always affordable," she says.

Further, she advises warriors to speak with their fertility clinic's financial services team for help in fully understanding their current coverage—and any and all opportunities to apply for additional discounts, like she did.

Ask Your Clinic

When I was up-front with my nurse about our financial circumstances, she revealed that patients often returned unused medications to the clinic, and they were then made available free of charge to future patients who expressed a need. (It is *illegal* to resell medication in the United States, so it's best to donate unexpired leftovers back to your clinic. Pay it forward!)

BUSTED

Myth: The cost of the medication will be astronomical.

Fertility medication *is* expensive. That's just a fact. But there are ways to lower your costs. There *are* ways to get deals on quality medications.

"Ask your doctor or nurse practitioner about their recommendations for medication," Tara from Minnesota advises. "We are starting injectables, and at a regular pharmacy, it runs about $1,900 per cycle. Our nurse practitioner told us of a specialty pharmacy that gives discounts if you're not using insurance, so we paid less than $600. So ask! Don't be afraid to talk to them about the concern of affording treatment."

My clinic collected unused—and (obviously) unopened and unexpired—medications from patients who no longer needed them. However, only patients who specifically asked had access to them. We were the beneficiary of free medication several times throughout our journey, for which we were extremely grateful.

Shop Around for a Pharmacy

The local pharmacy where you normally fill prescriptions is not usually the best choice for fertility medications. They either don't carry the drugs or charge an obscene amount of money for them. Your fertility clinic likely has a preferred pharmacy, but don't feel pressured to use it.

Shop around for the best prices on each individual prescription. You do not have to purchase all your medications from the same source. Plenty of specialty and online pharmacies are available to serve your needs. Some list their current prices directly on their website, while others require you to call. I kept a spreadsheet of all my prescriptions, filled it in with prices from each pharmacy, ordered the cheapest option of each medication, and updated the spreadsheet each cycle to reflect current costs.

Additionally, your insurance provider might have in-network specialty pharmacies or preferred medication brands. Call your insurance company in advance, and get any information provided in writing, if possible.

You can also check with pharmacy networks and pharmaceutical manufacturers to see what sort of discounting programs they may offer.

Go Generic

Brand-name medications are always more expensive than generic versions, so avoid them when possible. In fact, your insurance company may only cover generics. Michele Purcell, MHA, RN, director of specialty services at Shady Grove Fertility in Rockville, Maryland, says, "When planning to use insurance benefits to cover the cost of treatment, proactively speaking with your insurance provider to determine their preferred brands can help ensure your physician prescribes the most cost-effective medication."

Online Pharmacies

Many websites purport to sell fertility medications. They may offer enticements like discounts, free shipping, and no valid physician prescription required. However, be wary.

In 2017, a report from the National Association of Boards of Pharmacy (NABP)

WARRIOR TIPS
Finding a Safe, Reputable Online Pharmacy

Several tools exist to help you verify whether or not a pharmacy is reputable and the medication you're receiving is safe:

- **National Association of Boards of Pharmacy's Accredited Digital Pharmacies**

- **LegitScript:** A business certification service that allows you to check the legitimacy of any online pharmacy or medication.

- **Websites that end in the ".pharmacy" domain:** Established by the NABP, the .pharmacy domain verifies a website as being a safe digital pharmacy through which patients can purchase fertility (and other) medications.

- **Check My Meds app from EMD Serono:** A mobile app that authenticates the serial number on packages of most EMD Serono medications.

examined online pharmacies claiming to be from Canada and found that nearly 96 percent of these sites operated illegally and out of compliance with US state and federal laws. Additionally, also in 2017, the World Health Organization (WHO) estimated that more than 50 percent of medicines purchased from illegal sites were counterfeit. Unfortunately, the problem has become so pervasive that WHO no longer offers such estimates "because of the difficulty of providing accurate measurement," according to a report by the National Intellectual Property Rights Coordination Center.

To be considered reputable, a pharmacy should require a valid prescription from your doctor, display a US business address, receive a NABP Digital Pharmacy Accreditation, make a licensed pharmacist available to answer your questions, and offer 24/7 customer service.

Specialty Pharmacies

Specialty pharmacies operate much like your local pharmacy, except they exclusively offer medications that require something "special"—special storage, special handling, or specialized knowledge of a particular condition. These medications cost a lot of money and are often not available at your regular pharmacy.

I used a combination of specialty pharmacies throughout my journey. In addition to actually being able to obtain the medications I needed, I experienced a number of other benefits, including fast—and sometimes free—shipping, knowledgeable and compassionate pharmacists, and telephone support—sometimes available 24/7—to walk me through exactly how and when to take my medications.

Brianna also used specialty pharmacies for her prescriptions and was extremely pleased with the experience: "We used a fertility-specific pharmacy that worked directly with our clinic. The pharmacy staff was always so compassionate, very quick to rectify clinic mistakes, and continued to cheer us on. They also went above and beyond to ensure that we were taking full advantage of our insurance benefits, which was truly helpful."

Although the cost of the fertility medications themselves will often dictate which specialty pharmacy (or pharmacies) you choose,

WARRIOR TIPS
Beware When Purchasing Abroad

While it may be tempting to get your fertility medications from abroad, this can be risky. Other countries do not have the same regulations as the United States, and counterfeit or expired drugs are common. And because all medication must pass through US Customs, there are often delays, which is a problem for drugs that have a short shelf life or require refrigeration.

consider other benefits that might be helpful while you are undergoing treatment, such as 24/7 access to a pharmacist or nurse, free shipping, discounts, and a financing program to spread out the cost over a period of time.

If you have insurance coverage for fertility medications, lucky you! Many specialty pharmacies take insurance, help you with the preapproval process, and submit all the paperwork on your behalf. If your insurance caps the amount you can spend on medication, ask the pharmacist about the self-pay price versus how much they would bill your insurance. Self-pay patients often receive discounts, and you might be able to self-pay to get the discount, then submit the receipt to your insurance company for reimbursement.

⚡ If you don't have insurance coverage for your medications, ask pharmacies about discounts and financing programs. The pharmacists I spoke with were always up-to-date on the latest pharmaceutical company coupons.

The Bad Rap of Fertility Medications

More than 40 years ago, in 1978, Louise Brown—the world's first IVF baby— was born in England. Decades later, fear and rumors still surround fertility treatments, especially the medications used during the process and their possible long-term side effects.

Though it's natural to fear the unknown, Dr. Rodgers reassures us that fertility medications have no known long-term risks.

Amy also encourages—you guessed it— self-advocacy. "Talk to your doctor or pharmacist if you're worried at all," she says. "Be kind to yourself, too, because it's a big thing emotionally to inject yourself with a whole lot of drugs."

To put you at ease, let's tackle the most common misconceptions about fertility medication individually.

Blood Clots

Dr. Rodgers explains that estrogen levels rise during both fertility treatments and pregnancy, which can increase the risk of conditions like deep vein thrombosis. However, she says that for most patients, "the benefits of medication outweigh the rare risk of a complication."

She adds this warning: "If you are genetically predisposed to blood clots, it is important to speak with your doctor about how to reduce these risks when taking fertility medications and during pregnancy."

⚡ As you've hopefully noticed throughout this book, communication with your doctor is important every step of the way. "Rare" is not the same as "impossible," and everyone's situation is different. Feel empowered to better understand your body. If additional testing would make you more comfortable or help you make better decisions about your care, advocate for it before moving forward. Work alongside your doctor as a team to develop a treatment plan that's best for *you*.

Cancer

Infertility itself can increases the risk of uterine, breast, and cervical cancers, says Dr. Marut. "Naysayers have been trying to blame future illnesses on fertility drugs for years, and the data does not bear out that premise. Infertility itself is a risk factor for gynecologic cancers, and the use of fertility drugs may actually lower those risks. If the drugs have an adverse effect on certain individuals, which can never be proven, it would be small."

Ovarian Cancer

A review of studies from 1990 through 2013, which together included 182,972 women, was conducted to evaluate whether ovarian-stimulating drugs increase the risk of ovarian cancer. Published in the *Cochrane Database of Systematic Reviews* in August 2013, the review identified seven studies that found women with infertility had the same risk of developing ovarian cancer whether or not they used fertility medications. According to the authors, the studies that did find an increased cancer risk did not take into consideration what Dr. Marut explained about infertility itself being a risk factor, or the sample sizes were just too small to be statistically valid.

While the review did find a possible increased risk of borderline ovarian tumors in women who used fertility medications typically associated with IVF, the risk was not present for women using just Clomid or Clomid with gonadotropins. Further, a follow-up study published in *Human Reproduction* in 2015 found *no association between borderline ovarian tumors and the use of fertility medications.*

A 2018 study published in the *British Journal of Medicine* looked at 255,786 women who underwent fertility treatments between 1991 and 2010 and found no increased risk of breast or uterine cancer compared to the general population. It did, however, find a small increased risk of ovarian cancer, with 11 out of every 10,000 in the general population and 15 out of every 10,000 who underwent fertility treatments developing the cancer. This risk was higher in the first 3 years following treatment. However, again, the general consensus of the researchers was not that the fertility medications themselves caused the cancer but rather that the infertile women who needed them were more predisposed than the general population.

Breast Cancer

The largest study to date looking at the risk of developing breast cancer following ovarian stimulation was published in *Fertility and Sterility* in 2017. It looked at two cohorts of women, each comprising more than a million subjects. Both cohorts included women who had and had not given birth, had and had not received fertility treatment, and were and were not diagnosed as infertile. The researchers found *no increased risk of breast cancer among the women who used ovarian-stimulating fertility medications.*

Another large study published a year earlier in the *Journal of the American Medical Association (JAMA)* followed up with 25,108 women who underwent IVF between 1980 and 1995. These women were found to have *no increased risk of breast cancer compared to the general population.* Additionally, researchers found that the risk of developing breast cancer was even lower for women who had seven or more IVF cycles than for those who had one or two cycles.

Dr. Rodgers adds, "These studies show that 10 days of extra hormones from the stimulation portion of IVF—because the rest of it is just extra progesterone or the natural pregnancy that happens after—on average does not affect things long-term, even if you have to do it a couple times. So, I think this is really reassuring from a fertility doctor's perspective."

However, Dr. Rodgers does require that all her patients have annual breast examinations and that those who are at increased risk for breast cancer or are older than 40 have annual mammograms. "Sometimes I get a lot of pushback from patients about why. But if something's abnormal, I make them follow up on it before treatments. Even if you have breast cancer, going through IVF to freeze your eggs does not, over the long term, impact your survival. So, I tell patients the reason we want to do the screening is because if you have breast cancer, IVF may inflame it and we don't want to get you pregnant while you have breast cancer, right? We want to make sure you're healthy and safe."

Uterine and Cervical Cancer

In 2015, *Human Reproduction Update* published a meta-analysis of nine studies involving a total of 109,969 women who underwent IVF. Of those women, 76 developed ovarian cancer, 18 developed uterine cancer, and 207 developed cervical cancer. After considering that infertility itself increases the risk of developing cancer, the authors concluded that *IVF does not elevate a woman's cancer risk.*

Also in 2015, the *European Journal of Obstetrics & Gynecology and Reproductive Biology* published a meta-analysis of six studies involving a total of 776,224 patients. Of those subjects, 103,758 had undergone fertility treatment and 672,466 had not. The incidence of uterine cancer was actually lower in the fertility treatment group (0.14 percent) than in the group that had not received fertility treatment (2.2 percent).

To close out the conversation surrounding cancer and fertility medications, the American Society for Reproductive Medicine (ASRM) published a guideline on this topic in 2016, which can be summarized as follows: "Given the available literature, patients should be counseled that infertile women may be at an increased risk of invasive ovarian, endometrial, and breast cancer; however, use of fertility drugs does not appear to increase this risk."

Cardiovascular Disease

The *Canadian Medical Association Journal* published a study in 2017 of 28,442 women who received fertility medications between 1993 and 2011. Of these, 9,349 became pregnant and subsequently gave birth, whereas 19,093 did not. The researchers identified 2,686 cardiovascular events among the whole group over a median 8.4 years of follow-up. No link was found between cardiovascular events and the number of treatment cycles. However, those who did not become pregnant had a higher incidence rate—four additional events per 1,000 women—than those who did. Again, the authors contend that *fertility treatments themselves were not the cause* but rather the underlying infertility condition.

Subsequently, the same researchers conducted a meta-analysis of six other studies, totaling 41,910 women who received fertility medications and 1,400,202 women who did not. Published in 2017 in the *Journal of the American College of Cardiology*, their analysis found *no statistically significant increase for the risk of a cardiac event among the women who underwent fertility treatments.*

BUSTED

Myth: I have to take whatever medication my doctor prescribes.

You absolutely can decide not to take a medication your doctor prescribes. Medications can have side effects and carry certain risks, and if they make you uncomfortable, tell your doctor. Your decision might mean a course of treatment is no longer possible, but you *can* say no.

Just make sure your objection is founded. Dr. Rodgers says doctors and patients need to work together to get to the root cause of any concern. "Some patients are worried about something they read online or were told by a friend that may not be true," she says. "We live in an age where there is a story online for every possible scenario, whether good or bad. This is why it is so important to have good communication between doctors and patients in order to lay concerns to rest."

When it comes to coping with fertility medication, often the biggest hurdle is dealing with the side effects. You may experience mood swings that dredge up a laundry list of intense emotions. Practice self-care and have a coping plan in place—especially when you're in a public place, like at work.

Also, be open and honest with your partner or loved ones about what you're experiencing. Let them know about the discomfort you're feeling. And don't be afraid to ask for help with aspects of your daily life. If you've got nausea or intense headaches, don't strain your body any further by, say, vacuuming the living room.

WARRIOR ACTION STEPS
Making It Through the Side Effects

Remember, in most cases, you will not be taking these medications for long—and therefore the side effects themselves will not last long. This is one aspect of infertility where you *know* when the bad part will go away. To help you get through those uncomfortable days, take time to:

- **Log your symptoms.** Keep track of what you're feeling, when, and to what degree. When you talk to your doctor about side effects and possibly changing your dosage, this information will help them make the best decision for you.

- **Have a countdown calendar.** Like a kid waiting for Christmas, it can help to have a visual representation that your side effects are running out of time. Create a tear-off calendar that counts down the days and hang it where you'll see it regularly.

- **Complain!** Often infertility warriors feel they cannot vent. After all, you *want* to go through these treatments, so why should you complain about the tough parts? However, you have every right to whine and moan if you're experiencing negative side effects. Talk to other infertility warriors because they'll get it. They might even have suggestions to ease your discomfort.

WARRIOR WISDOM
Thinking of Medication as Hope

"There are some women who only require a simple fix—one round of Clomid or one IUI or something like that. So, I think it's just so important to remain hopeful." — Abbey, Wisconsin

→

WARRIOR CHECKLIST
Fertility Medications

❑ Know how to assess whether or not to take a medication your doctor suggests.

❑ Learn about the common fertility medications and what they are used to treat.

❑ Consider the different ways you might pay for medications and whether there are any discounts, savings programs, or other cost-saving measures you might use.

❑ Have a plan for how to deal with any unpleasant side effects of fertility medications.

❑ Dispel your misconceptions and fears about fertility medications. Remember, there are no long-term risks.

Add more items to your Warrior Checklist or jot down any notes here:

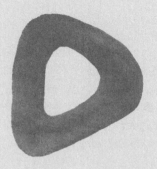

PART TWO

Paths to Parenthood

Timed Intercourse (TI) and Intrauterine Insemination (IUI) 101

IN AN ATTEMPT TO HELP US CONCEIVE on our own, I began charting my basal body temperature (BBT) and using ovulation predictor kits (OPKs) in September 2012. I'd heard about these methods in online forums as the best way to time intercourse. Sure enough, I became pregnant that first cycle—though I ultimately miscarried.

I continued BBT charting month after month and—to this day—never became pregnant again without medical intervention. While BBT charting is the beginning of the end for many, for me, it was merely the beginning. I was disheartened. It was time for a reproductive endocrinologist (RE) to step in.

But just because something didn't work for me doesn't mean it won't work for you. There are plenty of techniques and tools that might help you conceive on your own, even beyond what was available to me back then. And if those methods are unsuccessful, remember that you still have options. It's not the end!

Trying to Conceive on Your Own

Since you're reading this book, you're probably past the "it'll happen when it happens" stage of trying to conceive. For those who realize they may need to take a more targeted approach, the first step is getting to know your cycle. Because I had endometriosis, my cycles were all over the place. I bled more often than not, with often less than a week of reprieve before starting again. And still, for far too long, I assumed I was ovulating around cycle day 14, like books and Dr. Google said back then. Even once I began tracking my cycles, it was difficult to predict when exactly my husband and I should be having intercourse, so we simply had a lot of it—which eventually became an exhausting chore for both of us.

However, tracking your cycle can be an invaluable way to gain insight into your own body's particular rhythms. You can get a sense of your ovulation window, the length of your luteal phase, and any irregularities that may explain your trouble getting pregnant.

Basal Body Temperature (BBT)

Charting your BBT can help you identify your fertile window. Your BBT is your temperature after you've been asleep for several consecutive hours—and before you even so much as sit up in bed. The progesterone produced in your body following ovulation causes your BBT to rise and stay elevated. Then, when your period is imminent, your progesterone level drops, and so too does your BBT. Charting these temperatures throughout your cycle will (potentially) provide a snapshot of when you ovulate,

BUSTED

Myth: **If timed intercourse isn't working for me on my own, it won't work with a doctor.**

A doctor can prescribe medications and run tests to improve your odds.

Dr. Melissa Esposito, a board-certified reproductive endocrinologist with Shady Grove Fertility in Mechanicsburg, Pennsylvania, had a patient who was in her late 20s who, with her husband, had been trying unsuccessfully to conceive. Polycystic ovary syndrome (PCOS) was the couple's only diagnosis, but because the patient didn't ovulate on a predictable schedule, trying on their own was extremely difficult.

"I used Femara in this couple," Dr. Esposito says. "Since the husband had a normal semen analysis, we used ultrasounds and bloodwork to monitor the growth of a follicle and check that the uterine lining was appropriately thick, and we used a medication to make the patient ovulate at a very predictable time. We were then able to tell the couple when the best and most effective times to have intercourse would be to result in the best chances of conceiving. The couple was successful with this treatment."

WARRIOR TIPS
Measuring Your BBT
....

Here are a couple guidelines for ensuring an accurate BBT reading:

• **Be consistent.** Take your temperature at roughly the same time each morning—give or take 30 minutes. I know, this will stink on weekends! Also, use the same thermometer for the entire cycle. (One drawback to using a digital thermometer is that it can die partway through a cycle.)

• **Avoid ALL activity.** At whatever time you decide works best overall, you must take your temperature *immediately* upon waking up because any other activity will (albeit slightly) increase your temperature. That means no checking your phone, sitting up, or getting out of bed first. Make sure to leave your thermometer within reach the night before, and try not to knock it out of reach when your alarm startles you awake.

• **Get enough sleep.** You need to have at *least* 3 consecutive hours of sleep prior to taking your temperature. (As someone who has trouble both falling and staying asleep, this was a tough one for me!)

the length of your luteal phase, and when to expect your next period (or not, if you're pregnant!). You can do this either manually, or you can use an online or phone app (see page 96).

It is best to use a digital thermometer accurate to a hundredth of a degree (say, 97.52°F) or a tenth of a degree (97.5°F). Because my temperature did not fluctuate all that much and every little bit mattered, I preferred the former. However, you might do fine with the latter.

Other potentially helpful features on a thermometer include memory recall (so you don't have to record your temperature immediately), a backlit display (so you can read it in the wee morning hours), a beep to indicate the thermometer is finished, a quick read time, phone-syncing capability, and a built-in alarm to remind you to take your temperature. Plenty of options exist, so read reviews before shelling out too much money. I don't recommend spending more than $30 or $40, and as long as you can easily read the thermometer to the tenth of a degree, you can even use a cheap glass one—just make sure it's non-mercury.

When you're first starting out, it's best to chart your BBT starting on the first day of your period. After you have some experience, you might feel comfortable waiting until cycle day 5, 6, or 7. However, until you have a better idea of when you truly ovulate, it's best to chart the entire cycle. Although your temperature will likely rise and fall throughout your cycle (warning: drinking *any* amount of alcohol the evening before will raise your temp the next morning!), you're looking for an overall pattern. When you've had three or more consecutive days with an elevated temperature, you'll know that you likely ovulated on the day before the first one. While it doesn't happen every cycle, or even to every woman, occasionally your body will do you a solid and "notify" you that ovulation is coming with a sudden steep reduction in temperature prior to your temperature becoming and staying elevated. If this happens, definitely have intercourse that day.

BUSTED

Myth: Certain post-intercourse positions make pregnancy more likely.

"A common misconception is that infertility patients should assume a certain position after intercourse, such as elevating the pelvis to keep the sperm inside. Vaginal mucosal folds and the cervical canal will provide enough reservoir for the sperm," says Dr. Thomas J. Kim, a board-certified reproductive endocrinologist with Reproductive Medicine Associates of Southern California in Los Angeles.

What's more important is the *timing* of intercourse. After all, remember that sperm have 12 to 24 hours to fertilize an egg. You need to make sure the sperm make that deadline. How you position your body after intercourse has no impact on whether that happens.

Two huge caveats, one of which you've perhaps picked up on: BBT charting will not predict ovulation *before* it happens. If you're using an app, it may be able to make an educated guess once you've recorded enough cycles, but let's face it—you're not a machine, and if your body was functioning as expected, you wouldn't be reading this book! Further, a temperature shift does not guarantee you *did* indeed ovulate. While BBT is helpful in terms of learning more about your cycles, at best it's an imprecise method of predicting the best time to have intercourse—and at worst, it can cover up the fact that you may not be ovulating at all.

Brianna from Pennsylvania decided tracking her BBT was not for her. "In the beginning, I tried tracking BBT but found much room for error. I have busy mornings, so stopping to take my temp for several minutes at the same time quickly became an inconvenience." Her story is a great reminder that you're in control!

Cervical Mucus and Position

The only data points you must track for BBT charting to be successful are your temperature and the time you took it. However, monitoring your cervical mucus and position can also be helpful in optimizing your chances of conceiving.

Cervical Mucus

The condition of your cervical mucus can indicate when ovulation is imminent, which makes it potentially more helpful than basal body temperature in terms of hitting your fertile window. Cervical mucus should become more sperm-friendly as you get closer to ovulating. There are four stages:

- **Lowest fertility:** Mucus is minimal or absent; if present, it feels dry or sticky.

- **Low fertility:** The mucus appears thick, creamy, and white or yellow in color, and it feels damp.

- **Intermediate fertility:** The mucus begins to thin but increases in quantity and moistness.

- **High fertility:** The mucus is transparent, thin, and stretchy or elastic, like raw egg white, and feels wet, smooth, and slippery.

- **High, soft, and open:** During ovulation or the height of your fertile window.

- **Low, hard, and tightly closed:** During your luteal phase.

- **High, soft, and tightly closed:** During early pregnancy.

WARRIOR TIPS
How to Check Your Cervical Mucus

One option is to examine the toilet paper following urination or a bowel movement. You can also check your underwear for discharge. The final option is an internal examination, following the steps below.

Step 1. Wash and dry your hands.

Step 2. Sit on the toilet, squat, or stand with one foot up on the toilet—whichever feels least awkward.

Step 3. Place one finger—your index or middle finger typically works best—inside your vagina, getting as close to your cervix as possible.

Step 4. Remove your finger, and observe the look and feel of your cervical mucus.

WARRIOR TIPS
How to Check Your Cervical Position

It can take practice to accurately determine your cervix's position, and it will be more difficult to reach if you're nearing ovulation. To start, try after you've taken a shower or bath, and follow the steps below.

Step 1. Wash and dry your hands.

Step 2. Sit on the toilet, squat, or stand with one foot up on the toilet—whichever feels least awkward. Whichever position you choose, use the same one every time you check the position of your cervix.

Step 3. Place one or two fingers—your index and/or middle finger typically work best—inside your vagina, far enough to feel your cervix.

Step 4. Note the feel of your cervix, and then remove your finger(s).

Note: Don't check your cervical position during or immediately after sex because it will not be accurate and your cervix may be sensitive to touch.

Cervical Position

Like your cervical mucus, the position of your cervix should change as you approach ovulation, and it will become softer, higher, and more open. After you've ovulated, it will become firmer, lower, and more closed. Throughout your cycle and during pregnancy, the positions include:

- **Low, hard, and slightly open:** During menstrual bleeding to allow the blood to flow out.

- **Low, hard, and closed:** Once your menstrual bleeding stops and you enter your follicular phase.

- **High, soft, slightly open, and moist:** Entering your fertile window as your cervical mucus becomes more fertile.

Ovulation Predictor Kits (OPKs)

OPKs detect luteinizing hormone (LH) in your urine, which indicates that your body is gearing up for ovulation. You can either pee directly on the OPK test strips or pee into a paper cup and dip the test strips into the cup (my preferred method). Most women ovulate about 36 hours after their LH surge. However, OPKs can detect impending ovulation anywhere from 12 to 36 hours in advance, so you might not have a whole lot of warning—and women with conditions like PCOS may have multiple LH surges.

Looking back, Brianna says that she would have tried to conceive a bit differently and offers great advice: "I put an immense amount of pressure solely on myself at the beginning. I wish I would have asked my husband to minimally participate in the process to ease some of the mental strain. Tracking by myself for weeks—followed by quickly requesting intercourse—didn't allow my husband and me to connect. Bringing him into the conversation—simply informing him of my body's changes—allowed him to feel more involved and took some burden off me."

For conception, it's best to have sex the day before and the day of ovulation. Some women have also reported success having sex the day after ovulation, although it's possible they were simply wrong about their ovulation date. Regardless, don't have *too* much sex—twice a day won't increase your odds.

Dr. Allison K. Rodgers, a board-certified reproductive endocrinologist with Fertility Centers of Illinois in Chicago, advises, "Patients worry that the amount of intercourse they are having is too little. Sperm can survive for 5 days within the female reproductive tract, and with intercourse, 99 percent of sperm are left in the vagina. This means only 1 percent get into the uterus. It's not the quantity of intercourse you are having, but rather the timing of the intercourse in relation to ovulation."

One meta-analysis of studies found that for couples with infertility, intercourse timed with some method of ovulation prediction has a pregnancy rate of 14 to 23 percent, compared to just 13 percent without. Of course, as is the case with basal body temperature shifts, it's possible to have an LH surge and never ovulate. There are some women—like me—for whom these methods never work. For us, the only way to truly predict and confirm ovulation is through an ultrasound and blood work with an ob-gyn or reproductive endocrinologist. However, there's an upside to cycle tracking: You now have months of data to share with your doctor.

Using an OPK

Be sure to read the test's instructions, as they can vary. Some tell you to test first thing in the morning, when your urine is concentrated, whereas others say to test midday, when it's less concentrated. Regardless, you're looking for the test line to be at *least* as dark as the control line—unlike with a home pregnancy test, which is positive if any shade of test line appears.

I had a system back when I used OPKs to help predict ovulation. I began testing once a day around cycle day 7 (but I had short cycles—around 21 days—so most women can likely start a bit later). I used the cheap Wondfo brand you can buy online in bulk. Once I saw the test line become darker but not quite as dark as the control line, I began testing twice a day—in the morning and evening. My surges were always short, so if I didn't test twice a day, I would miss them. In hindsight, this was a sign that while I *might* have been ovulating, it was likely a weak ovulation and a potential indication of my poor egg quality. If this is happening to you, tell your doctor.

Because OPKs are notoriously difficult to interpret (is the test line *really* as dark as the control?), if I thought the Wondfo test was positive, I would confirm with a pricier digital test (using the Clearblue brand).

Brianna had a similar approach. "I purchased a bulk of OPK test strips on Amazon.

WARRIOR TIPS
OPKs Might Not Work If You Have PCOS

Women with PCOS either have high LH throughout their follicular phase or have multiple LH surges. So if you have this condition, you may get a lot of false positives.

They are inexpensive but work tremendously. I have been using these OPKs for about a year now, and every cycle they provide me with vital information to pinpoint my LH surge and ovulation. I like the inexpensive test strips over the expensive digital ones, because you can track your test line getting darker each day until your surge for a definitive timeline."

Fertility Apps and Devices

Back in 2012 when I began tracking my cycles, there weren't too many fertility apps available. (I used Fertility Friend to chart my BBT.) Now there are a lot more options. However, most of them are not accurate at predicting your fertile window. In fact, a 2016 study published in the *Journal of the American Board of Family Medicine* found that of the one hundred apps reviewed, only six had either a perfect accuracy score or no false negatives ("days of fertility classified as infertile"). But more independent research is needed as new apps enter the market.

Although certainly not cheap, the best apps today are paired with a separate device, but even they are far from perfect. Some of the better apps and devices at the time of this writing include:

• **Ava.** Ava is a nighttime wristband that tracks resting heart rate, skin temperature, and much more. The manufacturer claims the device is 89 percent accurate at predicting your fertile window up to 5 days before ovulation.

• **Daysy.** Daysy is an oral BBT monitor that becomes more accurate over time as it learns about your cycles. The manufacturer claims the device is 99.4 percent accurate at predicting your fertile window up to 5 days before ovulation.

• **OvaCue.** OvaCue is an oral and vaginal monitor that measures changes in your electrolyte levels as your body moves from estrogen dominance in your follicular phase to progesterone dominance in your luteal phase. The manufacturer claims the device accurately predicts your fertile window up to 7 days before ovulation.

• **OvuSense.** OvuSense is a vaginal BBT monitor that reads your temperature every 5 minutes overnight and averages out the data. The manufacturer claims the device is 99 percent accurate at predicting ovulation 24 hours in advance. And, unlike many other fertility wearables, it doesn't require two or three cycles to learn about you.

• **Tempdrop.** Tempdrop records your BBT throughout the night using a sensor that can be worn as an armband or tucked into a bra. It becomes more accurate over time as it learns about your sleeping patterns.

One final word of advice from Amy of Victoria, Australia: "If you feel better tracking everything, then go for it. But you can get very caught up in all the things you're 'supposed' to do. Ultimately, if you're already struggling to conceive, drop anything that's causing you stress!"

Moving On to Fertility Treatments

Deciding to take the step toward fertility treatment, and each subsequent step along the way—from timed intercourse to IUI to IVF and beyond—will likely trigger a grieving period. Remember, your feelings are valid, and it's OK to be sad or angry or whatever you're feeling. This is a big moment—a big change—in your life. Your dream of how you thought you'd start a family—how you'd tell your partner or your loved ones you're pregnant—slips further away. After all, no one *wants* fertility treatments. This is not what we envisioned when we first imagined becoming parents.

But if you have a diagnosis of fertility issues, or even if you're just having challenges with fertility, it's important to be honest with yourself. If a treatment is not likely to work for you, think long and hard about whether you want to put yourself through it, irrespective of how easy the treatment may seem.

Consider what Dr. Michael Grossman, a board-certified reproductive endocrinologist with CNY Fertility in Albany, New York, has to say: "I honestly believe people will find themselves gravitating toward a certain style of treatment, based on their own worldview and preference. The notions of cost, invasiveness, burden, and success are all directly related. They all increase together."

BUSTED

Myth: Timed intercourse isn't an option for "extreme" cases.

Often, certain fertility conditions are deemed too extreme or advanced for timed intercourse. But given the minimally invasive nature of TI, it may still be worth a shot. Dr. Rodgers admits that she's seen "hopeless" cases end well with timed intercourse.

She tells us, "A recent patient who was older and had serious diminished ovarian reserve saw me as a fourth medical opinion. She had been advised to go right to egg donor by several doctors, as this would have given her the best chance of success. I agreed with the assessment of the other doctors but moved forward with an ovulation induction and timed intercourse. She became pregnant with a healthy baby! I see miracles every day."

Timed Intercourse

You probably assume you've been having timed intercourse ever since you began trying to conceive. However, *true* timed intercourse can be difficult to achieve without help from a medical professional who can offer ovulation confirmation and a more accurate idea of timing than you can get from charting and OPKs.

Ultrasound Monitoring and Blood Work

The gold standard for properly timing intercourse with ovulation is ultrasound monitoring and blood work. While it's a pain to visit your ob-gyn or RE multiple times each cycle, the accuracy is unmatched by all other methods.

When your period starts, you'll call your ob-gyn or RE—assuming they are on board and have a transvaginal ultrasound machine—to schedule a baseline appointment for day 2 or 3—or at most, day 4—of your cycle. Using a transvaginal ultrasound, your doctor will examine your ovaries for an antral follicle count (AFC), which we discussed on page 42, and to make sure your follicles are all small and no cysts or lead follicles are present. Additionally, your doctor will measure your uterine lining to make sure it's thin. Your blood will also be drawn and checked for human chorionic gonadotropin (hCG) (<5 mIU/mL), estradiol (E2: 25–75 pg/mL), progesterone (P4: <1.5 ng/mL), and luteinizing hormone (LH: <7 mIU/mL). You'll be told the ultrasound findings immediately—I recommend asking for the AFC of each ovary and the thickness of your lining—but you'll receive a call later that day with the blood test results.

Assuming all looks good, you'll be approved to start the treatment cycle (we'll talk more about specific protocols on page 102). The timing of your next monitoring appointment depends on the doctor, but the routine will be the same as that of the baseline appointment. Your doctor is looking for at least one mature follicle (17–20 mm), a thickened uterine lining (7+ mm) that is trilaminar in appearance, and hormone levels that indicate your body is ready to ovulate (E2: 200+ pg/mL; LH: >20 mIU/mL; and P4: <1.5 ng/mL).

WARRIOR TIPS
When and When Not to Consider Timed Intercourse

People often think that seeking out medical assistance, especially from a reproductive endocrinologist, automatically means you're headed toward IUI or even IVF. However, that doesn't have to be the case! Timed intercourse is a great place to start if:

- Both the female and male patients have hormone levels in normal ranges.

- The female patient has at least one open fallopian tube.

- The female patient has good ovarian reserve but does not ovulate on her own.

- The female patient has no history of uterine abnormalities.

- The female patient produces fertile cervical mucus.

- The male patient's semen analysis is normal.

Unfortunately, as is the case for all treatment options, there are some patients who should not choose timed intercourse as an initial treatment. Timed intercourse is not a good option if:

- The female patient is older than 35 and interested in having more than one child.

- Both of the female patient's fallopian tubes are blocked.

- The female patient has severe diminished ovarian reserve and thus might not respond well to ovarian stimulation.

- The female patient has a history of uterine abnormalities or severe endometriosis.

- The female patient produces unfriendly cervical mucus.

- The male patient's semen analysis is abnormal, particularly in terms of sperm count, motility, and/or morphology.

- The male patient has any type of sexual dysfunction.

Stay informed throughout the process so you can advocate for yourself, if needed. Don't accept the blanket statement "Everything looks great!" Instead, ask for the specific hormone levels, follicle count and size(s), and uterine lining thickness and appearance.

Once your surge day has been identified, you'll likely be instructed to have intercourse that day and the following day—and perhaps a third consecutive day, depending on the doctor. You also might be given the option of "triggering" ovulation using a hCG injection to further ensure optimal intercourse timing. Ovulation typically occurs approximately 36 hours after this injection.

Amy went in for scans to monitor where she was in her cycle, sometimes triggered ovulation and sometimes ovulated on her own,

then timed intercourse accordingly. She found pros and cons to timed intercourse.

"It was boring and tedious, and I hated it!" she says. "But I had a chemical pregnancy from one of these cycles, which gave me some hope. However, that hope probably made me continue for longer than I should have."

WARRIOR TIPS
How Many Timed Intercourse Cycles Should I Try?

Assuming you are a good candidate for timed intercourse and you respond well to the treatment, most doctors recommend trying timed intercourse for three cycles before moving on to intrauterine insemination.

Intrauterine Insemination (IUI)

IUI is an early part of many infertility journeys. It is less invasive and less expensive than IVF, so for many, it's a logical next step. But know that you don't have to try IUI before proceeding to other fertility treatments.

With any fertility treatment, it's essential to know what the process entails so you can decide if it's right for you.

Before the Procedure

Before your first IUI cycle, your doctor will conduct transvaginal ultrasounds and blood work on day 2 or 3—or at most, day 4—of your of your period to establish baselines for the cycle. The sonographer will determine your AFC for both ovaries and the thickness of your uterine lining (it should be very thin at this point). The blood draw will test for h CG, estradiol (E2), progesterone (P4), follicle-stimulating hormone (FSH), and sometimes luteinizing hormone (LH) levels.

If everything is within expected ranges and you're undergoing a medicated cycle, you will go in for monitoring again around day 7, 8, or 9 of your cycle. At this point, your doctor is looking for at least one mature follicle (17–20 mm), a thickened uterine lining (7+ mm) that is trilaminar in appearance, and hormone levels that indicate your body is ready to ovulate (E2: 200+ pg/mL; LH: >20 mIU/mL; and P4: <1.5 ng/mL).

NOTE: You can conduct natural IUI cycles without in-person monitoring. You can monitor your basal temperature or use OPKs to schedule the procedure with your doctor. However, remember that these tracking methods aren't always accurate.

Once your LH surge day is identified, you may be instructed to take an hCG trigger shot to help time the insemination precisely—or you can opt for natural ovulation. Either way, the

WARRIOR TIPS
When and When Not to Consider IUI

There are certain factors that make you a good candidate for IUI. Give IUI serious consideration if:

- The female patient is younger than 35 and ovulates, with or without the help of medication.

- At least one of the female patient's fallopian tubes is open.

- The female patient is using donor sperm.

- The male patient's infertility is mild (motile sperm count more than 10 million).

- The female and/or male patients have unexplained infertility and have been trying to conceive for less than 2 years.

IUI is *not* a good option if:

- The female patient is of advanced reproductive age (38 or older).

- The female patient is older than 35 and interested in having more than one child.

- The female patient has severe diminished ovarian reserve and thus might not respond well to ovarian stimulation.

- Both of the female patient's fallopian tubes are blocked, partially blocked, or open but diseased.

- The female patient has a history of uterine abnormalities or severe endometriosis.

- The male patient has less than 10 million motile sperm.

- The male patient is unable to provide a semen sample due to sexual dysfunction.

IUI will take place approximately 36 hours later. Your doctor might also recommend that you have intercourse the day before the procedure.

You'll need to provide a semen sample on the day of the procedure (if you're using frozen or donated sperm, see chapter 10). The sperm sample can be collected at home or

IUI PREGNANCY SUCCESS RATES BY CARRIER'S AGE							
	<24	25–29	30–34	35–39	40–41	42–43	>43
Pregnancy rate per cycle	19.67%	12.94%	10.91%	8.84%	9.01%	6.25%	3.45%
Pregnancy rate per patient	37.50%	28.02%	26.20%	22.19%	21.28%	14.81%	8.33%

Source: Schorsch, M., R. Gomez, T. Hahn, J. Hoelscher-Obermaier, R. Seufert, C. Skala. "Success Rate of Inseminations Dependent on Maternal Age? An Analysis of 4246 Insemination Cycles." *Obstetrics & Gynecology* 73, no. 8 (August 2013): 808–811. https://doi.org/10.1055/s-0033-1350615.

in your doctor's office. If you are using fresh sperm and collecting it at home, it'll need to be taken to the office within 45 minutes and kept at body temperature during transportation.

After the sperm sample is collected, it will be washed. There's a solution in semen that helps them make that journey from the vagina to the uterus. Conditions in the vagina degrade or remove the compounds from this solution naturally, but when sperm is put directly into the uterus it needs to be washed to rinse away the solution, or else it may cause irritation and lower the odds of conception.

A lab technician will "wash" the sperm. This process begins by liquefying the sample on a warmer. The sample is analyzed based on several parameters, including volume, concentration (total count), motility (percentage of moving sperm), viscosity (thickness of the semen sample), total motile count (number of moving sperm), and morphology (shape and appearance). Then the semen is placed in a test tube with two liquids that act as a filtering system. The seminal fluid and nonmotile sperm are removed. The sample is resuspended in another liquid and reevaluated for those same parameters.

Insemination

Once you're ovulating, your doctor—or nurse—will use a speculum in your vagina to place a catheter into your uterus to inject the sperm, typically between 0.3 and 0.5 ml. As we learned earlier, during traditional intercourse, 99 percent

BUSTED

Myth: IUI is never successful.

Yes, success rates are low, but they aren't zero. Plenty of people fall into that 15 to 20 percent for whom IUI works. Take Liz from Florida. Despite being diagnosed with PCOS with insulin resistance, mild endometriosis, and mild motility issues, she and her husband, Will, decided to start with IUI. She took letrozole to stimulate her ovaries and triggered ovulation with an hCG injection, but unfortunately, the first cycle failed.

"The first IUI not working was a huge letdown. We thought in our heads that this would be the solution. My husband and I sat and cried like we never had before," she recalls.

Will convinced Liz to give IUI another try. She began taking supplements—CoQ10, L-carnitine, and vitamin E—to improve her egg quality and blood flow, and the second cycle worked.

"We tried to stay positive and know that pregnancy would happen, but seeing that it's really real was hard to believe. Here I am today with my 18-month-old son," she says.

BUSTED

Myth: IUI success rates are high.

While IUI assists infertility warriors in increasing the chances of conception, it's not perfect.

"The truth is that unfortunately, as humans, we are not very efficient at reproduction—so even though we can optimize the cycle by helping the patient develop multiple dominant follicles, time ovulation exactly, and wash the sperm prior to the timed insemination, it still may be unsuccessful," explains Dr. Shefali Mavani Shastri, a board-certified reproductive endocrinologist at Reproductive Medicine Associates of New Jersey.

This is important to understand because many infertility warriors choose to undergo multiple IUI cycles because they cost less than other options. But you have to weigh the price tag against the chances of success. As Emma from Colorado points out, you have to have the right expectations before pursuing IUI: "Think of it as a lottery ticket to potentially save you from the expense of IVF."

---

of the sperm stay in the vagina. IUI ensures that more sperm reach the uterus and have a chance to enter the fallopian tubes to fertilize the egg.

Warning: IUI is not always a comfortable procedure. Since insemination through intercourse isn't normally painful, many women assume that IUI won't be either.

"I wish someone had told me how uncomfortable it is!" shares Tara from Minnesota. "I had no idea it would hurt quite as much as it does."

Sometimes, during or after the procedure, women experience discomfort similar to menstrual cramps.

BUSTED

Myth: The sperm will fall out after the insemination.

Maybe this sounds silly to you—or maybe you've had the very same thought. Regardless, just like certain sexual positions don't keep sperm inside you at home, nothing is going to come back out after an IUI.

"In reality, the cervix serves as doorway of the uterus. Once the sperm is placed through this doorway and into the uterus, it does not reflux backward," says Dr. Aaron K. Styer, a board-certified reproductive endocrinologist at CCRM Boston.

After the Procedure

After the sperm is placed in your uterus, you will stay lying on your back in the doctor's office for about 10 minutes. However, there isn't a lot of research about whether this wait time increases the odds of conception. In most cases, you can go back to work after the procedure. There's a chance of vaginal leakage, but remember that this discharge isn't the sperm—it's your cervical mucus.

Some doctors recommend double insemination. This is when you undergo IUI twice in 2 days. Studies have found that this increases the chances of getting pregnant, especially if there is male factor infertility. If you are part of a heterosexual couple, your doctor might also suggest you have intercourse the day after IUI.

In the 2 weeks after the procedure, for the most part you can go about your life as you normally would. However, to avoid complications like ovarian torsion (when an ovary becomes twisted around its ligament and may require surgical correction), it's recommended you avoid high-intensity exercise.

For Lisa and her husband, Brad, from Illinois, IUI was exactly what they needed. "Our first round of IUI worked in 2016 and gave us our daughter, Anastasia. Once cleared at my 6-week checkup, we tried on our own

WARRIOR TIPS
How Many IUI Cycles Should I Try?

Dr. Rodgers points out that the chances of success with IUI are often low. After the first cycle, typically only 8 percent of infertility warriors get pregnant. Within the first three cycles, 25 percent will conceive.

"After the third cycle, less than 5 percent will get pregnant and it's best to move on to more aggressive treatment," she says.

Maria and her husband, Nathan, from Michigan originally planned to do only three IUIs. After the first two, unfortunately, her left fallopian tube was removed, making success even less likely. They did one more cycle with Clomid and switched REs after it was unsuccessful.

"[Our doctor] felt strongly that we should try one or two cycles with Gonal-F, as it may make better-quality eggs, so we decided to do a couple more in hopes that the medicine change would bring us success. It did not, so we moved on to IVF after that."

You might be thinking, *Lisa just got lucky*. Perhaps, but Meg and Zach from Georgia had the exact same experience—even with her low anti-Müllerian hormone (AMH) levels (see chapter 3). "After 2 years of trying to conceive, I did my first IUI at a fertility clinic with an RE. I didn't think the medicated IUI would work since I had low AMH. I had the insemination in April 2017 and took a pregnancy test the day before Mother's Day. It was positive! My first positive ever! My son was born in January 2018. We waited a year before we started the IUI process again for baby #2. I never dreamed the first IUI attempt would work again. We did the same IUI protocol in January 2019, and it worked again! Our daughter was born in October 2019."

Possible Protocols for Timed Intercourse and IUI

There are a lot of similarities in the protocols used for TI and IUI—the main difference being how the insemination takes place. You'll work with your doctor to determine which route is best for you, but knowing all the options will allow you to ask questions and advocate for yourself.

for a year with no luck. We then went in for another IUI. We used the same protocol and our doctor said, generally speaking, lightning doesn't strike twice and to not expect the first round to work again. It did, and we ended up with fraternal twin boys."

BUSTED

Myth: If my infertility comes from any male factor, IUI isn't an option.

Sperm have to overcome a lot of obstacles to fertilize an egg. Because of this, many people believe that if any factors prevent sperm from doing this naturally, IUI won't make much of a difference. But this isn't always the case. Inserting the sperm directly into the uterus instead of the vagina can be enough to give them an advantage to surmount certain male factors.

"Sometimes one could have a low morphology or low motility but still have adequate sperm for IUI if they have an adequate count. . . . [People] tend to think of sperm as all or none, when in fact it really depends upon the cross product of the factors," says Dr. Edward Ditkoff, a board-certified reproductive endocrinologist at CNY Fertility in Albany, New York.

Fertilization is a numbers game. Even if a portion of the sperm have morphology or motility issues, when there are enough sperm in a sample, the odds that one makes it to the egg improve with IUI.

Unmedicated

Perhaps you're against—at least for now—taking ovarian stimulation medication, or your doctor is reasonably certain you ovulate just fine on your own and simply need help with timing. Unmedicated TI or IUI is an option, albeit an uncommon one. In this case, your doctor may monitor your natural follicular and uterine lining development using ultrasound and hormone levels, as was described earlier in this chapter.

Oral Medication

Doctors typically prescribe one of two oral medications for ovarian stimulation: Clomid and letrozole/Femara. Although we covered the differences between the two, how they work, and potential side effects in chapter 5, let's go through the common dosages and timing in more detail.

Clomid

Clomid is typically taken for 5 days, from cycle day 3 through 7 or cycle day 5 through 9. The starting dosage is one tablet (50 mg) per day. It can be taken at any time during the day, but whatever time you choose, be consistent. You should be prescribed two tablets (100 mg) daily only if the 50 mg dosage failed to produce a mature follicle. Similarly, you should be prescribed three tablets (150 mg) daily only if 100 mg failed to produce a mature follicle.

In other words, if you ovulate on a low dose, increasing the dose has no benefit and will only increase the side effects you experience and your risk of conceiving multiples. In terms of the overall cycle timeline, you can expect to ovulate between 8 and 10 days after your last dose of Clomid—later than you might naturally.

Femara or Letrozole

Femara (letrozole) is typically taken for 5 days, from cycle day 3 through 7 or cycle day 5 through 9. The starting dosage is one tablet (2.5 mg) per day. You should be prescribed two tablets (5 mg) daily only if the 2.5 mg dosage failed to produce a mature follicle. Similarly, you should be prescribed three tablets (7.5 mg) daily only if 5 mg failed to produce a mature follicle.

In other words, if you ovulate on a low dose, increasing the dose has no benefit and will only increase the side effects you experience and your risk of conceiving multiples. In terms of the overall cycle timeline, you can expect to ovulate between 4 and 7 days after your last dose of Femara—similar to when you might naturally ovulate.

Femara is mainly known as a breast cancer medication. Many doctors will not prescribe it for a couple of reasons, including that the drug's manufacturer has not filed for approval from the Federal Drug Administration (FDA) for its use in treating infertility in the United States. (However, its "off-label use" when prescribed for ovulation induction is not illegal.)

The other big reason is a 2005 Canadian study suggesting that Femara may increase the chance of birth defects. But that study has received criticism for being small and improperly designed. Femara's short half-life leads some doctors to believe that it is out of your system prior to fertilization and therefore can't be responsible for birth defects.

It is possible to obtain Clomid or Femara from your doctor and complete the cycle entirely on your own from there. However, monitoring your cycle with ultrasounds and blood work can:

• Assess how well you're responding to the medication—or if you're responding at all

• Confirm when to have intercourse or perform insemination

• Identify when the cycle should be canceled due to overstimulation, which for most doctors is the presence of more than three mature follicles (both Clomid and Femara increase the chance of conceiving multiples).

In other words, monitoring by your doctor might provide important information about your fertility that could decrease the overall length and cost of your journey.

Injectable Medication

Injectable gonadotropins—Gonal-F or Follistim, for example—are also an option for timed intercourse and IUI cycles, although only in cases where women are not responding to Clomid or Femara. The dosage varies depending on your hormone levels and prior ovarian stimulation response—and it's possible you'll be prescribed a gonadotropin *and* Clomid or Femara.

Ultrasound and blood work monitoring are not optional with gonadotropin cycles because the risk of conceiving multiples and developing ovarian hyperstimulation syndrome (OHSS) are too great. Additionally, albeit rare, gonadotropin cycles put you at risk for ovarian torsion and ectopic pregnancy.

Most doctors begin monitoring after 3 days of injections, although some only perform a blood draw at that point. You can then expect another monitoring appointment—this time including an ultrasound—after 5 days of injections. Monitoring will continue daily or every other day until your doctor indicates that it's time to trigger ovulation. Although it's rare, some women ovulate prematurely with gonadotropins. If this happens to you, please know that every cycle is different and it's extremely unlikely to happen the following cycle.

COPING AND GETTING SUPPORT

Regardless of what treatment you choose, or if you decide treatment isn't right for you, remember that the decision is ultimately yours. You have control here. Even though timed intercourse and IUI are less invasive forms of fertility treatments, they can still be stressful. Make sure that you are addressing your emotional needs during these cycles, or you'll quickly get burnt out.

One point of tension among many infertility warriors is that sex loses its spontaneity. With both timed intercourse and IUI, you are planning out when you and your partner will be intimate, which honestly cancels out the fun. (Remember, in addition to the insemination, it's recommended that heterosexual couples have sex the day before and the day after the procedure.)

"We had been so used to the routine that, at times, it became a chore to schedule intercourse," says Beth from Utah.

When you're going through these treatments, pay close attention to your and your partner's intimacy needs. Find other ways to express your love and make a point to have sex outside of your most fertile days. And most importantly, keep the lines of communication open. Let your partner know what you need for you both to feel close and not like you're just going through the motions.

⚡ WARRIOR ACTION STEPS
Making It Through TI and IUI Cycles

When you're going through TI and IUI cycles, set yourself up for emotional success by taking the following steps:

• **Manage your expectations.** Remember that many people still don't conceive after timed intercourse or IUI. Try to be cautiously optimistic going into these cycles. It can also help to approach these treatments as fact-finding missions. After each one, you'll know more about what's going on with your body—and that can help you tailor future treatments.

• **Track, but try not to obsess.** It's easy to let tracking your ovulation—and your post-ovulation temperatures when you're looking for signs of pregnancy—become an obsession. There's a lot of information to look for and log. But given how imprecise the process is, don't let your ovulation cycle overtake your life. There are going to be some months when things don't happen as planned. Be flexible and understand you're doing the best you can. Obsessing will add stress, not increase the chance of conception.

• **Don't feel rushed.** Each month that passes without a pregnancy can be frustrating or heartbreaking. If you need to take time for your mental health, that's OK. Just because there's another ovulation cycle coming doesn't mean you have to spend another month tracking and trying. Take a break and tend to your needs.

WARRIOR WISDOM
Focus on the New Information You Gain

"Don't assume that it will go according to plan. Doctors do a lot of guessing about how you'll respond and sometimes get it wrong or your body swerves. The nurses make it sound like there is a routine and it's no big deal, but your body might not get that memo. Try to remember that while you may not have success, each cycle can give you valuable information or help you move to the next step for you." —Elise, Missouri

WARRIOR CHECKLIST
Understanding Timed Intercourse and IUI

❑ Know what options you have for tracking your fertility cycles.

❑ Learn what timed intercourse (TI) and intrauterine insemination (IUI) entail and whether you should consider those options.

❑ Understand how your doctor might track your ovulation during TI and IUI cycles.

❑ Become familiar with the common TI and IUI protocols and the medications and tests they may involve.

❑ Take proactive steps to deal with your emotions during TI and IUI cycles.

Add more items to your Warrior Checklist or jot down any notes here:

_____

_____

_____

In Vitro Fertilization (IVF) and Frozen Embryo Transfer (FET) 101

CHAPTER 7

URING MY IVF CONSULTATION, I remember that my doctor brought out a chart showing what to expect if, for example, fifteen eggs were retrieved. Fifteen eggs retrieved does *not* mean you will have fifteen embryos. Instead, there's an attrition rate at every step of the process. Not all of the follicles you see during ultrasound monitoring produce eggs. Not all of the eggs retrieved are mature enough to fertilize. Not all of the mature eggs fertilize. Not all of the fertilized eggs develop into day 3 morulas, let alone day 5 blastocysts. In other words, IVF is a numbers game—and it varies from person to person and cycle to cycle.

We briefly discussed the number of embryos to transfer. My doctor gave me that line about "Our goal is to have one healthy baby," which I ultimately misinterpreted as having a healthy baby by any means necessary. He said my nurse would discuss our protocol and next steps. And that was that.

My nurse handed me a list of medications and instructions on when to take them, and she directed me to online videos to show me exactly *how* to take them. She called in the prescriptions to a specialty pharmacy. I wrongly assumed that this pharmacy was our only option, and the medications put a serious ding in our wallets.

Although I was initially *terrified* at the prospect of being injected—by my husband, no less—the process was relatively painless. My husband was in charge of everything related to the medications, and he also attended monitoring appointments, which made him feel more involved. However, one person was missing from the monitoring: my doctor. Ultrasounds were conducted by nurses—and often, not my own.

The morning after my first egg retrieval procedure, we received a call from our nurse telling us how many eggs were mature and fertilized. On the third day, she gave me the date and time of our transfer. The transfer—performed not by my doctor but one with whom I was familiar—went smoothly.

You know the rest.

Overall, I went through my first IVF cycle in a haze—accepting every member of my treatment team at their word and just going along for the ride.

IVF and FET involve a lot of information that sometimes contradicts. Certain medications are used to suppress egg production in some cases and stimulate it in others. Sometimes women produce a dozen eggs during their first retrieval—and with the same protocol, only one in the second. It can be overwhelming and confusing, so set aside your preconceptions and go slow. Write down your questions as you go, then once you've finished reading this chapter, go back and look for clarification on things you're still not sure about.

You have a lot of options when it comes to IVF and FET cycles. I'll help you figure out what questions to ask so you get the information you need from your doctor. And be sure to manage your stress, as these procedures are not a walk in the park.

What Is IVF and When Might You Need It?

*I*n vitro fertilization means conception outside the body—that is, in a lab (*in vitro* is Latin for "in glass")—whereas methods like timed intercourse and IUI are considered *in vivo* ("in the body") conception. IVF involves stimulating a woman's ovaries to produce as many eggs as possible, then retrieving, fertilizing, and developing those eggs into blastocysts (rapidly dividing balls of cells; the inner group of cells becomes the embryo). If embryos develop, they are transferred into the uterus, hopefully leading to implantation.

Most often, doctors recommend moving on to IVF after three failed IUI cycles. However, some patients do more IUI cycles before IVF because they're much cheaper.

"We did four rounds of IUI. We got pregnant after the second but learned that the baby had Down syndrome. Our baby's heart stopped the day after we found out, when I was 11 weeks pregnant. We went on to do two more IUIs after that, which were both unsuccessful," says Natalie from California.

Those lucky enough to have insurance that covers IVF will likely have to follow a set of protocols.

Jessica from Hawaii had insurance that required her to complete three IUI cycles before it would cover IVF. "We ended up doing four

WARRIOR TIPS
When to Consider IVF
••

You should consider IVF if:

- The female patient has been unsuccessful with other fertility treatments like IUI and timed intercourse.

- Both of the female patient's fallopian tubes are blocked.

- The female patient is of advanced reproductive age (38 or older).

- The male patient has severe male factor infertility (total motile sperm count under 10 million).

- The female patient has an ovulation disorder.

- The female or male patient has a genetic condition that should not be passed on to a child.

- The female or male patient has lost their fertility but previously froze their eggs, sperm, or embryos.

- The female or male patient is planning to use a donor egg, sperm, or embryo.

cycles of IUI, with one canceled due to too many follicles. After our last cycle was unsuccessful, we were able to move on to IVF," she says.

Michelle from Maryland on the other hand, had insurance coverage for both IUI and IVF but still did five IUI cycles before moving to IVF. "Cost wasn't a consideration for us. However, after almost 2 years of trying on our own and our understanding of the relatively low success rate of IUI, more IUI cycles just seemed like asking for heartbreak."

The "Typical" IVF Cycle

OK, there is no typical IVF cycle. Each cycle can and should be customized to your situation, which means your protocols might change throughout your journey. But there is a general timeline and progression to the process.

Every step serves a purpose, so it's essential to learn what you'll be facing along the way.

Consultation

Before you start an IVF cycle (or any type of fertility treatment), you should have a virtual, phone, or in-person consultation with your reproductive endocrinologist. The goal of this appointment is to help you decide whether or not to proceed—and if so, what exactly "proceeding" will look like. Do not feel pressured to decide right then and there. Instead, use this as your opportunity to ask questions and get a good understanding of all your options. Assuming there aren't any specific time constraints, such as your period just starting or about to start, take all the time you need to consider the best way forward. Then, when you're ready, reconvene with your doctor.

Like many people, Andrea from Ohio found the IVF process confusing at first. But thankfully, her doctor did a great job of explaining the process. She says, "When we began IVF, our clinic provided us with a calendar that mapped out our schedule for the month of our egg retrieval, including office visits, blood work, ultrasounds, and medications. It was not until we had this calendar that the process of IVF became clear to me. Before that, I had only a vague understanding that there would be a lot of shots and office visits, but I didn't really grasp the process until I saw my own personalized calendar."

Other warriors aren't so lucky. Natacha from Maryland explains, "My doctor sent me a link with a couple of videos to learn more about the IVF process. I was not satisfied with this. I ended up leaning on friends and joining Facebook support groups to learn more. It would've been really helpful to have a full-blown 'guide to IVF,' but in hindsight, everyone's experience is so different, it would be impossible to have a one-size-fits-all guide!"

If only she'd had this book!

Mock Embryo Transfer

Your doctor may suggest a mock embryo transfer, especially before your first IVF cycle. The overall goal of this procedure is to avoid a difficult transfer, which has been shown to reduce pregnancy rates. More specifically, your doctor uses this opportunity to select the best catheter for your body, ensure there are no anatomical reasons—such as scar tissue on your cervix—that might prevent smooth catheter insertion, identify the best place to put the embryo in your uterus, measure the length from your cervix to that spot, and "map out" the best way to get there. Most often, mock transfers are done about a month (or longer, if your doctor is also taking a biopsy) before your IVF cycle during a saline infusion sonogram (SIS), hysterosalpingogram (HSG), or hysteroscopy.

You will be asked to arrive at your clinic with a full bladder, which improves the ultrasound guidance and enables an easier transfer. Similar to a Pap smear, you will be asked to lie on your back and put your feet into stirrups. Your doctor will place a speculum in your vagina to help guide the catheter through your cervix and into your uterus. Your doctor may push a dye through the catheter to ensure the same result with an embryo on the day of your real transfer.

Some women have no pain at all, whereas other women find mock transfers extremely painful as their doctors insert and maneuver the catheter—especially if there's any difficulty getting it through their cervix. However, there's no denying that having a full bladder throughout it all is extremely uncomfortable! With any luck, the cost of your mock transfer will be wrapped into the overall cost of your IVF cycle.

Endometrial Scratch

Although once a common procedure, the endometrial scratch—a small injury or tissue biopsy made to the uterine lining—is no longer a default for most fertility clinics. The idea is that the small injury to your lining triggers new lining to develop that may be more receptive to implantation. However, the science behind it is conflicting, with some studies showing an improvement in pregnancy and live birth rates and others showing no benefits. Have a discussion with your doctor about whether it's right for you.

Charity from Tennessee says, "Even though I'm a physician and I would pull the literature on interventions and know how little science there was to back some of these things, I found myself willing to try anything!"

The endometrial scratch is typically performed during your luteal phase in the cycle immediately preceding your transfer cycle. Endometrial scratches can be done right in the office while you are awake, or under light sedation.

I've had several, and the one time I was awake for it, I found the procedure *extremely* painful. (One study found that women rank the pain of an endometrial scratch as 6 out of 10, so I'm not alone!) I can see a scratch as something to try if you've had several failed transfers, but I recommend combining it with a sedated hysteroscopy so you're unconscious during the procedure.

Priming, Suppression, and Prep

When you're talking about IVF, the terms *priming*, *suppression*, and *prep* all refer to the same thing: an attempt to begin your cycle with hormones at the low end of normal ranges and antral follicles on both ovaries all roughly the same small size. You're suppressing your body's natural hormone production to ensure that each follicle has the same likelihood of maturing, rather than one follicle becoming dominant.

Dr. Rodgers explains, "Think about a horse race. They put the horses in their gates one at a time. They hold them there until the last horse is in, then they open the gates and all the horses run out at the same time. And that's what we want to do with the eggs. We want to hold them there and really get them synced up, and then let all those eggs run out at the same time."

Suppression begins days or weeks before your baseline appointment (see page 111), and there are multiple ways to approach it. However, please note that *not priming at all* is often the best choice. As Dr. Rodgers says, "Different patients will respond differently to different protocols and some of it is an art. This is where the art of medicine comes in, and some of it is understanding how these protocols work, which patients they're most beneficial for, and knowing the patient's levels. It should not be a rubber stamp where everyone gets the same protocol."

Let's take a quick look at the options for suppression protocols.

BIRTH CONTROL PILL

May be recommended for patients with:

- Polycystic ovary syndrome (PCOS)
- High anti-Müllerian hormone (AMH) levels
- No period or an irregular period
- Prior good response to ovarian stimulation without birth control pills

May not be recommended for patients with:

- A history of blood clots, migraines, or ovarian cysts
- Diminished ovarian reserve
- Endometriosis
- Prior poor response to ovarian stimulation and/or poor egg quality

How it works:

- Prohibits the production of naturally occurring estrogen and progestin to "quiet" or suppress your ovaries prior to ovarian stimulation
- Allows coordination of your cycle with your clinic's availability to perform your egg retrieval or embryo transfer
- You will likely be prescribed a monophasic type, which contains the same amount of estrogen and progestin in every active pill.

When and for how long you might take it:

- You will call on cycle day 1 and be instructed to start birth control pills.
- Your clinic may require that you come in for an ultrasound and blood work before you start birth control pills.
- You likely will take the active pills for a minimum of 10 days, but the average is 21.
- You may overlap the birth control pills with Lupron for the last few days before starting ovarian stimulation medication(s).

WARRIOR TIPS
When Birth Control Pills Are Not Recommended

More and more reproductive endocrinologists are moving away from priming with birth control pills, especially for women who have poor egg quality, diminished ovarian reserve, or a poor response to ovarian stimulation. These women's hormones tend to become so suppressed that once their IVF cycle begins, their ovaries have a hard time rebooting and have to work harder than expected to produce the desired results.

I fell into the "poor egg quality" category, and my ovaries responded *much* better during the one retrieval cycle when I was not primed with birth control pills, producing eight high-quality embryos during my third retrieval compared to six and one poor-quality embryos during my first and second retrievals, respectively.

Dr. Geoffrey Sher, a board-certified reproductive endocrinologist and cofounder of Sher Fertility Solutions in Las Vegas, says the problem lies with clinics transitioning patients from hormonal suppression with birth control pills straight into ovarian stimulation, which is the protocol my clinic followed during my first two retrievals. Instead, for the final 5 days of suppression, he suggests overlapping birth control pills with a gonadotropin-releasing hormone (GnRH) antagonist like Lupron. This, he explains, will increase your follicle-stimulating hormone (FSH) levels naturally prior to menstruation and properly prepare your follicles for recruitment.

ESTROGEN PROTOCOL

May be recommended for patients with:

- A history of blood clots, migraines, or ovarian cysts

- Diminished ovarian reserve

- Advanced reproductive age (38+)

- Prior poor response to ovarian stimulation and/or poor egg quality

- Regular, predictable ovulation

May not be recommended for patients with:

- Any other infertility diagnosis

How it works:

- Suppresses FSH by maintaining high estrogen levels

When and for how long you might take it:

- You will begin using estrogen patches after ovulation and continue through ovarian stimulation until the "trigger shot."

- You'll take a GnRH antagonist (such as Cetrotide or ganirelix) simultaneously—typically starting a day after patches—for 3 to 4 days to keep your eggs from growing.

- You'll stop the GnRH antagonist—and begin stimulation—when your period begins.

LUTEAL LUPRON PROTOCOL

May be recommended for patients with:

- Young reproductive age (less than 35)

- Prior poor response to ovarian stimulation and/or poor egg quality

May not be recommended for patients with:

- Advanced reproductive age (38+)

- Prior fair or good response to ovarian stimulation (with or without priming)

How it works:

- Lowers estrogen levels by triggering the release of FSH and LH from your pituitary gland

- Inhibits the pituitary gland's ability to control the ovaries

When and for how long you might take it:

- Used in combination with birth control pills for priming (see page 110)

- You will begin Lupron during the last few days of the cycle before starting ovarian stimulation medication(s).

No Suppression or Priming

As I mentioned, my most successful cycle involved no suppression or priming prior to beginning ovarian stimulation. However, just because it worked well for me doesn't mean it's the best for you.

⚡ If your doctor suggests only birth control pills, ask why. If the reasoning is mostly or entirely because the clinic needs to time your cycle with *its* schedule, consider advocating for a protocol customized to your body's unique needs instead. This process is too emotionally and financially expensive to cater to your clinic's needs over your own.

Baseline Appointment

Finally, the one time you actually want to see your period and it has arrived! You'll contact your clinic immediately, and it will schedule your baseline appointment on cycle day 2 or 3. At the appointment, your doctor will draw your blood to check your human chorionic gonadotropin (hCG), estrogen, progesterone, FSH, and LH levels; check the thickness of your uterine lining; and examine your ovaries for antral follicle count and to ensure that your follicles are all roughly the same size.

After this appointment, the course of treatment for the cycle might change. Taking into account the cost of an egg retrieval, your doctor might say your follicle count is too low and it would be more beneficial to switch to an IUI or timed intercourse cycle. But remember, ultimately the decision is yours.

Dr. Rodgers recalls recommending to a patient that she cancel the cycle, but the patient responded by saying, "Nope, I really just want to move forward." Now that woman has a beautiful, healthy son.

If you have a cyst, your treatment will be delayed until it resolves or your doctor drains it with a needle. You also may be temporarily prescribed birth control pills with the goal of eliminating the cyst more quickly. If all looks as expected, you'll be approved to begin ovarian stimulation.

⚡ Ideally, your reproductive endocrinologist will print out a tentative schedule of your medications, dosages, and instructions. If not, ask your doctor to do so. Having this information clear and readily at hand will make you feel more at ease about the cycle.

Ovarian Stimulation (Stimming)

The goal of "stimming," as it's known, is to retrieve as many healthy, mature eggs as possible. On average, IVF patients stim for 9, 10, or 11 days. Stimming for too long may damage your eggs and/or uterine lining (which is a problem if you're planning a fresh transfer). Additionally, eggs can be immature or overmature, so determining the best day to "trigger" is both a science and an art.

At each monitoring appointment, your doctor should be tracking your estrogen, progesterone, and LH levels; measuring your uterine lining thickness and noting its appearance; and counting and measuring your follicles.

Although you will not receive your blood work results until the afternoon, don't leave your clinic without a printout of the other information. Pro tip: Create a spreadsheet of all of this information so you can keep track of it throughout your cycle(s).

Do not compare your cycle to someone else's. I have clients who have gone in for monitoring six or more times, whereas I never went more than four. There's no "right" number of monitoring appointments. It depends on your body's response to stims and your doctor's strategy for how often—and when in the cycle—to take a look at how things are progressing.

EXAMPLE STIMULATION TIMELINE

Again, this is a broad overview, and the specifics of your cycle may vary.

TIMELINE	POSSIBLE RESULTS
Cycle day 1, 2, or 3	Follicles all ≤ 10 mm
Stim day 4	Most or all follicles still ≤ 10 mm
Stim day 6	Some follicles 12–13 mm
Stim day 7 or 8	Some follicles 14–15 mm
Stim day 8 or 9	Some follicles 16–17 mm
Stim day 9, 10, or 11	Some (preferably the majority) of follicles 18–20 mm
Trigger	Trigger with hCG and/or Lupron (a dual trigger with hCG and Lupron in the evening, followed by Lupron the next morning, has proven to be most effective in most situations)
Retrieval	Takes place 36 hours after the trigger

There are several different stimming protocols, and your doctor should make it clear why the one they are recommending is best for you. Also know that over the course of a cycle, your doctor will continue to monitor your progress and should adjust your medication according to your body's response.

ANTAGONIST (OR SHORT) PROTOCOL

May be recommended for patients with:

- Young reproductive age (less than 35)
- Unexplained infertility

- No prior ovarian stimulation with injectables
- Prior fair or good response to ovarian stimulation (with or without priming)

May not be recommended for patients with:

- Any other diagnosis, especially those with high baseline or otherwise premature LH levels

Typical stimulation timeline:

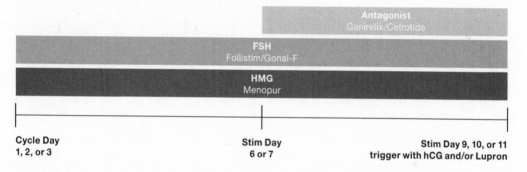

| Cycle Day 1, 2, or 3 | Stim Day 6 or 7 | Stim Day 9, 10, or 11 trigger with hCG and/or Lupron |

LONG LUPRON (OR LUPRON DOWN REGULATION) PROTOCOL

May be recommended for patients with:

- Young reproductive age (less than 35)

- Prior poor response to ovarian stimulation and/or poor egg quality

May not be recommended for patients with:

- Any other diagnosis

Typical stimulation timeline:

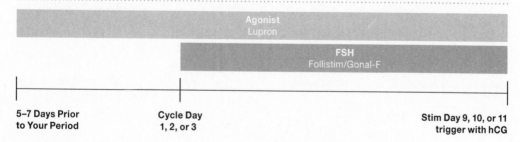

| 5–7 Days Prior to Your Period | Cycle Day 1, 2, or 3 | Stim Day 9, 10, or 11 trigger with hCG |

FLARE (OR MICRODOSE LUPRON) PROTOCOL

May be recommended for patients with:

- Advanced reproductive age (38+)
- Prior poor response to ovarian stimulation and/or poor egg quality
- A poor or fair response to the long Lupron (or Lupron downregulation) protocol

May not be recommended for patients with:

- Any other diagnosis

Typical stimulation timeline:

Agonist Lupron
FSH Follistim/Gonal-F

Cycle Day
1, 2, or 3

Stim Day 9, 10, or 11
trigger with hCG

MINI IVF

May be recommended for patients with:

- PCOS and at a severe risk of developing ovarian hyperstimulation syndrome (OHSS)
- Diminished ovarian reserve
- Cancer and hoping to preserve their fertility before treatment
- A poor or fair response to antagonist and/or Lupron protocols

May not be recommended for patients with:

- Any other diagnosis, especially those with high baseline or otherwise premature LH levels

Typical stimulation timeline:

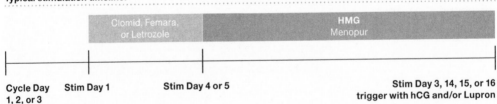

Clomid, Femara, or Letrozole	HMG Menopur

Cycle Day   Stim Day 1   Stim Day 4 or 5
1, 2, or 3

Stim Day 3, 14, 15, or 16
trigger with hCG and/or Lupron

LUTEAL PHASE PROTOCOL (WITH OR WITHOUT DUOSTIM)

May be recommended for patients with:

- Regular and/or predictable ovulation without medication
- Diminished ovarian reserve
- PCOS, as long as ovulation is regular and/or predictable without medication
- Advanced reproductive age (38+)
- Prior poor response to ovarian stimulation and/or poor egg quality

May not be recommended for patients with:

- No, or unpredictable, ovulation without medication

Typical stimulation timeline:

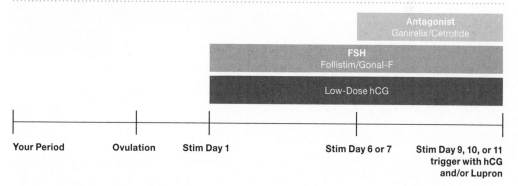

AGONIST/ANTAGONIST CONVERSION PROTOCOL

May be recommended for patients with:

- Advanced reproductive age (38+, especially 40+)
- Diminished ovarian reserve
- A poor or fair response to other protocols

May not be recommended for patients with:

- Any other diagnosis

Typical stimulation timeline:

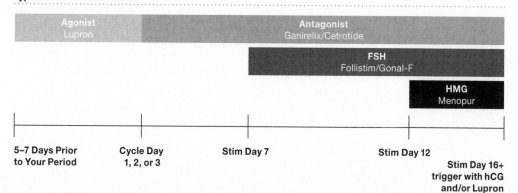

AGONIST/ANTAGONIST CONVERSION PROTOCOL WITH ESTROGEN PRIMING

May be recommended for patients with:

- Advanced reproductive age (38+, especially 40+)
- Diminished ovarian reserve
- A poor or fair response to the agonist/antagonist conversion protocol

May not be recommended for patients with:

- Any other diagnosis

Typical stimulation timeline

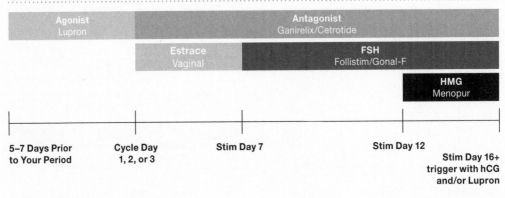

Warning: Your first IVF cycle is a bit of a crapshoot. Your doctor is making an educated guess about the best protocol for you, given what they already know about your body. But it's possible that this first cycle will yield information that causes your doctor to change recommendations for future cycles. And even then, the next cycle might not be as successful as you would hope, whether due to the protocol or to the fact that we all vary from menstrual cycle to cycle.

Take Natacha, for example. She recounts, "Rounds one and two were antagonist protocols with a Lupron trigger. The second round, they lowered the Gonal-F dose and increased Menopur because we learned that I am a high responder. The third round, I did a long Lupron protocol, starting Lupron injections for a week, then adding Menopur and Follistim, and triggering with hCG. Woof, that round sucked!"

Adrienne from New Jersey also changed protocols—and even switched clinics for her third round. "For our first two rounds of IVF, the protocol included Menopur, Gonal-F, and Cetrotide for stimulation and then a combination of low-dose hCG and Lupron for trigger. For our third round, we switched to a new clinic and a different protocol. At this point, we eliminated the Menopur and used Follistim and low-dose hCG for the stimulation and Provera [instead of Cetrotide] to suppress ovulation. We used a Lupron-only trigger. This was our best outcome of the three cycles."

"Triggering" Last-Minute Maturation

Once the majority of your follicles are 17+ mm and several follicles are mature (18–20 mm), (if you're doing a fresh transfer, your uterine lining should be thick [7+ mm] and trilaminar in appearance), and your hormone levels indicate your body is ready, you will be instructed to take a trigger injection. Unlike during a timed intercourse or IUI cycle, the goal here isn't to trigger ovulation. Instead, as has been described previously, the trigger shot helps your eggs reach final maturation—with the hope that the majority will be in the 18 to 20 mm range by the time of your egg retrieval. It's very important to inject the medication at the exact time provided by your clinic. Your retrieval will likely take place exactly 36 hours later—which means you might take this injection in the middle of the night.

There are four main types of trigger shots:

- Urinary-extracted human chorionic gonadotropins (hCGu), such as Novarel and Pregnyl

- Recombinant DNA-derived hCG (hCGr), such as Ovidrel

- Antagonists, such as Lupron

- A combination of hCG (5,000–10,000 IU) and Lupron

The type and dosage you're prescribed will depend on your estrogen level and risk factors for OHSS.

Egg Retrieval

The best advice I can give you going into an egg retrieval is to let go of expectations—or at least set realistic ones.

"My egg retrieval experience was largely positive," says Lindsay from Washington. "We went into the process knowing that I would have to do more than one retrieval, and this helped set my expectations. If we got more than one egg, we would consider it a success. The first cycle, we retrieved four eggs and we've never been more thrilled. It was the first time I had hope that I might get to have a biological child in the 3 years since I was diagnosed with diminished ovarian reserve."

WARRIOR TIPS
What Is DuoStim, and Why Might I Need It?
• •
If you have diminished ovarian reserve or premature ovarian insufficiency, or if you are about to undergo chemotherapy, your doctor might recommend a DuoStim—a double (or dual) ovarian stimulation within the same cycle. This means you'll do one round of stimulation and retrieval, often beginning stimulation during your luteal phase rather than your menstrual phase (see the luteal phase protocol on page 115). Then, about 5 to 7 days later, you'll stimulate *again*. Often the second retrieval is more successful than the first—something I've witnessed with many of my infertility coaching clients.

You will be under light sedation during the procedure, so you will be instructed not to eat or drink for 8 to 10 hours beforehand. (And you will need to bring someone to drive you home afterward.) Your reproductive endocrinologist may also prescribe antibiotics to lower the risk of infection. You'll need to provide a semen sample. The semen can be collected at home or in your doctor's office; if you're using frozen or donated sperm, see chapter 10. If you are using fresh sperm and collecting it at home, it'll need to be taken to the office within an hour and kept at body temperature during transportation.

A lab technician will "wash" the sperm and then evaluate it. (For more detail on this procedure, see page 100.)

Warning: Unless you've been in your clinic's operating room before, your egg retrieval will feel very clinical compared to your other appointments. This isn't a bad thing, but it's something to be prepared for.

"As I look back now, it was relatively manageable. At the time, however, it felt very extreme. I was surprised at how clinical and cold it felt," explains Michelle. "My egg retrieval took place in a different part of the clinic that looked much more like a hospital than the colorful, comfortable visit rooms of the floor below. The actual procedure took place in such a sterile, cold operating room . . . again, not what I'd expected relative to the rest of my experience at the clinic up to that point. But it wasn't all bad. My recovery was far easier than I'd expected, and it was a numerically great retrieval!"

You will remove all your clothes (including your underwear—I accidentally made the mistake of leaving mine on once, and the doctor and nurses had a good laugh!) and change into a surgical gown. I recommend leaving your jewelry at home, but if you have any still on, you will remove and store it. A nurse will take your vitals and explain the procedure and discharge instructions. You will sign a consent form. A nurse or anesthesiologist will insert your IV, and the anesthetist will review your medical history, including any previous bad reactions to anesthesia. (Because I had severe vomiting following a surgery many years ago, they always include an antinausea medication in my anesthesia cocktail. I highly recommend asking for this, but please note that it increases

the likelihood of constipation following the procedure. So, to avoid a call later, ask the nurse what's safe to take if you have constipation.) Your retrieval will be performed under light sedation rather than general anesthesia. This allows you to fall asleep and wake up quickly—and then continue your day as usual.

⚡ Depending on the size of your clinic, your reproductive endocrinologist may perform your retrieval, or you may have another doctor—possibly one you've never met before. This can be unsettling for some people, so when your retrieval is scheduled, ask who will be performing it. Looking up the doctor's bio in advance might help calm any nerves caused by unfamiliarity. The doctor performing your retrieval will discuss the procedure and confirm your plans for fertilization and the resulting embryos. If you have any questions, don't hesitate to ask!

The procedure doesn't take very long—about 20 to 30 minutes. Although it always *feels* like they are starting while you're still awake, don't worry! Once you're asleep, the doctor will locate your ovaries and examine your follicles using ultrasound. Under ultrasound guidance, the doctor will use a needle to remove the fluid from each follicle. At the same time, the embryologist examines the fluid under a microscope to identify how many eggs are retrieved. You're typically told the total number of eggs retrieved—and sometimes the number of mature eggs—before you leave, but assessing their quality takes a bit longer.

The time you spend in recovery varies from person to person, but the average is about 30 minutes. Most people return to work the next day. You will be told to avoid sex, swimming, baths, and tampons for a period of time following the procedure. Also, don't go home and immediately lie down, as that may result in complications. If you develop a fever above 101°F, severe abdominal pain or swelling,

BUSTED

Myth: IVF causes cancer.

Women who have undergone IVF do have higher rates of cancer, but not because of IVF. It's because infertility and related factors lead to a higher risk of cancer.

"There are no long-term risks with IVF, and a few weeks of hormones have no long-term effects on the body," says Dr. Rodgers. "Conversely, infertility will increase the risk of breast, ovarian, and uterine cancer. Typically, this is not due to the infertility itself, but the fact that pregnancy has not occurred. In cases of obesity or PCOS, there is an increased risk of uterine cancer."

While risk factors exist with IVF and FET, they are short-term. There are no long-term risks directly caused by IVF or FET.

BUSTED

Myth: Once IVF, always IVF.

Many people think of IVF as a point of no return—if it's the only way you've ever gotten pregnant, it's your only option from then on. But this is not necessarily true.

"Many think 'once IVF, always IVF,'" says Dr. Aaron K. Styer, a board-certified reproductive endocrinologist and a founding partner and co-medical director of CCRM Boston. "In reality, patients can get pregnant on their own while preparing to start IVF, immediately after a failed IVF cycle, or many years after getting pregnant with their initial IVF cycles."

IVF does not have to be the death of your hopes for spontaneous conception. And once you've been successful with IVF, that doesn't mean you can't return to less invasive treatments if you want to try for a second child. You still have a right to consider and advocate for timed intercourse, IUI, or other options.

---

heavy vaginal bleeding (more than one pad per hour), trouble breathing, severe shoulder pain, painful urination, or dizziness, call your clinic immediately.

Embryology

Now that your fertility team has your eggs, it's time to start making embryos. This is a complicated process involving science that always amazes me. Let's break down the process so you can understand what's going on with your precious gametes.

Day 0: Egg Retrieval and Fertilization

Approximately 6 hours after your egg retrieval, the embryologist goes to work. Attempts to fertilize your eggs can happen in one of several ways. One option is conventional or natural insemination—putting eggs and sperm in the same petri dish, enabling a natural selection process between the two. Another option is to inject a single sperm into each egg, a process known as intracytoplasmic sperm injection (ICSI). The "best" sperm are selected for injection based on a visual assessment of morphology and motility. Especially during their first retrieval, some couples opt to do half and half—half conventional insemination and half ICSI—to compare fertilization rates between the two methods.

"In our first two retrievals, we used conventional fertilization," says Adrienne. "We did inquire about ICSI, but our embryologist advised that they would make the decision on conventional versus ICSI based on the sperm sample collected. Our third retrieval was with a new clinic, which does ICSI as a standard for all fertilization."

WARRIOR TIPS
When to Use ICSI or PICSI

You should consider ICSI if any of the following apply to your situation:

- Low sperm concentration
- Low sperm morphology
- Low sperm motility
- Using frozen sperm
- Few eggs retrieved
- Eggs with a thick zona pellucida
- Previous failed or low rate of natural fertilization

You should consider PICSI if any of the following apply to your situation:

- Low fertilization rate with ICSI
- Male partner with high DNA fragmentation
- Previous poor embryo development between days 3 and 5 or a low blastocyst conversion rate

There is also a procedure known as "rescue ICSI." If none of your eggs fertilized using conventional insemination, ICSI can be performed the following day. However, it's not always successful, and it requires a fresh semen sample. All resulting viable blastocysts will be frozen for later use because these embryos are no longer developing on the same timeline as your uterine lining.

Technically, there is one more—but *much* less common—approach called physiological intracytoplasmic sperm injection (PICSI). This technique involves selecting sperm that bind to hyaluronic acid, which is part of the protective barrier that surrounds your eggs, when tested in the lab.

Day 1: Fertilization Report

Approximately 18 hours after attempting to fertilize your eggs, or 24 hours after your retrieval, the embryologist will check on their status. If two round pronuclei—one containing genetic material from the egg and the other containing genetic material from the sperm—are observed inside an egg, it has fertilized and is now considered a zygote embryo. You should receive a call telling you how many eggs were mature (if this was not communicated after your retrieval) and are now fertilized.

Of your mature eggs, unless there's known severe male factor infertility, approximately 70 to 75 percent should fertilize. If the fertilization rate was lower than expected, ask about the quality of the eggs and sperm—and if the embryologist has any other observations or theories about why the rate was low.

Here some reasons why an egg might not fertilize:

Conventional Insemination

- Sperm had poor concentration, morphology, or motility.

- Egg was not mature.

- Egg had a thick, hardened, or pigmented zona pellucida.

- Sperm had difficulty penetrating the cumulus cells surrounding the egg.

- Sperm could not fuse with the egg membrane.

- Sperm head lacked the ability to break through the egg's zona pellucida barrier.

- Sperm head failed to decondense, keeping the sperm's DNA inside its head.

- Egg and sperm did not form a pronucleus, or combined genetic material, inside the egg.

- More than one sperm entered the egg.

ICSI

- Egg was of poor quality, such as a hardened or pigmented zona pellucida.

- Egg was overmature.

- Egg matured just before ICSI was performed.

- Egg didn't "activate," or respond appropriately on a cellular level, when the sperm entered.

- Sperm head failed to decondense, keeping the sperm's DNA inside its head.

Day 2: The Embryo Begins to Divide

Although the embryo itself does not grow larger, the single cell that was formerly the egg divides into two cells and then four, each about half the size of the last. Because slight variations between embryos can be observed at this stage, it's possible for the embryologist to begin grading them. However, most clinics leave embryos alone on day 2 to avoid opening the incubator more often than necessary.

Day 3: Embryo Grading and Possible Transfer

The embryo should now contain about eight cells. The embryologist moves the embryos to a new petri dish that contains a solution similar to uterine fluid to help enable their next stage of growth. Each embryo is given a grade based on the number of cells (four to eight), amount of fragmentation (graded A through D), and symmetry of the cells (graded G for good, F for fair, or P for poor). A "perfect" day 3 embryo would receive the grade 8AG, meaning it has eight cells, there's no fragmentation, and the cells are all the same size. However, some clinics use their own grading system. Ask your doctor how your embryos will be graded so you know what to expect.

GRADING BASED ON FRAGMENTATION

Fragmentations look like cells within an embryo, but they are not. More fragmentation is linked to a lower chance of success.

FRAGMENTATION GRADE	DESCRIPTION
A	No fragmentation
B	Less than 30% fragmented
C	30–50% fragmented
D	More than 50% fragmented

GRADING BASED ON SYMMETRY OF THE CELLS

SYMMETRY GRADE	DESCRIPTION
G (good)	All cells are of equal size
F (fair)	Almost half of the cells are of different sizes
P (poor)	Most cells are of different sizes

Approximately 75 percent of embryos will develop to day 3, but there are no guarantees about which ones will continue to grow from there. If you have very few embryos, the recommendation might be to transfer rather than take the risk that they stop developing in the lab. However, in most cases, it's better to wait because embryos that do not continue to develop in the lab often are aneuploid (not chromosomally normal).

If you are planning to do a fresh transfer, you might receive a call on day 3 updating you on the status of your embryos and advising you when to come in—either that day or on day 5—for a transfer.

Day 4: Cleavage Stage to Morula

On average, about half of embryos develop beyond day 3. Most embryologists do not observe embryos on day 4—again, to avoid opening the incubator more often than necessary. On this day, embryos are in transition to become morulas with 10 to 30 cells.

Day 5: Blastocysts Are Graded and Transferred or Frozen

Embryos now contain 100 or more cells. The embryologist will grade them, typically based on the degree of embryo expansion (graded 1 through 6), the appearance of the inner mass cells (graded A through C), and the appearance of the trophectoderm layer of cells (graded A through C). A "perfect" day 5 embryo would receive the grade 4AA, 5AA, or 6AA, meaning it is an expanded blastocyst, it is in the process of hatching out of its shell, or it has already hatched, respectively; the inner layer has many tightly packed cells; and the outer layer has many cohesive cells. Again, some clinics use their own grading system, so it's best to ask rather than assume.

Unfortunately, grading is not an exact science. It's useful in terms of deciding which embryo(s) to transfer first, but viable embryos

GRADING BASED ON THE DEGREE OF EMBRYO EXPANSION

The cavity is the internal part of an embryo. The more it expands, the higher the likelihood that it becomes a blastocyst.

EXPANSION GRADE	DESCRIPTION
1	Cavity fills less than half of the embryo
2	Cavity fills more than half of the embryo
3	Cavity fills the embryo (full blastocyst)
4	Cavity is larger than the embryo, with a thin zona pellucida (expanded blastocyst)
5	Hatching out of the shell
6	Fully hatched out of the shell

GRADING BASED ON THE INNER CELL MASS

If implantation is successful and the pregnancy progresses, the inner cell mass will eventually become the fetus.

INNER CELL MASS GRADE	DESCRIPTION
A	Many cells, tightly packed
B	Fewer cells, loosely packed
C	Few cells

GRADING BASED ON THE TROPHECTODERM CELLS

The trophectoderm is the single cell layer of the embryo wall that makes the placenta.

TROPHECTODERM GRADE	DESCRIPTION
A	Many cells forming a cohesive layer around the embryo
B	Fewer cells forming a loose, thin layer around the embryo
C	A few large cells

of *all* grades have gone on to become babies. One of my first coaching clients successfully gave birth to a daughter who began life as a 4CC embryo. The best viable embryos are either transferred now, frozen, or biopsied for preimplantation genetic testing and then frozen. Some embryos need an extra day (or 2) before they are ready to transfer, freeze, or biopsy. This is normal, so don't panic! The embryologist will monitor their development until they can be properly graded.

Most doctors consider grading to be a prioritization system. Lindsay agrees, saying, "We knew that we had two [embryos] that had roughly the same implantation percentage (70 percent) and one that had a lower percentage (50 percent). This helped us decide which to transfer first." (Implantation percentage means the chance that the embryo will implant.)

When I started the IVF process, I didn't know about grading. Once I researched it, I inquired about my embryos and discovered they were very poor quality. It would have been nice to know that much sooner than *after* my second retrieval!

Natacha, too, had to ask for this information rather than having it readily provided. "My doctors were so tight-lipped, and it frustrated me to no end. You have to be your own advocate and ask for the information you want. Don't expect them to willingly give it to you!"

Day 6 or 7: Final Blastocyst Count
The embryologist will grade all embryos that are still developing. Most labs will discard

embryos that have not reached the blastocyst stage by day 7. The viable embryos are frozen or biopsied for preimplantation genetic testing and then frozen. You will receive a call with the final count and grades of your embryos.

Day 16–21: Preimplantation Genetic Testing Results

If you chose to perform preimplantation genetic testing (see chapter 4) on your embryos, you will receive a call anywhere from day 16 through 21 about the results. Most genetics companies say the testing can take up to 2 weeks, but many people receive the report within 7 days.

"My first and fourth reproductive endo-crinologist had completely different opinions about this," explains Lindsay. "The first wanted to transfer a day 3 embryo without genetic testing, while the fourth one wanted to do genetic testing due to concerns about my quality. He was really trying to focus on not just getting me pregnant, but also the end goal of making sure I had a healthy pregnancy that would lead to a healthy baby. He felt that the research now shows that if an embryo is not 'healthy' via genetic testing, it won't recover in the body."

Cryopreservation and Storage

Although it wasn't always this way, most clinics now use a process called vitrification to freeze embryos (and eggs and sperm). Vitrification cools the embryos quickly, transforming your embryos into a glass-like state and preventing the formation of ice. They are stored at −196°C in liquid nitrogen tanks that are constantly monitored with sensors and alarms—although if you have any questions about how your clinic approaches this process, you should ask.

The College of American Pathologists accredits approximately 350 reproductive labs around the United States. Although accidents happen, of course, an accredited lab means that it is inspected every 2 years for program compliance. In 2018, two clinics—the University

Hospitals Ahuja Medical Center's Fertility Center in Cleveland and the Pacific Fertility Center in San Francisco—experienced tank malfunctions that may have impacted the viability of thousands of embryos. Ariana Eunjung Cha of the *Washington Post* wrote a great article, "FAQ: Are my frozen embryos safe? Everything you need to know about the freezer malfunctions," a great resource if you want to better understand how your lab freezes and stores embryos.

It's unknown how long cryopreserved embryos will remain viable, but babies have been born from embryos frozen as long as 20 years ago. If you're concerned about your age because you're transferring an embryo frozen when you were younger, remember that your embryo is frozen in time and the age of your uterus is a much smaller factor in the end result.

Also, heads up, cryopreservation and storage fees are not always included in the cost of an IVF cycle. So be sure to ask your clinic how much they charge.

Believe it or not, some infertility warriors end up with too many embryos, and it's best to consider your options if that happens *before* your retrieval. Angela from Missouri advises you to research your options and do some soul searching. "I have a dozen frozen embryos, and while I'd have a dozen children, it's not reasonable for my family. I have some hard decisions to make that I didn't consider prior to my IVF cycle," she explains.

Michelle also wishes she had thought before she started the IVF process about what would happen if she had more embryos than she and her husband would need but for a different reason: her faith.

"A friend divided her eggs retrieved into two groups, some eggs to freeze and a small number of eggs to use to try to make embryos. Her church pastor had advised her about this option. We never spoke to our priest about decisions in our IVF journey, but I think doing

WARRIOR TIPS
What to Do with Remaining Embryos
....

With couples, most clinics make both partners sign a document prior to a retrieval cycle about what they want done with their embryos in the event that they separate, divorce, or one or both of them passes away.

There are four options when you have extra embryos:

1. Save them for a future cycle. You never know how you might feel down the road! Plus, women run out of eggs completely when they hit menopause, but believe it or not, they can still get pregnant and carry a child—although the pregnancy is extremely high-risk. This option requires an annual storage fee. However, your embryos will never "go bad" while they are cryopreserved, so rest assured that they're ready and waiting should you decide to use them.

2. Donate them to another couple. Whether the couple is known or unknown, donating your embryos is another option. This a very personal choice, and people have very different feelings about it. (See chapter 10 for more discussion of embryo donations.)

3. Donate them to science. This option gives you the opportunity to advance reproductive medicine in the future and help other infertility warriors have children. (My husband and I quickly decided this is what we wanted to do with any remaining embryos.)

4. Thaw and dispose of them. Depending on your local laws about human tissue, some clinics might even give them to you for burial. Clinics might also do what is known as a "compassionate transfer"—transferring the embryos during a time of your cycle when pregnancy is not possible. However, most embryos are simply thawed and disposed of in the embryology lab.

so may have changed our decisions, or at least invited us to think about the IVF journey through our spiritual lens. I had been scared to do this because I didn't want the spiritual lens to force me to change my mind."

Fresh Embryo Transfer

Whether your transfer takes place on day 3 or day 5, the procedure is the same. Remember the mock embryo transfer? Your fresh transfer will be exactly the same, except this time with a real embryo instead of dye!

⚡ You don't need anesthesia for the transfer procedure. However, if you are a sexual assault survivor for whom penetration could feel triggering, or experience severe pain when a speculum is inserted into your vagina, don't be afraid to ask your doctor about anesthesia. All seven of my transfers were done under anesthesia because I have vaginal scarring that makes placing a speculum difficult and traumatic.

Before and During the Transfer

To recap: Your doctor might instruct you to premedicate with Valium or a similar medication. Most people think it's to help them relax, but in reality, it's to relax your uterus and increase the likelihood of implantation.

You will be asked to arrive at your clinic with a full bladder, which improves the ultrasound guidance and enables an easier transfer. You'll likely have to sign some forms and confirm your name and date of birth, as well as the number of embryos you want to transfer.

You will be asked to lie on your back and put your feet into stirrups. Your doctor will place a speculum in your vagina to help guide the catheter through your cervix and into your uterus. Most women experience either no pain or light cramping. The embryo(s) will be transferred through the catheter. And that's it—you're officially PUPO (pregnant until proven otherwise)! The entire procedure is very quick.

My husband and I transferred two fresh embryos from our first cycle and became pregnant with twins. After they were stillborn, we transferred a single embryo in each of our following IVF cycles, totaling four FETs and two fresh.

AMERICAN SOCIETY FOR REPRODUCTIVE MEDICINE (ASRM) RECOMMENDATIONS FOR LIMITS TO THE NUMBER OF EMBRYOS TO TRANSFER				
	AGE (YEARS)			
	<35	**35–37**	**38–40**	**41–42**
CLEAVAGE-STAGE EMBRYOS (DAY 3)				
Euploid (genetically normal) embryos*	1	1	1	1
Other favorable embryos**	1	1	≤3	≤4
Embryos not euploid or favorable	≤2	≤3	≤4	≤5
BLASTOCYSTS (DAY 5, 6, OR 7)				
Euploid (genetically normal) embryos*	1	1	1	1
Other favorable embryos**	1	1	≤2	≤3
Embryos not euploid or favorable	≤2	≤2	≤3	≤3

*Demonstrated (through genetic testing) euploid embryos

**Other favorable = embryos meeting any ONE of these criteria:

Fresh transfer: expectation of 1 or more high-quality embryos available for cryopreservation, or previous live birth after previous transfer with a sibling embryo

Frozen embryo transfer: availability of vitrified day 5 or day 6 blastocysts, euploid embryos, first FET cycle, or previous live birth after an IVF cycle

Source: Practice Committee of the American Society for Reproductive Medicine and the Practice Committee for the Society for Assisted Reproductive Technologies, "Guidance on the Limits to the Number of Embryos to Transfer: A Committee Opinion." *Fertility and Sterility* 116, no. 3 (2021): 651–54.

Andrea and her husband, Sean, made a different decision. "We transferred one embryo because we knew it was chromosomally normal and had a higher chance of success. We only had two normal embryos to transfer and did not want to risk transferring them together and possibly having twins—or worse, having a failed FET and being left with no more embryos."

Adrienne and her husband, Matthew, took the same approach. "We have only transferred one embryo at a time. With PGT-normal embryos, we don't feel the need to transfer more than one at a time. For us, the risk of multiples and any potential complication is greater than the risk of a failed transfer."

Remember the goal: You can have as many babies as you want, but it's best to have one healthy baby at a time. And for you, that may mean transferring more than one embryo. Familiarize yourself with the American Society of Reproductive Medicine (ASRM) guidelines for the best chance of success.

After the Transfer

You should receive printed discharge instructions that will likely include things like avoiding intense exercise, lifting anything over 10 pounds, extreme temperatures, taking a bath or swimming, and having sex until your pregnancy test.

Your doctor also will probably direct you to continue taking estrogen and begin taking one or more medications, including progesterone. Because your progesterone level should be naturally high following an egg retrieval, you

WHAT TYPICALLY HAPPENS AFTER A DAY 3 TRANSFER	
DAYS PAST TRANSFER (DPT)	**EMBRYO DEVELOPMENT**
1	The embryo begins at 6–8 cells and further divides into 10–30 cells (morula). It floats in your uterus and derives nutrients from the egg and uterine fluid.
2	The embryo is a blastocyst with 100 or more cells. It continues to float in your uterus. Still growing, it begins to develop a fluid-filled cavity.
3	The growing cavity breaks the zona pellucida, and the embryo hatches out. It continues to float in your uterus.
4	The embryo attaches to a receptive portion of your uterine lining.
5	The embryo pushes into your uterine lining, initiating implantation. You may feel implantation pinching or cramping.
6	The embryo continues to implant. You may feel implantation pinching or cramping. The early placenta produces human chorionic gonadotrophin (hCG), although it cannot be detected yet.
7	The implantation process is nearly complete. You may feel implantation pinching or cramping, and implantation bleeding is possible. The placenta continues to develop.
8–11	The placenta continues to develop, releasing more hCG. It's now possible to detect hCG on a home pregnancy test. However, a negative test does not mean you are not pregnant—your embryo could have implanted later than expected.
12	Implantation is complete.

likely do not need more than vaginal gel or suppository progesterone for proper luteal phase support—although some doctors prefer progesterone injections because that type is more easily tracked via blood work. If there's any doubt, though, you can request a progesterone level check 7 days following your egg retrieval or 2 days following your transfer, similar to a cycle day 21 blood draw. If it's more than 15 ng/mL, you're in great shape—although I am very conservative with my infertility coaching clients and shoot for at least 20 ng/mL. One of the pitfalls of testing progesterone, however, is that your level varies widely over the course of 90 minutes, so you don't know if the time of your draw is during a peak or a trough.

And then there's bed rest. Some doctors advise it, and others don't. Studies have shown that bed rest following an embryo transfer is *not* advantageous and in fact may hurt your chance of becoming pregnant. Instead, it's recommended that you to get up immediately and go about your day. If you can arrange it, my recommendation is to take the next 5 workdays off—hopefully there's a weekend in there, too—to relax and practice good self-care, especially if your job is stressful.

Two-Week Wait (TWW)

You've had plenty of 2-week waits before, but when you're spending thousands or tens of thousands of dollars on IVF, the wait can feel that much harder. We will talk about some ways to make it through the TWW in chapter 8, but here are a few other tricks to maintaining your sanity during this time:

	WHAT TYPICALLY HAPPENS AFTER A DAY 5 TRANSFER
DAYS PAST TRANSFER (DPT)	**EMBRYO DEVELOPMENT**
1	The growing cavity breaks the zona pellucida, and the embryo hatches out. It continues to float in your uterus.
2	The embryo attaches to a receptive portion of your uterine lining.
3	The embryo pushes into your uterine lining, initiating implantation. You may feel implantation pinching or cramping.
4	The embryo continues to implant. You may feel implantation pinching or cramping. The early placenta produces human chorionic gonadotrophin (hCG), although it cannot be detected yet.
5	The implantation process is nearly complete. You may feel implantation pinching or cramping, and implantation bleeding is possible. The placenta continues to develop.
6–9	The placenta continues to develop, releasing more hCG. It's now possible to detect hCG on a home pregnancy test. However, a negative test does not mean you are not pregnant— your embryo could have implanted later than expected.
10	Implantation is complete.

- Meditate
- Practice positive visualization
- Journal
- Limit infertility talk

Pregnancy Test

To test or not to test? Nearly every fertility clinic, at least in the United States, will advise you not to test on your own and instead to wait for the clinic to give you a beta-hCG test, a blood test for human chorionic gonadotropin, estradiol, and progesterone levels, all of which can very accurately identify your pregnancy— or lack of it. Personally, I'm a POASer (pee on a stick–er), but my advice is to do whatever makes *you* feel the best. If you prefer to be in control and want to take a home pregnancy test, then test. If seeing a negative test will send you into a tailspin, then don't test.

To help you determine your preference, perhaps it would be helpful to understand what's happening in your body and when.

Your beta-hCG test may happen 11 to 12-plus days after a day 3 transfer or 9 to 10-plus days after a day 5 transfer. My clinic made us wait even more time—14 days after a day 5 transfer, and longer if the 14th day fell on a weekend.

If you're planning to test at home, here's what I recommend: Buy a large pack of cheap pink-dye tests, as well as one box of digital tests. (Stay away from the blue-dye tests—they are notoriously inaccurate, often giving false positives.) Begin testing the day after your transfer—not to detect pregnancy but because you need to test out the trigger shot. If you used hCG as your trigger, it can remain in your system for up to 14 days, although it's typically a much shorter time frame—it really depends on the person. Test every day until the test is clearly negative. Then, wait 2 days, or until *at least* 9 days past a day 3 transfer or 7 days past a day 5 transfer—whichever is longer. Test your urine both first thing in the morning and again in the evening after a 6-hour "hold" (stop drinking liquids at noon, and test at 6 p.m.). Some women, like me, test better in the evening. It's important that you pee into a paper cup and not directly on the stick because you might need to re-dip a different test strip if the result is inconclusive or you want to test again using a digital. If you get a result that *might* be positive (the pink-dye test doesn't look clearly negative), wait 48 hours and test again, this time with both a pink-dye test and a digital test. (Digital tests are much more expensive, so you don't want to waste them unless you think you might be pregnant.) If you're really pregnant, both will be positive by this point. Although many sources on the internet say digital tests don't detect hCG until it's at least 50 mIU/mL, I've seen some detect as low as 10 mIU/mL.

So there you have it. Test at home or don't. *You* are in control.

However, remember that home pregnancy test results may not be 100 percent accurate. A positive could mean a chemical pregnancy, and a negative may turn out to mean your hCG level was too low to detect at home but detectable in your blood. Two of my infertility coaching clients in the last 2 months had negative home tests on the morning of their betas, and both are now entering their second trimesters.

WARRIOR WISDOM
Consider Last-Minute Testing

I've seen people test at home on the morning of their beta-hCG test so they aren't surprised by the call they receive later that day. Charity from Tennessee says, "My general policy was to wait until the day of my hCG lab draw and do a first urine of the morning home test just so I would have an idea of what to expect on the phone call. I never liked the idea of getting a phone call that my hCG was negative when I could have known already."

Other In Vitro Options

What I've described so far in this chapter goes by several names—classic, conventional, or traditional IVF. However, there are other ways to approach in vitro fertilization, depending on your prognosis and preferences (see chapter 18). As is the case for all fertility treatments, your doctor will recommend a specific type, but educate yourself on the differences and speak up if you feel strongly about another option. Just keep in mind that some are newer and more experimental than others. As always, go in with eyes wide open—and don't be afraid to get a second opinion.

Natural Cycle IVF

Unlike traditional IVF, which relies on ovulation stimulation, natural cycle IVF takes advantage of your natural menstrual cycle, in which a single egg matures inside a single follicle. You are still closely monitored via ultrasound and blood work so you do not ovulate before your doctor can retrieve your egg. The one medication typically used during a natural cycle is a trigger shot. This helps your doctor time the egg retrieval procedure. If your egg fertilizes and an embryo—hopefully a blastocyst—develops, your doctor will transfer it back into your uterus.

Some women don't respond well emotionally and mentally to excess hormones. Others are against fertility medications for personal reasons. Regardless, if this method interests you, ask your doctor about your chance of success.

INVOcell

This unique method combines *in vitro* (in the lab) and *in vivo* (in the body). Following mild ovarian stimulation and an egg retrieval, the embryologist combines eggs and sperm in the inner chamber of a small device called an INVOcell. This chamber is locked and placed inside the outer chamber. The entire device is put into your vagina, held in place by a diaphragm. After 3 to 5 days, the INVOcell is removed and the embryologist observes the embryo(s). The best one(s) is chosen for immediate transfer back into your uterus. This option is popular among lesbian couples, as both partners can be involved in the process—one person's eggs, the other person's uterus. It is also a good option for those who want their embryos to spend more time in the body than in the lab. The carrier will likely need medication—potentially birth control, estrogen, and progesterone—to sync her cycle with the appropriate time to transfer the embryo into her body.

Not every clinic can or will do this version of IVF, so check out the INVOcell website to see which doctors near you perform the procedure.

Risks of IVF

IVF is generally considered safe, but there are some risks, some of which can seriously impact your health. Be sure to discuss your risk level with your doctor.

Ovarian Hyperstimulation Syndrome

OHSS is the main possible complication of IVF. Remember how your ovaries expand during treatment, and your doctor continues to monitor their size? The hormone hCG, which your body produces during pregnancy and is often used as a trigger shot, can sometimes cause the blood vessels in your ovaries to act abnormally, and leak fluid into your abdomen after your egg retrieval. Fluid can also come from your follicles, so the more follicles you produce, the larger your ovaries, the greater potential that they will leak fluid.

Symptoms may arise anywhere from 2 to 7 or more days after your retrieval. If your fresh transfer was successful and you are pregnant,

the symptoms will likely worsen. In the most severe cases, OHSS can be life-threatening, so be in tune with your body and don't be afraid to contact your doctor if you're concerned.

Mild symptoms include:

- Bloating and/or mild weight gain

- Mild pain or discomfort in the abdomen

- Mild nausea or diarrhea

Severe symptoms include:

- Severe bloating and/or rapid weight gain (2 or more pounds per day)

- Severe abdominal pain

- Severe nausea and/or dizziness

- Difficulty urinating

- Shortness of breath and/or rapid heartbeat

Some women are predisposed to developing OHSS. They include women who:

- Have PCOS

- Are 30 or younger

- Have high AMH levels

- Developed OHSS in the past

- Have a BMI that is too low or too high

I had OHSS in my first IVF cycle, and it was not fun. I was 29, at the high end of the normal BMI range, and newly pregnant with twins following my fresh transfer. My symptoms included severe abdominal pain, shortness of breath, and rapid heartbeat. I was weighed and had an abdominal ultrasound several times each week for at least a month to monitor my condition. Thankfully, the fluid went way on its own and I never had to have my abdomen drained.

Egg Retrieval Complications

In general, the egg retrieval procedure can cause cramping and/or light bleeding. But less common complications include bleeding from the ovary or pelvic vessels, a pelvic infection (this is why you will likely be prescribed an antibiotic in advance), or accidental puncture of the bladder, blood vessels, or bowel. If you develop a pelvic infection, you may be treated with stronger or intravenous antibiotics.

Embryo Transfer Complications

You may experience mild cramping during the procedure. However, in rare cases, some may experience cramping or bleeding *after* the transfer. As is the case for egg retrievals, it's possible—although rare—to develop an infection. If this happens, you will be prescribed antibiotics. The final risk of an embryo transfer is becoming pregnant with multiples—twins or more. The simplest way to reduce this risk is to transfer only one embryo.

Frozen Embryo Transfers (FETs)

FET cycles are relatively easy compared to fresh transfer cycles. The eggs have already been retrieved, and the embryos have already reached a certain level of development. All that's left is to transfer the embryo into your uterus and wait for implantation.

There are different ways to approach FETs, however. I provide a comprehensive overview of the options here, but your particular protocol might be different.

Consultation

As you probably know by now, every cycle starts with a consultation appointment. Expect your doctor to lay out the plan for your cycle, including a timeline, a list of possible medications you'll be taking, and possible success rate. It'll be very similar to the consultation appointment you had before your retrieval cycle, but of course now your eggs have already been retrieved and frozen.

WARRIOR WISDOM
Fertility Travel and Tourism

Given how complicated and expensive IVF is, you deserve to find a doctor and clinic that meet your needs—and sometimes that means seeking treatment outside of your area. Many infertility warriors decide fertility travel (having an out-of-state doctor where most of the routine parts of treatment occur long distance) or fertility tourism (traveling to another country to have fertility treatments) is their best option for IVF.

With fertility travel, many patients find an out-of-state clinic that provides a higher level of service or is more focused on the individual patient's needs.

Meredith from Alabama didn't like the options in her area. Because she knew people who had success with a clinic in Colorado, she decided to become a patient there.

"I had a level of comfort from my very first phone call," she shares. "So the advice that I would have for anybody else who's evaluating an out-of-area clinic

is to have the phone calls and see if you have a good rapport with the doctor. See if you feel comfortable with them, if you like what they have to say, if they have new ideas that you haven't heard before. I think you really know right off the bat if this is where you would feel comfortable pursuing this kind of treatment."

With fertility tourism, many patients decide to go abroad because certain European countries have more affordable treatments (sometimes they're up to 30 percent cheaper) and shorter waiting lists. Caroline Phillips, founder of Fertility Clinics Abroad in Edinburgh, United Kingdom, adds that there are many clinics that offer high-quality, highly regulated services.

"There are government bodies set up, and they come along and inspect the clinics every year or every 2 years. They need to meet certain criteria to continue as a clinic," she explains. "There are a lot of laws and safety measures in place."

When to Consider a FET

Some of the reasons you might have a frozen embryo transfer (FET) include:

- Your fresh transfer failed, but you had embryos remaining that were cryopreserved.

- Your fresh transfer was canceled due to a high risk of or confirmed OHSS.

- Your fresh transfer was canceled for another reason, such as your uterine lining was not ideal.

- You opted for preimplantation genetic testing.

- You did a "freeze all" cycle, where all of your embryos were frozen following your egg retrieval.

- You're using a donated embryo.

- You had a previous child via IVF and want to give them a sibling using a cryopreserved embryo.

Prepare a list of questions so you can better understand any changes to your protocols and the general differences with a frozen transfer. Before this appointment, check in with your emotions. If it's been a rough week or you're overwhelmed, you might want to make sure someone else—like a partner, friend, or relative—comes with you. They can absorb the information with a clear head, so if you have concerns or can't remember certain details later, they can let you know what the doctor said.

"Even though I've tried hard to self-advocate and ask questions, I wish I did *more*," explains Alexandra from California. "It's hard to remember every question I have when the doctor calls. I'm finally getting used to just emailing her when I have a question, and she usually answers."

Think, too, about the bigger picture. Andrea from Ohio regrets jumping into a frozen transfer too soon rather than "banking" embryos—going through as many consecutive retrieval cycles as it takes to get the number of embryos you might need for the number of children you want (typically you'll need two or three genetically normal embryos for every live birth).

Andrea says, "In hindsight, I wish we had done two consecutive retrievals before attempting a FET, since I was already 37 and our window for healthy embryos was closing, and we wanted two children. We were so anxious to get to that first positive pregnancy test that I

BUSTED

Myth: FETs are significantly less successful than fresh transfers.

Before cryopreservation, fertility clinics used a process called slow freezing. Initially, there was a lot of hesitation around the new technology but now most clinics use vitrification, which is an ultrarapid method of cryopreservation.

"With slow freezing, the success of embryos surviving the freezing and thawing process was maybe two-thirds," says Dr. Rodgers. "With vitrification, probably 95 percent plus of embryos survive the freezing-thawing. It is rare that they don't."

As the technology has improved, so have the the pregnancy success rates, which is important to remember from a financial perspective. Dr. Rodgers says that in the past it was common for couples to decide not to freeze leftover embryos because their chances were better with fresh cycles. However, the difference in cost is tremendous—a frozen cycle costs about one-third less than a fresh cycle. So now that FETs are becoming more successful, there's less need to do costly fresh cycles every time.

There are several ways to hopefully avoid OHSS altogether:

- Receive lower hormone dosages or follow a protocol specifically designed to reduce your risk of developing OHSS.

- Take a medication called cabergoline prior to your retrieval to help reduce fluid accumulation.

- Closely monitor your follicle count and estrogen level. If your follicle count is high and/or your estrogen is approaching 4,000 pg/mL, use a Lupron trigger shot, or one that combines Lupron with low-dose hCG.

- Cancel your fresh embryo transfer and freeze all resulting embryos for later use.

For her first retrieval, Adrienne was not given any specific instructions aside from drinking plenty of fluids and eating salty foods after the retrieval—both of which are recommended to reduce the likelihood of developing OHSS. For the second cycle, her hormone levels were higher, so her doctor was more concerned about this potential. But aside from the same advice and frequent follow-ups after the procedure, she was not given any other instruction. Then she changed clinics.

"With a different clinic for the third procedure, my doctor altered the protocol, triggering with Lupron instead of hCG in order to minimize the risk of OHSS. I found my recovery time to be much faster with this protocol."

There are additional steps you can take to either prevent or reduce the symptoms of OHSS following your retrieval:

- Avoid alcohol and caffeinated drinks. (Sorry!) Instead, drink plenty of fluids with electrolytes and *some* sodium and potassium—enough to make your urine pale or clear.

- Stay away from carbohydrates. (Sorry again!) Instead, maintain a diet high in protein.

- Maintain light, frequent activity while not overexerting yourself.

- If you're in pain, take an over-the-counter pain reliever like Tylenol.

couldn't really see past it. I wish we had taken a broader view of IVF as a tool for planning our family, and not just a way to get pregnant."

Endometrial Receptivity Analysis (ERA)

The quality of the uterine lining is a major factor in whether an embryo can successfully implant. Before implantation, your body produces progesterone as a signal for your uterus to prepare the lining for implantation, and the amount of progesterone determines the length of the implantation window. When there seems to be no clear reason why a previous embryo failed to implant, your doctor might suggest a uterine lining test like an endometrial receptivity analysis (ERA) to determine the exact timing of your implantation window. Those who are good candidates for an ERA include patients who have:

- Two or more failed embryo transfers

- A failed PGT normal embryo cycle

- A limited number of embryos

- Experienced recurrent ectopic or chemical pregnancies

With this test, you go through the prep steps of a frozen transfer cycle, but instead of transferring an embryo, your doctor will take a small biopsy of your uterine lining. This means it takes around 6 to 8 weeks to prepare for and complete the test and another 2 weeks before the results are back. An ERA is rarely covered by insurance (though it never hurts to ask). But the results are accurate and let you and your doctor know how many hours of progesterone you need prior to the ideal time to transfer your embryo. From there, your doctor will adjust your medication schedule to get progesterone levels that are more favorable and schedule future transfers in your specific implantation window.

Dr. Rodgers, who reports great success with pregnancies after this test, says it's important not to wait too long to have it if you are a good candidate. "If somebody has gone through four failed transfers, we do the ERA test, adjust the progesterone, and then hopefully see success," she explains. "But I can tell you that one of the biggest downsides about this particular test is that by the time patients are having this test done, we're putting in two embryos instead of one and my twin rate in this population is incredibly high."

Other Uterine Receptivity Tests

Your doctor might also suggest a ReceptivaDX test for endometriosis or Igenomix's ALICE (Analysis of Infectious Chronic Endometritis) test for inflammation of the uterine lining, which is treated with antibiotics (see chapter 3). The procedures are similar to an ERA but test the sample for different factors. However, because these are newer tests, currently there isn't a lot of research about how effective or useful they are in increasing your odds of getting pregnant.

Possible FET Protocols

With a FET cycle, two things need to happen: prevention of natural ovulation and preparation of the uterine lining. There's not a focus on stimulating follicular growth because you're not worried about needing an egg.

In general, less blood work is needed, too, but your uterine lining thickness and appearance will be monitored via transvaginal ultrasound throughout the cycle. In most cases, FET protocols also require less medication because you're not preparing for an egg retrieval. While some patients still do better with ovarian stimulation, it's rare.

Estrogen and Progesterone Supplementation

One of the most common ways to control ovulation while preparing the uterine lining is by using estrogen and progesterone supplementation. The estrogen is typically administered with a patch or pills for 2 to 3 weeks, then the progesterone is added at a specific time in your cycle, with either a shot or vaginal suppositories. Your doctor might also use Lupron and/or a GnRH antagonist to further control ovulation.

After the first day of your period, you will have a baseline appointment to establish your starting point. Starting at about day 8 or 9 of your cycle, your doctor will check the thickness of your uterine lining. Once the uterine lining reaches 7+ mm and is trilaminar in appearance, your doctor will have you start taking progesterone and schedule a day for the transfer based on what day the embryo was frozen (or your ERA results). Also know that appearance is more important than thickness. If you have a 6.5 mm thickness but it's trilaminar, you're going to be given the green light.

Natural Cycle

With a natural cycle, you don't use medication to suppress your ovulation cycle. While this can be a big pro for some infertility warriors, know that it also means more monitoring by your doctor. Your doctor isn't controlling when ovulation happens, so they will need to monitor the progression of your cycle and catch the moment when it's time to do the transfer. If you do not ovulate on your own, natural cycles aren't an option for you.

Sometimes your doctor will use an hCG trigger to stimulate the natural LH surge that causes ovulation on the day of your transfer to ensure ovulation. About 10 percent of women who attempt a natural cycle ovulate early. You might also be prescribed progesterone supplementation to help support your uterine lining post ovulation, especially if you have a known luteal phase defect.

Risks of FETs

There are significantly fewer risks with FETs. Since the ovaries are not being stimulated, there's very little risk of OHSS. Also, all the risks associated with the retrieval process aren't a consideration. However, there are still some risks involved:

- Multiple pregnancies if more than one embryo is transferred

- Embryos not surviving the thawing process (rare, but possible)

- Ectopic pregnancy

- Infection

- Side effects of the medications used in preparation for the FET

COPING AND GETTING SUPPORT

IVF and FET cycles are overwhelming because there are a lot of moving parts, your hormone levels are out of whack, and you're dealing with all the general pressures of trying to get pregnant. Take advantage of any sources of support you have during your cycles.

Also know that one of the biggest struggles with IVF is making time for all the appointments and medications. You might need to miss work, which means having a conversation with your boss about what's going on (see chapter 21). While you don't need to reveal everything about your infertility journey, you might be surprised by how supportive and understanding colleagues and employers can be. It can also help to talk to your friends and family about what's going on in your life. If they know when you have appointments and procedures, they can find ways to support you on those stressful days. Of course, if you don't want to be bombarded by phone calls or texts, it's perfectly fine to set those

boundaries as well. As always, it's best to be open and honest about what you need from others.

"Like many people, I never thought I would do IVF. It seemed too expensive, too much of a medical intervention, and too intimidating," explains Carynne from North Carolina. "But when the time came, it felt like the right decision and I haven't regretted it. It was not easy, but it also wasn't as hard as I expected. I was very open with my family and friends about what we were going through and asked for their love and support, which really helped give me strength to get through IVF. And being in touch with others who had done IVF or were in cycle with me was extremely encouraging as well."

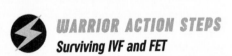

WARRIOR ACTION STEPS
Surviving IVF and FET

Coping with IVF and FET cycles requires a game plan. Much like you'll have a protocol for your course of treatment, you should map out how you're going to deal with the stress and emotions of the cycles. And be prepared to make changes. To get emotionally ready for IVF and FET, be sure to:

- **Have an organization system in place.**
These treatments are informational juggling acts. You'll need to remember when your appointments are, what the doctors say, when and how to take

medications, and more. Have a system that works for you to keep everything organized and minimize stress during the cycle.

• **Tune in to your body.** Given the different medications you might take during the cycle, you're going to physically feel different. But not all of these changes will be caused by the medication. Stress can manifest as tense shoulders or a queasy stomach, so when you're feeling these different sensations, consider whether they are caused by your emotional state. They may be telling you that it's time to get more support from the loved ones in your life.

• **Schedule self-care.** Self-care is always an important part of the infertility journey, but because of the hectic nature of an IVF or FET cycle, it can easily fall to the wayside. Make time in your schedule—at least 30 minutes each day—to do activities that you enjoy and that will help you relax.

Don't listen to anyone who uses the phrase "don't give up" on this journey. It is *not* giving up if you decide to cease pursuing fertility treatments or other paths to parenthood. But only *you* know when you're ready to stop.

Lindsay from Washington says her dad gave her some great advice: Do everything she felt comfortable trying so she wouldn't look back with regrets. "None of us was sure if I would ever be successful with my own eggs, but my dad encouraged me to keep going and seek the best treatment I could so that I would never wonder whether things would have been different if I had tried something else. I felt at peace following this path because I knew that if it didn't work out, I had truly exhausted all possible options."

WARRIOR WISDOM
Opening Up to the Possibilities

"When I first started on this journey, I thought there's no way we're ever going to do IVF. Out of the question. We can't afford it. I'm never going to be able to give myself injections, never going to be able to manage the stress of that. But we did do it. Keep your mind and your heart open to possibilities. Try not to take anything off the table."— Kara, North Dakota

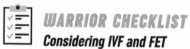

WARRIOR CHECKLIST
Considering IVF and FET

❑ Understand the basic process of both IVF and FET cycles, while knowing your individual experience might be different.

❑ Know who is and isn't a good candidate for each form of treatment, as well as the various priming and stimming protocols.

❑ Have prepared questions for your doctor to ensure you understand the plan and can decide whether it's right for you.

❑ Be aware of how stress can flare up during IVF and FET cycles and have a plan to cope with these emotions.

Add more items to your Warrior Checklist or jot down any notes here:

_____

_____

_____

_____

Preparing for Fertility Treatments

CHAPTER 8

I DIDN'T DO MUCH TO PREPARE for my two IUI-converted-into-timed-intercourse cycles, nor for my first fresh or first two frozen embryo transfers. I simply went along with whatever my reproductive endocrinologist instructed.

After two failed frozen transfers, I was ready for a change.

Leading up to my third frozen embryo transfer, I started weekly acupuncture appointments, including a session immediately before and after my transfer. That cycle, I became pregnant. Although it ended in an early miscarriage, I couldn't help but think that the addition of acupuncture might have helped with the initial implantation (we didn't test this embryo, so it's possible it was genetically abnormal). I continued acupuncture through my fourth frozen transfer and second and third fresh transfers. If nothing else, it relaxed me, and I often fell asleep during sessions.

Next, I decided to try visualization. I was inspired by my interview with Joanne Verkuilen, founder of Circle + Bloom in Andover, Massachusetts, who specializes in guided fertility meditation programs. Every night as I fell asleep, I visualized my child being born. At first the image was fuzzy and I couldn't focus on it for too long because it felt like an improbable, if not impossible, eventuality. However, over time, I was able to hear the music playing, see who was in the room, and perceive the exact moment my child was born. Of course, I knew the actual delivery would be nothing like what I envisioned, but having this positive image in my head—especially at bedtime—noticeably impacted my hopefulness.

Also, at least twice a day, I listened to Circle + Bloom's IVF mindfulness program. I'd never meditated before, so having a guided program specific to my IVF cycle was extremely helpful. Otherwise, I never would have known where to start!

I went into both my third retrieval and seventh transfer confident that everything would work out in the end, even if it took several more transfers. I'd *never* felt that before—not even during my first transfer. I *finally* felt some modicum of control over the outcome.

While no amount of preparation—physical or mental—can fully protect you from unexpected or unwelcome outcomes, it does allow you to start the journey from a place of strength and confidence.

What You Need to Know About Fertilization

Fertilization and implantation are *complicated*. Because we see others who (seemingly) get pregnant easily, we forget there are countless factors that must go right for pregnancy to occur. And when the stars don't align month after month, it's incredibly draining.

To prepare your body for success and to make the best decisions about which fertility treatment to pursue, if any, it's important to understand how fertilization is *supposed* to happen.

In order to fertilize an egg, sperm must have:

• **A favorable environment that will not destroy sperm.** Since the vagina is naturally acidic, after ejaculation, semen must form a protective gel that liquifies within 20 to 30 minutes, freeing the sperm to begin their journey toward the egg.

• **The ability to swim through the vagina and cervix.** Cervical mucus guards the entrance to the uterus, supporting sperm survival but allowing only the most motile to pass through.

• **The ability to penetrate the egg.** The first sperm reach the fallopian tubes within mere minutes of ejaculation, but those early arrivers are the least likely to fertilize the egg because slower sperm conserve energy and can better fight off competitors. Sperm that reach this point *may* survive for up to 5 days, but slower sperm tend to live on the longer end of the spectrum—and the egg is capable of being fertilized for only 12 to 24 hours.

As discussed in chapter 6, a woman's cervical mucus should become more sperm-friendly as she gets closer to ovulating. However, some women, like me, never produce "high-fertility" mucus. This can be a sign of a hormonal imbalance and, as you might imagine, greatly reduces the likelihood of fertilization.

Also, as Dr. John Rapisarda, a reproductive endocrinologist at Fertility Centers of Illinois in Chicago, explains, "the reality is that there is a 'fertile window' when the egg is present and capable of being fertilized. Having unprotected sex well before this fertile period or after this window is very unlikely to result in pregnancy."

Patients often falsely assume that it takes only one good sperm to fertilize an egg, says Dr. Lora Shahine, a board-certified reproductive endocrinologist at Pacific NW Fertility in Seattle. "Only one sperm gets into the egg for fertilization, but it takes millions to get to the egg in the fallopian tube and millions more to help break through the [egg's protective shell]. Some [people] have such low sperm count that they are not good candidates for IUI and need to go straight to IVF with Intracytoplasmic sperm injection (ICSI) in which one sperm can be placed into an egg with the help of the embryologist."

You've likely heard of some tricks that supposedly improve fertility, like certain sexual positions, foods, or activities that "guarantee" pregnancy. Perhaps you've even tried a few—I know I did! Here's the truth: although there are ways to *improve* your chances of success, this journey comes with no guarantees.

Fertilization

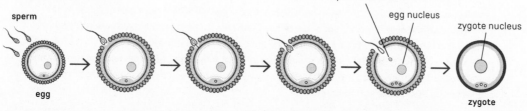

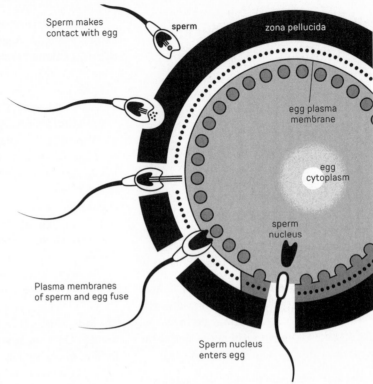

Detail of a single sperm fertilizing an egg

Dr. Naveed Khan, a board-certified reproductive endocrinologist with Shady Grove Fertility in Leesburg, Virginia, says, "There is little that one can do to boost this step in the process of trying to get pregnant, as long as the timing is correct. There are no 'extra fertile' positions, such as lying on your back or elevating one's hips. Use of any specific lubricants does not enhance fertilization, nor does eating any specific food."

BUSTED

Myth: Eating pineapples improves implantation.

There is a long-held belief throughout the infertility community that consuming pineapple—particularly the core—aids with embryo implantation. But in reality, pineapple core contains bromelain, a digestive enzyme that acts as a blood thinner. High levels of bromelain—or any blood thinner—may cause uterine contractions, thus *preventing* implantation.

Dr. Kat Lin, a board-certified reproductive endocrinologist with Sound Fertility Care in Seattle, sets the record straight, saying, "There are various 'old wives' tales' about foods to eat, such as pineapple core, or other substances/supplements to increase the likelihood that an embryo will implant. There is no scientific evidence supporting this advice."

Yes, there are many natural foods and supplements that may improve sperm and egg *health* and therefore increase the odds of implantation. But always do your research and make sure the claims are backed up by *credible scientific research*.

Getting Sperm Ready for Fertilization

A male partner can take certain actions to improve the likelihood of his sperm fertilizing an egg, regardless of the fertility treatment he and his partner pursue. And little changes can go a long way.

"The life span of sperm is 60 to 70 days, so changes made even 8 to 10 weeks prior to conception can improve sperm health," explains Meredith Nathan, a board-certified massage therapist at Pulling Down the Moon in Highland Park, Illinois. "Gentle methods of detoxification and improving lymphatic flow, as well as reproductive 'blood building' (increasing reproductive blood flow) can improve sperm quality, quantity, and/or motility."

Check Over-the-Counter and Prescription Medications

Some medications—such as calcium channel blockers, cimetidine (for heartburn relief), antibiotics, and steroids (like prednisone and cortisone)—reduce sperm count and motility. If you are taking any of these medications and have concerns about your male-factor infertility, you should contact both the prescribing doctor and a reproductive endocrinologist (or reproductive urologist, if you see one) to determine next steps.

Eat More Antioxidants

A 2016 study published in the *International Journal of Reproductive BioMedicine* found that certain antioxidants improved overall sperm health, especially for people with male factor infertility. The study found the following to be particularly effective:

- **Vitamin C.** High levels are found in oranges, strawberries, spinach, and peppers.

- **Vitamin E.** High levels are found in trout, olive oil, sunflower seeds, and almonds.

- **CoQ10.** Broccoli, oysters, liver, and cabbage all have CoQ10, but only in low doses, so CoQ10 supplements are often recommended.

Change Up Your Sex Life

A 2017 study published in *JBRA Assisted Reproduction* found that longer periods of abstinence improve sperm *concentration* but significantly decrease *motility* and *vitality*. Periods of abstinence also led to a higher percentage of DNA fragmentation and mitochondrial damage.

Although the World Health Organization (WHO) officially recommends 2 to 7 days of ejaculation abstinence before ovulation, recent studies conclude that frequent ejaculation—every day or two—is best for conception.

Take Prenatal Vitamins

Research has found low folic acid levels lead to sperm DNA damage and low sperm count and concentration. And vitamin D has been linked to increased sperm motility. Both nutrients can be found in men's prenatal vitamins. As always, consult your doctor before taking any supplements.

WARRIOR TIPS
Lifestyle Changes

If you'll recall from chapter 1, there are relatively easy steps you can take to optimize sperm health:

- Quit smoking and recreational drugs.

- Avoid prolonged exposure to toxins.

- Avoid prolonged exposure of the testicles to heat.

- Moderate your caffeine and alcohol intake.

- Maintain a normal BMI (18.5 to 24.9).

- Eat a balanced diet with plenty of antioxidant-rich foods.

- Get enough sleep.

- Don't overexercise.

Journey of an Egg

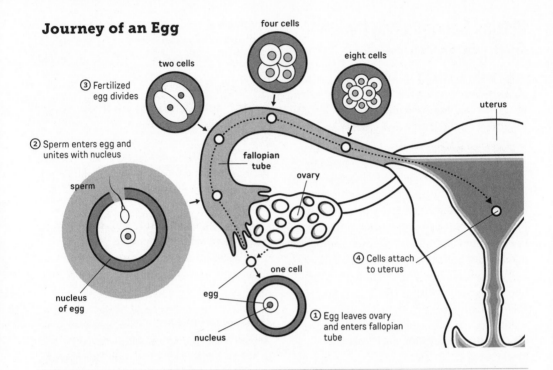

four cells

two cells

eight cells

③ Fertilized
egg divides

uterus

② Sperm enters egg and
unites with nucleus

fallopian
tube

ovary

sperm

④ Cells attach
to uterus

nucleus
of egg

one cell

egg

① Egg leaves ovary
and enters fallopian
tube

nucleus

What You Need to Know About Implantation

Fertilization of an egg does not guarantee pregnancy. Blastocysts may fail to implant; they may implant but fail to grow; or they may implant and grow but stop developing, resulting in a chemical pregnancy (see chapter 17) or miscarriage.

Reproductive endocrinologist Dr. Allison K. Rodgers with Fertility Centers of Illinois in Chicago explains it this way: "[The endometrium] exposes a Velcro-like substance we call pinopodes. The embryo has to stick to these pinopodes, and that window of implantation is often very short. So, if an embryo comes by too early or too late, it's not going to be able to implant. Or if the machinery of the egg is not normal, it's not going be able to implant."

If it's going to happen, implantation typically occurs between 6 and 9 days after ovulation. Successful implantation tells your body to produce human chorionic gonadotropin (hCG), which can be detected in your blood 3 or 4 days later and through a home pregnancy test (HPT) potentially 6 or 7 days later. This is the point when pregnancy officially begins.

Implantation Hinderances

Dr. Michael Grossman, a board-certified reproductive endocrinologist with CNY Fertility in Albany, New York, warns, "Making an embryo doesn't mean you made a baby. There are many steps left before a fertilized egg becomes a live-born child, and trouble can strike anywhere along the way."

Several factors impact whether a blastocyst implants. They can be broken down into two main categories: problems with the embryo and problems with the uterus.

Problems with the Embryo

There can be genetic issues with the embryo, which we discussed in chapters 3 and 4. Even

WARRIOR ACTION STEPS
Surviving the TWW

After you ovulate during a timed intercourse cycle, are inseminated during an IUI cycle, or complete an embryo transfer, there's the dreaded "two-week wait" (TWW) before you can take a pregnancy test. The amount of time you have to wait depends on the type of cycle, but those days may drag on—and your emotions might fluctuate from hope to worry to anger and everything in between. Make the time a little easier with the following:

• **Don't over-research.** You're going to be looking for signs that you're pregnant, and any new or different sensation will seem like it could be confirmation that the cycle was a success—or not. Do not go down the rabbit hole of googling every possible symptom. In fact, ignore any potential symptoms—or lack thereof—altogether, if possible.

• **Avoid social media.** Facebook, Instagram, and TikTok are full of triggering photos of people and their children. If your emotions are heightened during the TWW, don't torture yourself with scrolling.

• **Plan distractions.** Your entire life should not be about infertility, and the TWW is the perfect time to focus on your other interests and passions. Plan activities that excite you so your mind has something to look forward to beside the pregnancy test results.

• **Name your feelings.** Imagine you feel a pain in your hand. At first you don't know what's wrong or why it hurts, but when you examine your hand, you might see you have a paper cut or were stung by a bee. Identifying the pain allows you to treat it effectively. The same is true of your emotions—examining and identifying them will help you work through them.

• **Schedule obsession time.** Let's be real, you're going to have thoughts about what's going on with your body. There's no point in trying to suppress them all. However, you can limit when and how much time you spend with these thoughts. Set boundaries for yourself and hold yourself accountable. For example, you might give yourself 15 minutes at 7 p.m. each night—or, even better, 15 minutes only on Sundays at 7 p.m. Set a timer, and when that timer goes off, obsession time is over.

---

with genetically normal embryos, one wrong gene expression can prohibit implantation.

There could also be a metabolic issue—a complicated topic that has fascinated researchers for decades. Some genetics companies test mitochondrial DNA because embryos go through a tremendous growth process. This growth is accomplished by the mitochondria (a cell's energy factory) producing adenosine triphosphate (ATP—an energy-rich molecule). So, if there are issues with mitochondria or how mitochondrial DNA is expressed, it can keep an embryo from implanting.

The ability of the embryo to divide into more cells can also be impeded by being frozen and thawed multiple times. Dr. Rodgers says that sometimes an embryo, after being frozen and then thawed, can have normal preimplantation genetic testing (PGT) results

but metabolically can't continue to develop for reasons scientists don't yet understand.

Problems with the Uterus

When it comes to your uterine lining, there are many possible issues, including:

Polyps. Uterine polyps are growths that attach to the inner wall of your uterus and extend further into your uterus, sometimes descending into your vagina. They range in size from a few millimeters to several centimeters. Typically, although not always, they are benign (noncancerous). When patients have trouble conceiving, the American Association of Gynecologic Laparoscopists (AAGL) recommends removing any uterine polyps.

Fibroids. These are extremely common and almost always benign growths. Some studies suggest that fibroids may impact uterine receptivity, particularly when infertility is otherwise unexplained. There are five main types: *Intramural fibroids* are the most common, and they grow within the muscular wall of the uterus. *Subserosal fibroids* grow on the outer surface of the uterus—or outside of it altogether. *Submucosal fibroids* grow beneath the uterine lining and can crowd your uterus. *Pedunculated fibroids* grow on small stalks either inside or outside your uterus. *Intracavitary fibroids* grow within the uterine cavity.

Adhesions. Adhesions are scar tissue, and in the uterus, they may involve the layers of your endometrial lining, the smooth muscle of your uterus (myometrium), or the connective tissue within your uterus. These are typically the result of a physical trauma or procedure, such as a D&C performed after a miscarriage. *Endometrial adhesions* look very similar to your regular lining. A *myofibrous adhesion*—the most common type—looks like a thin layer over your lining. *Connective tissue adhesions* prevent uterine lining development and are distinct enough to easily recognize. As is the case for polyps, in patients who have difficulty conceiving, the AAGL and European Society for Gynaecological Endoscopy (ESGE) recommend treating any adhesions, citing multiple studies showing improved pregnancy rates.

Endometrial lining thickness. What thickness is best for the endometrial lining is somewhat up for debate. Most studies report that a lining less than or equal to 7 mm is too thin, whereas some say a measurement as low as 6 mm is acceptable. Dr. Khan and many other fertility specialists, including my own, cite 8 mm as the cutoff. Regardless, there is widespread consensus that your uterine lining should be trilaminar in appearance, which means that on an ultrasound, you can see that it has three distinct layers. In other words, the structure or

appearance of your lining is more important than its thickness.

Uterine receptivity. There is a very short period of time—between 12 and 24 hours, according to Dr. Rodgers—during which your uterus is receptive to implantation. Receptivity is largely controlled by hormones—estrogen and progesterone—so if either one is off even slightly, your embryo could miss its window. (If you plan to undergo IVF, there is now a test for receptivity; see page 133.)

Adhesion molecules. The endocrine system increases adhesion-promoting molecules and decreases adhesion-inhibitory molecules to ready the uterine lining for implantation. Implantation is a complex process that requires a lot of factors to be just right—down to the molecular level. Although the importance of these molecules is known, this is an ongoing area of study because exactly how they work and how they might be manipulated to improve implantation is yet unknown.

Inflammation. Inflammation can arise from conditions like endometriosis and chronic endometritis, a painful condition in which endometrial cells grow outside the uterus, often on your ovaries, fallopian tubes, and other pelvic areas. Researchers continue to debate the impact of endometriosis on implantation, with some studies showing no decrease in implantation rates and others showing a significant decrease. Chronic endometritis is an infection that causes uterine inflammation, resulting in pregnancy loss and implantation failure. Treating it, which is typically as simple as a course of antibiotics, has been shown to improve implantation, pregnancy, and live birth rates, although more studies are needed.

Hydrosalpinx. This is an abnormal distension of one or both fallopian tubes with fluid, which often spills into the uterine cavity. Some research has shown that hydrosalpinges reduce implantation rates, likely by suppressing the development of substances important to implantation or by the fluid flushing the embryo out of the uterus. One study found that these same receptivity substances return to normal levels in two-thirds of patients whose hydrosalpinges are treated by removing the affected tube(s).

Müllerian anomalies. Müllerian anomalies occur when the Müllerian ducts develop abnormally. These are congenital disorders, which means they form in utero and are present at birth. *Mayer-Rokitansky-Küster-Hauser syndrome* (MRKH) is a Müllerian anomaly in which the Müllerian ducts do not develop, resulting in a missing uterus and an underdeveloped vagina. *Uterine duplication* is an anomaly in which two uterine cavities develop; in some cases only one of these cavities has a cervix and vagina, but in other cases both cavities have them. With a *bicornuate uterus*, the uterus appears to be heart-shaped and has two conjoined cavities. A *septate uterus* occurs when a membrane (septum) divides the uterine cavity into two parts. A *unicornuate uterus* describes a uterine cavity that is smaller than normal; the cavity may have a "rudimentary horn," or incomplete attachment of one Fallopian tube, which renders the tube dysfunctional. An *arcuate uterus* occurs when the top of the uterine cavity is concave rather than straight. Of the Müllerian anomalies, only a septate uterus can be surgically corrected. However, you still have fertility treatment options—such as IVF with surrogacy for MRKH—that you should discuss with your doctor.

BUSTED ══════════════════════════

Myth: I only need to worry about the health of my reproductive organs.

Our bodies are complex. Countless factors play into fertility—many you wouldn't even think about. Various studies have found links between male factor infertilty, semen quality, and oral health.

"If you have inflammation in your mouth, that can cause fertility problems," says Rebecca Fett, author of *It Starts with the Egg*. "So just keep that in mind, get your dental checkups, and take care of your teeth."

I know it's hard when you're going through fertility treatments, but remember to take care of *all* aspects of your health. Don't put off non-fertility-related checkups, and always take the time to care for your mental health.

"It can boil down to being your healthiest and practicing self-care. We all know what we need to do—eat well, exercise in moderation, get sleep, and use stress reduction techniques," says Dr. Shahine.

Getting Your Body Ready for Implantation

There are a lot of things you can do to potentially improve your egg and uterine health. These include activities from holistic self-care to quitting your worst habits. Talk to your doctor about the best plan for you.

After beginning work with a reproductive endocrinologist, Brianna from Pennsylvania decided to make small lifestyle changes to promote fertility. "I limited my coffee intake to one cup in the morning, I kept up with my already established workout routine (strength training three times weekly), and I focused on a restful night's sleep. Just recently, after 6 months of treatment with my RE, I have implemented dietary changes to promote fertility and overall health. My husband and I started a partial Mediterranean diet for lunches and dinners."

Acupuncture

While research is divided about whether acupuncture helps with live birth rates following fertility treatments like IVF, there is evidence that acupuncture leads to higher pregnancy rates, especially when the treatment plan is customized to the patient.

Acupuncture is an ancient Chinese medicine practice, which centers on the idea that our bodies contain energy channels, and when our energy (chi) is unable to flow freely through the channels, health problems arise. Acupuncturists place needles on pressure points to clear the channels. And evidence shows that acupuncture can be used to increase blood flow to reproductive organs to improve their function.

Research also shows that, at the very least, acupuncture helps infertility warriors deal with the stress of treatments. As Stephanie Gianarelli, clinic director of Acupuncture Northwest & Associates in Seattle, reminds us, "Infertility is inherently stressful and acupuncture is very relaxing." I agree!

Christine Davis, a licensed acupuncturist at Pulling Down the Moon in Highland Park, Illinois, recommends one or two treatments a week for 3 months before trying to conceive. "This can be helpful to balance the body, regulate the menstrual cycle, reduce stress, and can help with many other physical, mental, and emotional concerns. It's not just about becoming pregnant, but creating balance and wellness wherein the body can sustain a healthy pregnancy and a healthy mama."

Stephanie from Kansas credits a holistic approach for her spontaneous pregnancy with her daughter after years of infertility and loss. "I'm incredibly, incredibly grateful for my acupuncturist, who was able to pinpoint what was going on and help me combat that with nutrition and acupuncture," she explains.

To find an acupuncturist near you who specializes in fertility treatments, check with the American Board of Oriental Reproductive Medicine (aborm.org).

Exercise

Get moving with strength training and aerobics. Aim to exercise for at least 150 minutes each week, ideally for 30 minutes a day for 5 days. Fertility yoga and walking are two great ways to improve circulation and increase the strength and flexibility of the muscles surrounding your uterus, but find exercises that keep you interested and motivated to continue. Don't forget to drink plenty of water each day—at least half of your body weight in ounces—especially once you step up your workout routine.

As Dr. Rodgers reminds us, maintaining a normal weight is essential to getting pregnant. "Being too heavy or too thin can decrease your chances of success," she explains. "The correct amount of fat cells are vital to keep the pituitary gland actively instructing the ovary to produce eggs. Fat cells also produce hormones, mainly estrogens that can change the chances of success if there are too many or too few."

After adopting their son Jackson, Michelle and her husband, Michael, from California wanted a second child. Michelle, who had polycystic ovary syndrome (PCOS), didn't ovulate or get a period, so she knew trying on their own would be difficult at best. But she had a plan: She forced herself to slow down—no more working out twice a day.

"I still ate healthy and incorporated lots of walking—and more high-intensity workouts when I could. A few months later, I got my period on my own for the first time since I was 21. I continued focusing less on my intense workouts and more on strength training. I cut down cardio from 6 days a week to maybe 3 days," she explains.

BUSTED

Myth: Lifestyle changes will overcome my infertility.

It is incredibly important to be healthy during your infertility journey, but getting in shape and eating right will not "cure" infertility. There are many other factors, some of which will be out of your control.

"A common misconception is that one's habits play a major role in whether implantation happens or not," says Dr. Rapisarda. "While lifestyle and environmental factors are important to optimize one's fertility, the most important factors are the 'health' or quality of the embryo and the uterine environment."

Taking care of your health will help you feel better during your treatments and give you strength during tough times. And you want to be in good shape when you do become a parent. But remember that lifestyle changes are just one piece of the puzzle.

Her menstrual cycles became shorter over time, until they were eventually 35 days. Michelle and Michael decided it was time to track her ovulation and try on their own to see what happened. The first cycle was unsuccessful, which didn't surprise them. But they tried again her next cycle. Michelle says, "The second month came, and I tracked my ovulation again. When my period was a few days late, I didn't think anything of it. Now, I am 18 weeks pregnant with my little boy!"

Fertility Massage

Fertility massage may increase blood flow to the ovaries, fallopian tubes, and uterus—and simultaneously helps old blood and tissue that was not expelled during a prior menstrual period leave the uterus. You can find a professional who specializes in fertility massage in your area, or you can learn to do it yourself—there are many tutorials available online.

Food and Supplements

First things first, some words of caution:

• *Never* take a supplement or make a major change to your diet without consulting with your doctor first. If you are working with more than one doctor, make sure they all know what supplements you're taking. Some supplements, even natural ones, can interact poorly with certain medications or exacerbate their effects.

• Quality counts, so do your homework and look for high-quality brands that contain pure, contaminant-free ingredients.

• Most supplements should be discontinued once pregnancy is confirmed, and some should be taken only through ovulation. The importance of close coordination with your doctor cannot be overstated.

• It's possible to oversupplement, so don't go crazy.

Now that the serious business is out of the way, let's go over some vitamins and hormones to discuss with your doctor. In some cases, you can increase your levels with slight diet changes, but in other cases, you might need to take a supplement.

Calcium. Calcium is a bone-building nutrient we consume through food, but if you're not getting enough through your food, it might be beneficial to supplement. Calcium is also believed to help sperm reach your egg and aid embryo growth. The typical recommended dose is 1,000 mg per day. Foods high in calcium include milk, yogurt, figs, spinach, and canned salmon.

Coenzyme Q10 (CoQ10). CoQ10 is a nutrient that naturally occurs in our bodies, acting as an antioxidant to protect cells—including egg cells—from damage. As we age, CoQ10 levels decrease, so supplementation may help. It comes in two forms: ubiquinol (125 mg per day) and ubiquinone (600 mg per day). Most doctors recommend ubiquinol because your body absorbs it better.

DHEA (dehydroepiandrosterone). DHEA is a hormone produced by your adrenal glands. When taken as a supplement, it impacts your testosterone and estrogen levels, potentially helping you produce more and better-quality eggs. However, DHEA should *not* be taken by people with high testosterone or anti-Müllerian hormone (AMH) levels because it will only increase those values. It is typically taken in three 25 mg doses throughout the day and should not be taken for more than 3 consecutive months. Be sure to get your DHEA-S levels tested before starting a supplement to ensure you don't already have a naturally high level for some other reason.

L-arginine. This amino acid increases blood flow. Recall from chapter 1 that low oxygen levels may result in immature eggs that don't fertilize, implant, or develop properly. However, L-arginine levels are typically low only if your protein intake is low. So if you are a vegetarian or vegan, consider taking 1 to 2 g as a supplement per day. Otherwise, you should be covered by diet alone. Foods high in L-arginine include turkey, chicken, peanuts, and chickpeas.

L-carnitine. This amino acid transports fatty acids into your cells to produce energy. Acetyl L-carnitine, in particular, has been shown to improve egg health. The recommended dose is 1 to 3 g per day. Foods high in L-carnitine are milk, cheese, chicken, and beef.

Magnesium. This mineral helps your body absorb calcium and regulates your pituitary gland. As you already know, the pituitary gland regulates hormones vital to healthy ovulation. Magnesium can also stabilize glucose levels, which is particularly important for people with PCOS and diabetes. The recommended dose is 320 mg per day. Foods high in magnesium include squash and pumpkin seeds, dark chocolate, mackerel, and raw spinach.

Melatonin. This hormone is produced by the pineal gland and regulates your sleep-wake cycles. It also acts as an antioxidant, and studies have shown it can improve egg and overall embryo quality. The recommended dose is 3 mg per day, taken 30 to 60 minutes before bed. Because you don't want your body to stop producing its own melatonin, don't use it as a supplement for long periods of time—between the start of your period and ovulation will do just fine. Don't take melatonin if you are being treated for a thyroid condition. Melatonin supplements make thyroid medications less effective, which negatively impacts ovulation and overall health.

Ovasitol. Ovasitol is a brand-name supplement containing a combination of the vitamin B–like nutrients myo-inositol (MI) and d-chiro-inositol (DCI). Current research shows the combination of MI and DCI to be most effective for the management of PCOS symptoms, improving how your body uses insulin and regulating your menstrual cycles and ovarian function. Each dose, taken twice per day, contains 2,000 mg of MI and 50 mg of DCI.

Vitamin B$_6$. Vitamin B$_6$ functions as an antioxidant and may regulate estrogen and progesterone levels, as well as improve egg quality. The typical dose is 10 mg per day, or 50 mg per day for a very short period of time. It's possible to take too much, so do not exceed 100 mg per day. Foods high in vitamin B$_6$ include sunflower seeds, pistachios, and tuna.

Vitamin C. Vitamin C functions as an antioxidant and improves blood flow. It may have a particularly positive effect on people with a luteal phase defect. The recommended dose is 500 mg per day, but because it increases heartburn, be sure not to take it right before bed. Additionally, do not take more than 1,000 mg per day because it can make your cervical mucus unfriendly to sperm. Foods high in vitamin C are oranges, strawberries, spinach, and peppers.

Vitamin D$_3$. Vitamin D$_3$, also known as the "sunshine vitamin," is produced in the skin. Although there is not a consensus about vitamin D's impact on fertility, some studies have found that people with blood levels of 30 ng/mL or higher had better pregnancy rates. If your vitamin D level is less than 24 ng/mL, the recommended dose is 4,000 IU per day. If your vitamin D level is 24 to 30 ng/mL, the recommended dose is 2,000 IU per day.

Zinc. Zinc promotes healthy ovulation by regulating your pituitary gland. The recommended dose is 15 to 25 mg per day, or 30 mg per day for vegetarians or vegans. Do not take more than 40 mg per day because it could negatively impact your immune system. Foods high in zinc include oysters, whole grains, lean beef, and beans.

Some supplements may help with fertility but are not yet routinely recommended because more research is needed. However, they are worth knowing about so you can discuss them with your doctor.

N-acetyl-cysteine (NAC). NAC acts as an antioxidant and may help prevent DNA damage in your eggs and help with ovulatory disorders like PCOS. However, more research is needed to explore its uses and effects. The recommended dose is 600 mg per day.

Pycnogenol. Pycnogenol, a compound derived from pine tree bark, acts as an antioxidant. It *may* be most beneficial for people with endometriosis or of advanced reproductive age, but it has not been extensively studied. The recommended dose is 25 to 60 mg twice a day. Consider increasing your natural antioxidant intake instead. Foods high in antioxidants are pomegranate, blueberries, green tea (though drink no more than 1 cup per day), and dark leafy vegetables.

Vitamin E. Vitamin E is a fat-soluble antioxidant that increases blood flow and *may*

WARRIOR TIPS
Making Dietary Changes

Aside from choosing to eat real, vitamin-rich foods, many infertility warriors decide to adopt a completely new diet. Research shows that certain diets, like the Mediterranean diet and ketogenic diet can improve the odds of success. (A keto diet is also particularly effective for people with PCOS.)

The Mediterranean diet is a low-sodium, high-flavor diet consisting mostly of vegetables, fruits, fish, and whole grains, with olive oil being the primary source of fat. The keto diet is a low-carb, moderate-protein, high-fat diet where each day you eat 1.5 grams of protein for each kilogram of your ideal body weight and keep your daily carbohydrate intake less than 50 to 75 grams.

improve egg health. However, more studies are needed. The recommended dose is 200 IU per day. Foods high in vitamin E include trout, olive oil, sunflower seeds, and almonds.

Lifestyle changes are not a cure for infertility, but they can help overcome some challenges that hinder fertility, such as abnormal BMI and overexercising. One option for customizing your diet to your unique body is purchasing a food sensitivity test from Everlywell, which analyzes which foods cause you inflammation and to what degree.

Brianna reminds her fellow warriors not to be overly restrictive with their lifestyle choices. "If you enjoy a glass of wine, have it! If you love to lay around on a Sunday afternoon instead of running on the treadmill, go for it! [You] have to remain happy during this time. You have to have a fulfilling life in between the wait."

Letting Go of Expectations

Humans are reward-seeking beings. Whenever things go well, we get a hit of dopamine that makes us feel great and want to repeat that experience. Subconsciously, we set expectations—often unrealistically high ones—because it'll feel *so good* if we meet that goal. But with infertility, when our expectations *repeatedly* aren't met, the opposite happens—we have a surge of hormones that makes us feel miserable.

Dr. Maria T. Rothenburger, a psychotherapist who specializes in infertility at Miracles Happen Fertility Center in Salem, Oregon, says the trick is to modify how you set your expectations. Find a way to keep working toward your goal of becoming a parent without trying to dictate every step of the journey. "I like the analogy of floating on top of waves rather than feverishly paddling for the shore. Instead of thinking 'Gotta get to the shore! Gotta get to the shore!' it's saying 'OK, I'm

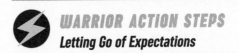

WARRIOR ACTION STEPS
Letting Go of Expectations

While it takes time to let go of the sense of control that expectations give you, Dr. Rothenburger suggests practicing the following steps:

• **Get quiet.** This might make you feel anxious at first, but finding a safe, quiet place will allow you to truly examine your expectations and whether you should hold on to them.

• **Ask yourself.** Does the expectation serve your end goal? Remember, you're trying to move forward toward the ultimate goal of becoming a parent. So, for example, what if you expect to become pregnant by a specific time—say Christmas—and you're not pregnant by then? How exactly does that expectation serve your end goal? (Hint: It doesn't!)

• **Consider alternative ways to achieve your goals.** If you can get comfortable with multiple paths to get to your ultimate goal, you will be more adaptable when one path doesn't go as planned.

• **Focus on a sense of ease.** Continue to check in with yourself to see if certain expectations are creating resistance. If they are stressing you out, it's time to let go.

going to start here and kind of ride that wave.' Eventually you make it there, but if you surrender, there's a lot more ease," she explains.

Know that sometimes letting go of expectations also means recognizing when the work you're doing to prepare for pregnancy actually creates more stress. Preparations are supposed to help you overcome obstacles, not create new ones.

Elyse from Minnesota realized that trying to prepare for treatments could be as overwhelming as the fertility treatments themselves. "I tried to relax a little more. I tried to be less regimented with acupuncture, yoga, and all these things that I was trying to fill my schedule with to make me feel more in control," she explains. "It actually just ended up stressing me out even more, so I tried to let go a little bit in the second round [of IVF] and not necessarily compare that round with the first one. The second round went way better."

Reaching Emotional Acceptance

Infertility warriors are notorious for avoiding their emotions. There's so much pressure to continually move forward that we push down our feelings so we can focus on taking the next steps. But make no mistake, your emotions will wait you out.

"Emotions just sort of sit and wait, and they fester," says Dr. Rothenburger. "They will look for a vulnerable moment, and then they will simply explode."

It's important to process and accept your feelings. This means being OK with experiencing some really negative emotions. The trick is finding *healthy* ways to move forward—not despite your feelings, but because of them. Dr. Rothenburger calls this gentle empowerment. "You begin treating yourself and others as you would your baby," she says. "It's very similar to your baby crying and you going over to her and picking her up and saying, 'I've got you. I've got this.' It's not like proclaiming, 'I'M GOING TO MAKE YOUR CRYING GO AWAY!'"

Taking this slightly different approach allows you to move from feeling emotions to processing them to accepting them and moving on.

You should consider waiting to start fertility treatments until you're in a good—or at least stable—place emotionally. These cycles are draining, and you cannot draw from emotional reserves that are already depleted. That's not to say all your thoughts have to be sunshine and rainbows, but know that you need to be prepared for additional strain.

Talking Through Possible Fertility Treatments

Once you feel ready, it's time to have a discussion with your partner (if you have one), support network, and doctor so you can weigh your fertility treatment options. Think of this as a way to consolidate and sift through all the details of your situation so you can get a customized course of treatment with which you feel comfortable.

This will be an ongoing process that won't happen in one sitting; you'll only end up frustrated and exhausted. If you can, break up the decision-making into smaller chunks. Continue to check in with yourself—and your partner, if you have one—about where you stand.

Before you meet with your reproductive endocrinologist, try to get clarity on the following questions:

- What fertility treatment(s) are you willing to do?

- What medication(s) are you willing to take?

- How much are you willing to spend?

If you can get comfortable with your answers to these questions (and if you can ensure that you and your partner, if you have one, are on the same page), you'll be in good shape for the treatment plan conversation with your doctor. This is also a good opportunity to deal with your emotions, rather than carrying them with you to the appointment.

After hearing the treatment plan, it's time for another conversation. The specifics of this discussion will vary depending on where you left things with your doctor—and whether you already agreed to move forward with treatment—but some questions to consider include:

- What are your worries and fears?

- What makes you feel hopeful?

- Do the chances of success seem promising?

- Does the treatment align with your beliefs and values?

- Can you honestly afford what's been suggested?

It's also important to discuss the risks and possible complications of the treatment plan. (You might want to do this in a separate sitting, depending on how long you've already been talking.) Have an honest conversation about what you would do if:

- You end up pregnant with multiples.

- The treatment ends in a miscarriage or pregnancy loss.

- The cycle fails or is canceled.

- There are unpleasant or dangerous side effects from the procedure or medication.

Discussing Fertility Treatments with Others

It's important to have friends and family you can turn to for support when you're preparing for treatments (for more on maintaining those relationships, see chapter 16). But for many infertility warriors, making treatment decisions and preparing for those procedures is the first time you'll lean on your newfound infertility community. These are the people who have been where you are and will hear you out without hesitation or judgment.

Still, it's not always easy to talk to new people about what you're considering or facing. Find your comfort zone, and ask your support system to meet you there. For instance, you might hear a fellow warrior share a story similar to yours in a support group. If you're not ready to talk to the group as a whole, ask if that warrior will meet you for coffee. You'll be surprised how open and welcoming most members of the infertility community are.

WARRIOR ACTION STEPS
Finding Your Allies Within the Infertility Community

Taking advantage of infertility resources and connections will make all the difference throughout your journey. But when you're still adjusting to your own identity as an infertility warrior, it can be hard to find ways to reach out to others. Here are some tips for establishing a support system in the infertility community:

- **Start small.** It takes time to establish trust with new people. And while many in the infertility community will step up to the plate, it's natural to want to start slow. You might not feel comfortable unloading everything you're dealing with at once, so maybe take small steps instead. Share one aspect of your journey, and take note of how it feels to get that off your chest.

- **Use "I feel" and "I need" statements.** In many cases, members of the infertility community will listen to you for hours on end. But they can still use some guidance about your current emotional needs. When you're having a conversation, focus your thoughts by saying statements like "Right now I'm feeling overwhelmed and I need advice" or "I feel scared and I need this treatment explained in more detail." These direct statements help others know how to better support you.

- **Pay it forward.** You're still learning and aren't an expert on all things infertility, but there are small ways you can start being a supportive member of the community. For instance, you might not know all the details of a complex IVF protocol, but you can still volunteer to make a meal for a fellow warrior going through treatment.

After realizing the physical impact stress and anxiety had on her body, Brianna decided to open up about her infertility journey. "I committed to weekly therapy, small gratitude practices, and being HONEST with friends and family about my feelings and struggles. I learned that holding things back only made me more isolated and upset, so I started voicing my thoughts and feelings in a healthy way to those close to me."

Discussing Fertility Treatments with Your Doctor

Unlike a fertility workup, this conversation will likely be a virtual meeting. (One less trip to the doctor's office!) Consider this your opportunity to define your relationship with your doctor (and the rest of the treatment team)—and vice versa. And according to Jody Madeira, author of *Taking Baby Steps* and professor at the Indiana University Maurer School of Law, your emotions can set the tone.

"If the patient is excessively emotionally needy, they might not get the information they need or ask the questions they should. If they are experiencing many negative emotions—such as anger or frustration, especially if they have switched providers several times—they are likely to be defensive and distrust their treatment team. If the patient is eager and optimistic, then she is likely to embark upon a productive partnership with her treatment team. The patient's emotional baseline—the 'norm' to which the patient returns—sets the groundwork for the relationship," Madeira says.

I know this is an emotional process. I've been "that patient" who's shown every spectrum of the emotional rainbow right there in the office. But if you go into this appointment knowing the treatment team's expectations, an understanding about how far you're willing to go in terms of treatments, and a clear plan for the conversation itself, you should be able

to keep in check the big emotions that might derail a productive conversation.

As for the conversation itself, if you didn't go over it during your initial consultation, make sure your doctor understands the family you want to build—i.e., the number of children you'd like to have. This is an important factor and may impact the entire treatment plan.

WARRIOR TIPS
Building a Good Relationship with Your Team

To promote a successful relationship with your treatment team, focus on the following:

- **Active listening.** Concentrating on, understanding, and responding to what is being said—being present in the conversation.

- **Active questioning.** Asking questions to elicit two-way dialogue and better understand what your doctor is saying.

- **Openness.** Being honest about what you're thinking and how you feel.

- **Cooperation.** Following the instructions you and your fertility treatment team developed together.

- **Trust.** Trusting your fertility treatment team to provide the best care after all the other actions above.

Some behaviors can hinder your relationship with your treatment team. To the best of your ability, try to avoid:

- **Defensiveness.** Negatively responding to a perceived personal criticism.

- **An unwillingness to listen.** Taking over the conversation with one-way dialogue.

- **Ignoring instructions.** Not following your fertility treatment team's instructions.

- **Anger directed toward a prior provider.** Proactively bringing up past negative experiences, especially using doctor and clinic names.

- **Distrust.** Not trusting your fertility treatment team to provide the best care.

Your doctor will likely drive the discussion from there. But, as always, come with questions—and hold your doctor accountable for answering them to your satisfaction. Recall from chapter 3 the treatment-related questions you might ask. If your doctor hasn't been able to answer them adequately before this, or if there's new information now, ask them again.

- What are my/our chances of conceiving without treatment?

- What type of treatment should I/we try first, and why?

- What does this treatment involve? Walk me/us through it step-by-step.

- What are your success rates with this treatment for patients like me/us? How do you define success?

- Are there any risks or side effects of your recommended treatment?

- How many cycles of this treatment should I/we go through before I/we try something else?

- What does this treatment cost? What if my/ our insurance doesn't cover certain aspects of this treatment? Do you offer financing plans?

- Do you truly believe you can help me/us build a family?

- Are there any other questions you think I/we should be asking?

⚡ Remember, you are a unique individual, and your doctor's answers should pertain to your situation. If your doctor speaks in generalizations or doesn't provide success rates for patients with similar conditions, you don't get all the information you need to make an informed decision.

"Some patients might not want to jump to the most sophisticated treatment and have a good chance of success with timed intercourse, while others might need to proceed directly to IVF because of advanced age or other diagnoses," says Madeira. "Patients should discuss any hesitations they have about particular options or inform their treatment teams of any constraints they think they have. For example, a couple might only be able to spend a certain amount of money. It's also important to clear up any areas of confusion before choosing an option."

Ultimately, whatever treatments are discussed, you should walk away feeling confident and informed. Do not walk out of the office until you have all information you need. Keep in mind that you don't need to make your decision by the end of this conversation if you're still unsure, but you shouldn't be left with questions.

"Before someone commits to expensive, invasive treatment, they need to know their realistic chances of success, the emotional and financial resources required, and review all options for moving forward," agrees Dr. Shahine.

Discussing Specific Fertility Treatment Protocols

Once you choose a course of treatment, it's imperative that you understand the protocol (medications, medication instructions, and timeline) beforehand. Most fertility treatments require medication, and there's little room for mistakes.

"It is important for the patient to understand the basics of why the protocol is designed in the way that it is so that she can help detect any errors in the administration of her medications," explains Dr. Lin.

Some medications require that you take them at the same time every day, but the exact time is up to you. Others require you take them at specific times as instructed by your doctor. Plan ahead and develop a system for keeping track of all the moving pieces.

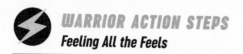

WARRIOR ACTION STEPS
Feeling All the Feels

There are going to be times before, during, and after fertility treatments when you feel terrible. Don't run from those emotions. Work toward acceptance with the following steps:

- **Pay attention to your physical response.** Often, before we realize we're emotional, we have a physical response. We have an ache in our gut or a tightness in our shoulders. Use your physical responses to stress as a reminder to stop and take a moment to accept and deal with your feelings.

- **Give yourself a safe place.** Often, we don't give ourselves permission to feel because we're not in a safe place. It's not "socially acceptable" to start bawling in the middle of the grocery store whenever you see a pregnant woman. But those emotions need to get out somehow. Find a place where you can be vulnerable and let everything out without judgment—including from yourself.

- **Find genuine positivity.** There's so much pressure to put on a happy mask during your infertility journey, but this is a form of denial, not acceptance. As you work through your feelings, look for smaller positive moments to celebrate. For example, if you're able to read a pregnancy announcement and don't feel guilty for your sadness, that's a positive sign. This shows you've made progress, and that deserves to be recognized!

WARRIOR WISDOM
Leaning on Your New Community

"I was lucky to have support on my journey, though community was the biggest factor for me. I met women at Pulling Down the Moon through their free patient education events and their yoga for fertility that have been with me every step of the way. We now have playdates with our rainbow babies years later!"—Michelle, Illinois

WARRIOR CHECKLIST
Preparing for Treatment

❑ Understand how fertilization works and how you can potentially improve the quality of your eggs and health of your uterus—or the health and quality of your sperm—and thus your chance of success.

❑ Recognize which physical and mental factors are in your control and which are not—and what actions to take.

❑ Learn how to discuss treatment options with your partner, allies, and doctor to make the best decision for your family.

Let's Talk Multiples

CHAPTER 9

"**O**UR GOAL IS TO GIVE YOU one healthy baby," my doctor said during our very brief conversation about transferring one versus two embryos.

Unfortunately, that sentence meant very different things to each of us. To him, it meant that we should transfer one embryo at a time. To me, it meant we should do whatever it took to ensure I became pregnant. But we never discussed it.

On transfer day, the doctor on call—not ours—asked how many embryos we wanted to transfer.

"Two. Definitely two," we told him. And that was that—he didn't object.

Looking back now, I am shocked at how little thought we'd given to such an important decision. But we'd just paid around $18,000 for the cycle and knew we couldn't afford another. We wanted the best chance at becoming pregnant, and to us, that meant transferring two embryos. Surely one—only one—would implant and this journey would all be over.

The transfer went smoothly and we headed home. The next several weeks were a blur. An ultrasound confirmed we were pregnant with twins—a possibility I thought would *never* happen. I began bleeding at around 5 weeks, heavily at times. I was told my uterus was expanding so rapidly that blood vessels were bursting. My heart rate and blood pressure continued to be all over the map, but I was told everything would resolve after I gave birth.

We "graduated" from our fertility clinic and began seeing a high-risk ob-gyn. At our 14-week appointment, I was told Baby A was too close to my cervix—resulting in a condition known as placenta previa—but given no information about what that meant, other than they would continue to monitor me.

By 16 weeks, they were able to confirm that Baby A was a girl, whom we named Alexis Rae, and Baby B was a boy, whom we named Eric David. Our 18-week appointment revealed that I no longer had placenta previa and the babies looked "perfect."

But then, at 20 weeks, I was hospitalized. Alexis and Eric were stillborn at 21 weeks. I finally understood what my doctor meant by "one healthy baby," and I'll never stop wondering about what might have happened had I transferred only one embryo.

The Truth About Twins and Triplets

"**T**he human body is designed to carry one pregnancy at a time," says reproductive endocrinologist Allison K. Rodgers with Fertility Centers of Illinois in Chicago. "I always tell patients that I will help them have as many babies as they want with the goal of one at a time."

I know how it feels to want the journey to end. I know how transferring multiple embryos or proceeding with an insemination when you have many follicles might seem like the best way to make that happen. I made my decision based on a combination of impatience and financial concerns—something I would not recommend. In this chapter, I'll walk you through the potential complications of carrying multiples. If you do end up pregnant with multiples, you'll also find advice on ways to cope should difficulties arise.

You Don't Know What You Don't Know

Surprisingly, many reproductive endocrinologists do not thoroughly educate their patients on the risks of carrying multiples. A survey conducted by FertilityIQ uncovered some interesting insights into the current state of this conversation—or lack thereof.

Many doctors still recommend multiple-embryo transfers. More than 90 percent of patients said that their doctor made a recommendation about how many embryos to transfer. *Roughly half (53 percent) recommended transferring more than one embryo.* That was true even for patients younger than 35, even though they already, thanks to their relative youth, have a higher chance of success. As you might imagine, patients followed their doctor's advice—of those who were advised to transfer more than one embryo, 82 percent did just that.

Cost seems to play a role. Perhaps due to the high financial cost of IVF, 60 percent of the recommendations for multiple-embryo transfers came in states that did not mandate some level of infertility insurance coverage.

Preimplantation genetic testing isn't weighted heavily enough. If embryos are confirmed to be genetically normal, there is not a reason to transfer more than one. However, 60 percent of doctors recommended transferring more than one (untested) embryo, even though genetic abnormality is the biggest cause of failed implantation or early miscarriage.

Conversations are poorly timed. Even though we made our decision on the day of our transfer, the brief discussion we had with my doctor took place during our IVF consultation. But others haven't been so lucky. FertilityIQ found that 21 percent of patients were counseled right before the transfer itself and 18 percent had the conversation during their first fertility clinic visit only—which, depending on the situation, could have been weeks, months, or even years earlier.

Risks of conceiving—and the challenges of raising—multiples aren't properly communicated. Turns out, I'm not alone, as 23 percent of patients were not informed about the risks to themselves, 39 percent were not informed about the risks to their babies, and 77 percent did not discuss with their fertility team the challenges of raising multiples.

Possible Complications for the Gestational Carriers

Many infertility warriors disregard their own health during their journey. It's not uncommon to trivialize certain risks as long as it means you end up with a healthy child. However, being pregnant with multiples can be risky for both you and the fetuses.

Let's start with potential complications for you.

Anemia

Bodies need oxygen. But when there aren't enough red blood cells to deliver it, you develop anemia. It's most often the result of iron deficiency, which is more common in multiple-gestation pregnancy and may be a precursor for preterm labor.

Bed Rest

When I was pregnant with Eric and Alexis, I was told early on that some level of reduced activity was common starting at 24 weeks due to the variety of complications that typically arise around then or soon after. Both the American College of Obstetricians and Gynecologists (ACOG) and the Society for Maternal-Fetal Medicine (SMFM) no longer recommend traditional bed rest, instead calling simply for reduced activity, whether at home or (if you require constant monitoring) at a hospital. However, your particular situation still may require traditional bed rest.

Bleeding

Approximately 20 percent of women experience vaginal spotting or bleeding during the first trimester, according to the American Pregnancy Association. This potential increases during a multiple gestation pregnancy. Bleeding during the first 12 weeks may be caused by having sex (my husband and I were told to abstain for the entire pregnancy), an infection, or changes in your blood flow, hormones, or cervix.

I bled on and off—heavily at times—from approximately weeks 5 to 10 with my twins. Unfortunately, the risk of bleeding doesn't end once you hit the second trimester. Later in your pregnancy, you may develop placenta previa (when one placenta covers the cervical opening) or a placental abruption (when the placenta prematurely detaches from the uterine wall), both of which can cause bleeding and even lead to the loss of one or more fetuses.

Finally, the risk of a hemorrhage during and after pregnancy is increased in women carrying multiples. This uncontrolled bleeding can be caused by the overextended uterus and large placental coverage area—and can sometimes put the mother's life at risk.

Caesarean Section

From the beginning of my twin pregnancy, I was told to expect a C-section. However, while more common in multiple gestation pregnancies, it's no longer the default. In fact, a study published in the *New England Journal of Medicine* found that in twin pregnancies of 32 to 38 weeks and 6 days of gestation, in which

---

BUSTED

Myth: The most challenging part of having multiples is the pregnancy.

Even if your multiples are born completely healthy, remember that raising two or more children at once is exponentially harder and more expensive. Infertility warriors need to understand what their lives might look like with multiples.

Also, many multiples are born premature—and prematurity doesn't cease to be an issue once your babies are released from the hospital. Dr. Meaghan Bowling, a reproductive endocrinologist with Carolina Conceptions in Raleigh, North Carolina, says that many patients are unaware of what it means to have a child born prematurely. But as the mother of twin girls born at 29 weeks, she always walks them through it.

"I ask parents to imagine their twins potentially needing years to a lifetime of treatment and assistance in the form of speech therapy, physical therapy, feeding tubes, and other support related to the medical problems associated with prematurity. While not everyone with twins will experience these scenarios, we can certainly limit the potential for premature birth by transferring a single embryo at a time," Dr. Bowling says.

the first twin is head down, "planned cesarean delivery did not significantly decrease or increase the risk of fetal or neonatal death or serious neonatal morbidity, as compared with planned vaginal delivery." But a lot of factors are at play, including the type of multiples, the position and size of each fetus, gestational age, and of course the skill of your ob-gyn. The caesarean section is so common now that it's often easy to forget that it's a major surgery and comes with the potential risks and complications of any major surgery, such as an extended hospital stay (typically 3 to 5 days), risk of infection, postpartum hemorrhage, blood clots, and increased risks during future pregnancies, to name a few.

Gestational Diabetes

Gestational diabetes is a form of diabetes that develops during pregnancy. The risk of developing it is higher for twin pregnancies than for single gestation pregnancies, according to studies. Once you develop gestational diabetes, your risk for preterm birth, preeclampsia, and a C-section delivery increases, as does your risk of developing type 2 diabetes later in life.

Intense Morning Sickness or Hyperemesis Gravidarum

Doctors still don't know exactly what causes morning sickness, though they suspect that it's tied to high and rapidly increasing hormone levels in the first trimester. Because hormone levels are especially high in multiple gestation pregnancies, it makes sense that the risk of developing intense morning sickness, or hyperemis gravidarum—in some cases so severe that it might require hospitalization—is increased.

Postpartum Depression

Postpartum depression is 43 percent more likely in multiple gestation pregnancies. It can make it difficult to care for your babies and participate in everyday life. And as you'll learn

in chapter 25, women who've gone through infertility are already at greater risk for postpartum depression.

Pregnancy-Induced Hypertension (PIH) and Preeclampsia

Pregnancy-induced hypertension, or high blood pressure, occurs in anywhere from 18 to 37 percent of twin pregnancies—three to four times more than in singleton pregnancies. Left untreated, it can develop into preeclampsia.

Preeclampsia results in high blood pressure and protein in your urine. It's accompanied by rapid weight gain and headaches, among other symptoms. You don't want to mess around with preeclampsia because, left untreated, it can develop into eclampsia and lead to seizures and even the death of both the carrier and fetus(es). This is part of the reason they make you pee in a cup at every ob-gyn visit—to test your urine for protein.

Pruritic Urticarial Papules and Plaques of Pregnancy (PUPPP)

Although it's relatively benign in that it poses no long-term risk to the carrier or child(ren), this condition is a very itchy rash that typically develops in the third trimester. The only "cure" is to give birth. One of the main risk factors is multiple gestation pregnancies.

Possible Complications for Fetuses

Now let's take a look at how multiple gestation pregnancies might impact your fetuses.

Birth Defects

Birth defects present at birth—such as cerebral palsy and heart, neural tube, and digestive system issues—are about two times more likely in multiple pregnancies than singleton pregnancies.

Discordant Twins

According to a 2011 report in the *American Journal of Obstetrics and Gynecology*, 16 percent of twins experience a discordance of 20 percent or more, meaning that one twin is 20 percent smaller than the other. The smaller twin is more likely to develop health issues both during pregnancy and after birth.

Intrauterine Growth Restriction (IUGR) and Low Birth Weight (LBW)

In the *best-case scenario*, according to the American Pregnancy Association, beginning at between 30 and 32 weeks of gestation, twins no longer grow at the same rate as singletons. This slowdown, or intrauterine growth restriction (IUGR), happens even earlier—at 27 to 28 weeks and 25 to 26 weeks—for triplet and quadruplet pregnancies, respectively. One possible reason for IUGR is that the babies begin competing with each other for nutrients late in the pregnancy.

Babies are said to have low birth weight (LBW) if they are born weighing less than 5 pounds 8 ounces, which understandably happens often in cases of IUGR. They are more likely to be born with health problems and to develop them later in life. LBW occurs in more than half of twins and nearly all higher-order multiples (triplets and more).

Miscarriage, Stillbirth, and Neonatal Death

According to the American Society for Reproductive Medicine (ASRM), the risk of miscarrying multiples is higher than singletons. However, in as many as 20 percent of multiple pregnancies, only one fetus continues developing and the other disappears (typically in the first trimester), which is known as "vanishing twin syndrome." And twins are 2 to 3 times more likely to be stillborn than singletons.

The difference between a miscarriage and stillbirth depends on when the fetus dies in utero. Before 20 weeks gestation, fetal death is categorized as a miscarriage. After 20 weeks, it's a stillbirth. My twins, for example, were stillborn at 21 weeks—although, technically, they died as a result of not being able to survive outside my body, rather than in my uterus. We heard their hearts beat for the last time immediately before delivery.

Stillbirth can occur as a result of many of the pregnancy complications listed in the previous section, including anemia, second- and third-trimester bleeding, and gestational diabetes. Other conditions that may lead to preterm labor—and ultimately stillbirth—include incompetent cervix and preterm premature rupture of membranes (PPROM), which studies show occurs in 7 to 20 percent of twin pregnancies.

A baby who dies within 28 days of birth is classified as a neonatal death, and this occurs most often following a preterm delivery—which is a considerable risk for multiple gestation pregnancies.

Premature Birth

Babies born before 37 weeks of gestation are considered premature. They may have short- or long-term health issues and/or require a longer hospital stay than full-term babies, potentially in the neonatal intensive care unit (NICU).

Potential health issues range from immature lungs, digestive system issues, and feeding problems to developmental delays, learning disabilities, cerebral palsy, and more. The Centers for Disease Control and Prevention (CDC) reports that:

- 19.2 percent of twins are delivered early preterm (less than 34 weeks).

- 59.9 percent are delivered preterm (less than 37 weeks).

- 8.8 percent are born at very low birthweight (less than 1,500 grams, or 3.3 pounds).

- 54.8 percent are born at low birthweight (less than 2,500 grams, or 5.5 pounds).

For comparison, the CDC reports that:

- 2.1 percent of singletons are delivered early preterm.

- 8.4 percent are delivered preterm.

- 1 percent are born at very low birthweight.

- 6.7 percent are born at low birthweight.

Twin-Twin Transfusion Syndrome (TTTS)

In some identical twin pregnancies, one twin takes the majority of the blood flow from the placenta, depriving the other twin. Depending on the severity, treatment options may be available, although if the twin-twin transfusion syndrome (TTTS), as it's called, is untreated or untreatable, the result may be the loss of one or both twins—or infant heart failure sometime after birth.

Dr. Rodgers says, "When you are feeling hopeless about your situation, twins seem like a great idea, but twins come with very serious risks. They are high risk for preterm labor, gestational hypertension, fetal death, and postpartum hemorrhage. No one thinks this will happen to them, but it can and it does. If you deliver at 22 weeks, you lose both babies. If you deliver at 26 weeks, you have two children with lifelong disabilities. These are not positions we want anyone to have to face."

Risk Factors for Increased Chance of Multiples

There are factors that increase the odds you will have multiple gestations. Knowing what risk factors you have will help guide your decision-making.

Risk of Conceiving Multiples Without Fertility Treatments

Some women are naturally at greater risk of conceiving multiples. As you might imagine, when these women use fertility treatments to achieve pregnancy, that risk increases even more.

Age

Although egg quality declines with age, the number of eggs released during a menstrual cycle may increase. Follicle-stimulating hormone (FSH) levels increase with age because more of the hormone is needed to develop eggs before ovulation. Sometimes, this results in the release of two or more eggs.

BUSTED

Myth: Ending up with multiples is a random twist of fate.

Yes and no. While there is not a "formula" for getting pregnant with twins or triplets, there are risk factors that increase your chances of ending up with multiples. Plus, with embryo transfers, you *choose* how many embryos to use, so you do have some control over whether you end up with multiples.

"The goal of fertility treatment is a healthy mother and a healthy child," says Dr. Alan Copperman, medical director of Progyny in New York. "This is really best achieved by minimizing the chance of twins."

Family History

A history of fraternal, or nonidentical, twins in the maternal family can mean that you have an increased chance of ovulating more than one egg and thus conceiving multiples. This chance increases if fraternal twins run on both sides of the family. There does not appear to be any genetic component to the occurrence of identical twins, however. A male partner's family history does not play a role in the likelihood of twins.

Race

As reported in *Scientific American*, women of West African descent are most likely to have fraternal twins, followed by Caucasians and those with Chinese or Japanese heritage. African Americans have a slightly increased risk compared to the general population.

Weight

Though we know that excess weight produces high levels of estrogen and lower levels of fertility, research published in *Obstetrics &* *Gynecology* showed that women with a BMI greater than 30 are more likely to conceive twins. This is because high estrogen levels may overstimulate the ovaries, causing them to release more than one egg.

Risk of Conceiving Multiples with Fertility Treatments

Most fertility treatments increase your risk of conceiving twins. (Although, as you'll read later in this chapter, it's possible to design a protocol that minimizes this risk.)

In the general population, the CDC reports a twin birth rate of 31.1 twins per 1,000 births (approximately 3.1 percent) and triplet birth rate of 79.6 per 100,000 births (approximately 0.79 percent).

Multifetal Pregnancy Reduction

Pregnancy reduction is an emotionally and ethically complicated topic, and one you might face along your journey. "Twins and triplets clearly can create risks to both

RISK OF CONCEIVING MULTIPLES WITH FERTILITY TREATMENT		
FERTILITY TREATMENT	**RISK OF TWINS**	**RISK OF TRIPLETS**
Clomiphene citrate (Clomid)	5 to 12 percent	1 percent
Letrozole (Femara)	3.4 to 13 percent	No available data
Gonadotropins	22.4 percent	9 percent
IVF	2.1 percent when transferring one embryo; 33.6 to 42.7 percent when transferring two embryos; 22 to 28.2 percent when transferring three embryos; 19.7 percent when transferring four or more embryos	Less than 0.1 percent when transferring one embryo; 0.6 to 1 percent when transferring two embryos; 3 percent when transferring three embryos; 2.1 percent when transferring four or more embryos

*Statistics on clomiphene citrate come from the American Society for Reproductive Medicine; those on letrozole and gonadotropins come from studies published in the *New England Journal of Medicine*; those on IVF come from the US Centers for Disease Control (CDC).

mom and child," Dr. Copperman says. "Some patients choose to undergo a procedure to interrupt one or more of the gestations in hope of having a healthier mom and a healthier baby."

Multifetal pregnancy reduction is defined by the ACOG as "a first-trimester or early second-trimester procedure for reducing the total number of fetuses in a multifetal pregnancy by one or more." Most often, it involves reducing a triplet or other higher-order multiple pregnancy down to twins. Reduction to a singleton is typically done for medical or financial reasons. For example, with my history of cervical insufficiency, if I ever became pregnant with multiples again, my doctor would likely recommend a reduction to a singleton.

Dr. Copperman adds, "Historically, it was not uncommon for a mom [undergoing fertility treatment] to conceive with two, three, or even four embryos. These days, it is far less common because rarely are fertility injections used with inseminations, and frequently, only a single embryo is transferred. When higher-order multiple gestations occur, the patient is referred to a high-risk specialist who explains all options and provides clinical support."

Avoiding Multiples

Let's be real: Avoiding multiples isn't always possible, whether in spontaneous pregnancies or when using fertility treatments. But there are actions you can take to reduce the risk.

Timed Intercourse

A timed intercourse cycle, as discussed in chapter 6, is when your doctor—either your regular ob-gyn or a reproductive endocrinologist—prescribes an ovulation stimulation medication, such as Clomid or letrozole, and you and your partner time intercourse with ovulation.

The best ways to minimize the chance of a multiple pregnancy in a timed intercourse cycle are as follows:

• Start with the lowest dosage of ovulation stimulation medication.

• Be closely monitored via bloodwork and ultrasound by your doctor, so you know if and how you're responding to the medication, exactly when to have sex, and whether or not the cycle should be canceled due to overstimulation.

• Avoid using a "trigger shot"—a medication that matures lagging follicles in addition to signaling that it's time to ovulate. This will help ensure that no additional follicles develop at the last minute.

Although you lose the spontaneity of sex with your partner, and scheduling and attending multiple monitoring appointments is a pain, this type of cycle can be done with your regular ob-gyn—no reproductive endocrinologist required. As long as your doctor is willing to prescribe an ovulation stimulation medication and monitor you for your body's response, there's no need to head to a fertility clinic just yet—*plus* you can work toward that goal of one healthy baby at a time.

Intrauterine Insemination (IUI)

An IUI cycle involves placing sperm directly inside a woman's uterus, bypassing the vagina and cervix. There are many possible variations of an IUI cycle (see chapter 6), but the important thing to note is that ovulation stimulation medication—*not* IUI itself—increases the risk of conceiving multiples. Knowing this, you can take precautions similar to those for a timed intercourse cycle—start with low doses,

BUSTED

Myth: Medical professionals always agree about how many embryos to transfer.

I think my story shows immediately that this isn't true. While I didn't understand it at the time, my reproductive endocrinologist clearly would've preferred that we transfer just one embryo. However, the doctor who performed the transfer didn't bat an eye when I said to transfer two embryos.

Be prepared to get dissenting opinions from members of your fertility treatment team.

Divya from Bodensee, Germany, experienced this firsthand. While her ob-gyn was worried about her ability to carry twins following a myomectomy (surgery to remove uterine fibroids), her reproductive endocrinologist was concerned that, at 37, Divya was of "advanced" age and encouraged her to transfer two embryos to increase the chances of success, which she did. "I think about it a lot because even though both embryos implanted and I made it to 8 weeks, we didn't see a heartbeat with one of them and I subsequently had a missed miscarriage," Divya says. "I sometimes feel that maybe the one that didn't make it would have done better on its own." (A missed miscarriage is when the fetus stops developing but the woman hasn't had any miscarriage symptoms, such as pain or bleeding.)

The final decision is yours, so be sure you know why each doctor has recommended transferring a certain number of embryos—and that you agree completely.

---

undergo bloodwork and ultrasound monitoring, and forgo any trigger shot.

If you've had multiple failed IUI cycles or simply aren't responding to ovulation stimulation medications like Clomid or letrozole, it's common to move to injectable gonadotropins. But gonadotropins *dramatically* increase your risk of becoming pregnant with twins or even triplets. Although IVF is far more expensive than IUI, if you find yourself in this position and don't want to chance a multiple pregnancy, IVF is the safer option.

Michelle from Illinois started her IUI cycles with Clomid. When she wasn't pregnant after several tries, she moved on to IUI with gonadotropins—and became pregnant with twins. Sadly, the end result was similar to my own. "We had cervical shortening at 20 weeks, followed by bed rest and preterm delivery at 21.5 weeks. It was very difficult to 'overcome' infertility only to then lose our babies," she says.

⚡ Advocate for yourself by having a conversation with your ob-gyn about your goals and your desire to reduce the risk of conceiving multiples through TI and IUI. If both you and your doctor are comfortable proceeding, great! If not, you will likely be referred to a reproductive endocrinologist.

In Vitro Fertilization (IVF) and Frozen Embryo Transfer (FET)

There are many possible protocols for IVF cycles and FETs, but there's really only one way to reduce the chance of conceiving multiples: Transfer the appropriate number of embryos for your particular situation.

Dr. Rodgers says, "The American Society for Reproductive Medicine guidelines are in place to decrease risk and increase success. . . . The number of embryos to transfer are determined by a patient's age, prior success, prognosis, the stage of embryo development, and if genetic testing was performed on the embryos."

The chart on page 125 walks you through ASRM's guidelines. (If you are using donor eggs, the guidelines should be applied to the donor.)

Things have changed since my first transfer of two embryos back in 2013. Dr. Bowling explains some of the newest updates to the ASRM guidelines: "First, ASRM increased the age in which physicians should only transfer a single blastocyst to include all women under 38. Second, ASRM states that all women who have done preimplantation genetic testing and have a euploid embryo, regardless of age, should transfer one embryo at a time."

Even though Dr. Bowling strictly adheres to ASRM guidelines, Dr. Rodgers points out that these guidelines are not laws. "Prior to treatment, each patient case needs to be evaluated by the physician and embryology team to determine what is best for the individual patient. Each physician also needs to determine whether they are willing to take on the liability and risk of going above the guidelines. Unfortunately, it's not just about what a patient's desire may be. We need to assess what is safe."

So, who should determine the number of embryos transferred—the patient or the doctor? Ideally, the conversation with your reproductive endocrinologist will take place during your IVF consultation—*not* your first clinic visit and certainly not when you're heading into the transfer room.

Mindi from Ohio found herself in this situation. She and her husband had two frozen embryos, both genetically tested and found viable. A week before the embryo transfer, she and her husband still had not decided whether to transfer both or just one. Ultimately, they transferred only one—and it worked. "It's not that we weren't comfortable with the idea of having twins," Mindi says, "but I wanted to make sure that we gave our embryos the best chance possible and that my body could sustain that. I did have lots of issues during my pregnancy, and I'm glad that we only transferred one embryo because I think things could have been a lot more difficult." They now have a son and one more frozen embryo that will hopefully become his brother in a few years when they're ready for another child.

Dr. Juan Alvarez, a reproductive endocrinologist with Fertility Centers of Illinois in Chicago, adds, "The final decision is ultimately up to the patient. I always counsel my patients based on ASRM's guidelines. After describing the risk of having twins or higher-order multiples with the transfer of more than one embryo, most patients agree to ASRM guidelines."

WARRIOR WISDOM

Transferring Two Embryos Does Not Increase Live Birth Rates

Dr. Rodgers explains, "Many patients think that putting in more embryos increases the chance of pregnancy. Interestingly, this is not usually the case. Transferring more embryos often does not increase chances of success but dramatically increases chances of multiples."

The data supports her claim. According to the CDC, across all fresh transfers with patients' own eggs, 36.2 percent of those who transfer one embryo and 40.8 percent who transfer two embryos have a live birth, respectively. Meanwhile, the chance of conceiving twins goes from 2.1 percent for a single embryo transfer to 33.6 to 42.7 percent for a double embryo transfer. *Is that 4.6 percent increase in a live birth worth the risk?*

It's Not All Doom and Gloom

Despite the risks, multiple gestation pregnancies can work out.

Lindsay from Missouriand her husband began trying to conceive a couple of months before their wedding. Thirty-one at the time, she already feared her age would negatively impact their chances. After 15 months of meticulously tracking her cycles and taking advantage of her fertile windows, she decided it was time to have a conversation with her ob-gyn.

Lindsay's ob-gyn conducted some of his own testing, including sending a sample of her husband's semen for analysis. His sperm count initially came back slightly low, but her doctor felt they were still good candidates for IUI. And because he performed them in-office, she didn't need a reproductive endocrinologist just yet.

The original plan was to try up to five IUI cycles before discussing IVF. Their first IUI cycle, which was unmedicated, was canceled because Lindsay ovulated very late—likely, she says, due to stress. The second cycle, which was medicated with Clomid, failed—devastating Lindsay and her husband, and not just because she wasn't pregnant.

"When they did the wash of my husband's sperm, before we even actually did the IUI procedure, my OB said to me, 'If this does not work, you guys need to move on the IVF.' After we started doing the IUIs, my husband's numbers dropped. And I don't know if that was stress-induced or if we just got lucky [during the original semen analysis]."

It was time to try IVF. Lindsay's first retrieval cycle resulted in six embryos to send for preimplantation genetic testing. Unfortunately, only one came back normal. Because she and her husband knew they ultimately wanted more than one child, they opted for another retrieval cycle. Although they sent only five embryos for genetic testing that round, three came back normal.

"We had four embryos and decided that we were comfortable at that point with moving forward with transfer. Everything went really well, and I am one of the very fortunate people that can say that we transferred two embryos and both of them stuck." Her son and daughter were born early at 34 weeks, weighing 5 pounds and 4 pounds 12 ounces, respectively. While they were in the NICU for 36 days, both are happy and healthy today.

In addition to the overwhelming joy you'll undoubtedly feel, a pregnancy with multiples comes with many challenges—physical, emotional, financial—and possible complications. You're going to need support.

Also, be aware of the triggers you might face while carrying multiples. For instance, it's not uncommon for people in your life to describe carrying twins as "twice the joy." You might feel that such statements discount the difficulties of your pregnancy, so don't be shy about voicing your objections or sharing that you're actually very anxious about having multiples.

Finally, be kind to yourself. After failed cycles, don't play the "what if" game. (What if we *had* transferred two embryos? Would the other have implanted?) The same goes for a successful cycle. (*Twins?* What if we had transferred only one embryo? Would it still have implanted and we'd be pregnant with a singleton?) You're making the best decision you can for your situation at that time.

Like all post-infertility pregnancies, try not to feel guilty about any negative emotions that come up. You do *not* have to feel extra grateful because you're carrying two or more fetuses. Multiple pregnancies can be hard, and it's important to recognize and process any negative emotions surrounding the risks and challenges.

WARRIOR ACTION STEPS
Deciding How Many Embryos to Transfer

As a member of your own fertility treatment team, take the following steps to determine the number of embryos to transfer:

Get educated. Request a copy of the latest ASRM guidelines. Note the recommendations specific to your (or your egg donor's) age.

Decide about PGT. Discuss with your reproductive endocrinologist whether or not preimplantation genetic testing is recommended for you. If the determination is yes, then talk to your partner (if you have one) about this added cost and whether or not it's feasible or right for your situation.

Get real about the risks. Talk with your partner about possible risks to you and the fetuses should you indeed become pregnant with multiples. Think about what you would do if complications arise and whether you're prepared for the emotional toll complications might cause.

Learn about raising multiples. Discuss with a doctor (your reproductive endocrinologist and/ or ob-gyn or pediatrician), twin parents, and parenting coaches the challenges of raising multiples—ones you haven't even imagined. They'll have a unique perspective of what it's *really* like to have multiples, from pregnancy through the teenage years. Then, alone or with your partner, consider the feasibility of that scenario.

Make a decision. Together with your doctor and partner, decide *prior to* your transfer day how many embryos you will transfer—and be prepared to be adaptable should any of the variables change.

→

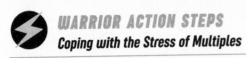

WARRIOR ACTION STEPS
Coping with the Stress of Multiples

Whether you're discussing ways to lower your chances of multiples or are pregnant with twins or triplets, there are steps that can help you cope.

Prepare for the multiples stigma. Guidelines for embryo transfers and fertility treatments have changed over the years. But there was a time when doctors and infertility warriors weren't as conscious of the risk of multiples. Because of this, society started associating fertility treatment with pregnancies of five, six, seven, and even eight babies. If you are out about your infertility and end up pregnant with multiples, some people may not have empathy for your situation. They may imply that you deserve the challenges you're facing because you underwent fertility treatments. Have prepared responses for less sensitive comments people may make. And know that a completely valid reaction is to just walk away.

Mourn all your losses. If the worst happens and you lose one or more of your babies, grieve your children as individuals. We'll talk more about grief in chapter 14, but as you create memorial traditions, make sure to honor all of your children.

WARRIOR CHECKLIST
Understanding the Reality of Multiples

❑ Know that being pregnant with multiples may not be like you imagine.

❑ Understand the possible complications of multiple gestation pregnancies for both carrier and fetuses.

❑ Determine whether you are at higher risk for a multiple pregnancy. Know what you can do to reduce the odds of getting pregnant with multiples.

❑ Acknowledge that reduction might be suggested by your doctor and think through what your decision would be in that situation.

❑ Remember that it is possible to have a safe pregnancy and end up with healthy twins or triplets.

❑ Be prepared to cope with the added stress of multiples.

Add more items to your Warrior Checklist or jot down any notes here:

Donor Eggs, Sperm, and Embryos 101

ONATED EGGS, SPERM, OR embryos are not a part of every infertility journey, but they are for many warriors, like Alicia and Pablo from Florida. They tried to conceive on their own for almost a year before they found out about Pablo's severe male factor infertility. They were told that IVF was their only option, so they pursued it with high hopes. However, after two failed cycles, they were advised to not attempt IVF with Pablo's sperm again.

"We completely understood and agreed," Alicia shares. "This was a blow, but we still couldn't see a future without a kid. We couldn't entertain the idea of a donor until our IVF options felt exhausted—and we reached that."

At the beginning of their journey, their first reproductive endocrinologist had wanted to discuss donor options, but Alicia completely shot him down. "Knowing we tried our hardest at IVF helped us move on to other options," says Alicia. "Time heals and time helps you accept things that you might not have initially accepted. This was true for us as far as the idea of using a donor to build a family. We also had a donor option that felt comfortable to us. My husband has a brother. Based on their relationship and personalities, this seemed like something that could work."

To Alicia, it was important to get a donor as close to her husband genetically as they could. "It was scary when my husband asked his brother the question, but his quick and sincere response was a relief," Alicia says, looking back on their decision. "If we hadn't had the option of a brother, I imagine we might have adjusted to something different, but it's hard to say. We feel very thankful, especially after what we had already been through."

With Pablo's brother's full-hearted support, they froze his sperm sample. They faced other bumps in the road, such as Alicia having ovarian cysts and not responding to ovarian stimulation with Clomid. But after a few exhausting months, Alicia and Pablo were finally able to try an IUI cycle. On the very first try, they were gifted their beautiful daughter, Georgie.

The Basics of Using Donated Eggs, Sperm, and Embryos

When you are unable to use your own eggs or sperm to create an embryo, you enter into donation territory—a land where it's easy to get lost. There are so many options and choices to navigate. By going through the individual nuances and considerations of each of meant to be a useful map to help you navigate the donor landscape, with tips and insights to help you cope and make good choices along the way.

Though it's difficult, try to maintain perspective as you consider donation. As Michelle from Illinois explains: "Keep your eye on the prize. I have two of the most beautiful children ever. I am biased for sure. But truly, I was not sure this day would ever come and now I am 5 years into this. Also know you will love your child regardless of the genes. Genes are overrated!"

Before you begin your parent-via-donor journey, know that your fertility clinic may suggest you undergo a psychological assessment. This is "not an evaluation and it is not my job to decide whether or not they are worthy of becoming parents," says Carole LieberWilkins, a marriage and family therapist from Los Angeles. Instead, she and other therapists like her represent the unborn child.

"The children resulting from all the procedures have no voice in how it all happens," says LieberWilkins. "Most of the time, patients are as qualified to parent as anyone off the street—only now, because they have been required to see a professional, they are much better educated about certain aspects of family-building and parenting."

Choosing the Right Attorney

Using donated sperm, eggs, or embryos can be a complicated process. Multiple people are involved, each with their own needs and intentions. There are contracts to sign and laws and regulations to follow. When you're already facing the stress of infertility, there's no reason to try to navigate the legal waters by yourself.

Even if you have the best personal attorney in the world, I recommend seeking out a lawyer who specializes in reproductive law.

the three forms of donation—eggs, sperm, and embryos—you can begin to determine which may be the best fit for you. This chapter is

"Reproductive law is really complicated," says Catherine Tucker, an attorney at New Hampshire Surrogacy & Fertility Law. "A lawyer must be able to draw from many different legal fields including family law, estate planning law, health law, immigration law, and employment law, to name a few."

Experience with Your Situation

Try to find an attorney who can match your needs as closely as possible. For example, just because a lawyer has 25 years of experience with adoption and surrogacy law doesn't mean they understand the legal issues involved with using donor embryos.

Do your research, using resources like RESOLVE's Professional Services Directory. Focus on attorneys near you who understand your specific third-party reproduction issue.

Aside from the attorney's education and years of experience, here are some other things to consider:

• **Mediation experience.** If you're using a donor you know personally, you don't want to ruin your relationship while hashing out contractual fine print. An attorney who knows how to mediate these sensitive conversations can ensure everyone's needs are respectfully addressed.

• **Understanding of the latest American Society of Reproductive Medicine (ASRM) and US Food and Drug Administration (FDA) recommendations.** From helping you choose a fertility clinic or donor bank to translating their legal paperwork, it's important for your attorney to know the current best practices. This will help ensure the safety of everyone involved—including your potential child.

• **Up-to-date knowledge of confidentiality concerns.** There are many methods of communication today, and no one knows what the future holds. If you decide that you don't want your donor—known or anonymous—to have future contact with your child, your contract needs to address new communication forums and pathways that may develop in the future.

• **What states they're licensed in.** If there's a chance that your donor or fertility clinic will be in a different state from the one you live in, you'll want an attorney who knows the laws of every state involved.

When Emily and Matthew from Indiana decided to use a known sperm donor, they knew they needed to find an attorney to represent their interests. "If any clinic says it's not necessary and you can 'just use their forms,' they are only protecting themselves," Emily says.

Luckily, her clinic provided a list of experienced attorneys. After she and Matthew chose one, they asked their donor and his wife to select another. This way, both sides could feel confident that someone would be focused on their interests. "It also made it easier to ask hard questions that are a little uncomfortable because you know they are going from your attorney to the other attorney. It feels less personal and less dramatic," Emily says.

The attorneys encouraged both couples not to discuss the agreement between themselves. At first this seemed odd to Emily. But after going through the process, she saw it was best to leave the discussion of nitpicky details to the attorneys.

Your Level of Comfort

Every aspect of your infertility journey is personal. Whoever helps and supports you along the way needs to be not only knowledgeable, but also a good fit for your personality. While your attorney shouldn't be part of your emotional support system, you need to feel comfortable with them.

Consider what you'll need from a lawyer. Do you need someone who can clearly explain legal jargon to you? How available do you want them to be for your questions? Do you want someone with an established relationship with your fertility clinic? How experienced is their legal support staff?

Once you have a list of potential attorneys, take the time to meet with a few of your top options. Go in with a list of concerns and questions and pay attention to how their responses resonate with you and your needs. It might take more time, but given how frustrating the legal process can be, it's better to wait and find the right fit.

When to Hire an Attorney

Legal costs can add up quickly. Because of this, you might be tempted to wait until you absolutely need a lawyer before you hire one. But if you wait too long, some legal wheels might already be in motion by the time you bring your attorney on board.

"Building your family is the most important thing you will ever do," says Tucker. "Don't get caught up in the many possible legal loopholes—have an attorney right from the start to protect your family and your future."

When you're considering using a donor, the sooner you can secure legal advice, the better. Even when you're using a fertility clinic or donor bank, a lawyer will give you confidence that the establishment's business practices and regulations will fit your needs.

Choosing the Source

Egg Donors

Unfortunately, there is no one-stop shop for egg donation and fertility treatments that will meet everyone's needs.

One thing that should give you peace of mind is knowing that egg donations are highly regulated by the FDA. Both known and anonymous donors are screened for diseases that may be passed to you or the baby. These include communicable diseases like HIV and genetic conditions like cystic fibrosis. ASRM also recommends that the donor be between 21 and 35 years old, undergo a thorough medical history for risk factors, and be evaluated for their emotional ability to understand the donation process.

It is important to remember that no matter how you choose your donor, there may always be complications. Angela from Ontario, Canada, explains "The first one we chose for health. She had three kids of her own, so we thought her eggs had a higher chance for success." Unfortunately, that wasn't the case, and Angela and her husband got zero embryos. However, the egg bank offered a replacement batch of eggs. This time, Angela asked for the bank's help selecting a donor. "They were amazing! They found someone the same size, red hair, left-handed—just like me! It made the experience of using donor eggs so much easier knowing we were getting someone so similar to me. She was a proven donor, meaning her eggs had worked for two other pregnancies, which was important to know."

WARRIOR TIPS
Communication with Donors

Many people decide to use anonymously donated eggs and therefore never meet their donor. This is a valid choice, but it can be helpful to at least have a communication intermediary for the future. For example, while donors are medically screened, it is possible for them to develop a genetic disease years later. Having that information will help you make better health-care decisions for your child. With an intermediary to communicate between the parties, the donor can update you about their medical history while retaining everyone's anonymity.

⚡ Depending on your situation, you may have to work with a variety of medical professionals—possibly at multiple locations. Don't be afraid to research different options to find the team that makes you feel comfortable.

Using Your Fertility Clinic

Depending on who you want to use as a donor, you might be able to work solely through your fertility clinic. For instance, if you have a friend or relative donating eggs, sperm, or embryos, there's no need to go through an outside source. And some fertility clinics handle donations in-house. Others will facilitate the process of choosing an anonymous donor from another program, which can make the process a lot less stressful. It's just important to do your research.

Where you need to be careful is keeping track of the costs of the services you choose. Some clinics offer packaged services with clear prices and guarantees. However, if you have a treatment plan that requires more than what's laid out in the packages, you could end up spending more than you expected.

Nichole from Tennessee explains how she and her partner concluded that working with her fertility clinic was better for them than the banks and databases. "It was important to me to find a clinic with an in-house egg donor program. I found agency fees to be cost-prohibitive, and I thought the large databases would have overwhelmed me," she says.

Her clinic's egg donor pool was smaller, but she liked that her coordinator knew each of the donors because she had been involved in the screening process. "Her 'insider knowledge' about their personalities was invaluable to me, and really made our choices come to life from their 'on paper' appearances in pictures and profiles," Nichole says.

Using an Egg Bank

Most fertility clinics don't have egg donor programs. Instead, they partner with or recommend organizations with a list of available donors. In most cases, egg banks offer frozen eggs that can be fertilized with your partner's or chosen donor's sperm.

When evaluating which egg bank to use, consider the following factors:

• **The screening process.** Most egg banks have a rigorous screening process and accept only a small percentage of donors. But what they screen for might not match your needs, so it's important to find out if they're asking the right questions for you.

• **The size of the donor pool.** The more options you have, the higher the chances you'll find a donor that meets all your needs and priorities.

• **The available donor information.** Each bank has regulations about what you can learn about donors. Some provide only basic information, like the donor's race and medical

---

WARRIOR TIPS
Options for Male Couples

In a couple in which both partners are male, you will, of course, need a donor egg, and you will also need someone to be a surrogate (see chapter 11). You will then need to choose which partner will be the biological parent. Or you might let fate decide and both provide sperm samples; after IVF, your doctor can choose the embryo with the strongest chance of success.

Whichever route you decide, know that the plan is never guaranteed. Be sure to talk with your partner about different possible outcomes.

FERTILITY CLINIC vs. EGG BANK vs. EGG DONOR AGENCIES			
	FERTILITY CLINIC	**EGG BANK**	**EGG DONOR AGENCIES**
Success rate (percentage of egg cycles resulting in live births)*	Frozen donor egg cycle: 36% Fresh donor egg cycle: 50%	Frozen donor egg cycle: 36%	Fresh donor egg cycle: 50%
Size of donor pool	Varies, depending on the clinic	Large, and not limited to your region	Large, though your choices vary depending on donor availability
Number of eggs	With fresh eggs, there's no guarantee of the number; with frozen eggs, you'll know ahead of time how many you'll receive.	You'll know ahead of time how many eggs you'll receive.	You'll receive all the eggs from the donor's cycle, but there's no guarantee of the number.
Timing	Frozen eggs are available immediately. Matching with a fresh egg donor and preparing for the procedure can take from 6 months to a year.	Frozen eggs are available immediately.	Matching with a fresh egg donor and preparing for the procedure can take from 6 months to a year.
Cost**	$35,000–$40,000	$16,000–$20,000	$25,000–$50,000

* Source: Centers for Disease Control and Prevention, "2019 Assisted Reproductive Technology Fertility Clinic and National Summary Report," 2021, online.

**Price ranges subject to change.

history, while others give you the donor's personal account of why she decided to become a donor. Depending on how much you want to know, the availability of this information could influence your choice.

Using an Egg Donor Agency

Egg donor agencies deal only with freshly donated eggs. For couples concerned about using frozen eggs, they are a great option. Like with an egg bank, you get to choose from a wide range of donors. The major difference is the logistics once you've chosen a donor.

With frozen eggs, the retrieval has already happened. The donor's part is done. For a fresh transfer with an egg donor agency, your chosen donor will have to be available at the time during your cycle when you would have ovulated. Both you and your donor will have to set aside a good chunk of time to sync your cycles and medically prepare for the retrieval process.

Sometimes this gets complicated. Your number one choice may not be available, or she may back out. If she doesn't live in your area, you will likely have to pay for her to travel and stay while undergoing the procedures.

When evaluating egg donor agencies, consider:

• **What happens if the donor backs out.** Will you have to wait before being matched again? Can the process be rescheduled, and if so, how long will you need to wait?

- **Relationships with your doctors or clinics.** After a fresh egg retrieval, there's only so much time to fertilize the egg. If the agency can't easily work with your fertility team, it might not be the right choice.

- **The number of eggs you'll receive.** With a fresh cycle, there's no guarantee on the number of eggs retrieved. If you get only a few eggs, you may need to go through the process again.

Choosing Your Donor

The FDA requires all gamete—eggs, sperm, or embryos—donors to go through a screening process that involves screening for HIV, Hepatitis, Gonorrhea, Chlamydia, and other communicable diseases. Egg donors require testing no more than 30 days before the donor's retrieval cycle. Similarly, sperm donors must be tested no more than 7 days before intended use or freezing for later use. Donors also have to give an extensive medical history and undergo a physical examination.

Going through an embryo placement agency provided Kelli from Oregon with a three-generation health history for Chris and Becky, her embryo donors. This was important to her, she says, because she lost her sister to breast cancer, and she wanted to minimize the risk of that condition being passed on to her children.

Beyond these details, you need to determine what additional information you want about the donor, as it can influence who you choose and what source you use. Here are some considerations to discuss:

- **The depth of medical history.** There are no regulations on testing for genetic diseases. If your family has a history of certain health problems, you want to be sure your donor doesn't increase the risk of your child inheriting the disease.

- **Physical appearance.** For some, it's important that the child somewhat resembles the intended parent(s). While most organizations provide information about a donor's race or ethnicity, they might not provide photos or further details.

- **Interests and talents.** You might like to imagine what hobbies your child will have. Knowing if the donor was musical, intelligent, or athletic could then influence your decision.

- **Availability for future children.** If you plan on having more than one child and would like them to be full genetic siblings, you'll need a source that has more of the donor's gametes on reserve.

Further, consider the following factors before deciding to use donated embryos:

- **What information you want about the donors.** If the embryo donor used donated eggs or sperm, you only have access to the information they know about the initial donors of the genetic material.

- **Quality of the embryos.** In most cases, the embryos that people freeze and later donate were unused for a reason. Often, but not always, they were of lower quality than the embryos the donors themselves used. However, this does not mean the embryos aren't viable or won't produce a healthy child.

- **The age of the female donor when she had her egg retrieval.** Generally speaking, the younger the donor was when an egg was retrieved, the more likely that egg is to lead to a successful pregnancy.

- **Location of the donor.** Your choices may be limited to donors in your area, or you may need to travel outside of your area to transfer the embryo.

BUSTED

Myth: I'll be judged for choosing a complicated medical treatment rather than simply adopting a child.

With a donated embryo, neither you nor your partner has a biological connection to the child. The resulting baby is as genetically related to you as an adopted child. Because of this, many infertility warriors wonder if they'll be judged for not giving a living baby a home.

First, you are under no obligation to tell people you used a donated embryo. So if this is a concern of yours, you can keep the story behind your pregnancy to yourself. Second, you are allowed to want to be pregnant. Carrying a child is a meaningful experience for many people. If that's part of your parental plan, go for it!

Third, using donated embryos often has a shorter timeline than adopting a child. Many people sit on adoption waiting lists for years, while having a child through the use of a donated embryo can be much quicker. As an embryo recipient, you may also have greater legal empowerment and access to more information about the biological parents.

Kelli notes, "Dan and I had several friends burned by adoption when mothers changed their minds. With embryo donation, we valued a clear transfer of ownership of the embryos. We wanted to pour our hearts into these precious little ones without the risk of them being taken away."

When you're deciding whose gametes you want to use, it's important to prioritize your needs. Do you feel more comfortable with a donor you know or someone who's anonymous? Do you want access to the donor's medical history before making your choice? Having these types of answers will help you make the right choice for you.

Be honest with yourself. It's okay to say you want your donor to be a gorgeous genius. If music is a passion of yours, look for donors who have musical talents. If you love sports, look for donors with some athletic talent. But remember, no one can ever be sure that they'll pass their talents on to their children; there are no guarantees.

"Choosing an egg donor was much harder than expected," says Natasha from New Hampshire. She and her husband, Nate, had to agree on a list of must-haves, like appearance, medical history, and life achievements. And even when they thought they had their priorities set, new considerations would pop up. "At times, we would even get stuck on an above-average shoe size, delaying our final decision on a donor," she admits.

Ultimately, it comes down to what you want for your child. As Cassie from Florida explains, "I wanted to find a [sperm] donor who fit the qualities I would want my child to have. Emotional intelligence, healthy body weight, average height, healthy grandparents—stuff like that. Race and religion did not matter to me."

As with most aspects of this journey, cost also went into consideration. "The prices for different donors can vary, depending on the type of profile they have with this [sperm] bank. So, I went with a donor who met my needs and was more affordable than other donors," Cassie says.

Anonymous Donor

With an anonymous donor (also known as a "nonidentified donor"), you have limited access to the donor's personal information.

They also will not know you or your story. For many people, not knowing the donor makes it easier for them to see the child as completely theirs.

Anonymity, however, does not mean you have no data about your donor. Most organizations will provide you with basic information like the donor's medical history, level of education, physical appearance, and whether their gametes have been used before. If these factors are important to you, you can use this information to choose a donor that meets your needs. Do know, however, that the stricter your criteria, the longer it will take for you to find a donor.

Nichole worked with her fertility clinic to choose an anonymous egg donor—but she was thrilled about the amount of information she was provided about the donor. "Most importantly," she adds, "I chose a donor who was open to contact when our child reaches age 18. It was crucial to me to preserve that channel if my child chooses it."

Most sperm banks use anonymous sperm donors. Be sure to research what information sperm banks are willing to divulge about the donor if you'd like the possibility to learn more about your donor or contact him in the future.

Hillary from Tennessee chose an anonymous sperm donor with consideration of future possibilities. "I used an anonymous donor through a bank, but the donor is open ID, so my son can reach out to him when he turns 18," she explains.

Cassie, on the other hand, chose an anonymous sperm donor based on time. "I was going to use a known donor, but the process for a known donor to donate and have the sperm ready for insemination could take at minimum 6 months. I did not want to wait that long, so I went with an anonymous donor instead."

When a person or couple decides to donate their unused embryos, they can choose to do so anonymously. While you'll still have access

BUSTED

Myth: If the baby doesn't look like me, people won't believe the baby is mine.

Depending on who you choose as a donor, your baby may end up having little or no physical resemblance to you. This can lead to awkward questions from people who do not know your story. Even hearing a well-meant comment like "She looks just like you!" can be painful.

However, remember that no parent has control over what their child looks like. There are parents with biological kids who look nothing like them. A family resemblance is not what makes a family. While it might take some time to adjust, try to let go of what your child "should" look like and embrace their unique identity.

to information about the donors, it could be limited. This issue is further complicated if the embryo was created using donated eggs or sperm because the donor's information is protected by their original agreement with the egg or sperm bank. When researching donated embryo options, ask questions about what details you'll be given.

Also, many embryo banks use a matching program that considers the needs of both the donors and the recipients. This is different from egg and sperm donation because the donors can set stipulations on who can receive their embryos. If they want the resulting child to be raised by parents of a certain race, religion, or other criteria, you must meet those requirements to be considered as a recipient.

Before choosing an anonymous donor, consider the following factors:

• **How will you handle your child's questions about their donor?** If you tell your child you used a donor, they may have a lot of questions.

ANONYMOUS vs. KNOWN DONOR CONSIDERATIONS		
	ANONYMOUS	**KNOWN**
Future relationship with donor	Some donors are completely anonymous—no contact will ever be established. Others are open to some contact (usually by letter, facilitated by a mediator) with the family. Some are open to being contacted by the child when the child is older.	The donor may be a part of your life. You and the donor will have to agree upon the level of contact you are both comfortable with and whether or not you want the child to know that your donor is the child's biological parent.
Information about the donor	Varies depending on the source. Most organizations provide at least basic information (appearance, race or ethnicity, interests).	In-depth information about the donor's life, personality, and medical history.
Chance of biological siblings	The availability of a specific donor's gametes is not guaranteed for the future unless you purchase extra.	While a known donor is willing to donate now, there's no guarantee they'll agree again in the future. So you may want to ask if you can freeze extra gametes for later use.

With an anonymous donor, you won't always have all the answers.

• **Do you want to have more than one child?** Some families feel it's important for their children to be biological siblings. This isn't always possible if you use an anonymous donor and then decide to have another child later on but have no remaining gametes.

• **How quickly do you want to get pregnant?** Sometimes using frozen gamates from an anonymous donor is the quickest way to start. On the other hand, if you're using fresh gametes, the process can take a while (because there's a future egg retrieval cycle involved, and there might be a waiting list), and with an anonymous donor, there is a higher chance of the donor dropping out (because they don't know you personally).

• **Do you want any contact with the donor?** Depending on the organization you use, you might be able to send the donor appreciation letters or other forms of contact. This is not always guaranteed, however.

Known Donor

You may have a known donor (also known as a "directed [identified] donor") in your life who is willing and able to donate to you. If this route is right for you, it can be faster than using anonymous donors. At many organizations, there are long waiting lists for anonymous donors. Having a friend or family member as a donor allows you more control over your timeline.

You also might just feel more comfortable using someone you know as your donor. Having a connection with your donor and knowing who they grew up to be can give you more confidence about what your child might be like.

The legal side of using a known donor may seem more straightforward than dealing with an anonymous source, but Nicole Sodoma, managing partner at Sodoma Law in Charlotte, North Carolina, points out that without the right contract, a known donor could face unexpected legal rights or responsibilities, such as owing child support. "Both parties really need to address their intentions as it relates to the donation. Then go through

ANONYMOUS vs. KNOWN DONOR: ADDITIONAL CONSIDERATIONS		
	ANONYMOUS	**KNOWN**
EGG		
Length of process	Frozen eggs are available immediately. Fresh eggs require syncing up your cycles with that of the donor, which can take 3 to 5 months. Also, there can be a long waiting list for fresh donor eggs, and fresh egg donors can always drop out unexpectedly.	While there are no waiting lists for known donors, there is a chance unforeseen circumstances in your donor's life will cause delays. If you are doing a fresh cycle, you will need to sync up your cycles, which can take 3 to 5 months.
Compensation for donors	Most egg banks have an agreement established with their donors even before you choose them.	In most cases, it's up to you and your donor to create a contract that details how the donor will be compensated for her time and discomfort.
SPERM		
Overall cost factors	Sperm banks usually have set fees or fee schedules that you can look up online. There may be shipping charges, and the sperm bank may charge additional fees if you want to know more about the donor.	You will need to pay for testing and preparing the sperm sample, plus possible freezing and storage fees if you're saving sperm for future use.
EMBRYO		
Chance of biological siblings	Most embryo banks have packages that include a certain number of embryos. If you become pregnant following your first transfer, you can use the remaining embryos later. However, if you have no remaining embryos, there's no guarantee you'll be able to get more from the same donor later for a sibling.	As long as there are enough embryos, chances are a known donor will have no issue with you using them to get pregnant multiple times. But this is a legal issue you'll want to clarify in your contract.
Length of process	Due to stipulations donors may have about who can use their embryos, the matching process can be lengthy and some embryo banks have long waiting lists.	Since known donations are directed to you, this route tends to be quicker. However, if you're getting embryos through a bank and want to know your donor, the matching process could take a long time.

and waive obligations that would otherwise exist," Sodoma advises.

Consider what part the donor will play in the child's life. Will they be present at important milestones? Will your child know that this person was the donor? You and your donor should discuss these issues to avoid complications later on.

Jannette from Ontario, Canada, decided to use donor eggs after several failed IVF cycles. Her doctor explained that her age was likely a factor in her lack of success, which made the decision easy. However, in Canada, donor eggs cannot be purchased. Instead, recipients must rely on a friend or relative to gift them a chance for a family.

"I have a sister who is 7 years younger than me, and she very generously offered to give her time and body for this. She had to undergo all the needles and painful process of egg retrieval. I felt so bad for her!" Jannette says.

As a result of several surgeries in his teenage years, Matthew from Indiana was left with a low sperm count that made conceiving unlikely. He underwent a testicular sperm extraction (TESE) for the first round of IVF with his wife, Emily, but it was unsuccessful. After weighing their options, they decided to use a known sperm donor.

"I put myself in my child's shoes, and I would want to know where I came from genetically, if possible," Emily says. "I felt using a known donor would give the child the ability to know who helped us create them and that [the donor's] a good person. Then hopefully we could move on."

It was also important for Emily and Matthew to be able to give their child as many answers about where they came from as possible. With an unknown donor, they didn't feel they'd have enough information to satisfy themselves or the child.

"[Having a known donor] can be easier and better," says Marie Davidson, a licensed clinical psychologist at Fertility Centers of Illinois in Chicago. "But it can be complicated due to relationship history or not agreeing about disclosing the truth to children."

If using a known donor is the right choice for you, know that most fertility clinics recommend you and your donor attend counseling sessions together before you get started. A counselor can help you work through potential complications and ensure that you both are ready for how sperm donation could change your relationship.

Financially speaking, using a donor you know is the least expensive option. You're only responsible for the testing and preparation of the donated sample, which in most cases costs around $300. But there could be additional storage fees if you want to freeze sperm to preserve the possibility of having another child in the future. Depending on your fertility clinic, you might also have to cover the medical screening processes your donor undergoes.

With embryo donation, "knowing" the donor is different from knowing an egg or sperm donor. When you use a known egg or sperm donor, that person may be someone already in your life, an acquaintance, or a connection you made through someone. That is not necessarily the case with donor embryos.

Some donors are willing to give their embryos to strangers, but they want to meet the recipients before saying yes. This does not mean that the donor wants to be a part of the child's life. They just want to get an idea about who will be raising the child.

Embryos can also be directly donated. When you are part of the infertility community, chances are you know someone who has frozen embryos. If these individuals have decided they don't want any more children, they can pass their remaining embryos to you.

Just know that using directed embryos can come with complications. Be sure everyone is on the same page. Discuss whether or not the child will meet the donors and come to a legally binding agreement.

Here are some other things to consider before choosing a known donor:

• **How your relationship will change.** Donating gametes is a huge commitment. This can change the dynamics of an established relationship because there's a sense that you're indebted to your donor. It's important to address how this can impact your relationship and whether it's something you're both ready for.

• **The time commitment of donating.** Especially for donor eggs and embryos, there's a lot of preparation that goes into the donation process—starting with a fertility workup and ending with the egg retrieval. The whole process can take 3 to 5 months. While your donor might be completely willing to go through all the steps, factors in their life might cause issues. For example, what are the chances they'll have to travel for work, causing unexpected delays? And what if they need to donate more than once?

• **How you will feel if your child looks like the donor.** There is a chance your child will look or act like your donor. Because you know this person, it can be complicated to see reminders of them in your child's face. So, it's important to think deeply about this possibility and be honest about how it will impact you.

Using Donor Eggs

According to the US Centers for Disease Control (CDC) and the Society for Assisted Reproductive Technology (SART), there were 27,131 cycles—roughly 9 percent of all cycles tracked—involving donor eggs in 2019. And for people 35 or older, donor egg cycles were reported as the most successful fertility treatment. Here you'll find tables comparing the success rates of donor cycles to that of using your own eggs.

2019 DONOR EGG TRANSFER CYCLES (ALL AGES)			
	FRESH	**FROZEN**	**THAWED EMBRYOS**
Number of transfers	1,630	2,726	17,199
Live births	53.9%	45.8%	48.8%

Source: Centers for Disease Control and Prevention, "2019 Assisted Reproductive Technology Fertility Clinic and National Summary Report," 2021, online.

2019 PATIENT'S OWN EGG TRANSFER CYCLES					
AGE	**35**	**35–37**	**38–40**	**41–42**	**> 42**
Number of cycles	41,269	20,156	14,433	5,048	2,532
Live births	46.7%	34.2%	21.6%	10.6%	3.2%

Source: Centers for Disease Control and Prevention, "2019 Assisted Reproductive Technology Fertility Clinic and National Summary Report," 2021, online.

Legal Issues and Considerations

Complications of Parental Rights

Your fertility clinic will have consent forms and legal documents designed for your treatment plan. But in many cases, those documents will address only events and risks directly related to what happens at the clinic. Depending on your individual situation, you may be in a legal gray area regarding your parental rights.

When going over the paperwork—hopefully with a lawyer—be sure to discuss the following factors:

• **The state's definition of "biological parent."** If you have a partner, and you and your partner were to separate in the future, the custody of your child could be impacted based on who is or is not the child's biological parent. Legal agreements made ahead of time can prevent this circumstance.

• **Parental rights.** Depending on what state you live in and whether your egg donor is known or anonymous, you may have to go through a legal process to secure parental rights.

• **Where the birth could take place.** If your child is born in a different state or country than what you have planned, there might be issues establishing the parental rights for a

BUSTED

Myth: If my baby is not biologically related to me, we will never bond.

When you use a donor—whether for eggs, sperm, or embryos—you and/or your partner will not be genetically related to the resulting embryos. You might worry that without that biological connection, it'll be harder to bond with your child. But the relationship between you and your child is built on more than shared genes.

You may find that your feelings change throughout the process. Nichole was excited once she and her husband decided to use young, healthy donor eggs because they made her feel like there was a better chance of success. But then, she explains, "I was really surprised to find myself feeling very detached once our donor started her retrieval cycle. I was very aware that another woman's eggs were being mixed with my husband's sperm in a lab. I felt a little lost. But once I got the call with the embryo report, my excitement came rushing back. I feel 100 percent like those embryos are mine."

Even with a donor egg, sperm, or embryo, pregnancy affords a powerful connection to the developing child. Scientifically speaking, your baby begins to bond with you as they develop in the womb. In fact, a 2015 study from the University of Dundee found that fetuses react to both their mother's voice and touch. The fetuses were more likely to move after feeling their mother's touch. They also calmed down and moved less at the sound of their mother's voice.

In addition, the sound of your voice can impact your child's memory and learning. A 2014 study published in *Infant Behavior and Development* had mothers speak the same phrase to their baby over the last term of their pregnancy. By 34 weeks of gestation, the babies showed signs that they were learning what their mother said. At 38 weeks, the development of memories was evident.

"Many of my patients hope to experience pregnancy, feel their baby move inside them, deliver their child, and nurse their baby. With donor eggs, patients still get to have all those life experiences they are hoping for themselves," says Dr. Allison K. Rodgers, a reproductive endocrinologist with Fertility Centers of Illinois in Chicago. "They still have a biological connection to their child even if the egg didn't come from their body."

Of course, if you struggle with the loss of the possibility of having a genetic connection with your child, know that your grief is perfectly appropriate. When you realize that you will need to work with an egg, sperm, or embryo donor, or you turn to surrogacy (see chapter 11) or adoption (see chapter 12), or you have made the choice to have no children at all (see chapter 13), feelings of loss are natural—and can be overwhelming. If that is the case for you, Dr. Rodgers says, "please consult with a mental health professional, who can help you grieve and come to terms with your loss."

---

partner or a nonbiological parent. Legal agreements made ahead of time can prevent this circumstance.

• **Death of a partner.** If you are part of a couple and one of you dies, the surviving partner may still want to use the donated eggs. Perhaps the partner who died did so before the implantation could take place, or perhaps you have extra donated eggs stored for later use. Either way, the surviving partner's legal right to the eggs needs to be established, so consider creating a living will that includes this information.

Compensating the Donor

From the beginning, it's important to understand that a donor is not paid for the number of eggs retrieved from her or the viability of the embryos produced from her eggs. Legally, she is being compensated for her time, medical discomfort, and willingness to accept the risks of the procedure. Whether your donor produces many eggs or only one, your cost will be the same.

Given the amount of time the process takes and the nature of the medical procedures, they deserve financial support. It's a common myth that egg donors are only in it for the money. Many understand that they are helping to start families and don't take on that responsibility without serious consideration.

Good egg banks and fertility clinics have rigorous screening processes. Potential donors fill out mountains of paperwork and have to be cleared medically, after which they undergo in-depth interviews and psychological evaluations. This weeds out anyone who might be motivated solely by money.

A Donor Egg Cycle with IVF

While many aspects of traditional IVF are the same when you're using a donor egg, key differences will impact the process. Whether you decide to use fresh or frozen eggs will change the costs, the medical processes you undergo, and the possible outcomes.

Fresh Egg Cycle

When using fresh eggs for a fresh transfer, you will need to sync your menstruation and ovulation cycle with that of the donor. You will need to take medication to suppress your natural cycle. You'll likely also take some form of estrogen to prepare your uterine lining for the egg transfer.

Your donor will undergo ovarian stimulation to increase the number of eggs she produces. As soon as the eggs are retrieved, your reproductive endocrinologist will fertilize them with the sperm sample you have provided. Typically, 5 days later, your doctor transfers at least one embryo.

With a fresh egg donation, there's no guarantee on the number of eggs you will receive. But in general, this method of egg donation is most successful in terms of live births.

Using fresh eggs is typically much more expensive than a frozen egg cycle. According to WINFertility, a family-building benefits company, the egg retrieval alone can cost between $5,000 and $10,000, and then you have to add on the typical price of a transfer cycle. In most cases, your insurance company will not cover these expenses. (For more about insurance and paying for procedures, see chapters 19 and 20.)

2019 PREGNANCY SUCCESS RATES WITH DONATED FRESH EGG CYCLES			
	ALL	SINGLETONS	TWINS	TRIPLETS OR MORE
Percent of live births	53.9%	88.2%	11.5%	0.3%

Source: Centers for Disease Control and Prevention, "2019 Assisted Reproductive Technology Fertility Clinic and National Summary Report," 2021, online.

Frozen Egg Cycle

One of the biggest advantages of using frozen eggs is more flexibility for both you and the donor. The donor undergoes the retrieval whenever it's convenient for her. When you're ready—and that can be years later—the eggs are thawed and fertilized. This leads to a lower chance of cancellation due to unforeseen complications in either of your lives.

After the egg retrieval, the clinic or egg bank uses vitrification—which prevents the formation of ice crystals in the cell—to preserve the eggs. When you're ready to use the eggs, they are thawed and then fertilized using intracytoplasmic sperm injection (ICSI)—the sperm is injected directly into the egg (see chapter 7). From there, the transfer is similar to other forms of IVF.

Using frozen donated eggs is often more affordable than using fresh ones, and it comes with a guaranteed number of eggs. Different clinics and banks structure their pricing

differently, but in most cases, the cost is about $1,000 an egg or around $15,000 per cycle. Because frozen eggs can easily be transported, going this route opens up your donor pool, as well. Depending on your source, you could have access to eggs from all over the country.

Denise from Connecticut decided to use an egg bank because her clinic had a very small donation program. And, even though her doctor recommended against it, she decided to go with with frozen donor eggs because the wait time was much less than with fresh eggs, and she wanted to keep moving forward. She became pregnant after transferring an embryo that had matured on day 7, but the pregnancy ended before her first ultrasound (chemical pregnancy). Because her egg bank offered an additional egg batch if the cycle didn't result in embryos that matured by day 5, she was able to get an additional batch of frozen eggs at no extra cost. "This time, two embryos made it to maturity [by day 5]. We transferred both, and one implanted and developed properly. We were pregnant!"

2019 PREGNANCY SUCCESS RATES WITH DONATED FROZEN EGG CYCLES			
	ALL	SINGLETONS	TWINS	TRIPLETS OR MORE
Percent of live births	45.8%	91.9%	8%	0.2%

Source: Centers for Disease Control and Prevention, "2019 Assisted Reproductive Technology Fertility Clinic and National Summary Report," 2021, online

Disposal of Unused Eggs

Sometimes people complete their families before using all of their donated eggs. If this happens, depending on your doctor and clinic, you may have options about what to do with unused eggs.

FRESH vs. FROZEN DONOR EGG CONSIDERATIONS		
	FRESH DONOR EGGS	**FROZEN DONOR EGGS**
Success rates*	53.9%	45.8%
Number of eggs available	There's no guarantee on the number of eggs that will be retrieved. This can limit how many cycles you go through.	Often, you can choose how many frozen eggs you'd like to acquire based on how many transfers you can afford or plan on trying. (Keep in mind that there is no guarantee that any of the frozen eggs will become viable embryos).
Medical procedures	If you are doing a fresh transfer, both you and your donor have to take medication to sync your cycles. Five days after her egg retrieval, your embryo transfer will take place. Alternatively you, can opt for fresh donor eggs that are then frozen for preimplantation genetic testing (PGT) and transferred at a later date.	The donor undergoes retrieval on her own schedule. When you're ready, you undergo a typical transfer cycle.
Chance of cancellation	Unexpected circumstances in the donor's life can cause delays or for her to drop out completely. This means you might have to go through the preparation process multiple times.	Since the eggs have already been retrieved, there's no chance of cancellation.
Overall cost factors	Cost incurred from donor vetting, egg retrieval, and a transfer cycle. Total costs can be $25,000–$50,000.	Cost incurred for egg processing and thawing and a transfer cycle. Total costs around $16,000–$20,000.

* Source: Centers for Disease Control and Prevention, "2019 Assisted Reproductive Technology Fertility Clinic and National Summary Report," 2021, online.

Here are some options to consider:

- Donate them to an egg bank for another infertility warrior to use.

- Freeze the eggs to preserve the possibility of having another child in the future.

- Donate the eggs to scientific research.

If you know your donor, it's important to include her in this discussion. Trachman says that while your donor may be willing to give *you* her eggs, she may not want a stranger to use them. If this is the case, you need to agree on how to dispose of the unused eggs.

Trachman also says that if the donor *does* want unused eggs to go to another infertility warrior, it's up to you—not her—to do your best to follow her wishes.

Using Donor Sperm

According to data in the Donor Sibling Registry, nearly 50 percent of those who used a sperm donor were single, heterosexual females. Another 33 percent of the parents were members of the LGBTQ+ community, and 17 percent were heterosexual couples with fertility issues.

A 1987 survey from the US Office of Technology Assessment estimated that 30,000 children were born using sperm donation in the United States that year. Given that the process has only become more popular since then, experts have begun extrapolating to get more current figures ranging from 30,000 to 60,000 per year, but to date there is no system or survey in place to provide accurate information about the success of sperm donation.

Still, as with every form of fertility treatment, it's important to know what you're getting into so you can make the right decision for you and your body.

BUSTED

Myth: If I use a sperm donor, my child will have hundreds of siblings.

Sperm banks do not have to inform you whether your child has any half siblings (also known as donor siblings) resulting from other people using the same sperm donor as you. But if this is a concern for you, you can find a bank that will limit how many times a donor's sperm can be used or ensure that one donor's sperm isn't given to two people who live in the same region. You can also find resources like the Donor Sibling Registry, where you can see if your selected donor's sperm has already led to successful pregnancies.

Remember that it's not necessarily a bad thing for your child to have donor siblings. Many children conceived with donated sperm choose to meet their siblings and develop meaningful relationships with them.

Legal Issues and Considerations

Parental Rights

In most states, sperm donors who make their donation anonymously through a sperm bank or clinic waive their parental rights. If their sperm is used, they receive no information about the people who used it. And if a child is born, in most cases, donors have no legal right to know about the child.

Where parental rights can get difficult is if you use a donor you know and make arrangements on your own, without the help of a sperm bank or clinic. Without a written legal contract in which your donor agrees to relinquish his parental rights, he will be the legal father of the child, which could impact child support, custody, inheritance, and citizenship. In these cases, you will want to work with an attorney and file paperwork stating that the donor relinquishes his parental rights.

Tucker strongly advises against giving a known donor a parental role, even if you have a written agreement about parental rights. "Even if you set everything up right at the outset, you can destroy all your hard work by letting the donor take on a parental role in the child's life," she says. "It's fine to have contact with a known donor—after all, that's why many parents chose known donation—but it's not acceptable to let him act as a father figure." This can set a legal precedent that's difficult to undo. Dean Hutchison, the director of legal services at Circle Surrogacy and Egg Donation in Boston, advises, "The legal issue is always that of parentage. You want to make sure you are following proper procedure to fully insulate yourself from a parentage challenge by the donor. Some states will have statutory schemes to follow—others, you just use best practices like having a written agreement and doing procedures in medical offices."

WARRIOR TIPS
Getting Information
••••••••••••••••••••••••••••••••••••

When you work with a sperm bank or clinic, the donors go through medical screening before giving their sample. If a donor develops a medical issue later in life, it could be necessary for you to know about it in order to determine whether your child is at risk. But not all sperm banks have a system in place to convey this information. When considering the source of your sperm donation, ask if there's a way to access updated medical information. Also, find out how your and the donor's anonymity is protected in these situations.

A single mother by choice, Cassie was trying to use a friend as a sperm donor. "During the process of trying to conceive by hooking up with this friend," she explains, "I learned that it's quite difficult to prevent the friend from coming for parental rights in the future, which is not something I wanted to be an option for my donor. I decided to stop using my friend, and switched to using a donor sperm bank."

If you are using a sperm bank, Tucker advises that you understand your parental rights from the beginning by going over the service agreement with your attorney. "Sperm banks are businesses," she reminds us. "They have lawyers working for them who write these agreements to protect the sperm banks."

Establishing Legal Parentage

When using a donor, you or your partner—if you have one—will not be a biological parent. In many states, this will not matter, and you will be recognized as legal parents. However, some situations can complicate things.

For couples, for example, if you move to a state with different laws or get divorced, the nonbiological partner might lose parental rights. The same is possible if the biological parent passes away; the nonbiological parent may lose custody of your child. Consult a lawyer about how this could impact you and ways to protect yourself in your state.

While it might take extra steps and money to ensure that you or your partner are always recognized as your child's parents, regardless of biology, it can be a good idea for the nonbiological parent to formally adopt the child. Tucker says this provides an extra level of legal protection and avoids legal issues later on.

Fresh Sperm Donations

One advantage of using a fresh sperm sample is an increased number of viable sperm cells. According to Dr. Rodgers, usually half of the frozen sperm do not survive the thawing process. But unless your chosen donor already has a low sperm count—which would be extremely unlikely when you're working with sperm banks or clinics, which screen for sperm health—this is rarely an issue.

BUSTED

Myth: My child will favor his or her biological parent over the nonbiological parent.

Many people who use sperm or egg donors worry that their child will prefer their biological parent over their nonbiological parent. This is not the case. Sometimes children seem to connect more deeply with one parent than another; sometimes they do not; sometimes they do and then switch, forging a stronger connection with their other parent. This happens in all kinds of child-parent relationships, whether they are biological or not. Genetics play no part in this behavior. It's simply what happens as children and parents grow and evolve.

If you want to use fresh sperm, you'll likely need to know the donor. Sperm banks offer only frozen sperm due to the required 6-month waiting period to test the donor for infectious diseases and the high-volume nature of the business.

Alicia used her husband's brother's sperm. "It helped ease the blow of realizing we wouldn't have a biological child together. It would be as close to a biological child as we could get. We would know his medical history, and his family history would be the same as if we had conceived with my husband's sperm."

However, even though it was an easy choice, it wasn't without potential pitfalls. But in Alicia's case, it worked out in the end. "Even with what could be seen as [the] complicated nature of using a relative as a sperm donor, it felt right and we were lucky."

Frozen Sperm Donations

After it's collected, soon-to-be frozen sperm is stored in a vial with a solution that prevents crystallization from damaging the cells. It is then stored in subzero conditions until it is ready to be used.

If you are purchasing a frozen sperm sample from a sperm bank, it will be shipped to you and can stay frozen and viable for several days—or your fertility clinic can store it in its freezer indefinitely, as long as you continue paying storage fees. Depending on your location and the sperm bank you use, you could face shipping fees. The overall cost of the sample varies depending on the source but ranges between $300 and $4,000. The difference in price tends to depend on the amount of additional screening the sperm bank puts donors through.

If you're planning to get your frozen sample from a sperm bank, do your research about different financial options. Some banks have additional fees if you want more information about your donor. There can also be variations in price for washed versus unwashed sperm. If cost is an issue, some sperm banks have buy-back programs where you can return unused frozen samples and get part of your money back.

Melinda from New York says her sperm donor cycle was very easy. She used a sperm bank located blocks from her fertility clinic, so the frozen sperm was sent via messenger rather than shipped. "The fertility clinic has to have your source of sperm before your IVF cycle starts," she advises. "But as soon as the sperm came, I was ready to go! It was actually very exciting to have that piece all sorted out. The outcome is that I have three beautiful children from that same sample of sperm."

A Donated Sperm Cycle with Intracervical Insemination (ICI)

With intracervical insemination (ICI), the sperm sample is deposited inside the vagina but on the outside of the cervix, similar to intercourse. Often, you'll have to stay lying on your back for about 20 minutes to give the sperm time to enter through the cervix. You may also need to insert a small medical sponge into your vagina, as close to your cervix as possible, and leave it there for 2 to 3 hours. This increases the odds that the semen will stay in place.

Many people choose ICI because the necessary sperm sample and procedure are less expensive than other options. The procedure can also be performed at home without the aid or cost of a doctor.

However, ICI is generally less successful than other methods. The sperm still need to make it into the uterus and fallopian tubes for fertilization. If your sperm sample was frozen and then thawed, the sperm are less motile and have a shorter life span, and other methods, which insert the sperm closer to the egg, can be more successful.

ICI vs. IUI PREGNANCY SUCCESS RATES AFTER 6 CYCLES	
	RESULTING PREGNANCIES
Intracervical insemination (ICI)	37.9%
Intrauterine insemination (IUI)	40.5%

Source: Kop, PAL, M. van Wely, B.W. Mol et al. "Intrauterine Insemination or Intracervical Insemination with Cryopreserved Donor Sperm in the Natural Cycle: A Cohort Study," *Human Reproduction* 30, No. 3 (March 2015): 603–7. https://doi.org /10.1093/humrep/dev004.

the washed sample is prepared, your doctor will place the sperm directly into your uterus using a catheter and speculum.

While success rates are higher with IUI than with ICI, it can cost four times as much as ICI. You will have to weigh whether the increased chance of getting pregnant outweighs the price. (You can learn more about IUI in chapter 6.)

A Donated Sperm Cycle with Intrauterine Insemination (IUI)

With IUI, the sperm first goes through a washing process. This removes seminal fluid that can cause cramping when introduced to the uterus. The sample is also often spun to separate healthy sperm from less viable cells. Once

A Donated Sperm Cycle with IVF

With in vitro fertilization (IVF), the eggs can be yours (fresh or frozen) or from a donor. The process itself is similar to other IVF cycles—likely using ICSI, especially if your sperm sample is frozen.

While IVF success rates are good, the process is extremely expensive. In most cases, one cycle of IVF will cost ten times more than IUI—and that does not include the price of obtaining your donated sperm sample.

ICI vs IUI vs. IVF CONSIDERATIONS			
	ICI	**IUI**	**IVF**
Success rates	38% resulted in pregnancy after six cycles.*	41% resulted in pregnancy after six cycles.*	In 2019, 54% of transfers resulted in a live birth when a fresh egg was used, and 46% resulted in a live birth when a frozen egg was used.**
Invasiveness of procedure	Can be performed at home. Sperm is deposited in the vagina just outside the cervix.	Must be performed by a doctor. Sperm is deposited in the uterus.	Must be performed by a doctor. The embryo is deposited in the uterus. Might require you to do an egg retrieval if you're not using a donor egg.
Overall cost factors	Largest cost is the sperm itself.	Can cost four times more than ICI.	Can cost ten times more than IUI.

*Source: Kop, PAL, M. van Wely, B.W. Mol et al., "Intrauterine Insemination or Intracervical Insemination with Cryopreserved Donor Sperm in the Natural Cycle: A Cohort Study," *Human Reproduction* 30, No. 3 (March 2015): 603–7. https://doi.org/10.1093/humrep/dev004.

**Source: Centers for Disease Control and Prevention, "2019 Assisted Reproductive Technology Fertility Clinic and National Summary Report," 2021, online.

Using Donor Embryos

Donated or adopted embryos are a great example of how people in the infertility community support one another. Donated embryos are an option only because some infertility warriors understand how difficult it can be to have a child, so if they have remaining embryos, they pay it forward and help other people start a family.

BUSTED ═══════════════════════

Myth: If I have a child using a donated embryo, the biological parents will always be a threat.

Especially with known donors, you may worry that the biological parents will compete for your child's love. This is completely untrue. People do not take donating embryos lightly. They've decided their family is complete and want to give someone else the gift of a child.

Most donors just want to know that the child will be taken care of and don't want any more contact. What's important is working out an agreement that everyone is happy with.

For some infertility warriors, like Maya from California, it is important to have an open relationship with the donors. But, as she points out, many people don't think this is an option. "There isn't enough education around embryo donation, so patients often feel unsure about their rights or what the relationship with another family might be. Some people assume it's just better to keep everyone separate."

If you'd like to have a relationship with the donor, for yourself and your child, Maya recommends counseling and solid communication. "With the right support, everyone can move forward in a relationship that feels comfortable for all."

Because this fertility treatment involves viable embryos, there may be some ethical and moral distinctions that you will want to explore.

Embryo Donation vs. Adopted Embryos

Medically speaking, there is no difference between a donated embryo and an adopted one. The difference comes in how both the donor and recipient view embryos.

Fertility clinics and organizations that offer donated embryos approach the process the same way they do with donated eggs or sperm. In most cases, once the donor has given the embryos, they are done. As with sperm and egg donations, the donor may agree to be open to meeting the child in the future, but often the donor receives no information about the recipients.

Organizations that offer embryo adoption usually do so based on their belief that life begins at conception. From that perspective, the process of receiving an embryo is similar to that of adopting a child. In this case, donors may play a bigger part in deciding who can use their embryos and frequently want to meet the recipients before agreeing. Also, many organizations require more than a medical screening; potential recipients may be required to go through home inspections or to be of a certain religion.

To avoid confusion and for the sake of consistency, the rest of this chapter will refer to embryo donation rather than embryo adoption.

Legal Issues and Considerations

Because donated embryos come from other forms of fertility treatments, the legal issues are more complicated. Before deciding to use a donated embryo, be sure to discuss all your options with an attorney who specializes in family law.

Transferring Ownership

In most cases, donated embryos are remaining embryos from another person's fertility treatment. But depending on how those embryos were created, you might have to go through extra steps to acquire parental rights. Here are some things to know:

• **Frozen embryos from IVF.** Most often, couples use their own eggs and sperm to create and freeze embryos for use with IVF. They later decide to donate the embryos they aren't going to use. Depending on your state, you might need to have very specific legal paperwork showing a couple completely released their parental rights.

• **Embryos from donated eggs.** When a person donates her eggs to another person, there is often a legal agreement in place between her and the original recipient. Make sure that the preexisting agreement allows for the embryos to be donated to a new recipient.

• **Embryos from known sperm or egg donors.** Sometimes people receive egg or sperm donations from a close friend or family member. While that donor was willing to have someone they know raise a child with their genetic material, they may not want anyone else to. If there was a preexisting legal agreement, make sure it allows for the resulting embryo to be donated to a new recipient. If there was no legal agreement, have one drawn up.

Kelli says, "The longest part of the process was getting approval to travel to the embryos and become a patient at the clinic where the embryos were created, which took a month. Once approved, there was another round of clinic paperwork to complete, additional test, and then we traveled to Virginia Beach, Virginia, for our first embryo transfer, resulting in the birth of our son, Trevor. The total time from my infertility diagnosis to Trevor's birth was 18 months."

Reimbursing Donors

It is illegal to sell or buy embryos in the United States. If any clinic or medical facility says they are selling you embryos, they are not a reputable organization.

However, donors are typically reimbursed for certain aspects of the embryo donation process. For instance, you might be required to pay for the donor's legal fees or preservation costs. Don't forget to take into account what the donor originally paid to create the embryos. However, if their insurance covered most aspects of the process, they can't receive reimbursements that lead to a profit.

Contact with the Donor

With embryo donations, there are two people out there who are full biological parents for your child. Some embryo recipients see this as a plus; if your child has questions about their genetic family, the biological parents are available for answers. In some cases, knowing your embryo donors might even allow your kid to have a relationship with biological family. But other recipients think involving the donors in their child's life is too complicated or problematic.

Donating an embryo is a great gift. But that does not entitle the donor to any right to have contact with your child without your consent. You get to decide, and your attorney will help you draft a contract to lay out an agreement with the donor. Never enter into a legal agreement if you're not comfortable with it. Even if, for example, the donor says they just want the option to contact the child, stand your ground if that's not something *you* want. If you can't reach an agreement, don't be afraid to look for another donor.

Kelli and her husband, Dan, wanted an open embryo donation where they could know their donor family and vice versa. "This was in the best interest of any future children who would have questions," Kelli says. "If Dan and I couldn't answer their questions, then they would have the additional resource of their donor family."

A Donor Embryo Cycle

The process of using a donor embryo is similar to the standard frozen embryo transfer process. You'll take medication to create an ideal environment for implantation in your uterus. Then, once your body is ready, the embryos will be thawed and transferred into your uterus via a catheter.

Unfortunately, as is the chance with any frozen embryos, there's a small chance that donated embryos will not be viable once thawed. If this happens, you will most likely not be able to recoup any of the fees you paid.

At most fertility clinics, using a donated embryo costs between $2,500 and $4,000, but some services with higher standards for accepting donations can be more than $10,000. Still, using a donated embryo is less expensive than a normal IVF cycle because the egg retrieval, fertilization, and blastocyst development have already occurred.

in—transferring more than one embryo. The hope is that by transferring more than one, the chance of at least one of the embryos implanting is greater. But it's always possible for more than one embryo to begin gestating in your uterus—especially if the donor was younger than 25.

Carrying multiple fetuses at once can put a lot of stress on a body, which can lead to a higher-risk pregnancy. In some cases, you might be encouraged to terminate one or more of the fetuses in order to carry a healthy one to term. Seriously consider what you would do in this situation before transferring multiple donated embryos. Then you'll have a clear game plan if complications arise. (For more on the risks of multiples, see chapter 9.)

It's also important to note that the ASRM and SART recommend that the number of embryos transferred should be limited to one in most cases, especially for patients younger than 37. This decision was based on data from a 2017 report showing an increased risk of complications for women carrying multiples.

2019 PREGNANCY SUCCESS RATES

	RESULTING IN LIVE BIRTH
Fresh donated eggs	53.9%
Frozen donated eggs	45.8%
Frozen donated embryos	48.8%

Source: Centers for Disease Control and Prevention, "2019 Assisted Reproductive Technology Fertility Clinic and National Summary Report," 2021, online.

CHANCE OF MULTIPLES WITH DONOR EMBRYOS

	LIVE BIRTHS PER THAW RESULTING IN TWINS	LIVE BIRTHS PER THAW RESULTING IN TRIPLETS OR MORE
All transfers	4.5%	0.2%
Single embryo transfers	0.4%	0%
Double embryo transfers	14.5%	0.3%
Triple+ embryo transfers	12%	8%

Source: Centers for Disease Control and Prevention, "2019 Assisted Reproductive Technology Fertility Clinic and National Summary Report," 2021, online.

Risk of Multiples

We talked about this in chapter 9, but as a reminder, when you are using donated embryos, your reproductive endocrinologist may suggest—or you might be interested

Talking to Your Child

In the past, families sometimes thought it would be best not to tell their children if they were conceived through an egg, sperm, or embryo donation. That's no longer the case, however. As a general rule, researchers now agree, it's best to be honest with children about how they came into a family. ASRM released a formal statement about it in 2013, saying (in very stiff language): "While ultimately the choice of the recipient parent, disclosure to donor-conceived persons of the use of donor gametes or embryos in their conception is strongly encouraged."

A 2017 article in *Human Reproduction* by Susan Golombok, a professor of family research and director of the Centre for Family Research at the University of Cambridge, dug into the current research about telling children that they were conceived by donors. In her conclusion she writes, "As the research that exists so far suggests neutral or positive psychological consequences from disclosure, and possible psychological harm from non-disclosure, this leads to the conclusion—based on empirical evidence rather than an implicit moral judgement—that it is generally better to tell."

In terms of how to talk to your child about it, ASRM recommends the following approach:

- Begin the conversation early, so that the story of how your child came to be seems, to them, to have always been a part of their personal history. Waiting until your child is older to tell them about it can damage the bonds of trust they have with you.

- Explain the details in a loving context.

- Use age-appropriate language.

- Allow the child to have his or her own feelings, no matter what they are.

- Leave the door open for questions throughout the child's life.

- Do not ask the child to keep the information secret; the implication of a secret means something is wrong and can create shame.

When talking to your child about their origins, Maria T. Rothenburger, a psychotherapist who specializes in infertility at Miracles Happen Fertility Center in Salem, Oregon, stresses the importance of the child understanding the general concepts underlying their conception and not feeling like they are out of the ordinary. "Age-appropriate disclosure is essential, if a family [decides to talk about it]," she says. "A healthy discussion with family is a great place to start, so the child grows up feeling the normalcy of how they were conceived."

Also, understand that it's natural for children to be curious about their donor. When they ask questions about how they were conceived, they're not looking for a reason to love you less. Parents who support their child's curiosity tend to have better relationships with their child. In fact, a 2015 report from the *Journal of Reproductive and Infant Psychology* found that when parents were open and positive about their child's IVF conception, it correlated to a better-quality relationship.

Nichole plans to start sharing the facts of her child's conception from the beginning. "I don't want to wait for some big 'reveal.' I want it to be something they always know about themselves—no secrets or shame. I will tell them that we wanted them so badly, but that we didn't have all the parts we needed to build them, so a nice lady 'helper' gave us some of her eggs."

Hillary's son, who was conceived via a sperm donor, is only a year old, so they haven't had a conversation about it just yet. But she thinks telling him stories that represent different kinds of families is important. "We have some books that we will read as he gets older that represent his family, like *The Pea That Was Me* and *Mommy Chose Me*. We also have *What Makes a Baby* to explain that babies are made in different ways. I expect that it will not be a one-time conversation but a natural process of telling him his story."

No matter what your decision about how much to disclose to your child, know that with some donation banks, a child has the legal right to basic information about their donor once they turn 18. Keep this in mind when choosing where to get your donated sperm, eggs, or embryos.

Identifying Your Needs

If you are faced with losing a genetic connection with your child, think about what the link means to you. What are your current assumptions about how that impacts who you could be as a parent? Are you worried your child will have a harder time relating to you? Will it be hard to look at your child and not see any of your features? Are you afraid your child will feel there's a hole in their life because they don't know their biological parent(s)?

Once you've figured out how *you* believe genetics impact parenting, think about what you need in order to let go of those assumptions. In its most basic form, parenting is about simply loving and nurturing your child. Some infertility warriors focus on what their parents did to make them feel loved and safe as a child because it reinforces that behaviors and relationships, not genetics, create great parents.

Sarah-Jayne from Kent, United Kingdom, drives this message home. "Nothing beats becoming a parent. No matter how your baby got there, they become yours and only yours. The moment they are in your arms, whose genes they are become irrelevant. They are yours."

Communicating Your Needs

Communication is the foundation of an infertility journey involving donors. You will have countless conversations with your partner, support team, attorney, and doctor about your preferences and wishes. If you don't communicate your needs, your journey will be rougher. Keeping quiet will just cause more stress.

To hone your communication skills, start by expressing your needs about smaller aspects of your life unrelated to fertility. For example, say you need to go to the grocery store. How can your partner or others in your life help with that? You can ask your partner to make a grocery list. You can ask a friend to recommend a new recipe. You can ask your mom if she's heard of any stores that are having two-for-one specials. Of course, you can successfully buy groceries without any help, but it gets you into the habit of telling people what support you'd like them to offer.

Angela found support in her spouse, Adam, and several online communities.

"My husband was a rock for me," she shares. "He always reassured me that if we didn't have kids, it was OK and we would find other interests and hobbies. He never pressured me or made me feel like I wasn't enough."

WARRIOR TIPS
Find Support

Emma from Ohio admits that she found the sperm donation process isolating. "Your partner is struggling, and so are you. You can't talk about it with anyone except him out of respect for his privacy, but you are just falling apart and have nowhere to turn."

She advises people to find support outside of their partners. "You need each other," she explains, "but you also need to have another outlet."

Emma met someone through a RESOLVE support group online. "We began emailing because our stories were so similar, and she also was going through the donor sperm process. We quickly became friends— even though we lived in different states! We relied on each other a lot through our journeys."

Other sources of support include Parents Via Egg Donation, Donor Conception Network, and the Embryo Adoption and Donation Support Group on Facebook.

Throughout this chapter, we've seen tips and tricks to help you work through the tough choices and logistics of using donors. But now let's look a big-picture issue that pains many infertility warriors: the fact that you need to use a donor in the first place. It means losing a genetic link to your child. When you first started dreaming about your family, that wasn't part of the picture. Take the time to work through your feelings surrounding your loss.

Dr. Davidson advises that you seek out counseling. "[Losing a genetic link to your child] takes time, both to absorb and then to adjust to what it means. Don't rush into it," she says. "For couples, it is best to be sure you are on the same page. This won't work out well if the partner losing a genetic link feels coerced or if either partner is too uncomfortable with the idea."

Melinda came to terms with needing a donor quickly, as she was anxious about her age. "I knew that I would have to consider any option that made motherhood a reality for me. I do not think that children are 'ours' just based on genetic material. Additionally, my IVF doctor made it seem very normal. She took away a lot of the stigma for me and allowed me to see that it was just a means to an end, nothing more."

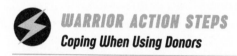

WARRIOR ACTION STEPS
Coping When Using Donors

When it comes to making it through tough times, you can take a few simple steps to minimize the pain and process your emotions. If donor sperm, eggs, or embryos are part of your journey, be sure to:

- **Play the "Worst-Case Scenario" game.** If you're a fan of the television show *This Is Us*, you're familiar with the Worst-Case Scenario game that the characters Randall and Beth, a married couple, play when they're facing a stressful situation. They simply say all their worst, most ridiculous fears out loud, without interruption or rebuttal. Do the same. If you're worried your child will run off and join the circus because they learn their sperm donor knew how to juggle, vocalize that fear. There's something about saying and hearing the words that's cathartic and takes away the power of your worries.

- **Meet a donor.** Have coffee with someone who has donated eggs, sperm, or an embryo.

Choose someone who is not in consideration to be *your* donor and pick their brain. Ask why they decided to donate, how it's impacted their life, if they'd do it again, and so on. Hearing the other side of the situation will help you better understand the road before you.

- **Write a letter to your future child.** Put down on paper your hopes and dreams for your child. Describe what you wish they'd look like and what their interests would be. Write about your relationship and the memories you want to make. After a day or 2, reread the letter. This will help you identify your preferences when choosing a donor and show you where you do and don't have control over shaping who your child is, regardless of genetics.

→

WARRIOR WISDOM
Don't Overthink

"We looked at it this way: We were getting ONE CELL from someone else, one cell from my husband, and all the rest from my body as I grew the baby. So while I didn't provide the egg or DNA, I was able to provide a huge part of my son." — Angela, Ontario, Canada

WARRIOR CHECKLIST
Using Donor Eggs, Sperm, and Embryos

❑ Understand what it's really like to use donated eggs, sperm, and embryos and the fertility treatment options available.

❑ Identify what traits you're looking for in a donor and what type of relationship you want with them.

❑ Consider all the different factors that can help determine your choice of where to obtain donated eggs, sperm, and embryos.

❑ Be aware of the legal pitfalls of using donated eggs, sperm, and embryos.

❑ Know what you need to consider before hiring an attorney to help you on your journey.

❑ Practice coping techniques that help you identify and communicate your needs so you get the support you need.

Add more items to your Warrior Checklist or jot down any notes here:

_____

_____

_____

_____

_____

_____

_____

_____

_____

_____

_____

_____

_____

Surrogacy 101

AT THE AGE OF 16, NANCY FROM Massachusetts was diagnosed with Mayer-Rokitansky-Küster-Hauser (MRKH) syndrome (see the appendix). From that moment on, she lived with the knowledge that she would never be able to carry a child. As a result, she and her husband, Tom, started a "baby savings fund" immediately after they were married. When they were ready to build a family, they decided to pursue surrogacy.

"Before moving forward with gestational surrogacy, you need to be emotionally prepared to trust the woman who will assist you," Nancy says. "It is not easy, but the carriers are looking to help, and you must be ready to accept that help with an open heart and all the gratitude you can give."

Nancy and Tom have two kids—now teenagers—born via two different surrogates. Nancy describes the process as rewarding for all—but not without its challenges. Both of her surrogates didn't immediately get pregnant, and each carrier went through multiple rounds of IVF. "You are not only experiencing the ups and downs, negative test results, positive results, et cetera, with yourself and your spouse, but also with your carrier. It is important to consider her feelings along the way, and important to seek support for yourself from loved ones."

Once the treatments worked, however, the pregnancies were, as Nancy says, "like a dream."

She stayed in constant contact with her carriers and attended their doctor appointments whenever possible. She particularly enjoyed shopping for baby items so she could feel more involved with the pregnancy.

That dream took on a different feeling when the due date arrived. "Seeing someone else in agony to help you is very difficult. My husband and I felt lost to some degree," she explains. She wasn't sure what she should do to help. "We just kept providing support, back rubs, offering ice chips, and pacing the hospital halls."

She recommends having an open and honest relationship with your gestational carrier from day 1. "We are very lucky in that we have a great relationship and see each other often, even years after the journey ended."

In the end, Nancy and Tom were very happy with both of their surrogacy experiences. She says, "I would not have my two miracles if not for the unselfish and giving women who helped us. Words cannot accurately describe how thankful we are to our carriers for making our dream come true!"

Surrogacy may not be right for everyone, but if you or your partner are unable to successfully carry a child to term, it can be a wonderful option. As with any path to pregnancy, it's important to start from a place of openness and willingness to research the pros and cons of the method you choose.

Traditional Surrogacy vs. Gestational Surrogacy

There are two ways to involve surrogates with building your family: traditional surrogacy and gestational surrogacy. With traditional surrogacy, the gestational carrier—commonly known as the surrogate—is also the biological mother of the child. It is her egg that gets fertilized via artificial insemination. She carries the child to term, and after giving birth, she gives the baby to the intended parent(s).

With gestational surrogacy, the gestational carrier is impregnated through IVF with the intended mother's egg, a donated egg, or a donated embryo. The surrogate is not genetically related to the child. After giving birth, she gives the baby to the intended parent(s).

One method is not inherently better than the other, but gestational surrogacy is currently much more common than traditional surrogacy. This may be because traditional surrogacy carries additional legal and emotional complexities. After all, the carrier agrees to become pregnant with a fetus that is biologically hers, carries the child, and then gives him or her to another parent. Also, traditional surrogacy agreements are not legally recognized in every state. Thanks to advances in IVF, gestational surrogacy mostly avoids these issues.

For the sake of simplicity, this chapter will focus on *gestational* surrogacy. The terms *surrogate* and *gestational carrier* will be used interchangeably, but with the understanding that the gestational surrogate is *not* biologically related to the child she carries.

Before we get started, below is a quick snapshot of things to consider with traditional versus gestational surrogacy:

TRADITIONAL vs. GESTATIONAL SURROGACY CONSIDERATIONS		
	TRADITIONAL	**GESTATIONAL**
Genetic factors	The gestational carrier's egg is fertilized, making her biologically related to the child.	The gestational carrier is not biologically related to the child. The embryo is formed using the gametes of the intended parents or of separate donors.
Legal standing	Not every state allows traditional surrogacy, especially when gestational surrogacy is an option.	Most—although definitely not all—state laws are in favor of gestational surrogacy.
Medical procedures	Typically, the surrogate is impregnated using artificial insemination (IUI).	The gestational carrier is impregnated using IVF.
Costs	Tends to be less expensive because the medical procedures are less invasive. There typically is no egg retrieval. However, you will still have to cover legal fees, compensate the surrogate, reimburse her for her pregnancy-related costs, and pay for her medical procedures. Depending on your agreement, the total could be between $50,000 and $100,000.	Cost depends on a variety of factors, including agency fees, number of IVF cycles, and whether or not you need to use donated eggs, sperm, or embryos. But on average, the process costs $100,000 to $200,000.

Legal Issues and Considerations

Surrogacy can be a wonderful journey to parenthood, but it can also be legally complicated. Laws and regulations can vary greatly from country to country and even state to state. The journey of a friend or acquaintance will not necessarily be your own, so due diligence is of the utmost importance, not to mention getting as much information and guarantees as you can in writing.

Location

Start your research during the early stages of your surrogacy journey so you know what you're up against legally—and location may have the biggest impact. Make sure you understand what the law requires in your state (and possibly in your gestational carrier's state) from the very beginning.

In agreements for what is called compassionate or altruistic surrogacy, the carrier is reimbursed only for direct expenses. In compensated surrogacy agreements, on the other hand, the carrier is compensated for her time and effort in carrying the child in addition to being reimbursed for direct expenses. Laws governing both vary by state. At the time of this writing, Michigan, for example, under the Michigan Surrogate Parenting Act, does not allow compensated surrogacy, and parents who enter agreements other than compassionate or altruistic surrogacy are subject to criminal penalties. (Thankfully, Michigan is one of only a handful of states with such strict anti-surrogacy laws.)

Each surrogacy agreement needs to be created in accordance with the laws of the state in which the surrogacy is happening. Depending on the state, this could mean that you or your carrier needs to temporarily relocate in the days leading up to the birth to a state where surrogacy is legally recognized, which can be an inconvenience for your surrogate and adds to your total costs.

Also, consider how location will impact your surrogacy experience. If your surrogate doesn't live near you, you might have to choose between traveling to doctor appointments or getting updates via video chat and phone calls.

Jen from New York had regular contact with her carrier, including weekly video calls and text messaging. "She had me on speaker phone for all medical appointments. We went to one appointment in person to meet the doctor. We felt very connected to her and what was happening."

She advises putting in the time to communicate regularly with your carrier—and being prepared for the mixed emotions you will experience at various times during the process. "Though you will be excited, you possibly will also have periods of fear, anxiety, sadness, and grief," she recalls. "I think many intended parents aren't prepared for uncomfortable feelings during the pregnancy, as they just want to be excited and positive. However, it is all part of their process, and it's okay to have some sadness."

To better understand the surrogacy laws in your state, Surrogate.com and ASRM.org are great places to start. You should also consult a reproductive attorney.

Finding an Attorney

No surrogacy agreement should be entered into without the assistance of an experienced attorney. Stephanie Brinkley, an assisted reproduction technology attorney at Brinkley Law Firm in Charleston, South Carolina, recommends that you start looking for an attorney as soon as you decide a gestational carrier is right for you. "[Having an attorney] will allow you to make an informed decision about factors like finding a gestational carrier and understanding standard compensation values for their state," she says.

Given that each state's laws are different, it's important that you find someone who is experienced with not only reproductive law but also surrogacy law specifically, and more specifically, surrogacy law in your state. Both you and your surrogate will need legal representation that can help with the following steps:

- Drafting a surrogacy contract that outlines responsibilities, expectations, and compensation

- Filing a pre-birth order that establishes you as the legal parent once the child is born

- Navigating legal situations like procuring donated eggs, sperm, or embryos

Shawn Kane, executive director of American Surrogacy and American Adoptions in Overland Park, Kansas, encourages intended parents to interview prospective attorneys so they can be sure they have a good fit. "Look for attorneys who have years of experience, can work with you where you live, are transparent about their fee schedule, and provide the sort of attention and support you are looking for as an intended parent," he says.

Reproductive law attorneys have a unique understanding of the complicated issues involved with gestational surrogacy, including even factors that don't relate to the law.

Through their years of experience, they will have navigated the legal side but also come into contact with other specialists and resources that can help you on your journey.

Melissa B. Brisman, a reproductive law attorney based in Montvale, New Jersey, points out that your attorney should be able to help you with questions about finding a carrier or managing associated funds. "Prospective parents will find it useful and financially efficient to hire an attorney who has developed contacts in the industry and can connect them to an escrow agency, an insurance agent, and a [surrogacy] agency," she says. "This type of 'one stop shopping' can be invaluable in reducing the stress and uncertainty that a prospective parent may encounter."

BUSTED

Myth: I'll be a bystander during a surrogate pregnancy.

There are a lot of milestones during pregnancy. The first maternity outfit. The first kick. The baby showers. When you're not the one who is pregnant, you can feel left out of these important moments.

But if these rituals are important to you, work them into your surrogacy agreement. You can ask to attend childbirth classes and doctor appointments with your gestational carrier. Just because you don't have the physical experiences yourself doesn't mean you can't be an active part of the journey. For Jen, whose gestational carrier lived across the country, even the distance couldn't disconnect her from the pregnancy.

"Our experience was wonderful. It was easier than expected," she shares. "Of course, it would have been nice to have been present for some more appointments and spend more time with her while pregnant, but we had great communication and I felt very much connected to the pregnancy."

WARRIOR TIPS
Your Child's Citizenship
• •

Any child born in the United States has American citizenship, no matter their parents' nationality. Typically, a child with foreign nationals for parents also gains the citizenship of their parents' country. However, this is not guaranteed if you have a child via surrogacy, which could mean your parental rights might not be recognized in your home country.

If it's important for you and your child to have the same citizenship, consult with an experienced surrogacy lawyer to get a sound understanding of the surrogacy laws in your home country. This will help you prepare for any issues before trying to travel back to your home country with your child.

Insurance Coverage for the Gestational Carrier

Chances are that your health-care insurance will not cover any medical expenses for your gestational carrier. (Although you should still check! You never know.) In most surrogacy agreements, you will be responsible for health-care costs. This includes the carrier's premiums and co-pays for any treatments related to the pregnancy.

Depending on what type of insurance your carrier has, it might be more affordable for you to purchase supplemental coverage or a completely different policy for her, rather than paying her medical costs out of pocket. Due to the restrictions of enrollment periods, this path could impact how long you have to wait before beginning the pregnancy.

When choosing insurance options, be mindful of the following factors:

• **Cost.** If purchased through the US Affordable Care Act, gestational carrier policies can cost $10,000 to $15,000—and that's before out-of-network health-care payments. Another option is a surrogate maternity liability insurance plan. These are more expensive; they start

at around $25,000 for gestational carriers with a single child and $42,000 for those carrying twins.

• **Using the surrogate's own insurance.** Your surrogate may be able to use her own health insurance plan to cover some of the costs. But even so, remember that her insurance can change if she changes jobs or her employer changes the plan.

• **Possible complications.** Even healthy gestational carriers can have complications, so don't choose a plan that just covers the pregnancy basics. This can leave you on the hook for expensive medical procedures if they become necessary.

• **Coverage for the baby.** You'll need to make arrangements so that once the child is born, they are under your insurance, not the surrogate's.

Discuss your options with your attorney *and* your surrogate so you can legally obtain the best coverage for your situation.

BUSTED

Myth: A gestational carrier will abuse our financial support.

Aside from the medical costs, a gestational carrier is often given allowances and stipends to compensate her for pregnancy expenses, time, and energy. Sometimes, intended parents worry that the money they're spending is being used inappropriately.

In most cases, the surrogate's compensation goes into an escrow account. This means that an objective third-party ensures that all the money is used appropriately.

Gestational Carrier Options

At this point, things get real and you need to begin looking for a carrier. In general, there are three sources to turn to:

• **Independent carrier.** Someone not already known to you whom you find without the assistance of an agency

• **Surrogacy agency.** An agency whose mission is to match you with a surrogate who meets your needs, while offering other support, like scheduling medical procedures or counseling

• **Known carrier.** Someone you know who has agreed to serve as your gestational carrier

Independent Carrier

Using an independent gestational carrier can make the process less expensive, but there are considerably greater risks without the guidance, support, or vetting authority of an agency.

Chrissy from Maryland posted on Facebook that she and her husband, Lee, were looking for an "extreme babysitter." Eighteen people shared their post. At a gathering, a friend of a friend casually offered to be their carrier.

"I didn't believe her at first," Chrissy recalls, "but then we scheduled a dinner with her and her spouse, talked about it, and agreed."

Before Chrissy and Lee found their eventual carrier, they had tried various Facebook groups and "classifieds" sites. They even video chatted with several prospects and were tentatively matched with someone from another state. "The week before we were planning to drive to meet her is when the friend of a friend offered, so we canceled our trip," Chrissy says.

Kelly and her husband, Tom, from Michigan unfortunately live in a state where there are no surrogacy agencies. Especially in these situations, she agrees with Chrissy—start with social networks and social media.

Here are some additional things to take into consideration with independent carriers:

• **The carrier.** An independent carrier does not work through an agency. All agreements are made independently through lawyers—one for you and one for the carrier. It is not uncommon for an independent carrier to have done previous surrogacies.

• **Finding your carrier.** Sometimes your lawyer or fertility clinic can help you connect with independent gestational carriers. If your attorney is familiar with surrogacy law (and they should be), they might already know someone who is interested in becoming an independent surrogate. Your clinic can screen the carrier, arrange for you to meet to check compatibility, and care for her medical needs during the IVF cycle.

• **Relationship with your carrier.** It is up to you and the independent carrier to come to terms about what your relationship will be like.

• **Cost.** Costs depend on the agreement you reach, but in general, you will pay for all medical procedures (which can start at $25,000), doctor appointments, legal guidance (around $3,000), and compensation for the gestational carrier (depending on their experience, this can come to $40,000 to $70,000, plus reimbursement for pregnancy-related expenses).

Surrogacy Agency

An agency is constantly looking for potential carriers, and reputable agencies follow strict guidelines when evaluating them. According to Surrogate.com, typical qualifications to be a surrogate include:

• Age between 21 and 40 years old, with at least one previous successful pregnancy

• No diseases that could be passed to the child during gestation

• No serious health issues during a previous pregnancy

• A healthy weight, usually meaning a BMI between 19 and 33

• Financial stability (to ensure the carrier will not spend money intended for the pregnancy on things like credit card debt)

• Completion of a mental health assessment to show the candidate is prepared for the commitment of surrogacy

• Completion of a home inspection to ensure the candidate lives an environment that is safe for her during the pregnancy

• Proof that she will be able to abstain from drinking, drugs, and smoking during the course of the pregnancy

While surrogacy agencies vet potential carriers, you should vet the agency itself. Namely, any reputable agency will be up-front about their pricing. With few exceptions, there shouldn't be additional costs once the surrogacy begins.

Lauren and her husband, Robyn, from California, wanted to work with an agency so they could have someone guiding them who had been through the process. She says, "We were able to work with their legal team, and our contract was all-inclusive, so we wouldn't have to pay again to be rematched or pay new legal fees. Most people, myself included, can't imagine switching surrogates during this journey, but the statistic is that 25 percent of people end up switching surrogates for a variety of reasons."

Here are some additional factors to take into consideration with agencies:

• **The carrier.** Surrogate candidates are screened based on a predetermined set of guidelines. They are then matched with potential intended parents.

• **Finding your carrier.** The agency recruits people willing to be gestational carriers and then selects the best match for you based on your needs and those of the gestational carrier.

• **Relationship with your carrier.** While the details will be ironed out after you are matched with a carrier, in general, agencies will take into consideration what level of involvement you want with your carrier before they match you.

• **Cost.** Total costs depend on a variety of factors. Agency fees cover background checks, medical screenings, and so on ($10,000 to $20,000). Some agencies have a sliding scale for carrier compensation based on the surrogate's health and experience as a carrier. But many agencies pay first-time surrogates between $40,000 and $60,000. You may also be subjected to additional costs if there are medical complications or the surrogate is carrying multiples. Finally, while an agency might be involved in organizing medical procedures and checks, the costs of procedures like IVF cycles are not usually included.

Known Carrier

A known carrier could be a friend, family member, or acquaintance who is willing to make a commitment to carrying your child. While this a great gift, it also means you are responsible for organizing most aspects of the surrogacy. This includes arranging for medical and psychological testing to ensure your carrier is a good candidate. However, similar to working with an independent carrier, you'll also have the support of lawyers and your fertility clinic.

Here are some additional things to take into consideration with known carriers:

• **The carrier.** If the carrier is friend or family, they will continue to be in your life after the child's birth.

• **Finding your carrier.** Finding a friend or family member who is willing to be a gestational carrier depends on your current relationships. Sometimes you might have to ask, or someone might volunteer if they know you're considering surrogacy.

• **Relationship with your carrier.** If you already have a relationship with your carrier, it's important that both of you examine how that relationship might change as a result of surrogacy.

• **Cost.** As with an independent gestational carrier, you cover all the costs. However, sometimes known carriers are willing to donate their time and effort by waiving compensation. This is called compassionate or altruistic surrogacy.

Raya and her husband, Dave, from Australia quickly moved on to IVF after a year of trying to conceive on their own. Multiple miscarriages and several fertility clinics later, she was diagnosed with Asherman's syndrome—a buildup of scar tissue in her uterus (see the appendix). Multiple attempts to thicken her uterine lining failed.

"I said to Dave, 'I think my body's not going to be able to do this,'" she recalls.

But then Dave's sister Lara offered to be their surrogate. "We had been keeping [Lara and her husband] in the loop, and she'd offered [to be our surrogate] a long time ago," says Raya. "She called me one day and said, 'Raya, my offer is still on the table. Please let me do this for you. I'm ready and I'm willing, and you've already been through enough. Let's just get your baby.'"

Interestingly enough, Lara herself had had the first two of her three children via IVF. "You hear these stories about people's bodies adjusting and fixing themselves. And you always think, 'Oh, well, that's nice for somebody else,'" Lara says. "But miraculously, I fell pregnant naturally with my third child. I realized that my body had improved."

And it worked. Lara carried and delivered a healthy baby for Raya and her husband.

WARRIOR TIPS
Avoiding Surrogacy Scams

From unreliable gestational carriers to unscrupulous "agencies," there are, unfortunately, people who will take advantage of your desire to have a child through surrogacy. You can take certain precautions to verify that a gestational carrier or agency is legitimate:

• **Do not rely on unregulated websites like Craigslist to find a gestational carrier.** For many individuals struggling with the cost of surrogacy, this might seem like a way to save money. But it's more likely that you'll regret the decision than benefit from it. At a very minimum, if you use a site like Facebook to find a surrogate, as several warriors mentioned in this chapter did, your first step should be to perform a background check.

• **Ask for references and recommendations.** When you're considering agencies, ask people in your infertility support network if they've used the organizations you're considering. This will give you a better picture of what it's like to work with each agency.

• **Listen to your gut.** There are plenty of honest, caring surrogates and agencies out there. If any part of your instinct tells you something isn't right, move on to another option.

Choosing a Gestational Carrier

Once you've determined whether or not you want to work with a surrogacy agency, the next step is determining what factors will guide your choice of the gestational carrier herself. Since the surrogate will not be the biological mother of the child, these considerations have less to do with her genetics and more to do with finding a gestational carrier who is looking for the same surrogacy experience as you.

The matching process often involves you and the gestational carrier working together to create a surrogacy plan and coming to an understanding about what you want your relationship to be like. Knowing your own answers to the following questions will help you determine what type of person will best meet your surrogacy needs.

• How involved do you want to be with the medical aspects of the pregnancy? Do you want to attend ultrasound appointments? Would you like to be in the room during the birth?

• Do you want a long-term relationship with your gestational carrier? Would you like her to be a part of the child's life?

• How much do you want to share with the gestational carrier? How much do you want her to know about your life?

Just as the surrogate has to meet certain criteria, know that you, too, likely will undergo a similar evaluation before you are matched with a gestational carrier. A surrogacy agency will verify that you are fit to care for the child once it is born. Some will visit your home to ensure it's a safe and financially stable environment. You might be asked to undergo a psychological evaluation to ensure you're mentally prepared for the difficulties of surrogacy.

The information the agency gathers continues to be useful even after you've been given the green light, as it helps the agency match you to the best gestational carrier for your journey.

"My husband and I met with a social worker both at the agency and with the IVF clinic to discuss our plans," says Jen. "We also had criminal background checks."

Creating a Surrogacy Agreement

Once you've chosen your gestational carrier, you'll need to hammer out the details of the surrogacy contract, which you should do with help of an experienced surrogacy attorney. "Putting things in writing is the best way to make sure everyone is on the same page," says attorney Catherine Tucker of New Hampshire Surrogacy & Fertility Law. "When it comes to surrogacy, there are no good surprises—well, except for gender reveals. It's important to have a written document to set out everyone's intentions."

Believe it or not, the financial aspect of a surrogacy contract can actually be the most straightforward. If you're using an agency, the organization will have already agreed upon compensation payment with the gestational carrier. However, it will likely need to be decided when the payment is made, how it's distributed, and whether or not the intended parents will cover any additional expenses. Both parties should be clear on these details before moving forward.

The more challenging parts of the contract are those questions with more flexible answers. How late into the pregnancy can the gestational carrier travel? How often will she contact the intended parents? Who gets to choose which doctors to use? It cannot be overstated how important it is to have open communication among all parties about the expectations throughout the process—the more detailed, the better.

Lauren and Robyn wanted to make sure that they could be included at doctor appointments and present for the birth. "Our contract says that if only one person is allowed in the room at birth, that person will be me and not our surrogate's husband. We also decided that weekly text updates would happen once a pregnancy started. As my surrogate and I have grown close, we text weekly and sometimes talk on the phone."

Here is a list of topics—by no means complete—to discuss with your gestational carrier:

• **The number of transfer cycles.** Embryo transfers are not always successful on the first try. But given that each round involves medication and invasive procedures, you can't expect your carrier to be available for unlimited cycles. It's best to have an agreement about how many times you will try and over what time period.

• **Health and diet.** Aside from the obvious abstinence from drinking, drugs, and smoking (all of which should be in the contract), you will also need to decide what constitutes a "healthy" pregnancy. Most intended parents and gestational carriers tend to put into their contract a clause that says the carrier will follow the suggestions of her ob-gyn, but you can also put in specifics as long as they are reasonable requests and your gestational carrier agrees to them.

• **The birth plan.** Of course, there's always a chance that a birth plan won't go as planned. Babies come early. There are complications that require unforeseen procedures. But there still needs to be a basic agreement that covers issues like whether the gestational carrier will receive an epidural, whether to use a midwife or doula, and who's allowed in the room during the birth.

• **The transfer.** The end goal of a surrogacy agreement is having the carrier hand a healthy baby over to the intended parents. But this looks different to every couple. Some intended parents want their carrier to provide breast milk for the child. Others want her to occasionally see the child during the first few weeks to help the child transition to their care.

WARRIOR TIPS
Wanting Multiples

Especially if you transfer more than one embryo, there's always a chance of multiples. But for some intended parents, this is part of the plan.

For example, male couples need to decide which partner will supply the sperm to fertilize the egg. If both partners wish to have a genetic link to their children, the intended parents can choose to have two embryos (each created with a different father's sperm) transferred into the gestational carrier.

If you would like multiples as part of your family's journey, there are additional considerations to be made, financial and otherwise. To begin, there are additional fees. In most cases, each additional child adds $5,000 to your overall cost. Also, finding a match could take longer. Not every gestational carrier is willing to carry multiples—and with good reason (see chapter 9).

You will also need to discuss what will happen if the pregnancy does not go as planned. If the transfer cycle results in only one viable fetus, but sperm from two donors was used, do you want to know who the biological father is? What happens if carrying multiples poses a threat to the gestational carrier's health? There is always a chance that the pregnancy will have to be reduced to ensure the safety of the carrier and/or at least one of the fetuses.

These are difficult situations. But it's best to discuss them before the issue arises so that the intended parents and the gestational carrier are prepared to deal with the fact that the surrogacy did not go as planned.

Building a Relationship with Your Gestational Carrier

The relationship between a gestational carrier and the intended parent(s) is unlike any other, so it can be difficult to navigate both the personal and impersonal aspects of sharing the surrogacy journey. The relationship requires trust and commitments from all parties, but it can be difficult to establish healthy expectations and boundaries. With a guiding principle of patience and willingness to assist each other, you can create a meaningful connection with your gestational carrier that meets both of your needs.

The first step is acknowledging the emotional minefield you're entering. Your mental health should be your priority as you navigate the ups and downs of your surrogacy journey. Lauren Ashlock Lane, a counselor with Bright Star Counseling in Bedford, Texas, emphasizes the importance of therapy. "[Emotions are] going to hit every time you go to the doctor's office. And every time the carrier talks about feeling movements and kicking or how she's eating," she points out. Having a safe place to vent those emotions makes it easier to interact with your gestational carrier. It also ensures there are no unresolved issues that impede bonding once the child is born.

Early on, you and your gestational carrier need to discuss your preferred methods of communication and a realistic frequency of contact. If one of you is an all-day texter while the other prefers weekly updates by email, you both need to find a way to feel supported throughout the surrogacy process. Working together—possibly with a counselor—establishes expectations for your relationship.

Once you've got a good foundation, understand that the situation can evolve over time. What was working at the beginning of the process might cause tensions later on. Check in with your gestational carrier about the process at the beginning of each trimester. Be honest about what's working and what's not. Focus on communicating your needs in a way that doesn't imply your surrogate has done something wrong. This is a new relationship and experience for both of you, so there needs to be room for growth and change.

"We built a relationship from the start quite organically," explains Lauren. "Our agency hadn't officially given us each other's email addresses and phone numbers, yet my surrogate stalked me on Facebook and sent me a message. From that moment I knew we were going to get along, as I can be a bit of a rebel when it comes to following the rules. We set up our first FaceTime with our husbands, and from that point on, she has become a close friend."

Transfer Cycles

There are many different transfer cycle options when you're using a gestational carrier, including:

- The eggs and the sperm (fresh or frozen) come from the intended parents.

- The intended parent's sperm (fresh or frozen) fertilizes a donated egg.

- The intended parent's egg (fresh or frozen) is fertilized with donor sperm.

- Donor eggs and donor sperm (fresh or frozen) are used to create a new embryo.

- A frozen donor embryo is used.

If you will be using your own fresh eggs for a fresh transfer, you and the surrogate will have to medically sync your menstruation cycles. The same holds true if you are using a fresh egg donor for a fresh transfer. This ensures that once the egg is retrieved and fertilized, your gestational carrier is ready for the transfer.

With donated embryos, your surrogate doesn't have to adjust her cycle. She most likely, however, will take hormones to increase the odds that she'll become pregnant. Your reproductive endocrinologist will transfer the agreed-upon number of embryos.

For more details on transfer cycles, refer to chapter 7.

Legal Preparations for the Birth

In many states, the person who gives birth is automatically considered the legal parent so you and your attorney will need to file paperwork to ensure that you and your partner (if you have one) are the legal parents of the baby as soon as the child is born. In most states, this is accomplished with a pre-birth order that:

- Declares the intended parent/s are the child's legal parents

- Allows the hospital to list the intended parent/s on the birth certificate

- Places the child under the intended parent/s' insurance

- Gives the intended parent/s the right to make medical decisions for the baby

- Ensures the child will be discharged with the intended parent/s

If your state does not allow pre-birth orders, your gestational carrier—and her partner, if she's married—will instead need to sign documentation relinquishing her parental rights when the baby is born. Because babies often come on their own schedule, it's wise to prepare these documents well ahead of your gestational carrier's due date.

Unfortunately, things might not go as planned and you may need to be prepared for a fight. After experiencing three miscarriages, the last of which were triplets, Kelly and Tom froze three embryos that were biologically theirs. Eventually, they decided gestational surrogacy was the best option.

Medically, the process was fairly uneventful. However, they lived in a state where compensated surrogacy was illegal, and they needed a pre-birth order to have their names placed on the birth certificate instead of their gestational carrier's. "We started the process to obtain the pre-birth order as soon as the first trimester was over," Kelly says. Though they applied for the order well in advance, the judge denied their petition days before their daughter was born.

"It was definitely a moment that took away some of my happiness as we waited for our surrogate to go into labor," Kelly says. "After years of infertility and then using a surrogate, it was such a stab to the heart to have to go through the adoption process for our own biological daughter."

Surviving the Pregnancy

Gestational surrogacy requires you to trust your carrier with the health and well-being of your child, but that doesn't mean that *your* health and well-being are unaffected. Not being able to experience the pregnancy firsthand can be emotionally stressful. Just as surrogates need to listen to their bodies and find the habits that work best for them, you, too, need to have a reliable support system.

Dr. Alice Domar, an expert in mind/body health and infertility, notes that it's normal to feel jealous of the person carrying your child. "I had a patient who really struggled during her surrogate's pregnancy because she was really envious that her carrier got to feel the kicks and got all the attention of being a pregnant woman," she says. "But know, once you get that baby, it's your baby."

Sometimes you may feel removed from the process. Depending on the location of your gestational carrier, you may not be able to attend doctor appointments, so if there are complications, you may not be the first to find out. Again, this is why a surrogacy agreement is so important. It allows you to lay out expectations on how involved you will be in the pregnancy. You need to find a balance where your gestational carrier does not feel micromanaged but you don't feel left out.

You can build your involvement in the pregnancy by adding these interactions into the surrogacy agreement:

- Receiving ultrasound photos

- Attending childbirth classes with your gestational carrier

- Hosting a baby shower

- Meeting your gestational surrogate's ob-gyn and other health-care providers

- Downloading pregnancy tracking apps

- Having your surrogate play recordings of your voice so your baby is familiar with you when they're born

Dr. Domar also likes to remind intended parents to keep things in perspective. "Sometimes you have to be practical," she says. "If you want a genetic child, this might be the only way. And 9 months is a very short period of time in your child's life."

Chrissy was diagnosed with MRKH at 14 and knew that if she wanted a child, another person would have to carry it. When setting out on her surrogacy journey, however, she didn't want to feel like she and her husband were just "getting a baby." It was important for her to find a gestational carrier who understood her desire to be actively involved.

"It was 'my pregnancy' in every way possible," she says. "When our carrier felt the first kicks, her spouse got excited and went to put a hand on her belly. Our carrier said 'No! Chrissy and Lee have to be the first to feel it.' While I wouldn't have been upset in the slightest if we weren't the first to feel the kicks, it just made everything feel more special and ours to know she felt that way."

Chrissy admits that, in the beginning, there was awkwardness—especially at appointments when the midwife would address only the surrogate. But eventually the pregnancy fell into a groove. Chrissy attended prenatal yoga classes with her carrier and they had weekly dinners together.

In order to find a gestational carrier who would be fine with this arrangement, Chrissy and her husband were careful not to rush. They asked questions and thoroughly outlined

BUSTED

Myth: The baby will not bond with me.

It is true that babies begin to recognize the touch and voice of their carrier while they are still in the womb. But that doesn't mean you can't be a part of that process.

Ashlock Lane says it's common for parents working with gestational carriers to worry about bonding with the baby, but once you have the child, that worry melts away. "It's hard to see before it happens," she explains. "It's hard to see when the fears are all kind of clouding the ability to make that decision and move forward, but I don't see people who are on the other side that ever regret going through that process at all."

There are other ways to ease the emotional transition and ensure your child recognizes you as his or her parent. While it won't happen overnight, if you focus on your child's needs and feelings, that precious bond will develop.

their expectations. "Before the pregnancy, we talked about what type, method, and frequency of communication we wanted," she says. "I wanted to know ALL the things at first—every bout of nausea, kicks, funny stories, etc. I was worried it might trigger me, though, so I told her I would tell her to stop if needed. But thankfully I really enjoyed all the updates and the daily videos of her belly moving and growing."

If you are fortunate enough to have a warm relationship with your carrier, it might be other people who complicate your emotions and provoke your triggers. People will ask awkward questions. They'll put their foot in their mouth because they aren't educated about surrogacy. Have coping mechanisms prepared so you can deal with stress in a healthy way.

The Birth

If your gestational carrier does not live near you, you or she will relocate once her due date approaches. This should all be planned based on your carrier's ability to travel and the surrogacy laws in your state.

When she arrives at the hospital, it's important for the gestational carrier to inform staff of her surrogacy agreement. This way, your rights will be recognized when you arrive. Often, you'll get the call that it's go time once her labor is confirmed.

Depending on your surrogacy agreement, you may or may not be in the delivery room. During the delivery, it's most important for you to be supportive of your gestational carrier and her needs.

Then, finally, you get to the part you've been waiting for: you get to hold your baby in your arms. But it's an incredibly emotional time—for both you and your gestational carrier. Her body has just given birth, and her hormone levels will be affected.

"Recognize that you may feel intense emotions, including immense joy, confusion, excitement, ambivalence, and fear," says Tiffany Edwards, a clinical psychologist at Fertility Centers of Illinois in Chicago. "Acknowledging that you and the gestational carrier may experience a range of emotions beforehand will help you all during the birth and transition period."

It's also important to have a plan regarding the baby. Many couples prefer a multistep process where the baby first has skin-on-skin contact with the gestational carrier and then with you to ease the transition. Other intended parents wait to hold their baby until after it's fed. If the gestational carrier agrees, some intended parents are the first people to hold the child. It's important to work out these details as part of your surrogacy agreement.

Surrogacy often means juggling a lot of emotions and responsibilities—the complexities of the legal process, weighing your surrogate considerations, entrusting the act of carrying your child to someone else, and much more. Look at your loved ones and determine whom you should lean on in which situations.

For example, a more practical friend can help you make legal decisions, while an empathetic person would be best to turn to when you are overwhelmed by a lack of control during the pregnancy. Just be sure to let your support network know why you're coming to them; they're going to need guidance, so identifying their strengths will help them know what to do.

WARRIOR ACTION STEPS
Coping During the Surrogacy Process

• **Keep track of what you do daily for your coming child.** Maybe you pick out the nursery color, fill out some legal paperwork, or make a list of potential names. You may not be carrying the baby, but you are readying your world for them and it's important for you to recognize what you're doing to shape this child's life. Writing down what you do every day in preparation will help you feel connected to the pregnancy.

• **"Grow" something.** Plant a garden. Knit a baby blanket. Raise money for a good cause in your child's name. You might not be able to carry your child, but you can create meaningful additions to the world. Finding ways to nurture and build will help channel your emotions during the surrogacy process.

• **Enjoy your last days without a child.** With a traditional pregnancy, women—and, to an extent, their partners—spend their last pre-baby months tired and uncomfortable. Take advantage of the fact that you can still travel, take long walks on the beach, or have a glass of wine. Your child is about to change your life, in both amazing and trying ways, so savor the days in ways you won't be able to once you're a parent.

WARRIOR WISDOM
The Beauty of Surrogacy

"There is a lot of worry and fear about this process because it isn't familiar. Get educated, trust your providers, and get support. If your dream is to become a parent, you will get there. The road just might take you on a different path than you expected. If you can open yourself up to surrogacy, it can truly be a beautiful experience."

— Jen, New York

WARRIOR CHECKLIST
Weighing Surrogacy as an Option

❑ Understand your different surrogacy options (traditional vs. gestational carrier, independent carrier vs. surrogacy agency vs. known carrier).

❑ Allow yourself to grieve the loss of the possibility of carrying your child.

❑ Learn about the surrogacy laws in your state, and research how they can impact your plan.

❑ Find an attorney who specializes in surrogacy.

❑ Determine what you want from a gestational carrier.

❑ After being matched, draw up a surrogacy agreement with the assistance of an attorney.

❑ Find ways to be involved with the pregnancy and birth that are meaningful for you.

Adoption 101

CHAPTER 12

RACHEL AND HER HUSBAND, KIT, from Illinois started trying to build their family just a couple of months after they were married. Although Rachel quickly got pregnant, she miscarried. Over the years, they would have two more miscarriages and lose their daughter at 39 weeks for unknown reasons. They eventually attempted IVF, but the cycle was canceled due to an ovarian cyst. At that point, fate—or whatever you want to call it—stepped in.

"I feel guilty, but adoption fell in our laps," Rachel shares. "We had no desire to adopt at that time, but the opportunity presented itself at the most perfect time. Looking back on it

now, it was divine intervention. He was always meant to be ours."

Their son's birth mother was getting ready to go to prison. She was pregnant but didn't want to keep the child. Rachel and Kit met her 3 weeks before she gave birth. "She was so sweet and gave us advice on bottles, diapers, schedules, et cetera," says Rachel. "I think that helped her feel a part of the process, and it was helpful to us. We didn't push her for information. We were just very grateful for anything she was willing to tell us."

Six weeks after her canceled IVF cycle, Rachel's son was born. However, the birth mother chose not to name the father on the

---

BUSTED

Myth: Adoption is a quick, easy process.

Not everyone's experience is like Rachel and Kit's. After years of wearying treatments and losses, adopting a child may sound easy, but the process is its own version of stressful, emotional, and complicated—and you need to be prepared for that before deciding to adopt.

Jenna and her husband, Patrick, from New York decided to adopt after having stillborn twins. Their doctor said that Jenna's medical history suggested a high chance she'd have another stillbirth. After going through the adoption process, Jenna says she hates when people say things like, "Why don't you just adopt?" as if it's the easier option.

"Adoption is beautiful," she says. "Adoption is love. But adoption is hard."

Chuck Johnson, a social worker and president and CEO of the National Council for Adoption (NCFA) in Alexandria, Virginia, says that many couples mistakenly think it will be easy to find a child. After all, the latest data from the US Children's Bureau reports that more than 123,000 children in the foster care system are waiting to be adopted. "However," Johnson says, "the reality is that the average age of a child in foster care is 8, and many have siblings that we hope to see remain together." This makes it more difficult for couples looking to adopt one newborn child.

birth certificate, which did create some problems for the adoption. "The first month of our son's life was very stressful waiting to see if a potential father would come forward [to claim custody]."

Rachel describes this as "the scariest time in our entire lives."

While they finalized the adoption, Rachel and her husband also moved forward with fertility treatments. She had her first egg retrieval when her son was 8 weeks old and did her first frozen transfer after his first birthday. Unfortunately, the cycle failed. They're currently planning their second retrieval, but for the time being, Rachel and Kit are just enjoying being parents. They have found their community very supportive. "Our son is biracial and we are white, so it is pretty apparent he is adopted," Rachel says. "We have people tell us almost every day how adoption has shaped their family. I can tell it helps them feel a connection to us and us to them."

Adoption After Infertility

There are many reasons to consider adoption after going through—or instead of—fertility treatments. It helps many infertility warriors finally build their family. We'll hammer this point home throughout the chapter, but know that adoption *isn't* a consolation prize. It's not a second-tier option. There are complex emotions involved—and the needs of the child *always* have to come first.

In this chapter, we'll go over the general adoption process, the choices you'll have to make, how to best approach those decisions given your infertility experience, and how to work through the intense emotions involved. But there are entire books about adoption that *still* don't cover every detail, so understand that what's included will be far from comprehensive.

> ### WARRIOR TIPS
> #### When to Consider Adoption
> You might consider adopting if:
>
> - You are unable to successfully carry a child.
>
> - You have been unsuccessful with fertility treatments and don't want to pursue them any longer.
>
> - You are single or part of an LGBTQ+ couple and don't want to use reproductive technology (sperm or egg donors, surrogacy, etc.) to have a child.
>
> - You simply want to adopt.

Legal Issues and Considerations

While your end goal is finding a child to love unconditionally, you first need to navigate a complicated legal system. Adoption laws differ among states and countries. Parental rights have to be reassigned. And through the entire process, the well-being of the child needs to be prioritized.

Finding a Lawyer

As soon as you start seriously considering adoption, contact an attorney who specializes in the process. While you may not need to retain their services right away, it's helpful to have someone give a general overview of the process and the challenges you may face.

"An attorney can give [prospective adoptive parents] a better idea of what requirements are needed in their state and what kind of state laws will affect their upcoming family-building journey, assuming the birth mother is from the state they live in," says Shawn Kane, executive director of American Adoptions and American Surrogacy in Overland Park, Kansas.

Take your time and do your research about an attorney's credentials. As Stephanie Brinkley, an assisted reproduction technology (ART) attorney at Brinkley Law Firm in Charleston,

WARRIOR TIPS
Where to Start with Your Research
···

- **National Council for Adoption.** This organization provides information for everyone involved in the process: prospective adoptive parents, birth parents, and adopted children.

- **American Adoptions.** American Adoptions is one of the biggest adoption agencies in the country. As a result, they have resources about almost every type of adoption situation. Their hotline is open 24/7 to answer questions.

- **RESOLVE** provides the unique perspective of what infertility warriors can expect with adoption.

South Carolina, points out, any lawyer can *claim* to specialize in ART and adoption law. But those who truly do will often be recognized by the American Bar Association's ART division and/or the Academy of Adoption and Assisted Reproduction Attorneys (AAAA). Above all, look for an attorney with demonstrated experience in the field of surrogacy law.

Ask for this information from your attorney up front:

- **Fee structure.** Legal costs can get out of hand quickly if you don't understand how or for what your attorney is billing you.

- **License location.** Depending on where you plan to adopt your child, your attorney may need to be licensed to practice in multiple states.

- **International experience.** International adoption is its own unique journey. If you desire to adopt abroad, you'll need an attorney who specializes in the particular country you would like to adopt from.

- **Relationships with adoption agencies.** Having an attorney who is associated with particular agencies can make the process easier. At

the same time, it can limit your choices when choosing which agencies to work with.

- **Caseload.** An attorney who is working with dozens of prospective adoptive parents may be stretched for time, which could possibly decrease the attention and energy you receive.

Using an Adoption Consultant

Adoption consultants, who coach and provide guidance to prospective parents, are becoming more popular. These individuals are great resources because they are educated about the adoption process, but it's important to know that they are *not* certified or held accountable by any licensing authorities. However, be prepared to pay them around $3,500 to $4,000.

Emma and Joe from Ohio decided to use an adoption consultant because it allowed them to avoid the long wait lists of most agencies since consultants work with multiple agencies. Having someone to hold their hand through the process also gave them a sense of comfort.

"There is so much information to weed out, but the adoption consultant was very

BUSTED

Myth: Our lack of a biological connection with our child will be an issue.

If you yourself were not adopted, it can be difficult to understand how true and beautiful the bond is between adopted children and their parents. You might worry that you won't be able to connect with a child who isn't biologically yours. But in reality, this concern is unfounded, says Lauren Ashlock Lane, a counselor with Bright Star Counseling in Bedford, Texas. She has worked with many parents who do not have a genetic connection with their child, and she's never had one who couldn't connect with their child.

helpful in educating us, helping calm our fears, and answering our questions along the way," she says. "I am a very organized and 'to-do' list kind of person, so I actually liked having a checklist of everything we needed to get done."

Creating an Adoption Agreement

While legal considerations dominate a lot of the process, there's no such thing as an "adoption contract." This means that before a person gives birth, there is no enforceable type of document that surrenders their parental rights and legally makes the child yours.

If you are in direct contact with the birth parent(s), you can—and should—create an *agreement* about everyone's expectations. The main purpose of an adoption agreement is outlining if and how there will be contact between birth parents and the child in the future. These agreements can be informal or written legal documents. Currently, this kind of agreement is only enforceable in some states and countries, but Kane points out that even if adoption agreements aren't enforceable in your state, it's important to have the discussion.

"This shows both parties have something to look to when it comes to their contact after the baby is placed," he says. "Each family should discuss this with an adoption attorney that represents them before signing so they understand the full impact of the agreement."

Securing Your Child's Citizenship

Once you have your child, it can be tempting to procrastinate on paperwork in order to focus on enjoying your new family. You should definitely allow yourself to live in the present and enjoy all of the beautiful little moments of life with a new child, but looking to the future will prevent an unwanted setback later. Staying on top of paperwork can be especially important if you adopt a child from abroad, as the wrong documentation can have serious implications for their citizenship.

Catherine Tucker, an attorney at New Hampshire Surrogacy & Fertility Law, suggests parents enlist a lawyer's help to secure their child's citizenship right away. "There are a lot of highly technical rules involved with the adoption process," she says. "By the time the child grows up and discovers the issue, it's too late. Adopted people have actually been deported based on such inadvertent failures to make sure the T's are crossed and the I's are dotted."

Types of Adoption

Like nearly every other aspect of this journey, adoption is far from straightforward. There are several types of adoption and each one has pros and cons.

Open Adoption

Many domestic adoptions are, to some degree, "open"—that is, the birth mother and the adoptive family agree to have some level of connection and/or contact. However, there are many options. Whether you meet the birth mother only once or she becomes a part of your child's life, you need to decide what level of contact you're comfortable with.

Chuck Johnson, president and CEO of the National Council for Adoption (NCFA), reminds prospective adoptive parents that they shouldn't feel threatened by or scared of the birth parents. "[The birth mom] is making a difficult but loving sacrifice to ensure that her child is adopted by a family that will love and care for the child as much as she wishes she could if her circumstances were different," he says. "Many families find that ongoing contact with the birth families (including biological grandparents) can be very helpful to getting greater and more robust health and family history information."

Beth and Sean from New Hampshire knew from the beginning they wanted an open adoption. "We were excited about the potential of having more people to love our child in our life," she says. When deciding whether to have an open adoption, she advises that you consider what both your life and your child's life will look like after 5, 13, and 18 years. "Be honest with how adoption will thread its way through your lives in ways you might not foresee."

Johnson also says it's important to make sure everyone's expectations are the same. You have to clearly define what "future" contact means. Will the child meet the birth mother? Or will they just exchange letters? How often will they have contact? Discussing these expectations early on leads to healthier relationships in an open adoption.

Closed Adoption

In a closed adoption, identifying information is not shared between the prospective parents and birth parent(s), and from the moment the child is born, all contact with the birth parent(s) is cut off. In theory, this type of clean break should simplify the adoption process, but mostly it just limits your agency and birth parent options.

While some birth mothers prefer a closed adoption, it's rare. They want to meet the prospective adoptive parents so they can have peace of mind about the child's chances at a happy life. Some agencies specialize in closed adoptions, but most don't.

Above all else, consider how a closed adoption will impact your child. With a closed adoption, you won't be able to answer their questions about their birth family. Even beyond issues like family medical history, this can lead to some unresolved feelings. For many children, having access to information about their birth family helps them process their own emotions about being adopted.

"I think we need to remember that our children's stories belong to them," says Dawn Friedman, a clinical mental health therapist.

BUSTED

Myth: Babies put up for adoption are high risk.

Depending on how you decide to adopt, you may have very little information about the child's health. Many people considering adoption imagine drug-abusing birth mothers who abandon their babies, but this is not the norm.

Most birth mothers are happy and healthy in their current lives and know that keeping the child isn't the right choice for the baby. These women seek prenatal care and do whatever they can to ensure the baby is born healthy.

However, also remember that there *are* children born with health problems for a variety of reasons. There also are older children who have special needs or have been traumatized. This doesn't mean these children are "damaged" or "unadoptable," but you should consider carefully whether you have the financial and emotional ability to support a high-needs child.

"When we're going through the adoption process, it feels like it's all about us. But the minute that child arrives to our family, it is not about us anymore. They have a right to that information. It belongs to them."

According to *Considering Adoption*, an online adoption magazine, children of closed adoptions may feel disconnected or struggle with their identity. These unresolved feelings may cause them to act out. However, not every child responds this way, and they may feel differently over time in their adult years.

Private Adoption

Most couples looking to adopt an infant use a private adoption agency or attorney. Generally speaking, although there are always exceptions, there are several differences between the

ADOPTION ATTORNEYS vs. ADOPTION AGENCIES		
	ATTORNEYS	**AGENCIES**
Qualifications	Don't restrict clients to only people of a particular marital status, sexual orientation, religion, or age.	Might restrict clients to only people of a particular marital status, sexual orientation, religion, or age.
Time to adoption	Quicker because they don't have long wait lists.	Require more paperwork and have longer wait lists due to limiting the number of clients at any given time.
Services	Require clients to hire additional professionals, such as a social worker for the home study.	More "all-inclusive," offering guidance and professionals—except an attorney, in many cases—for every step of the process. The role of attorneys in an agency setting is minimal, however. They mostly file paperwork to finalize the process rather than handling it start to finish.
Costs	Fees vary greatly depending on a variety of factors. If you already know the birth parent(s), the attorney needs to complete only the relinquishment, placement, and finalization legal steps. If not, then you pay higher fees due to the additional steps involved.	Most have set, up-front fees outlined in advance. Additional fees depend on the situation of the birth parent(s).
Support and education	Don't offer prospective parent(s) support and education.	Offer prospective parent(s) support and education. Sometimes education is even required.

two (see the chart above). But for the sake of simplicity in the rest of this section, I'm going to refer to both private agencies and attorneys as "agencies."

Once a birth mother determines that adoption is the best choice for her and her child, she either will get a referral to an agency from her doctor or seek out an agency on her own. Then the expectant mother typically undergoes counseling to ensure she understands all her options and is confident about—not coerced into—the decision to pursue adoption. The agency will ask her to create an adoption plan that outlines what type of family she wants to adopt the child, whether she wants an open or closed adoption, and what she wants for her birthing experience.

In the case of an open adoption, the birth mother will review prospective parents' profiles herself. If she prefers a closed adoption, the agency will find a couple based on the birth mother's adoption plan.

Once the birth mother delivers, she signs away her parental rights and the child goes home with the adoptive parents. How long the birth mother spends with the child before transferring parental rights should be agreed upon before the birth.

For those looking into private agency adoption, the major factors will be:

• **Cost.** On average, private adoptions cost $40,000, but your total will depend on the agency you choose, their fee breakdown, and how much financial assistance you provide the birth mother.

• **Your timeline.** Depending on how many birth mothers an agency represents, it might take time to get matched. Sixty-three percent of adoptive parents are matched within their first year of working with an agency.

• **Meeting the birth family.** If you want an open adoption with continuous contact with the birth mother, you'll need to make sure your agency can support and accommodate that.

• **Privacy policies.** Each agency has its own policies about how much information it shares with involved parties. In some cases, birth mothers might get more information than you realize if you are not familiar with your agency's privacy policies.

• **Dropout rates.** While a birth mother can always back out of an adoption, if an agency has a high dropout rate, it's a sign that something is wrong with their overall process.

Placing a child for adoption is not a decision someone makes lightly, and it's important for you to remember and respect the birth mother's perspective. The agency you choose plays a big part in how birth mothers are treated and supported.

After Mary Beth and her husband, John, from Colorado decided to adopt a child, they wanted to make sure the birth mother was never placed in a situation where she felt pressured to go through with the adoption. "Agencies should provide support to birth mothers first," Mary Beth says. "The first goal should be helping them understand every option and resource available, and only then, if the expectant mom is still confident adoption is the best option, should they be introduced to hopeful adoptive parents."

Jenna also was particularly sensitive to the birth mother's experience before she started the adoption process. The issue was particularly personal to her because her sister, as a teenager, had placed a child for adoption. This gave Jenna an intimate view of what adoption is like from the other side.

"I knew well how hard and how painful and how breathtakingly beautiful it could be," Jenna says. "When looking at each agency, I had one question that I would always ask myself first: Would I trust this agency to treat their birth families the way that I would want an agency to treat my family? I refused to work with any agency that I did not feel was treating their birth families with the dignity and the respect that they so richly deserve."

Jenna advises prospective adoptive parents to pay close attention to how agencies talk about and to expectant mothers. She says to check out the agency's webpage addressed to expectant mothers and to ask yourself:

• Does the agency present resources that educate expectant mothers about all their options?

• Does the agency use adoption-negative language, like "giving up your baby," or does it seem to genuinely respect expectant mothers?

• Does the agency have a dedicated point of contact (sometimes called an adoption specialist) for birth mothers?

• Does it offer counseling and other forms of support, both before and after the adoption is finalized?

• Does it provide professional guidance but promise complete personal control over all decisions?

• Does it have positive reviews and testimonials from other birth parents?

Knowing these answers will show you whether birth mothers are treated right.

Intercountry Adoption

In the United States, all intercountry adoptions have to be in accordance with the Hague Convention on Protection of Children and Co-operation in Respect of Intercountry Adoption. This agreement among 90 countries sets guidelines on international adoption to protect the rights of all involved parties. Even if you adopt a child from a country that hasn't signed on to this convention, if you are adopting a child into the United States you must use an agency that works in agreement with the convention's standards.

This means all intercountry adoption agencies have to be certified by the US State Department, and the agency must:

- Have considered local placement of the child first

- Provide counseling for biological parents

- Secure legal consent from the biological parents

- Ensure the child is properly cleared for adoption in the United States (that is, the child clears the guidelines established by the convention, or is an orphan in a country not signed on to the Convention)

These regulations were established in 2008, and though today there are fewer intercountry adoptions, these laws have made the process more positive for all parties. According to the US Department of State, most intercountry adoptions now happen with China, accounting for 202 adoptions in 2020 (compared with 2,231 in 2016).

In addition to finding an agency that works in accordance with the Hague Convention, here's what to know about intercountry adoption:

WARRIOR TIPS

Intercountry Adoption for LGBTQ+ or Single Parents

In 2017, a US Supreme Court decision overturned an Arkansas law that banned same-sex couples from adopting. This set a precedent that secured the right for members of the LGBTQ+ community to adopt within the United States. However, some countries will not approve intercountry adoptions involving same-sex prospective adoptive parents. Other countries will not allow single parents—regardless of their sexual orientation—to adopt. Any agency you use should have up-to-date information on other countries' restrictions. For additional resources on intercountry adoption rules and regulations, consult the US State Department's website.

- **Cost.** There are additional fees associated with intercountry adoption (like securing your child's visa and citizenship). On average, intercountry adoptions cost between $30,000 and $50,000, depending on the country.

- **Your timeline.** It takes time to arrange an intercountry adoption and ensure all documentation is in line. As a result, the process can take longer.

- **Meeting the birth family.** In most cases, you will not meet the birth family. You will probably receive very little information about them.

- **Medical care.** In some less developed countries, the child may not have access to the best medical treatment or nutrition, which could affect their health.

- **Traveling to meet the child.** If you want to meet your child before bringing them to the United States, be mindful of the cost of traveling to and from their birth country.

Foster Care System Adoption

Foster care is meant to be a *temporary* solution for children whose families can't—for whatever reason—take care of them, as well as those who have been abused or neglected. Public agencies handle these cases, and in most cases the goal is to reunite children with their birth parent or family. They are placed in the state's care until their home environment becomes a stable, safe place to live. If that can't happen and the parent loses or relinquishes parental rights, the child becomes eligible for adoption.

Adoption through the foster care system is the most popular avenue for adoption. In 2020, it accounted for more than 56,500 adoptions. In most cases, public agencies handle foster care adoptions.

Many people decide to become foster parents before adopting. This allows them to establish a relationship with the child and can ease the child's transition. According to the US Children's Bureau, 51 percent of children adopted from the foster care system in 2017 were adopted by their foster parents.

A child is put into foster care by a social service agency or the state after it has been determined that their family is unable to care for them. Typically, a foster child's legal guardian maintains parental rights, which are managed by the state, but does not get a say in where the child is placed. The length of time a foster child remains in a foster home may be weeks or years.

If you want to go straight for adoption, after completing the home study and background check process (more on that later), a foster child will be placed with you while the adoption process is finalized.

Foster care adoption demands the same level of consideration as any other:

• **Cost.** Due to government subsidies, adoption through the foster system is by far the least expensive option. On average, it costs less than $3,000.

• **Your timeline.** Many children in foster care are ready for immediate placement. But the wait time depends on your preferences. Fifty-nine percent of prospective adoptive parents are matched within the first year.

• **Meeting the birth family.** If you foster the child first, you will likely have some contact with their birth family. If your child has siblings still in the care of their birth parent, this can also influence your contact with the parents.

• **Age of the child.** The average age of a foster child waiting to be adopted is 7.6 years.

• **Child's siblings.** Often multiple children from the same family are available for adoption. The state prefers to keep siblings together, so if you'd like to adopt more than one child, foster care adoption provides the option to build a family with biological siblings.

• **Parental rights.** Children in the foster care system can't be adopted until their parents have legally relinquished or lost their parental rights. If you start by fostering a child, you'll have to wait for this to happen before beginning adoption proceedings.

PRIVATE vs. INTERCOUNTRY vs. FOSTER CARE ADOPTION		
	PRIVATE ADOPTION	**INTERCOUNTRY ADOPTION**	**FOSTER CARE ADOPTION**
Cost	Average: $40,000	Average: $44,000	Average: $2,938
Marital status	Some private adoption agencies with religious affiliations will only work with straight, married couples. However, this is not the norm.	Depending on the laws of the birth countries, LGBTQ+ or single parents may not be able to adopt.	Both couples and individuals can become licensed foster parents. However, Alabama, Illinois, Louisiana, Mississippi, and Utah require couples to be legally married (or, in some cases, to be in a civil union).
Length of time	63% of prospective adoptive parents are matched within a year and 82% within 2 years.	Depends on the birth country, but with the most popular country, China, 75% of prospective adoptive parents are matched within a year and 90% within 2 years.	59% of adoptive parents are matched within a year and 71% within 2 years.
Contact with the birth parents	If the birth mother wants an open adoption, there is typically at least one meeting.	It's very unlikely you'll meet the birth family.	If you foster the child before adopting, it's highly likely you'll know and have contact with the birth parents.
Age of child	82% of adopted children are under 2 years old.	Depends on the country, but between 25% and 70% are under 2 years old.	50% of adopted children are under 2 years old, 67% are under 5, and 85% are under 10.
Health of child	Barring genetic disorders, most of the children are perfectly healthy.	The quality of medical care in the birth country can vary; so too will the child's health.	Due to their previous living situation, many children have experienced some degree of trauma.
Additional concerns	A birth mother does not surrender her parental rights until after the child is born, which means she might decide to keep the child.	You'll need to find agencies that work in accordance with the Hague convention on intercountry adoptions.	Many kids adopted out of foster care have siblings who are also available for adoption.

Source: Much of this information comes from Adoptive Families, "Adoption Cost and Timing in 2016-2017," 2018, online.

Overview of the Adoption Process

There are many intricate steps to adopting a child. When you look at the entire process at once, it can be overwhelming. While each adoption journey is different depending on your choices, let's break down the general process—and the challenges and decisions you'll face along the way.

Coming to Terms with Adoption

To paraphrase Johnson, there's an important difference between viewing adoption as a "plan B" and as a "second choice." "I was a social worker for many years, and I worked with many families toward an adoption after infertility," he says. "I didn't expect every family to

have resolved all the grief and loss associated with infertility, but I did want to ensure that they didn't see adoption—and by default, the child—as second best."

For every prospective adoptive parent who has first struggled with fertility issues, this is the first step: accepting that adoption isn't admitting failure, nor is the child a consolation prize. It can take time to achieve such acceptance, and working with a mental health professional familiar with both adoption and infertility can help.

It's not always easy to predict when you'll realize that adoption is right for you. But you'll know when it happens. For example, Emma and Joe began considering adoption after a failed round of IVF. The two were watching TV when a sports analyst on ESPN began talking about adopting a son from Russia. "Something changed that day," Emma says. "I finally went from wanting to be pregnant to wanting to be a mom. I let go of the 9 months that I wouldn't experience and turned my attention to the rest of my life and every other experience I knew we would still get to have as parents."

Choosing an Adoption Avenue

Once you've decided to adopt, it's research time. You'll have to choose between a private agency, intercountry adoption, or the foster care system.

"I can't overemphasize doing your homework," says Johnson. "Become a lay expert on types of adoption, the legal issues, [and] how the process works and start preparing by reading about adoptive parenting."

At this stage, as you weigh your options, think about how you envision your adoption experience. Outline what's important with regard to:

• Cost

• Length of timeline

- Contact with the birth family

- Availability of information about the child and birth family

- Support from members of your adoption team

- Willingness/ability to travel to meet the child and/or birth mother

You'll also have to think about characteristics or qualities in a child you want to prioritize, like:

- Age

- Gender

- Race

- Nationality

- Siblings

- Health of the child (Are you willing and able to adopt a child with special needs or medical disorders?)

Your thoughts will help you narrow down your options. For example, if contact with the birth family is a big priority, international adoption isn't the best route. If finances are an issue, adopting through the foster care system is most likely to fit your budget.

Evaluation and Home Study

After choosing your route, you'll start filling out initial paperwork that will help you get matched with a child. Most agencies use profiles to help birth mothers decide who they want to adopt their child. You'll provide information about your background and create an adoptive parent profile.

When TJ and her husband were notified by a friend about a birth mother who was looking for a family for her baby, who was due in a few months, they immediately sent over their profile. "We included pictures of us and our family. We also included pictures of our neighbors, church, and family vacations," she said. "We included information on our occupations, our educational backgrounds, and what we would want to give our child. Lastly, we included why we were seeking to adopt."

No matter how you plan to adopt, in the United States, you will have to go through a thorough evaluation to ensure you are able and ready to care for a child. Many prospective adoptive parents have issues with the invasive nature of this part of the process, but know that it's not about finding fault with you or your life. These regulations are in place to protect children.

The evaluation process includes:

- Criminal background checks

- Medical histories

- Character references

- Financial information

- Home study

The home study in particular can be stressful for parents trying to adopt. You'll meet with a licensed social worker in your home and answer questions. While in your home, the social worker will want to see that your house is clean and not in disrepair, there is room for a child, and the neighborhood is safe. While it can feel like every aspect of your home is being judged, know that the social workers have reasonable standards. They are not going to fail you if there's dust on your blinds.

During the home inspection and throughout the evaluation process, your social worker will ask about your life, family, and relationships. They'll pose questions about the type of parent you want to be and make sure you're pursuing adoption for the right reasons. If you're arriving at adoption after struggling with infertility, they might ask some questions about your emotional health to ensure you've come to terms with your infertility.

The fees for these evaluations typically range from $1,000 to $3,000, and once they are completed, parent training may be recommended. Meanwhile, the social worker compiles all of their observations and makes a recommendation on whether or not you are ready to adopt a child. Normal processing time ranges from 3 to 6 months before you receive an approval.

The Waiting Period

After you're approved, you wait. (That's right, more waiting!)

Your agency or attorney will start looking for birth mothers or children who would be a good match. Depending on what you're looking for, it could take a while to find an adoption opportunity. If you're willing to adopt any child, regardless of age, race, or location, you'll probably be matched quickly. But if you want a newborn of a specific background, it could take a while.

Waiting can be frustrating. You've spent months undergoing evaluations, and then you're told to do nothing. While some couples try to busy themselves with preparations like setting up nurseries or hosting baby showers, others enjoy their final days of being adults without children.

"We tried to do everything we wouldn't be able to do with a baby," says Beth, who adopted a newborn boy. "We went out for fancy meals. We opened a bottle of wine on a Tuesday afternoon in the summer. We went to a lot of movies. It was easy to stay at home and wait by the phone, but we figured that if we busied ourselves, the call would come when we least expected it."

Getting Matched with a Child

The adoption method you choose determines what happens once you're matched with a child. But in general, this is how the different processes go.

In most private adoptions, birth mothers go through the profiles of prospective adoptive parents. Based on the type of life they envision for the child, they will choose the people who best meet their expectations. Once you're chosen by a birth mom, you will most likely meet her to ensure it's a good match. If everyone agrees to move forward with the adoption, once the child is born, he or she is your child.

Intercountry adoptions vary depending on the country and the agency you're working with. In most cases, the child is already born and living in a foreign orphanage. You may receive pictures or information about the child. Some people are able to travel abroad to meet the child. It is very rare that you will meet the birth family.

With foster care adoption, the process depends on the child's situation and the status of the birth family's parental rights. Many prospective adoptive parents are foster parents first and then decide to formally adopt the child. People who do not foster first are matched with a child who's currently under the care of the state. They could be in a foster or group home, and if you decide to adopt the child, they will be moved to your home while the process is finalized.

Dealing with "False Starts"

Unfortunately, even with adoption, the unexpected can happen and an adoption arrangement that is underway doesn't work out. Sometimes biological parents change their minds, intercountry adoption agencies shut down, or a child in foster care is reunited with their birth family. When something this important to you falls through, it can be devastating.

After nearly 10 years struggling to get pregnant, Heidi and her husband, Ruben, from Maryland started the adoption process—something they thought was a "sure thing."

They were successful in their first attempt and adopted their 7-month-old son, Xavier, through an intercountry agency.

In 2006, they decided to adopt again, this time a baby girl from Guatemala. While they were working out the details, they flew to Guatemala several times to see their daughter so that they wouldn't miss out on her first months of life. "We were once again in love and had bonded with the newest addition to our family," Heidi says.

But changes to adoption regulations kept them from bringing their baby home. "My heart was once again broken," Heidi remembers. "I can't begin to describe the agony associated with every month that passes knowing that your baby is getting bigger and yet still not home."

They persevered and continued to keep all their adoption files and applications up-to-date. Two years passed, and they were still waiting for their daughter to leave Guatemala.

During that time, Heidi and her husband decided to try IVF again with donor eggs. It worked, and 4 years after starting the adoption process in Guatemala, Heidi gave birth to twins. Meanwhile, their "waiting daughter" had become a preschooler.

Finally, they received official notice that the daughter they had visited, hoped for, and loved would never come home with them.

"While it is hard to lose a child who you have held in your arms and called your own, it is even harder to have never had the opportunity to begin with," Heidi says. "In the days that followed, I held my children a little tighter and thanked God that I have them in my life."

It's common to feel grief and sorrow when an adoption falls through. Take time to cope with your loss, and if necessary, take a break from the adoption process.

Petitioning for Adoption and Post-Adoption Check-Ins

After a child is placed in your care, you'll have to petition family court to finalize the adoption. Over the course of about 6 months, a social worker will do more home visits and meet with you and the child. The focus is on the child's adjustment and the overall health of the environment.

Later, there will be a court hearing in front of a judge. The judge will review the home study and reports from the social worker. You will have to prove that the birth parents relinquished (or permanently lost) their parental

WARRIOR TIPS
Understanding the Interstate Compact on the Placement of Children (ICPC)

Before a judge can approve an ICPC agreement, there are several steps that must happen first:

- **Step 1:** The child is assigned a state caseworker, who gathers information about the child's educational, medical, and social history, court cases in which the child is involved, and the intended parent or parents in the receiving state.

- **Step 2:** The information packet is sent to the ICPC office in the intended parent's state. If the information is sufficient, the office will send it to the social services agency local to the intended parent. The agency will send a representative to the intended parent's home to determine if the child should be approved to live there.

- **Step 3:** This home study is sent back to the state's ICPC office for approval.

- **Step 4:** The information collected thus far, as well as the approval from the intended parent's state ICPC office, is sent back to the ICPC office in the child's state.

- **Step 5:** If both the child's and intended parent's state ICPC offices approve, the child can be placed in the home.

WARRIOR TIPS

Spotting Scams

Unfortunately, some people will try to take advantage of people struggling to build a family. It could be a fraudulent agency that withholds information about the child, impeding adoptive parents from making an informed decision, ultimately leading to the adoption falling through—and the agency keeping the adoptive parent's money. In other cases, an expectant mother might promise multiple couples that they can adopt her child, take money and other support from them, and then back out of the adoption at the last minute.

Most states do not have fraud laws written with adoption in mind. As a result, it can be very difficult to prosecute these cases. Avoid getting caught up in an adoption scam by looking for the following red flags:

- Agencies, attorneys, or birth mothers insisting that the entire process be done over the internet

- Agencies or attorneys pressuring you to sign documents you don't understand

- Unsolicited contact to start the adoption process

- Agencies that have negative or no reviews online

- Anyone not providing contact information or being unresponsive to multiple attempts to reach them

- Anyone refusing to show proof of pregnancy

- Anyone making guarantees that are "too good to be true"

- Agencies that repeatedly refer to the child as "your child" before the adoption is finalized—an emotional tactic to create a connection and keep stringing you along

Always use an accredited and well-respected attorney during your adoption process. They will help you find an honest, legally operating adoption team.

rights. If you adopted your child from another state, you'll also need a completed Interstate Compact on the Placement of Children (ICPC) approval.

Should the judge approve everything at the hearing, your child is officially and legally yours!

Post-Adoption: More Paperwork

Once you've established your parental rights through adoption, there is more paperwork to fill out and bureaucratic hurdles to jump over. Here are some additional legal processes you might have to complete:

- Amending your child's birth certificate to list you as the legal parent(s)

- Changing your child's last name

- Getting a Social Security card (for children adopted via intercountry agencies) or getting a new one with your child's new name

- Establishing your child's citizenship (if they were not born in the United States)

Talking to Your Child

Ultimately, it's your decision whether to tell your child that they were adopted. But most experts agree that it is best to be open and honest. And in some cases, like when you adopt a child of another race, or a child who is old enough to have memories of the time before they came to live with you, you'll have no choice but to talk about your family's adoption story.

Dr. Angela Palmer-Wackerly, assistant professor of health communication at the University of Nebraska in Lincoln, says it's best to start talking about adoption when your child is young. That way, the truth isn't a surprise but instead becomes a part of who they are. "Don't wait for your child to ask questions about adoption," she says. "Ask them questions as you tell them their story to let them know that adoption is open for discussion and that you're supportive of their emotions, no matter how negative or positive they are."

Penny Joss Fletcher, a licensed marriage and family therapist in California who is herself an adoptive mother, says it's best to start simple. Share details that are appropriate for the child's age and maturity. As they get older and ask more questions, add more details.

Telling Others

Joss Fletcher, a transracial adoptive mother, says it can be tricky talking to others about adoption. She gets a lot of questions: "That isn't your child, is it?" "Where did you get your child?"

"[You] always [have] a choice as to how to respond, whether to talk about the adoption or just to say, 'Yes, this is my child!'" she says. And while it's not a stranger's business to know your child's adoption story, the trick is balancing sharing details with giving your child control over their story.

Dr. Palmer-Wackerly agrees, saying parents should keep specific details to themselves. "That way, your child will feel ownership over their own story and will share details as they want, to people that they want, in line with their own personalities and privacy preferences."

Have a conversation with your child about what they want to disclose. Let them be the one who shares the information with their friends or people they meet. That way, they can create an identity that includes being adopted without being defined by it. North American Council on Adoptable Children, Creating a Family, and The Child Welfare Information Gateway by the US Department of Health & Human Services offer fantastic resources about adoption.

BUSTED

Myth: Adoption "heals" infertility.

Infertility has kept you from having what you want most: a child. Adoption allows you to have that child. But don't think adopting "cures" infertility or makes all your grief go away. If you're considering adoption to ease your infertility pain, it's not fair to you or the child.

After a miscarriage, Beth and Sean decided to adopt. All that mattered was becoming parents; biology didn't need to be a factor. But she knew the emotions of their losses weren't going to magically disappear. "I had a newborn baby in my arms when I saw a friend's pregnancy announcement. It still stung," she admits.

For most of your infertility journey, you've envisioned creating a new life. But with adoption, you transition to bringing into your family a child that you had no part in creating. While adoption is incredibly meaningful and fulfilling, it doesn't necessarily make the process of building your family any faster or easier. Plus, many couples decide to continue with fertility treatments while adopting, which can compound the emotional stress.

Having the support of other adoptive parents helped TJ and her husband through the process. She reflects, "Fortunately, we had the support of having close friends who adopted so they helped us through it."

Your adoption agency most likely has many resources for prospective adoptive parents. Don't be afraid to use those sources of support. Joining a support group specifically for adoptive parents will connect you with others you can lean on and who can offer tricks they've picked up along the way.

If you have a partner, it's also essential to have ongoing open, nonjudgmental communication.

When couples conceive naturally, they don't have control over factors like what their children look like or how old they are. With adoptions, these decisions need to be made beforehand, and partners don't always agree. When you're talking about your hopes and priorities for the adoption process, take the time to explain the thought process behind your choices. And give your partner's preferences fair consideration. Maybe they've thought of something you haven't or have different concerns. It's best to get everything out in the open early.

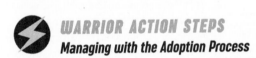

WARRIOR ACTION STEPS
Managing with the Adoption Process

While it's natural to get overwhelmed during the adoption process, organizing your thoughts and timeline can help you cope.

• **Set up a check-in schedule.** There's a lot of waiting during the adoption process, and it's hard balancing doing nothing with constantly asking your adoption team for updates. Before you start the process, think about how often you'd like to hear from different people involved. Then let them know your expectations. For example, when you're going through the home study, you might want the social worker to send you a general agenda the day before a meeting. Or while you're waiting to be matched, you might want to hear from your agency at least once a month—even if there's no new information.

• **Establish adoption discussion breaks.** It's easy to let conversations about adoption take over your and your partner's lives. Given

how emotional these discussions can be, you'll both need breaks from time to time. Establish a signal you both can use when your emotions are too heightened to continue the conversation. And respect each other's boundaries, no matter how much you want to keep talking. Walk away when the signal is given, and come back to the topic when you're both feeling calmer.

• **Put together an adoption book for your child.** This can be a scrapbook or a series of letters you write at different parts of your journey. The idea is to record what you did and felt while waiting for your child to arrive. This will help you focus on the positive and can be something that can help your child understand their story when they're older.

WARRIOR WISDOM
Discovering a Love You Never Imagined

"Be patient. Keep your eye on the prize. Never in a million years did we think we would be sitting here today with an almost 15-month-old. He has answered so many of our prayers and been such a blessing to us. I had worries I wouldn't be able to bond with him, but from the moment I laid eyes on him, he was mine. I can't imagine loving him more than I do right now. He may not share my blood, but boy does he have my heart." — Rachel, Illinois

WARRIOR CHECKLIST
Considering Adoption

- ❏ Understand that adoption does not cure infertility and an adopted child is not a "second best" option.
- ❏ Research the different adoption options and decide which best aligns with your vision to create a family.
- ❏ Find an attorney who specializes in adoption.
- ❏ Decide your priorities when it comes to finding the right child to adopt.
- ❏ Undergo the evaluation and home study part of the adoption process in order to be matched with a child.
- ❏ Finalize the adoption legally.
- ❏ Have a plan for how you will discuss the adoption story with your child and others.

Add more items to your Warrior Checklist or jot down any notes here:

Living a Happy, Full Life Without Your Own Children

CHAPTER 13

IF YOUR INFERTILITY JOURNEY ends with a decision not to have a child by any of the different paths to parenthood, you haven't "given up." Don't let *anyone*—including yourself—convince you of that.

In fact, for many infertility warriors, *choosing* to be child-free can be liberating. For Tia and her husband, Mark, from Illinois leading a child-free life was the best route in the end. They spent 6 years trying everything they could to get and stay pregnant. In the beginning, Tia bought every test she could find and tried every trick she came across. Eventually, her ob-gyn suggested they meet with a reproductive endocrinologist. "He recommended we move forward with our first IUI, and we jumped at the chance," Tia shares.

However, after undergoing genetic testing, she and Mark found out they were both carriers for medium-chain acyl-CoA dehydrogenase deficiency (MCADD), a metabolic disorder that can lead to seizures, breathing difficulties, liver problems, brain damage, coma, or sudden death. "Although our chance of conceiving a baby with MCADD was only 25 percent, we believed the risk [of that outcome] was too high," Tia says. So she and Mark decided to move forward with IVF and preimplantation genetic testing.

Luckily, the state of Illinois mandates infertility insurance coverage, so after getting Tia the right policy for their situation, they started IVF in 2016. She had back-to-back egg retrievals to get enough embryos to test. Although they found out Tia had poor egg quality and abnormal hormone levels, she and Mark ended up with two genetically normal embryos ready to transfer.

"Our first transfer was a complete failure, not even a hint of a positive," Tia remembers.

For the second transfer, Tia had an endometrial scratch and used a different suppression protocol. She became pregnant and had promising beta-hCG levels. "I watched, week after week, our baby boy growing right on track. It was simply a miracle."

But then, the day after Christmas, Tia had a miscarriage. "In a haze of grief and depression, I immediately refilled all my prescriptions and demanded we try again in 2017, but at a much slower pace," she says. "I needed to heal, which required a lot of therapy and understanding to grasp what had just happened."

They did a final retrieval in the spring of 2017 and ended up with one normal embryo, which was transferred in the fall. She got pregnant again, but Tia knew in her heart the pregnancy wouldn't last. After the positive pregnancy test, she miscarried within the week.

"My husband has always been my cheer-leader, even when I pressed to keep going. But after that third transfer failed, I knew I was not destined to be a mom," she explains. "The grief, worry, financial and emotional stress that comes with trying to find success with IVF was too much for me. I couldn't imagine starting from square one again."

They decided other family-building options weren't right for them, and Tia and Mark moved forward as a family of two (with mul-tiple bulldogs). While Tia admits that at first she questioned whether she'd made the right choice, she ultimately found a new purpose. She converted the intended nursery into an office and now works as an advocate and speaker for the child-free community.

"I don't regret how anything unfolded," she says. "My life was supposed to have this set of hurdles to learn and grow from. My life went exactly how it was supposed to go. I learned and failed and thrived through all of it."

Considering a Meaningful Child-Free Life

When you're doing everything possible to build your family, the idea of hav-ing a happy, fulfilling life without your own children is inconceivable. But for some cou-ples it's the right choice, freeing them from the stress and continuing pain of infertility. Still, deciding to be child-free isn't easy. It requires

consideration of multiple factors, a grieving period, and a new perspective on life.

BUSTED

Myth: I'll never be a whole person without children.

People often say having a child "completed them." But what does that really mean? Having a child does not make you a more valuable individual. And having a child does not guarantee a happier, more fulfilled life.

"Personal happiness is an elusive concept and also far-ranging for every individual," points out Marie Davidson, a clinical psychologist at Fertility Centers of Illinois in Chicago. "Research on the happiness of couples or individuals with and without children does not support that not having children leads to greater unhappiness, or that having children leads to greater happiness."

Stephanie from Kansas says it took a few years, but she eventually realized that with or without children, she is a valuable person. "That gave me more confidence," she shares. "That gave me a peace about my life and who I am. I really started to live, pursuing things that I love and bring me joy."

Terminology of a Life Without Children

Let's talk about the verbiage around not having children.

Most people decide to identify as *child-free* because they view the traditional term, *child-less*, as too negative. Others feel that *child-free* discounts the emotional gravity of the decision to stop trying to build a family—that it denies that they ever wanted children. Still others use the phrase "childless not by choice" because they don't believe they had or made a choice—that it was forced upon them due to their circumstances. Justine Froelker, the author of *Ever Upward: Overcoming the Lifelong Losses of Infertility to Define Your Own Happy Ending*, prefers to say she has a "child-full" life—in other words, there are many ways to have children in your life.

There is no right answer. You can choose whatever words you'd like to describe your situation. If you find any term hurtful, take the time to explain to others why you prefer other adjectives so they get a better understanding of what it's like to have to make the decision to be child-free after infertility.

For this chapter, we're going to use *child-free* and *without your own children* (which is *not*, to be clear, meant to imply that genetics plays a role in whether a child is "your own"). These are the terms most commonly used within the infertility community, but this in no way means you have to use them. The terms that feel most accurate and personal to you are the most important. In that regard, when quoting other infertility warriors, I defer to the terms they prefer in their circumstance.

Breaking Up with Infertility

Breaking up with infertility means that *right now*, fertility treatments or other options are not for you and you are embracing a child-free life. You are freeing yourself from the control and power that the attempt to try to build your family has had over your life and your relationships. And if your circumstances or feelings change, you can revisit your options down the road. Deciding to be child-free does not necessarily close the door forever. It may not always feel like it, but you are allowed to change your mind.

"Look at the things you do now that you love that would be harder or impossible with kids, and think about the possibilities that would open up—the financial pros and cons, emotional, physical, all of it. Look at it from all angles," advises Ariane from Minnesota. "You can make a decision at any time, and it doesn't have to be a permanent decision. Us deciding to be child-free doesn't mean we're going on birth control. We're deciding that we're not pursuing treatments and we're not pursuing other options right now, but we can change our minds."

Before we discuss *how* you work through the emotional decision to be child-free, let's look at the different infertility situations and their nuances.

WARRIOR TIPS
When to Consider Living Child-Free

You should consider living child-free if:

- You are financially unable to pursue or continue fertility treatment.

- The emotional toll of fertility treatment and its impact on your life is too great.

- Your health is being negatively impacted by the risks associated with fertility treatments or recurrent pregnancy losses.

- Certain or more invasive fertility treatments are not right for you or do not align with your beliefs.

- Adoption or surrogacy isn't the right choice for you because of your finances, emotions, or other reasons.

BUSTED

Myth: Without a child, I will always feel the pain of infertility.

Infertility is painful, plain and simple. But whether you end up with a child or not, the pain never fully disappears. Tia and Mark realized they were in so much emotional distress that their perspective on having a child changed.

"A baby doesn't automatically guarantee a happy ending," Tia says. "For a long time, I believed having a baby would automatically make all the sacrifice to myself, my marriage, and my career worth it, but I learned through all the failure that a baby would never be a cure-all for any sort of lingering anxiety or depression I held onto."

The only way to ease your pain is to work through it. The scars will always be there, but the antidote to grief isn't a child; it's time, developed coping skills, and processing your traumas.

Not Pursuing Fertility Treatments

Some couples decide to forgo fertility treatments as soon as they are diagnosed with an issue. It is common—and, more important, valid—for couples to decide right away that being child-free is the best option.

• **Financial constraints.** Fertility treatments are expensive, and many are not covered by insurance. It does not make you a quitter to decide against treatment because you are unable to afford it. Doing what's best financially for yourself and your loved ones is admirable.

• **Personal beliefs.** Your religious and ethical beliefs are important and personal. If fertility treatments do not align with your beliefs (see chapter 18), that's your choice and no one else's.

• **Emotional health.** Fertility treatments can be devastating, and having a stiff upper lip is not enough to get you through. Be honest about your mental health and whether pursuing treatment is something you're currently able to handle.

• **Health risks.** Some infertility diagnostic tests and treatments require surgery, and there's always a chance of complications. Pregnancy itself can be very high-risk for some people. No one should have to take on those risks if they don't want to.

BUSTED

Myth: I'd be a fool to stop trying after everything I've been through.

Choosing to be child-free is using your current situation and the information you've gained along the way to do what's best for you. Still, as psychotherapist Dr. Maria T. Rothenburger, who specializes in infertility at Miracles Happen Fertility Center in Salem, Oregon, points out, overcoming the fear of feeling silly or foolish for deciding to be child-free is a big hurdle for many.

Nobody makes this decision lightly. If you've worked through your issues, been honest about your emotions, and done your due diligence when weighing options, you're not being foolish. You're making an informed choice.

In fact, I'd argue that continuing to pursue treatment or to go through the adoption process when it is not conducive to your health and happiness is a little foolish. Trying to build a family was the right choice in the past, but once your circumstances change, it's okay to change your mind.

• **Not agreeing with the suggested treatment.** Depending on your situation, you might only have options that aren't right for you. For example, some couples want a biological connection with their child. If that's not negotiable, but your only options are to use egg, sperm, or embryo donation, you have a right to decide against treatment.

Discontinuing Fertility Treatments

At some point, many infertility warriors find themselves saying, "Enough is enough." You've undergone fertility treatments or other family-building options, and you no longer think continuing is best. Even if you've spent years trying and have persevered through undeniable pain, it is more than reasonable to move on from treatment if it's affecting your life negatively.

• **Damage to your relationship.** Infertility is hard not only on individuals, but also on partnerships and families. If your relationship is suffering because of the treatment you're going through, don't be afraid to stop and focus on rebuilding what you have.

• **Financial constraints.** Again, you don't have to bankrupt yourself by continually trying different treatments.

• **Emotional exhaustion.** If you continue with treatments until you're an emotional shell of your former self, what would your quality of life be?

• **Physical exhaustion.** Starting down the road of fertility treatments does not mean you have to keep going if the physical toll is too high.

• **No longer recognizing your life.** Infertility has a tendency to take over people's lives. Everything from your relationships to your career to your dreams outside of building a family can be damaged. When you find you're no longer leading a life you want because of infertility, consider stopping treatments.

"We need to never give up on *ourselves*, which for some of us—and, in reality, needs to be for more of us—means that we must let go of a dream before the pursuit of it destroys everything good about us," advises Froekler.

 WARRIOR ACTION STEPS
Taking a Break

You should never feel rushed into making a decision about any aspect of family building. Taking a trial break from treatment is a healthy way to figure out if you're ready to move on from having a child. If you'd like to try life away from fertility treatments or the adoption process, remember the following:

• **Don't run from your feelings.** Try new hobbies or return to old interests. But don't use them as a way to avoid your feelings. If you don't use the break to feel and cope, you won't be in a better place to make a decision when it's done.

• **Track changes in your emotions.** Are you happier or do you feel more despondent? Do you find yourself getting excited about certain events? Now that your life isn't focused on infertility, get perspective on your feelings so you can see what a child-free life would be like.

• **Don't set time-based deadlines.** Many people say they'll take a yearlong break, but making this decision is a process. So instead, look at milestones as a way to determine the length of your break. For instance, if you have a partner, you might decide to reconsider treatments when you both feel your relationship has recovered sufficiently.

Deciding Not to Adopt

As mentioned in chapter 12, it's important to remember that adopting a child is not a consolation prize. You should pursue it as an option only if it's right for you *and* you're putting the child's needs first.

Some reasons adoption might not be the route include:

• **The emotional toll.** The adoption process is not an easy solution to infertility. It's emotional and complex and shouldn't be entered into lightly.

• **Financial constraints.** Many couples underestimate the cost of adoption, especially after fertility treatments, so they don't have the resources required to adopt when the time comes.

• **Wanting a genetic connection with your child.** Adoptive parents bond with and love their children, but they have to come to terms with the absence of a genetic connection with the child. If you haven't reached that acceptance, it's best not to adopt.

Ariane offers a shift in perspective that made a big difference for her. "People often talk about starting their family, but the truth is, you already *have* a family—a family of two with your significant other."

For singles, I would add something my dad always says: Your family is who sits around your table. Family does not have to be a significant other or a blood relative. Family is who shows up when you need them.

Checking in with Your Feelings

The decision to be child-free comes with a lot of complications, but Dr. Rothenburger says the process can be compared to something simpler: shopping for jeans. Every brand has different styles, coloring, and fit, so you have to try on different pairs. When you put on *the pair*, you know.

"You pull them on and they snap perfectly, there's no gap in the back, and the length is great," she says. "And there's this feeling like a sigh of relief."

When deciding whether to continue trying to build your family, be honest with yourself about how each option makes you feel. If another round of treatment gives you a greater sense of comfort than being child-free, you might not be ready to change your plan. But if deciding not to have kids feels lighter and like a better fit, it's probably time to move on.

Tia describes her decision as finally listening to her heart. It didn't happen right away. Even as she saw the chaos infertility was bringing to her relationships, career, and finances, she kept prioritizing her treatments.

"My brain always wanted to keep pushing forward to 'get my money's worth' or to show everyone else I could succeed if I just kept trying," she says. "But my heart knew better. My heart and my intuition told me no matter how hard I tried, I was just digging a deeper hole. And what's the point of having a child if you lose your husband, you get fired, and you lose your own identity?"

Coming to a Decision with a Partner

It's incredibly scary to tell a partner that you want to consider a child-free life, or vice versa. But as with many aspects of infertility, being open and nonjudgmental is essential to the process.

Justine encourages everyone to determine their "enoughs" for themselves. "How far are you willing to go? How many losses can you endure? How much money can you spend? How much can your relationship take?"

BUSTED

Myth: Being child-free is failing.

Psychologist Julie Bindeman, co-director of Integrative Therapy of Greater Washington in Washington, DC, says society ingrains the message that a child-free couple has broken a societal "pact" to procreate. But you do not owe children to society or even to your family. If being child-free is right for you, you're honoring yourself (and your partner, if you have one), which is a success, not a failure.

Tia says she completely disagrees with the idea that being child-free is "giving up." After sacrificing for years, choosing to move on only made sense. "Dreams shift. Plans change," she explains. "Staying stagnant in a recurring circle of failure, sadness, and depression for one facet of your life is going to get you nowhere."

For Ariane and her husband, Ben, the key was redefining being child-free so it *was* a choice. "Infertility had all the control before when I felt like it was taking choice away from me. But once we reframed that, it feels like we are back in control. We are choosing not to pursue other options, and we are choosing to remain a family of two."

When you are a child-free adult, people will probably ask you about your plans for kids. That's problematic in and of itself, but unavoidable. You can't control what people ask you. However, when you are asked if you have kids or if you are planning to, find ways to refocus the conversation on other life purposes. You can simply say, "No, I don't have kids." Then switch up the conversation. Ask the individual about their non-child-related interests.

Once you've gained an understanding of your own feelings, you should approach this conversation with the following guidelines:

• **Talk when emotions aren't heightened.** Both you and your partner need to feel safe expressing your emotions and fears. That's not possible if either of you is feeling particularly angry, stressed, or sad. You'll be more likely to take things personally or inadvertently react in a hurtful way.

• **Have flexible checkpoints.** Many couples set deadlines about when to stop fertility treatments. You'll move on after three rounds of IVF or when you turn 35 or after trying for 5 years. But when you set those deadlines, you don't know how you'll feel when they arrive. It's better to designate times throughout your infertility journey to evaluate your situation and make decisions based on your feelings and circumstances at that point.

• **Compromise.** It may feel hard to compromise without one of you giving up something significant, but you can make an agreement to take a break or try less invasive or stressful treatments so both of you can continue to process the idea of choosing to be child-free in the meantime.

• **Consider seeking professional help.** If you and your partner are unable to discuss being child-free without using hurtful or blaming language, there's most likely an underlying issue. Consider meeting with a therapist to first address those problems, and *then* move on to the child-free decision.

Deciding to be child-free is a big change that means shifting your energy, focus, and time away from infertility. It may take some time to know what to do instead. Be patient and give yourself permission to make mistakes. And, of course, never be afraid to ask for help.

Grieving Your Loss

We'll dig deeper into grieving your losses throughout your infertility journey later on (see chapter 14). But as you go through your own emotions, be kind to yourself and try to remember the following:

• **Grief comes in waves.** There are going to be some days when your grief about being child-free will hit hard. On other days, you'll feel so fulfilled by your life that it won't cross your mind. It's important to recognize that this is natural and honor your feelings when they pop up.

• **There's no set timeline.** Everyone grieves at their own pace, and there's no one right way to process your feelings. It only matters that you are working through your emotions.

• **Partners grieve differently.** Each person has their own way of managing grief, and you and your partner will likely have different tendencies and processes. You may not recognize your partner's grief if it doesn't look like your own. Be respectful of how your partner may be feeling or dealing with their grief in ways you don't understand.

Even though deciding to be child-free is a healthy, valid, and liberating choice, it doesn't make all the negative emotions surrounding infertility vanish. Dr. Bindeman says it's not uncommon for infertility warriors to suppress their emotions to quickly move on to the "next phase." But this isn't coping.

"Just because emotions are pushed to the side doesn't mean that they aren't impactful or that they are actually 'gone,'" she reminds us. "They're just deferred to be dealt with at a future time."

Identifying Your Needs

"Grief is going to come up, likely at inopportune times," advises Tia. "Sit with it and understand where your triggers are. It's the only way to keep moving forward."

Over time, pay attention to how your feelings change. It can be helpful to take inventory of your life and determine what aspects may have suffered from neglect because of your focus on infertility. Look at what you've missed, and think of what you need to do to restore those parts of your life to their former glory.

Do this evaluation with kindness and forgiveness. Don't feel guilty about what you let fall to the wayside. Instead, remind yourself that you needed to put down some interests and responsibilities to go on your infertility journey. You made sacrifices to prioritize other important parts of your life. Those choices were the right ones at the time, and they've allowed you to eventually accept and embrace a child-free life.

Communicating Your Needs

Because of the existing taboo surrounding not having children, it's not easy to explain your needs to your family and friends once you've decided to be child-free.

A great first step is explaining that you're making a choice, not admitting defeat. You can lead them to your perspective by asking them to list any changes they've noticed in your personality, mood, and behavior during your infertility journey. Chances are they've seen your pain and struggle, and having them recount the issues aloud will help them understand why you've decided to shift your focus to endeavors that will get you back to being happy and fulfilled. Then, let them know what they can do to help you out.

If your relationship has been hurt by infertility, meet them halfway and ask what *they* need from *you* to strengthen your connection. For Tia and Mark, learning to support each other was a bumpy road. Both of them are extremely independent by nature—and in the past, they worked through

→

their own issues independently, seeking guidance from one another only as needed. "The need to just be present while one of us vented our frustrations or cried and screamed became a new scenario. It was a huge learning curve to take a step back and not try and solve the other one's problem, opting instead to just be there and listen," she explains.

"We finally found a groove with the feelings that stem from grief and loss. When one of us starts to get overly cranky or short-tempered, chances are grief is right around the corner. We are now aware of the signs of this and stop what we're doing, calm down, and let the other one speak about their concerns and allow any other emotions to flow. It's not about stifling our emotions from each other, worrying we will be 'too much' for the other to handle. This is our new normal, and it has brought us closer together on an emotional level than ever before."

Supporting Other Infertility Warriors While Erasing the Taboo

Societal pressure is a big part of what makes the decision to be child-free so difficult. When a friend tells you they've decided to be child-free, you may feel, on some level, the need to offer them pity. But what they really need is empathy and acceptance.

Whether or not you yourself are child-free, according to Dr. Rothenburger, how you interact with others in the infertility community is the perfect place to start undoing the taboo. "Consider congratulating them," she says. "It's freedom. They're done with the pain and the struggle, they've reached that conclusion. And who doesn't want to be there? It's a huge thing to celebrate."

Whether you've already decided to be child-free or it's still a consideration, every time you take on the taboo, it weakens its hold. It allows you and your fellow infertility warriors to be more comfortable with the choice.

"Going with your gut and staying true to your own convictions—not outside societal pressures—is key to finding happiness and fulfillment in your life," says Tia. "There is a *much* larger community of women without children than we are giving ourselves credit for. Reach out. Find your people. Lean on the good ones, and dismiss the naysayers."

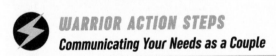

WARRIOR ACTION STEPS
Communicating Your Needs as a Couple

As your relationship as a child-free couple evolves, communication is key to strengthening your partnership. But good communication is more than just talking; it's showing your openness through your actions.

- **Share your triggers.** Talking with your friends about their kids, attending baby showers, seeing cute baby videos on social media—triggers are everywhere. Make sure you and your partner discuss your triggers so you can offer each other support when the need arises.

- **Find new ways to nurture.** Many people feel they've given up their chance to use their nurturing skills when they decide to be child-free. But this can place an unspoken stress on your relationship. There are thousands of ways to nurture without being a parent. Plant a garden. Babysit your nieces or nephews. Volunteer for

people in need. In other words, direct your loving nature into something productive that will help you cope.

- **Listen; don't fix.** If one of you is struggling with the decision to be child-free, don't try to "fix" each other's feelings. It's better to make your partner feel heard and unjudged and to allow them to feel the full range of emotions, from grief to happiness.

- **Reaffirm that your partner is your priority.** It's common for people to have doubts about whether their partner has truly accepted being child-free. This is particularly true if one of you (and not the other) is the source of the infertility issue. Look for ways to remind your partner of why you chose to be with them. For example, Tia says it always helps when her husband, Mark, says, "I married you. You come first in my world. Everything else is secondary."

Living Your Best Life

Once you've worked through your initial grief, you're ready to start living your best life. For couples who have spent years on the infertility journey, planning treatments and scheduling appointments, your first inclination might be to start mapping out the rest of your life.

"You have the freedom to make a lot of choices," says Dr. Alice Domar, an expert in mind/body health and infertility. "But you don't have to decide right now what you're going to do."

Start by defining what child-free means to you. For some couples, being child-free means not enduring another high-risk pregnancy or painful miscarriage, and they decide to go back on birth control. Others take the "we're not trying, but we're not preventing" route. Figure out which path is right for you.

WARRIOR WISDOM
A Journey of Acceptance

"After deciding to be childfree, I took a trip by myself, and it turned out to be the best possible thing I ever could have done. I covered a little over 6,300 miles, 11 states. I stayed at and hiked in 10 national parks. I saw friends and family. I camped. I stayed in Airbnbs. Essentially, it was the time alone that was incredibly introspective and meditative. I drove most of the trip in silence. As soon as the landscape started to change, I couldn't listen to anything, and I would just be present. It was the most mindful experience that I've ever had in my life, where I was able to really just sit with the way I was feeling. I could sit in the moment and experience awe and wonder."

— Ariane, Minnesota

WARRIOR CHECKLIST
Living a Happy, Full Life Without Your Own Children

- ❏ Understand that being child-free is a valid choice. It is not a sign that you are incomplete or a failure.
- ❏ Consider all of the factors at play when deciding to not pursue or continue fertility treatment or to not adopt.
- ❏ Take time to clarify your own feelings about the right choice for you.
- ❏ Discuss being child-free with your partner, if you have one.
- ❏ Grieve your loss and have coping mechanisms in place to help you deal with emotions.
- ❏ Embrace all the possibilities of a child-free life.

PART THREE

Big Feelings

The Emotions You Might Feel

CHAPTER 14

INFERTILITY ISN'T JUST A PHYSICAL journey. It's an emotional one, too.

Brianna from Pennsylvania, came from a large family and was the oldest of four. Her own mom inspired her to want to become a mother, but she and her husband, Chad, decided to wait until they had stable careers, bought a house, and were truly ready.

She knew she might face challenges in conceiving because her periods were always heavy and painful. After 6 months of trying, though, she was already frustrated and desperate. Her mom had conceived all four of her kids easily, and no one in Brianna's life could relate to her worries about fertility.

Brianna met up with a friend who, coincidentally, was also trying to conceive. While talking, the two women discovered that their periods were scheduled to start the same day, so they promised to check in on each other then.

Brianna got her period as expected. "Like an idiot, I texted her asking if she got her period," she says. "Did I actually want the answer I feared?"

Indeed, her friend was pregnant. "I remember that instant gut punch," she explains. "This was the first time I realized that I was going to be left behind. People around me were going to find sweet joy and happiness, while I suffered and waited. It all became so real."

Brianna was initially brushed off by doctors, who told her she was young and not to worry. "It made me so angry," she says. "Am I supposed to hurt less just because I am young?"

Eventually, testing revealed that she had a septate uterus and only 1 percent of her husband's sperm was normally shaped. "I was so scared for what this news would bring to our journey," Brianna remembers.

They went on to try several IUIs, all of which failed. It was time to bring out the big guns and try IVF. But first, after undertaking research and educating herself, Brianna advocated for her septum to be surgically removed. Her doctors agreed.

After Brianna's surgery, she began IVF, and her first egg retrieval cycle ended in 13 frozen embryos. "I was on a cloud. I was so damn happy," she says.

Next up: a frozen embryo transfer. Unfortunately, one of her routine uterine lining scans showed that the septum had returned, and the transfer was canceled. She was told she would need a second surgery. "Just when I started to see light at the end of the tunnel, the rug was ripped out from under me. I cried. I had many mental breakdowns, even dark thoughts. I mourned."

But Brianna got back up, brushed herself off, and decided to stay the course. After a second septum surgery, she finally had her frozen transfer—and is cautiously optimistic about the future.

Wading Through the Emotions of Infertility

Many infertility warriors struggle with this idea that they are supposed to feel a certain way. But there are no "correct" emotions, and punishing yourself for how you feel only creates more negative emotions.

Angela from Missouri experienced crippling depression during her infertility journey. When her niece was born, she couldn't bring herself to visit, and her father just couldn't understand. "He called me and used words that he never used before or since, including calling me disgusting. I was already in bed crying before the call so it didn't hurt as much, but I agreed. I was disgusting," she says.

Not all emotions you'll feel on this journey will be negative. However, expect to oscillate between positive and negative. "With treatment cycles, it's a constant swing between hope and grief as you try to stay positive each month—only to be disappointed when the cycle is unsuccessful," shares Adrienne from New Jersey.

Adrienne also struggled with recurrent pregnancy loss, making the hope-grief cycle even more complex. "As much as you're hopeful to become pregnant, after one or more miscarriages, you're equally terrified to see that positive pregnancy test. And once you do, every day is a polarizing battle between fear and hope."

Sheri from New York also experienced emotions that were all over the map. "Our 5-year journey with infertility has been incredibly emotional," she says. "We've experienced hope and optimism with each new idea or next step and extreme sadness with each treatment that didn't work, embryo that didn't take, and early pregnancy that was lost."

"Emotions are an inherent part of nearly all medical decisions and impact decision-making in several ways, both good and bad," Jody Madeira, author of *Taking Baby Steps*, explains. "If emotions get too intense, they can hamper our decision-making by making it hard to listen and process information that can be vital to making treatment decisions."

Sometimes, intense negative emotions catch warriors off-guard. This was the case for Nune from California. "I've had every emotion throughout this journey, but two emotions that have surprised me are fear and shame. I have been scared that . . . all this is just not meant to be and I don't deserve to have children. I have been feeling shame for not being able to be a real and complete woman."

An infertility survivor herself, Madeira says it's crucial to understand and accept all your emotions so you can seek support when you need it. "I think it's really important for individuals to know just how normal emotions are—they might even feel contradictory emotions at the same time. It's very important to be good to one's self—to be honest with one's self even if the infertility journey proves to be far harder, more painful, and longer than anyone expected."

Even once you've accepted that your emotions aren't right or wrong, it's common to feel completely isolated. How could anyone else feel this badly? How could anyone else understand?

BUSTED

Myth: There are acceptable levels of grief.

There's this (false) notion that some events are more "grievable" than others—you should feel more grief after a miscarriage than after an unsuccessful IVF cycle, for example. As a result, many people dealing with infertility feel like they don't have a right to feel as bad as they do for events and situations that other people might classify as "not a big deal."

Maria T. Rothenburger, a psychotherapist at Miracles Happen Fertility Center in Salem, Oregon, who specializes in infertility, warns that not acknowledging and experiencing the grief that surrounds infertility is dangerous. "Losing the potential for growing a baby in any given cycle is to lose the dream of a new soul coming into one's life," she says. "Expecting one to grieve infertility losses in any other way than 'normal' death is disheartening, painful. In my opinion, it serves to drive one further into isolation and [raises] the potential for major depression and even suicide."

After a failed frozen embryo transfer, Brandy from Idaho didn't feel like she had a right to grieve. There was so much else in her life to be thankful for. But eventually she realized that because she was denying herself permission to experience her loss, her depression was getting out of control.

It didn't help that she knew the gender of the baby she might have had thanks to genetic testing. For some warriors, all the information they can know about an embryo—because of the high-tech methodology of fertility treatments—makes the loss of the embryo feel more real. "While he didn't implant, I knew more about my little boy for the 2 weeks he was inside me than most people know their entire pregnancy," Brandy shares. "How could I not grieve that loss?"

As I've repeated throughout the book, you are *not* alone in your infertility journey. There are people currently in your life—and waiting to meet you via a support group—who will stand by your side.

While it can be scary to ask for help, it's an important part of your emotional health. Lisa from Illinois admits that she was extremely anxious about opening up. So she started with an online message board. From there, she found the strength to talk to her close friends and attend support group meetings. "It was unbelievable the stories that were shared with me, and I realized I was not alone."

As for me, I cried—a lot. I cursed—a lot. I recognized that I was in emotional trouble and needed to make a big change *fast* or risk losing myself completely. So, I made a choice—a choice to go out and seek positivity, to seek hope. My solution was to host the

Beat Infertility podcast. It started as a bit of a selfish venture—interviewing people who'd "beaten" infertility to help *me* regain a sense of optimism.

Working through your emotions is a process, and some feelings you've worked through will pop back up later. Even if it's two steps forward and one step back, focus on overall, long-term progress. Just remember: *You do not have to work through all your issues before moving forward.*

"Most of my patients seem to believe that they should work through their feelings of shock, disappointment, denial, anger, bargaining, and depression and find acceptance before they can move forward emotionally along their infertility treatment journey," says Georgia Witkin, director of psychological and wellness services at Reproductive Medicine Associates of New York. "But research finds there are no neat stages of recovery from loss. We each move at different rates, and we can experience and deal with more than one feeling at the same time. That means we can be sad, worried, or frightened about past fertility results and yet hopeful and excited about the next steps."

Riding the Emotional Roller Coaster

Over the course of 8 years, Krista from New Jersey suffered six miscarriages. After each loss, grief and sadness took over. Feelings of depression were particularly intense after she miscarried twins.

"It's deep and dark," she says. "There was a time, after I miscarried my twins, when I literally had to pull myself out of bed and force myself to do one thing a day that made me feel like a human."

Krista struggled with basic daily tasks. Some days, all she could manage was brushing her teeth. Other days, she felt stronger and could go to the grocery store. Eventually, as a way to cope with her grief, Krista worked to expand her mind, body, and soul. "I looked at my obstacles as a way to open myself spiritually. Meditation and energy work have been valuable tools in my self-care."

When Krista finally did give birth to her son, all the pain seemed worth it. "The second he was born, I said to my husband that I'd do it all over again if it meant having him. He was my last embryo after my first round of IVF."

Many of the emotions you'll feel during your infertility journey are negative, but I truly believe in acting on and making the most of the *positive* emotions.

But before you can do that, you need to learn to recognize and name the hard feelings.

Guilt and Shame

Dr. Rothenburger says, "Guilt and shame are the crux of infertility—and really, the baseline for all these other emotions."

The difference between guilt and shame is nuanced. Guilt focuses on behavior—how we feel about an action or actions. Shame focuses on the self—how we feel about ourselves.

Nune explains both perfectly: "I feel guilty for not trying to have children in my 20s. Instead, I played around and had fun. I

BUSTED

Myth: You deserve to feel pain.

It's common for people facing infertility to feel tremendous guilt. Because there's no one else to blame, they turn their disappointment and anger inward. And if the infertility is "your" fault, you deserve the resulting pain, right? *Wrong.*

There is no fault when it comes to infertility. It's a medical condition. The emotional pain you feel isn't a punishment for you to endure. It's a natural reaction to a difficult situation.

For Rachelle from Maine, her grief and guilt were complicated by the fact that she'd had two children in her 20s with her first husband. When she remarried in her 40s, her new husband, Nick, had no children and they wanted to build a family together.

After a year of trying, they discovered both of them had fertility issues. Rachelle began to feel terrible that she couldn't give her husband a child. "I had this horrible guilt that because he fell in love with me, he wasn't going to get to be a dad," she admits. "Then I had horrible guilt after I was actually relieved when we had our fertility diagnosis and found out it wasn't just my age—that he, too, had issues."

Rachelle understands how easy it is to fall into the guilt trap, but she also says it can crush you. It took a lot of long, open, honest conversations with her husband for them both to forgive themselves. "His constant love and assurance that he was in it forever, with or without a baby, was something I needed to hear and feel and know," she says.

---

feel shame that my body can't perform like it should. I'm not fully a woman, and I don't yet belong to the mother's club. I haven't lived up to my womanhood."

Guilt and shame are really powerful. You feel defective. You feel helpless. Those feelings are the ultimate vulnerability. They can even bleed beyond. These feelings can lead to self-doubt in areas of your life that aren't necessarily touched directly by infertility. You may start to feel unworthy or less-than in areas where you used to feel strong and proud.

"The guilt comes, too, when you think about other people," says Dr. Rothenburger. "I felt such guilt when my parents paid for a portion of our [IVF] cycle and the cycle failed. It's almost like I really, really did not want to tell them what happened because they invested and it didn't work out. They were not only out money, but they were not going to be grandparents through us."

And I hate to say it, but successfully having a child does not eliminate guilt. After Colleen from Colorado had her daughter, she still felt guilt often. "Any time I was tired or frustrated or overwhelmed by being a new mom, I was brought to tears because I felt so guilty for having those other emotions. We struggled to have a child. . . . Why was I complaining about lack of sleep? Why did I feel overwhelmed instead of grateful that I had a baby to overwhelm me? I felt like I should never have those emotions because we were the lucky ones."

Adrienne, who felt ashamed because, as she says, "there was no one else to blame" but herself for her miscarriages, healed mostly with time. "[Letting time pass] allowed me a bit more perspective on the situation. I did seek therapy, which helped to some extent. Listening to similar stories from other women was also extremely helpful because it helped me feel less isolated."

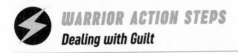

WARRIOR ACTION STEPS
Dealing with Guilt

- **Learn your triggers.** Identifying your triggers helps you not only avoid them in the future but also transfer your feelings to an external source. You're not feeling guilty because you're "less than" but because you've seen twenty-five pregnant people today.

- **Realize that infertility happens.** Infertility is a physical reality that can have a lot of explanations, but failure as a human being is not one of them.

- **Fight your inner critic.** Thoughts tend to dictate our next behavior or action. If a thought is negative, your action will likely be self-sabotaging. Every time you hear a voice of guilt or shame in your head, answer it with a comeback. To form a comeback, write down the negative thought and look at it objectively. Then think about how you would respond to it if you were your most confident self.

Envy

Envy is one of the most difficult emotions to acknowledge because it carries with it so much shame. When you are envious, you desire someone else's good news—you want what they have. When you hear or see that someone is pregnant, whether it's someone you know or a complete stranger, you think, "I'm happy for her but sad for me." In fact, you might even *not* feel happy for the other person and instead just sad for yourself—and that's okay!

One of my triggers is Kate Middleton, the Princess of Wales. I'm sure she's a perfectly lovely person, but it felt like every time I had an appointment at my fertility clinic, she was on the waiting room TV announcing either a new pregnancy or the birth of her latest child.

Sheri had several friends who got married around the same time that she did, so she wasn't surprised when they announced their first pregnancies. She was happy for them and excited to share this part of their lives with

them. But when her friends started announcing they were pregnant with their second child and Sheri saw no end in sight to her journey, it was hard on her.

"I was still happy for them, of course, but also envious," she recalls. "[I] felt like I was stuck in time while watching everyone else move forward. I distinctly remember one evening sitting on my couch and seeing a friend's name pop up on my phone. She and I would usually text or plan a phone date in advance, so it was unusual for her to call out of the blue. I turned to my husband and said, 'I bet she's pregnant again.' I ignored the call. It took me a couple days to gather the strength to call back and be supportive and genuinely (I hope!) happy for them when she shared the news."

Dr. Rothenburger says, "Sometimes the initial thought is of harm. So, 'I want something bad to happen [to that person].' And then comes the guilt and the shame for even having those thoughts. I know it's a tough topic, but you are absolutely normal if you have those thoughts. The worst thing that you can do is beat yourself up for them. There are no *have tos* when it comes to envy, or really any of these emotions. It's just an emotion."

"If your behaviors begin to match those thoughts of harm," she continues, "then that's a whole different topic. But for the most part, most people will have that kind of thought but never have an intention or a thought of actually carrying anything through. It's just an initial shocked response to the trigger."

Recognize that it is *normal* to feel this way. Allow yourself to feel envious in the moment, but don't let it consume you. Again, know your triggers and avoid them when possible. Don't hide from the world, but give yourself permission to stay away from baby showers, birthday parties, and other gatherings if they might overwhelm you.

Adrienne recalls the day when she learned she and her husband would have to move on

WARRIOR ACTION STEPS
Dealing with Envy

Envy is about a loss of control, so regain and harness that control in the following ways.

• **Tackle something you enjoy.** Doing something you are really good at redirects that negative energy. It can also remind you that while you may struggle to have a child, you possess qualities and gifts that others might envy.

• **Separate your envy from the person.** Remind yourself that you don't want to *be* that person or have exactly what they have (their specific child). What you want is a child of your own. That will help you process your feelings in a more objective way.

• **Don't seal yourself away.** Avoid your envy triggers when possible, but don't become a hermit. Feelings of isolation will just dredge up more negative emotions.

---

to IVF. "I came straight from my fertility clinic to work, trying to wrap my head around the enormity of that. When I got to my office, a coworker announced her pregnancy, and I just couldn't stop that envious feeling from welling up. I tried hard to put on an excited face, but inside I was crumbling."

You might be surprised to learn how she worked through her envy: by talking to that coworker. "Ultimately, I decided to share my fertility struggles with her. Because we were friends, I was concerned that as much as I may try to hide it, she may have been picking up on my envy. I thought that at least if she knew where I was coming from, she might understand my reactions better."

Alicia from Florida followed advice I give to my infertility coaching clients all the time: Take a break from social media. "I didn't like feeling so envious, but it seemed to eat me alive at times. I was surprised at how envious I was of people I cared the most about," she says. "I decided to be as honest as I could about my

feelings and take breaks from people when I needed to. I am lucky enough to have very caring and understanding friends who were not offended when I was candid about these emotions. A support system, being honest, and time helped [me] through this emotion."

Grief

Chapter 17 is devoted to pregnancy loss and the grief and more serious mental health problems it can cause. However, as you already know, infertility itself is a loss—the loss of being able to conceive spontaneously. There's no such thing as an infertility journey without grief. The grief can hit you suddenly in a single moment—such as when you receive a new diagnosis—or gradually build up over time.

Infertility can cause other losses, too—the loss of control over your own body; the loss of physical, mental, and financial wellness; the loss of friendships and familial relationships; and so on. Grief and the surrounding emotions may even develop into other issues, like depression and anxiety.

As Penny Joss Fletcher, a licensed marriage and family therapist in Tustin, California, succinctly put it, "Our society is not good with grief."

Grief is hard. Nobody wants to experience it, and few know how to deal with it. As a result, we often don't have a good understanding of grief. This can make our feelings even more difficult to process, leading to additional painful emotions like frustration, guilt, and shame.

The Five Stages of Grief

You are probably already familiar with the five stages of grief—denial, anger, bargaining, depression, and acceptance—first introduced by psychiatrist Elisabeth Kübler-Ross.

Over the years, there have been criticisms and objections to the five stages model. In practice, many mental health professionals

BUSTED

Myth: A successful pregnancy will solve everything.

When you've spent years trying to build a family, that end goal starts to feel like the solution to every problem in your life. Once you have a baby, you and your partner will no longer fight. You'll be able to rebuild strained relationships with your friends and family. All the stress and negative feelings will disappear.

But this isn't the way mental health works. As Julie Bindeman, a psychologist and co-director of Integrative Therapy of Greater Washington in Washington, DC, notes, issues can still bubble up. "The pain associated with some of these emotional experiences can last for a long time—even through a successful pregnancy and birth," she says.

Instead of pushing pain aside, deal with it head-on. Otherwise, your pain will continue to negatively impact your life—whether you are able to have a child or not.

For years, Ris from Minnesota went through multiple rounds of IUI and IVF. Eventually she gave birth to her daughter. But her negative emotions didn't go away. "I know I waited too long to address my grief and depression," she admits. "I let it get to the point where it was almost out of control before going to a therapist. It wasn't until my daughter was almost 2 that I finally realized I couldn't handle this on my own anymore."

remember two things. First, everyone experiences and responds to grief differently. Second, grief isn't linear. This is important, so let me repeat it: *Grief isn't linear.*

Dr. Rothenburger explains, "You can go through all five components of grief in 5 minutes, and then start all over again—or go back and forth, back and forth, between two of them. And there are times when people feel stuck in one of these parts of grief."

Even though Samantha from Delaware had grieved her unexplained infertility diagnosis, once she started IVF treatments, the waves of grief began crashing over her again. "Looking back, it felt like each month I went through the five stages of grief," she admits. "And each month I had to pick myself up and do it all over again."

DENIAL

Denial is almost the absence of a feeling because you refuse to admit something is truly happening—*you* couldn't possibly have infertility.

Katherine Hannon, a psychotherapist in Bethesda, Maryland, who specializes in infertility, points out that most people have a hard time accepting that they have infertility. "In the beginning, many ask, 'How can this happen to me/us?'" she says. "They think they have done 'everything right' and should be able to reproduce fairly easily."

Even people who know infertility is a possibility—or have already experienced another facet of it—are still shocked when they get new information, Hannon says. This was true for Brianna, who, after months of trying to conceive, reached out to her ob-gyn. When reviewing the initial lab work, her doctor noted Brianna had low progesterone. "I figured this was the answer to our problems! Such an easy fix. . . . I was confident. I remember saying to myself, 'I worried for nothing. *This* is my answer!'" Brianna explains. "Then I went in for an HSG and hysteroscopy—two

are moving away from it. But culturally, it is familiar, and it can ring true for many people. The experiences surrounding grief are complicated—especially with infertility. It can be difficult to organize your feelings in a coherent way. So, I'd like to use the five stages, not scientifically, but as a framework to help us delve into a difficult topic. But I'd like you to

⚡ WARRIOR ACTION STEPS
Dealing with Denial

Denial is brought on by the unexpected, so it can be tough to plan for. But if you think you tend toward denial, here are some steps you can take.

- **Recognize the signs.** Get to know your body really well and what it's trying to say. Listen to and process the information you're told so you can see when physical signs contradict what you "know" to be true. For example, perhaps you never get fertile cervical mucus or your cycles are shorter than 25 days. These are two of many possible signs that you should see a fertility specialist.

- **Never say never.** It's certainly okay to say no for now, but when the power of denial leads you to say never to a particular treatment or diagnosis, you close off many possible avenues to success. Open your heart and mind. I was a never IVFer, mainly because I didn't think I'd need it—I was in denial. But once I shed my denial, I ended up doing three retrievals and seven transfers, which gave me my amazing daughter!

- **Replace denial with knowledge.** Being a voracious researcher will help you see warning signs. It won't always stop denial from happening, but it will likely pass much more quickly because you'll recognize the reality of your situation sooner.

---

extremely painful procedures for me. During my hysteroscopy, a uterine abnormality was discovered. I was puzzled, concerned, and so heartbroken all at the same time. I started to cry under the dark light of the ultrasound room."

Perhaps you're reading this book because you have several of the signs of infertility, but you still feel it's not yet time to see a reproductive endocrinologist. Or maybe you've just received a diagnosis that explains your infertility struggles, but it's too overwhelming to possibly feel true.

"My own denial stemmed from the fact that I did get pregnant on our first cycle after birth control pills [but I quickly started bleeding]," says Dr. Rothenburger who is now a parent by way of adoption. "So, I went to the doctor, and he said, 'Oh, it's probably chemical pregnancy. You're just fine, just keep trying.' And then, I looked up the actual definition of infertility, and if you're younger than 35, it's when you've been trying for 12 months but still haven't succeeded."

Similar to Dr. Rothenburger, my denial initially set in because I became pregnant—twice, in fact—during my first year of actively trying to conceive, though in both cases the pregnancies ended in miscarriage. Looking back, even before these two early miscarriages, the signs of infertility were there—my diagnosis of endometriosis, and the fact that I'd had unprotected sex without pregnancy for years—but my brain (or perhaps my heart) refused to acknowledge them.

Alicia was in denial after she and her husband, Pablo, received their initial diagnosis. She even sought a second opinion because she didn't believe IVF could possibly be their only option. "During one of our initial consultations, I held my hand up in the stop motion to the doctor who delivered our diagnosis when he was discussing donor sperm and embryos. I looked at him and said, 'I don't just want to have a baby. I want to have my husband's baby.'"

Ultimately, Alicia and Pablo did use donor sperm. But first Alicia had to exhaust the opinions of all the doctors in her area to understand that their diagnosis was real. Time—combined with ample research, even if it didn't result in the answers they wanted—helped her pass through denial to reach acceptance.

ANGER

Anger is the most obvious emotion. It's in your face. It often comes when you feel a sense of vulnerability—of being wronged. Vulnerability comes from feeling out of control, and infertility is all about a lack of control.

Dr. Rothenburger says, "You see this all the time in the animal kingdom. When an animal is injured, for example, they tend to want to go into their cave, lick their wounds, and if any other animal comes in, they attack.

"Within the context of infertility," she continues, "we think, 'If I do step one, step two, and step three, I will always get the result I want. That's exactly how it's been my whole life.' But that is not what happens with infertility because you can do absolutely every step every single time and still not get the result that you want. It's a very disconcerting and a very vulnerable place, not to mention all of the triggers that are outside of you."

In other words, when we're faced with a problem, we're used to putting together a plan for solving it. When the plan doesn't work out, we get frustrated and angry.

Your anger might be triggered when you drive by the baby supply store, when you're invited to a baby shower, or when you see all the happy parents on your Facebook newsfeed. Anger also can come out of the blue. You might develop a short fuse. You might lose your filter during conversations, blowing up at people. When you keep anger bottled up, eventually that energy has to go somewhere. The lid blows off and the anger explodes outward.

Alicia was angry about the unfairness of it all. "I felt angry when I'd think about people getting pregnant on accident who didn't really want to be parents, about people who abuse their children, about people who are unfit to be parents but keep having babies, etc."

"I think it's best to deal with anger by acknowledging that it is completely normal, even if it is seemingly not 'rational'—like anger at a partner who has a medical condition that causes infertility," says Madeira. "Often, the worst thing one can do is try to push through the anger without acknowledging it—talking about it was definitely helpful."

Adrienne explains that she only felt anger once during her infertility journey, though she believes it may have been a blessing. "After our third miscarriage—this time with a genetically normal embryo—my first reaction was sadness and probably a bit of shock. Within a day, though, this turned to extreme anger. I

WARRIOR ACTION STEPS
Dealing with Anger

Anger is *exhausting*, mentally and physically. Not only is the emotion itself draining, but so, too, is trying to keep it inside—trying to control it, rather than it controlling you. While the solution looks different for everyone, try the following anger-release valves.

- **Exercise.** There's a ton of scientific research on how exercising releases hormones that can improve your mood. Plus, channeling your energy on an action rather than a fight will help you work through pent-up frustrations.

- **Meditate.** It's not easy to mediate when your anger is in full swing. But making meditation a part of your routine

helps ground you and gives you perspective so that, when you do get upset, you have the mental foundation in place to acknowledge and move past your feelings.

- **Go out into the woods and yell.** Scream like a crazy person. With anger, it's better out than in. And if nothing else is working, direct your fury at a tree instead of a loved one.

was angry at the doctors, at the IVF process, at myself, and yes, at God, too. My brain was trying so hard to find logic in the situation but just couldn't. There was no explanation to be had. In some ways, I'm grateful for the anger, because I think it compelled me to make a change in my treatment."

Sometimes we don't realize how much anger we hold within ourselves. Learn to recognize your external triggers, and avoid them when possible. It definitely will *not* always be possible, but at least you should be able to recognize that some big, hard feelings are coming on.

For Natascha from Arizona, anger surfaced only occasionally, typically as moodiness during PMS. But decades later, she realized she had never processed the invisible grief of infertility—and she became angry for no apparent reason. "When no one was at home, I would smash old flowerpots or beat up a bag of potato chips," she admits. "If I had lived alone, I would have smashed every single plate in the cupboard."

My triggers changed throughout my infertility journey, and yours likely will, too. You know how you barely noticed pregnant people or families with children before you started trying to conceive, but now you cannot open your eyes without running into them everywhere you go? This is a psychological phenomenon known as selective attention—and it reared its ugly head after I lost my twins.

Suddenly, twins and other higher-order multiples were *everywhere*. It seemed anyone and everyone was capable of carrying multiples to term *except me*. Surprisingly, this didn't make me envious—it made me *angry*. Angry that I was the "cause" of our infertility that led to us transfer two embryos in the first place. Angry that my cervix was incompetent. Angry that my body went into preterm labor—especially since the twins were otherwise perfectly healthy. Angry that my husband moved through the grief process faster than

me. And most of all, in the 7 months following the delivery, angry that—even with the transabdominal cerclage—my reproductive endocrinologist would never again allow us to transfer two embryos because he felt strongly my body would fail again when faced with carrying multiples.

One day, after a frustrating exchange with a difficult landlord about how our dog had to go, I just lost it on my husband. This was *the* fight to end all fights. *Have I not lost enough? Now I have to choose between my dog and my home?* But in my anger, I had forgotten everything that had happened to me also happened to *him*—to *us*, as a couple.

Thankfully, anger doesn't need to—and probably shouldn't—be a constant during your journey.

"I had to face my anger and express it to or with my husband to feel relief and bring us back to the goal—have a baby," says Alicia. "I had to remind myself that staying in this anger isn't a positive place to be and not good for my body. No one else could get us out of our anger but us, and we did."

Nune, on the other hand, meditated. "When I felt my anger coming up, I'd start to think about being present."

And Natascha? "I needed to scream, cry, and allow my body to move. Exercise and spending time in nature helped me to process the anger," she says. "And the occasional old flowerpot thrown on the backyard concrete."

There is no one right way to process anger (or any emotions, for that matter). Work through them in a way that works for you.

BARGAINING

Here's Dr. Rothenburger's example of bargaining: "If I take all the supplements, if I exercise, if I follow the fertility diet, and if I twirl around three times and sing 'Kumbaya,' then I'll get pregnant."

You know you've been there—we all have.

BUSTED

Myth: I just have to put up with people's hurtful comments.

After being diagnosed with endometriosis, Natalie from Florida told the news to those closest to her. Many of her friends and family responded with empathy and support, but she admits that some comments stung.

"These comments were not meant to be hurtful, but they were," she says. "For example, some people expressed excitement that we'd be doing IVF—as if IVF was something I should be happy about, would certainly guarantee a baby right away, and I should celebrate that."

These painful comments piled up, and when Natalie's first IVF cycle failed and people told her to "just relax," she decided enough was enough.

"I chose not to brush those comments away and started speaking up when a comment caused me pain." Stand up for yourself and ask people to change their behavior.

In the anger stage, I blamed my doctor for somehow messing up. But once I hit the bargaining stage, I began to wonder what *I* could have done differently. *Was I on bed rest for too long? Was I not on bed rest long enough?* (Back then, some level of bed rest was encouraged, so I took 5 days off work and lounged around, watching pregnancy-related movies like *Baby Mama, Father of the Bride Part II,* and *What to Expect When You're Expecting.* Ridiculous, I know.) *Should I have encouraged a mock embryo transfer? What about an endometrial scratch?* Suddenly, the failure became mine to own—and mine to bargain for so I could fix it.

Additionally, I strongly felt that our situation was *my fault.* Our infertility, like this latest cycle failure, was *mine.* I know you know this deep down, but I'm going to say it anyway:

You've done nothing wrong. You did not cause your infertility. You have a medical condition—simple as that. But these feelings of guilt often arise with the bargaining stage of grief—especially when you are part of a couple and only one of you has infertility.

DEPRESSION

Do not confuse the depression stage of grief with clinical depression (explained later in this chapter). Joss Fletcher adds, "[Clinical] depression is an overwhelming sadness that goes beyond that life event." Such depression becomes so far-reaching it impedes your ability to work or complete basic daily activities.

Grief-related depression is when your pain—*in response to the scenario*—deepens and becomes intense sadness.

Once I stopped blaming myself and others, I was just sad. And I sat with that sadness, together with my husband. We both had so much hope, and it all came crashing down unexpectedly. *Will we ever have a family?*

There's a difference between depression being common and depression being normalized. Yes, many people struggling to build a family experience clinical depression. But that doesn't mean it should become your new emotional baseline.

"While emotional ups and downs are normal to experience, you do not need to accept a constant and oppressive depression," says Lisa Stack, support coordinator at CNY Fertility in Syracuse, New York.

If you're clinically depressed, you *must* address the issue with a licensed mental health professional. (And you know I don't say "must" often.) Dealing with infertility can be hell, but that doesn't mean you're condemned to a life without joy.

"Trust your gut feeling and find someone who understands what you are going through," says Natascha about depression during the journey.

ACCEPTANCE

Acceptance is often confused with being okay with the situation. *It happened, and I'm cool with it now.* However, that's not the case. You may never be "over it." Instead, you've learned to cope. You're ready to develop a game plan for the next step in your infertility journey—whatever that step may be.

Dr. Rothenburger, who's also an infertility warrior, shares her experience: "Again, these things can go back and forth. I remember one day having total acceptance. *OK, next thing. I'm going to do it.* Then that day driving to work, I broke down in total depression at a stoplight. You never know where you're going to be. It is unpredictable, which of course mirrors the uncontrollable feelings in infertility in general."

I planned our second frozen embryo transfer as a version of acceptance. There was a fear that, if we didn't keep moving forward, I'd stop altogether.

WARRIOR ACTION STEPS
Coping After a Failed Cycle

Whenever you have a failed cycle, there's a good chance grief and its negative emotions will make an appearance. Work through your feelings by taking the following steps:

- **Prepare ahead of time.** Many infertility warriors are afraid that if they try to mentally prepare for a failed cycle, they're putting bad energy into the universe and increasing the odds of the cycle failing. However, if you refuse to prepare yourself, the emotions can be even more intense when they come. Dr. Rothenburger recommends focusing your thoughts on both possibilities while you're waiting to take a pregnancy test. It's okay to acknowledge another failed cycle will be devastating, but temper those thoughts and fears with reminders that you and your partner (if you have one) have done everything to increase the odds of success.

- **Feel all the feels.** It's not uncommon for infertility warriors to push aside their feelings because they want to move quickly into their next cycle. But know those feelings aren't going anywhere. They will wait you out, and if you don't take the time to address them, they will pop up eventually—sometimes when you least expect it.

- **Pay attention to your body.** With many fertility treatments, you're placed on medications that drastically alter your hormone levels. This can make your emotions more erratic after a failed cycle. It takes time for your hormone levels to return to normal, so be kind to yourself while you heal.

- **Don't play the blame game.** One of the hardest parts of infertility is accepting that a failed cycle isn't necessarily anyone's fault. When you can't point your finger at a reason and fling all your emotions at it, there seems to be a general sense of meaninglessness. But when you blame yourself, your partner, or your doctor, it strains your relationships, especially the one you have with yourself.

- **Prepare for your follow-up appointment.** After failed cycles, you'll meet with your doctor to discuss what happened. (Never schedule these appointments sooner than 48 hours after getting pregnancy test results.) This is your opportunity to ask questions and get answers. Every failed cycle is a chance to learn more about your diagnosis. Sometimes, there's no reason a cycle failed. No matter which is the case, view it through a positive lens. Finding out why the cycle failed can help you improve your treatment plan. When everything was perfect but still unsuccessful, take solace in the fact that you've discovered the best medication and protocol for you and now it's a numbers game.

- **Pay attention to your partner.** Even if things seem like they're a mess, it's still important to check in with and pay attention to your partner. You're both hurting, but you need to take the time to show you're still focused on each other as a priority.

For Nune, acceptance came without intentional trying. She explains, "Honestly, it was something that happened one day, and I felt like I had graduated from depression into what I call 'this is not unusual.' It's not something to be happy about, but it's something I can't change."

Other Types of Grief

You might experience one form of grief at one point during your journey and another later on—and there may be periods when you feel many kinds of grief all at once.

CHRONIC SORROW

According to *Infertility Counseling: A Comprehensive Handbook for Clinicians* by Sharon Covington, MSW, LCSW-C, and Linda Hammer Burns, to experience chronic sorrow, all of the following must take place:

- **A loss.** This loss triggers a sadness with no predictable end.

- **Recurrent sadness.** Sadness comes in waves over and over because the loss remains present. (*Continuous* sadness would fall under clinical depression.)

- **External or internal triggers.** A variety of factors can bring the loss—and the resulting sadness—to the forefront.

- **Progressive sadness.** Over time, the sadness intensifies rather than dissipates.

Covington, now director of the psychology team at Shady Grove Fertility in Rockville, Maryland, says that it's the continuous nature of grief and infertility that leads to chronic sorrow.

"With acute grief, such as with the loss of a loved one, there is a process of grief with feelings of shock, suffering, and eventual recovery," she says. "However, infertility creates a cycle of uncertainty with numerous losses over time.

Thus, grief becomes a 'chronic sorrow,' which is difficult to fully mourn, transcend, or integrate into one's life."

Adrienne says chronic sorrow definitely affected her—especially after her miscarriages. "I've been surprised by how even months later at the most unexpected times that sadness can creep back in. There is definitely trauma associated with these experiences—I often find myself reliving moments from each loss. Miscarriage is such a physical process, whether you choose to proceed naturally, medically, or surgically. There is a lot that the body and mind hold onto from those experiences."

DISENFRANCHISED GRIEF

When a person intensely grieves a loss that others do not recognize, they can feel disenfranchised grief (a term coined by grief expert Dr. Kenneth J. Doka). The loss is not socially or publicly acknowledged or mourned and is seen as insignificant or minor, thus not deserving of grief. In other words, the community that would rally around you if a loved one died are nowhere to be seen.

Unfortunately, the impact doesn't end there. Covington says that when grief is more invisible and less tangible, you feel less "entitled" to your emotions.

"When there are no ways to acknowledge a loss or no socially acceptable avenues to mourn, one feels disenfranchised from the right to grieve, which makes it very difficult to work through," she says.

Because of this, disenfranchised grief often leads to suffering silently. Once I was officially diagnosed with infertility, no one seemed concerned. *You're young,* they said. *You have plenty of time.* I loathed those words.

Nune knows all too well about grieving for something others do not recognize as a loss. After transferring two genetically normal male embryos, neither implanted.

BUSTED

Myth: Grief has to be tied to obvious "loss."

Most people associate a loss only with something ending or being taken away. When someone dies, we say they were taken too soon. After being let go, we say we lost our job. If something or someone was tangible, once they're gone, it's a loss people recognize.

But with infertility, a loss can mean gaining something (like a new diagnosis) or when things stay the same (like failing to get pregnant).

"Every month that a pregnancy does not happen is a loss," says Joss Fletcher. "And the depression and anxiety that can come from the strains of infertility treatment are real. Just because the loss cannot be seen by others does not mean that it is not real."

Give yourself permission to feel grief and loss. "You can grieve something that hasn't been definitively lost," says Samantha. She and her husband were so ready to have a baby that she started taking prenatal vitamins before their wedding. But after almost a year without success, she went to a fertility specialist.

"When it became apparent that we would need medical help, I grieved the possibility that I may never have biological children," she says. "Or maybe children at all."

"I feel like I have lost someone, and I can't ever have them back. Others won't see this as a loss because they'll say it was just a bunch of cells," she explains. "But it was my future baby (or babies). I had conversations with the embryos in my heart. I will always remember them. In my heart, they were both boys and they were sweet and kind men."

People Grieve Differently

I want to drive a point home: **people grieve differently**. Knowing this and *accepting* this is key to sustaining your relationship along your infertility journey. Dr. Rothenburger says there's a general rule when couples deal with loss: Do *not* expect your partner to grieve as you grieve. Refrain from judging when they act or respond differently than you would.

Often (but not always), these differences can run along gender lines. Whatever your gender identity (or your partner's), you may see some of these differences play out in your own experience.

MASCULINE APPROACHES TO GRIEF

Dr. Alice Domar, an expert in mind/body health and infertility, describes grieving men as stoic.

"They are suffering, but they don't tend to talk about it," she says. "They feel like they have to be strong and support their wives."

When they have male factor infertility, they can feel ashamed or embarrassed. Dr. Domar points out that men associate masculinity with their sperm count and virility. Suffering in silence while supporting their partner protects them from feeling more vulnerable.

But that doesn't mean the emotions don't exist. Men just tend to find less vocal ways to deal. Jamie Kreiter, LCSW, PMH-C, a maternal mental health therapist at Jamie Kreiter & Associates Therapy in Chicago, says it's not uncommon for men to channel their feelings into activities and planning. They exercise. They schedule appointments. They research treatment options. For women, it's important to recognize that these activities are their male partner's way of dealing with grief.

In Nune's case, "He is dealing with it by cleaning the shed and backyard."

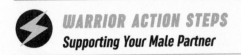

WARRIOR ACTION STEPS
Supporting Your Male Partner

Your partner may not come to you for support so you may have to get proactive.

• **Notice his coping behavior.** If you see him regularly going on hikes or watching his favorite team, join him. Don't try to bring infertility into this time (unless he wants to), but be there with him as he processes.

• **Allow for grief breaks.** Sometimes men need to step away from their grief. Taking a break allows them to recharge and unconsciously process what's going on. If your male partner needs a day away from grief and infertility, respect his boundaries.

• **Value vulnerability as a form of strength.** It can take a lot of courage for some men to express their emotions. When your partner *does* cry, thank him for his strength and willingness to be vulnerable.

KEENING SYNDROME

As Covington explains, "keening" is a traditional Irish custom in which women and men bury a loved one together but behave differently emotionally: the women openly weep and wail, while the men watch in silence.

In *Infertility Counseling*, Covington and her coauthor suggested that a so-called "keening syndrome" could also apply to infertility-elated loss—women cry, and men remain stoic about the couple's shared loss. Women take on the role of the primary mourner, carrying the emotional burden—as well as physical burden, depending on the situation—alone. And when men aren't able to express their emotions as openly as their female partners, inevitably their relationship suffers.

"Keening syndrome of infertility reflects the emotional burden women assume as the primary mourner," explains Covington. "Because the focus of treatment is primarily on women and their bodies, men are kept at a medical distance, needing primarily to show up and produce semen. This scenario creates a physical and emotional distance whereby men are often 'forgotten' in their grief and mourning."

For the most part, my husband seemed unaffected by our infertility and other losses. Throughout our journey, I asked my husband this question over and over: *Do you even want children?* He didn't initiate conversations, and he didn't really participate in conversations that I initiated. I envied his inability to feel the pain I was in. In reality, he felt it all—just didn't share it.

Neda from Norway explained how her husband just didn't seem as sad as she was after their fourth miscarriage.

"It was so heartbreaking. We had quarreled a lot in a 2-month period, and it was the first time I was afraid that infertility had affected my marriage. I started blogging without telling him because I thought he didn't understand my feelings. I also started listening to the *Beat Infertility* podcast, which was the lifesaver for me. Then one day, my psychologist said that maybe my husband is trying to complement me by balancing the emotions in my relationship. This sentence was life-changing for me."

FEMININE APPROACHES TO GRIEF

In general, women need to express their grief. Whether it's through talking or weeping uncontrollably, there's a need to get the horrible feelings out. As Covington describes it, "a feeling shared, is a feeling diminished."

The need to expel grief can happen after big events like a negative pregnancy test or an initial diagnosis. But women's grief is often triggered by smaller things—a pregnancy announcement from a friend, a baby on the street. Other times, it will seem like the grief came completely out of left field.

"The problem with grief is that it is a constant moving target," says Aviva Cohen, a psychotherapist, founder of The Blossom Method,

⚡ **WARRIOR ACTION STEPS**
Supporting Your Female Partner

Men tend to be doers. If something is broken, their instinct is to fix it, but this isn't the best way to help your female partner. "Women need to let it out without looking at grief as a problem to be fixed," says Dr. Bindeman. "When they ask to talk or when they cry, they aren't looking for a solution, but rather for their pain to be heard."

Here are a few things you can do to support your partner without going into fixing mode:

• **Listen.** It can be hard to sit and do nothing when you see your partner in pain. But think of it as her taking control of her narrative. She's telling you her story—give that attention and respect.

• **Learn her triggers.** It's always good to have a heads-up about when grief might pop up. If you know your partner's triggers, you know when she might need more support.

• **Set a 20-minute rule.** Covington suggests couples spend 20 minutes every day talking about emotions without distractions. When that time is up, the discussion ends and anything else goes on a shelf until tomorrow.

and a perinatal loss coordinator at Northwest Memorial's Prentice Women's Hospital in Chicago. "What a woman needs to hear on a Monday may not be the same thing she wants or needs to hear on a Tuesday."

Nune said that just sitting in silence with her partner was nice. "He didn't offer some bogus solutions, which was incredibly nice of him."

Clinical Depression

Infertility and mental health issues go hand-in-hand. A 2019 report published by the American Psychiatric Association found that 39.1 percent of women and 15.3 percent of men in the infertility community have a major depressive disorder. Comparatively, in the general population, just 8.4 percent of women and 5.2 percent of men are depressed.

Infertility warriors are so focused on their physical body that they often forget to care for their mind. Learn the signs and symptoms so you and your partner can get help if necessary.

SIGNS AND SYMPTOMS OF CLINICAL DEPRESSION

Again, clinical depression is different from the depression stage of grief. According to the American Psychiatric Association's *Diagnostic and Statistical Manual of Mental Disorders*, the symptoms of major depressive disorder include:

• Feeling sad or empty throughout the day on most days (or every day)

• Lack of interest in activities you used to find pleasurable

• Feeling guilty or worthless

• Feeling irritable, restless, or agitated

• Sleep changes

• Extreme fatigue

• Weight and/or appetite changes

• Inability to concentrate or make decisions

• Suicidal thoughts or actions

Dr. Rothenburger clarifies, "You have to have at least five of those markers for at least a 2-week period of time for it to be considered clinical depression."

It's also important to remember there's often a sense of numbness that goes with depression. This is not the same as suppressing your emotions, which is something you actively do. Numbness in depression is a general absence of any feelings without making a decision to remove the feelings. It's important to understand the difference when considering you or your partner's symptoms.

Nune describes the moment she knew she had clinical depression. "I remember going to the psychiatrist and telling her that food doesn't taste the same way it used to and that I can't get out of bed except to go to work." She's now on medication to help manage her condition.

In addition to knowing when you *have* to get help, Dr. Rothenburger says that prevention is the best medicine. "Do not wait. If you happen to notice the recurrent thoughts of death, particularly, definitely seek help now—like right now."

I became clinically depressed after the loss of our twins. My sisters-in-law (twins, as luck would have it) had flown in for my 30th birthday. They had planned to surprise me at the hospital, but we all know how that turned out. However, I had no desire to celebrate or even acknowledge my birthday.

One thing you should know about me: I used to see birthdays as the most important day of the year—a time to reflect upon all the accomplishments you've had, recognize everything for which you are grateful, and shower yourself with self-love and compassion. When I had employees, I always gave them the day off on their birthdays and money to spend on themselves. So, declining to participate in my own birthday was far from normal.

Beyond the birthday celebration, the visit itself was fairly normal—until everyone left for the airport. I locked myself in our bathroom—with access to everything I needed to kill myself. Yes, I contemplated committing suicide. I remember crying so hard that I could barely breathe, let alone talk. But what little I choked out was about how I deserved to die for causing their deaths.

We were seeing a grief counselor who specializes in loss, so my husband called her out of desperation and asked that she come to our house. Thankfully, she was able to talk me out of the bathroom before anything happened, and I eventually worked through my emotions enough to move out of clinical depression.

Sadness

"I think the experience of infertility is in itself about sadness," explains Dr. Madeira. "The depth of sadness that individuals may experience is interconnected with guilt, shame, and anger. Infertility, after all, is experienced (like other chronic medical conditions) as a loss—loss of privacy, loss of an idealized expectation of conception and pregnancy, loss of comfort, even loss of autonomy."

Give yourself permission to be sad. Recognize that it's *normal*. Denise from Connecticut describes her mental state after experiencing five miscarriages: "I was devastated. Each one was just as devastating as the last."

Alicia felt deep sadness when she found out their first IVF cycle resulted in zero embryos. "I was on the ground on my knees, leaning on the blowup mattress we had put up in our living room to camp out on while I was recovering from OHSS (ovarian hyperstimulation syndrome) when we got the call. After the call was over, I just laid there and cried and so did my husband. It was just complete and total sadness."

These deep feelings of pain and sadness are normal. You just don't want to stay stuck there. If your sadness turns into clinical depression, get help *immediately*.

Dealing with deep sadness can be particularly difficult for men. They don't think they can or should feel this emotion.

"Many men don't allow themselves to feel pain or vulnerability. Despite feeling deep sadness, fear and frustration, men oftentimes don't let themselves experience the intensity of the pain their wives will allow themselves to feel," says Hannon.

Alicia's husband, on the other hand, handled things a little differently than her, but he was still openly sad. "I am not sure if this was because he was carrying a lot of guilt knowing he was the source of our issue or if it was something else."

My failed cycles, especially the one in April 2015, made me sad. Target, malls, and other crowded spaces likely to contain pregnant people made me sad. My period in general made me *extremely* sad. I was sad—deeply so—after each of my miscarriages. But it was after the loss of my twins that I tipped into clinical depression. Our grief counselor eventually

WARRIOR TIPS
The Difference Between Grief, Depression, and Sadness
....

Although nuanced, there are subtle differences:

- **Grief.** A direct response to loss—even a loss that others cannot see.

- **Depression.** May not have a direct cause and instead be brought on by chemical and biological responses in the brain.

- **Sadness.** A symptom of depression but an otherwise normal emotion (as long as it doesn't last more than 2 weeks). Sometimes considered an adjustment disorder—a feeling of overwhelm brought on by change or a stressful trigger.

helped me—and both of us—get back on track.

Natascha didn't work through her sadness until a few years ago, but now she finds power in owning her story. "In my mind, I was not allowed to work through it because it was a sadness that did not exist in reality. I was always told to count my blessings and to take it as fate. I never had anyone who I could talk to and relate to what I was experiencing. I eventually realized that my feelings are real and that I do not need validation from anyone else."

WARRIOR ACTION STEPS
Dealing with Sadness

- **Have a sadness mantra.** It's important to allow yourself to feel sad. But at the same time, you need to remind yourself that being sad is not your new normal. Find a mantra that works for you, like "This too shall pass" or "My sadness is mine, but I am not my sadness."

- **Learn what makes you happy.** While you shouldn't ignore sadness, you can take steps to combat it before

it takes over. If you feel sadness coming on, engage in a happy activity.

- **Know the signs of clinical depression.** Depression is no joke. Learn what the signs and symptoms of clinical depression are so you can get the help you need and deserve early.

Anxiety or Stress

Stress and anxiety are an inherent part of infertility. Not only is there the lack of control and not knowing what will happen next, but also societal pressure that constantly reinforces that something about your situation is "wrong."

"Our society communicates subtly—and sometimes overtly—that motherhood is part of being a woman, so some infertile women may feel that they are not fulfilling what it means to be a woman," says Marci Lobel, PhD, a professor of social and health psychology at Stony Brook University in New York

---

BUSTED

Myth: If you just relax, everything will be better.

It's one of the most frustrating pieces of "advice" for people dealing with infertility and depression to hear: If you just relax, you'll feel better and you'll be able to conceive. But your depression is not causing your infertility.

Tara H. Simpson, Psy-D, a licensed psychologist at Shady Grove Fertility in Baltimore, points out that fertility treatments are stressful. *Of course* they could possibly impact your mood, and denying this adds undue burden to be serene at all times.

Viewing clinical depression as an exacerbating factor for infertility is the wrong approach. Depression is not another item on the list of things "wrong with you" preventing you from starting a family. It's a serious condition that can result from extreme stress and the pain you're feeling. Simply relaxing will *not* make depression go away. It needs to be taken seriously and addressed with the help of a mental health professional.

---

and director of the Stress And Reproduction (STAR) Lab.

This creates a stressful discord between what's expected and your reality. Being able to manage stress during infertility is essential.

As common as anxiety and stress are among women experiencing infertility, they can show up in a lot of different ways. In moments of acute anxiety, your heart rate might increase. You might start to sweat. You might feel a weight or slight pain in the pit of your stomach. Chronic anxiety can lead to trouble concentrating or remembering things, difficulty sleeping, rapid weight fluctuation, extreme mood swings, or persistent headaches or backaches.

When my first RE officially diagnosed me with infertility, I quickly moved from denial to stress. *Does infertility define me now? I've always wanted three kids . . . Should I now hope I even can conceive just one?*

Adrienne felt the same way. "There is a lot of 'unknowing' that you have to live with day to day. Will this cycle be successful? Is this the right protocol? Am I eating the right things? Am I exercising enough/too much? Will I ever achieve my goal of having a family? This constant questioning is mentally exhausting."

But when you're stressed about infertility, it takes over your entire life. You feel like you're failing at everything, even though you're not. So my *main* source of anxiety became work. At the time, I was the owner of a small public relations agency with about fifteen or so clients at any given time and ten employees. Entrepreneurship was wonderful in many respects and afforded me flexibility both in when and where I worked, but the responsibility was a heavy burden to carry. I often felt guilt for taking any time away from work and devoting time to self-care activities (and vice versa), which in turn led to a tremendous amount of stress.

⚡ WARRIOR ACTION STEPS
Finding a Self-Care Routine

For some people, self-care means getting a mani-pedi. For others, it's training for a marathon. Use the following steps to see what works for you:

- **Think about how you learn.** Tactile learners might find taking a pottery class, cooking, jewelry making, or playing in a sandbox to be therapeutic. Auditory learners might find listening to soothing music helpful. Visual learners might find comfort in walking in nature, painting, or coloring.

- **Revisit your moments of joy before infertility.** Find something that strikes the same emotional note as what made you happy in the past. If you have an analytical brain, then think about what works for you and fine-tune it. Note the times when you are resistant and when something doesn't work. People often discount their psyche's need for self-care.

- **Identify the path of least resistance.** Do the things that make you happy. If you like yoga, tie it to something that you do every day. When you're brushing your teeth,

just strike a downward dog for 10 seconds. Keep your self-care simple!

- **Define your non-negotiables.** In other words, in order to feel like your best self, what absolutely must happen every day or every week? For me, it's at least 30 minutes of reading each day and a date with my husband at least twice a month. No matter what's going on, these things are top priorities. Think hard on this one! Your list should be as long as is necessary to achieve your self-care goals.

- **Find self-care resources.** This can be anything from books, like *Present over Perfect: Leaving Behind Frantic for a Simpler, More Soulful Way of Living* by Shauna Niequist; to podcasts, like *Beat Infertility* or *Happier with Gretchen Rubin*; to guided meditations, like those from Circle + Bloom; and everything in between.

Know that you're going to feel anxious and stressed many times throughout your infertility journey. Discover your personal warning signs that your stress level is getting too high. Pay attention to what your body is telling you. Dr. Madeira points out that ignoring your stress levels is dangerous.

"Left unaddressed, stress can turn into anger and might jeopardize the very relationship in which one hopes to start a family. It helps to blow off stress through engaging in a favorite activity or hobby, whether it is exercise, reading, or knitting."

And most important, be kind to yourself. Learn what best counteracts stress for you and do it before the stress becomes overwhelming. This will be different for everyone, but practice self-care.

Alicia agrees that self-care was essential to making it through the hard times. "Therapy,

staying busy, self-care, and focusing on ourselves as a couple helped find positivity and lessen the feelings of anxiety and stress."

Signs and Symptoms of Clinical Anxiety

Dealing with infertility is stressful. Mix in feelings of intense grief, guilt, or powerlessness, and severe anxiety issues frequently arise. In a paper published by *Dialogues in Clinical Neuroscience*, Dr. Domar found that 76 percent of women and 61 percent of men in the infertility community have significant anxiety symptoms.

To put the level of stress caused by infertility into context, consider another of Dr. Domar's studies published in the *Journal of Psychosomatic Obstetrics and Gynecology*. The study found women with infertility experienced levels of stress and anxiety similar to cancer patients and people recovering from a heart attack.

Left unchecked, this can result in panic attacks or other panic disorders. Generalized anxiety disorder is one of the most common diagnoses and is defined in *Diagnostic and Statistical Manual of Mental Disorders* as:

- Having excessive anxiety and worry about a variety of topics for at least 6 months

- Feeling the worrying is very challenging to control

In addition to excessive anxiety and worry, having at least three of the following symptoms:

- Edginess or restlessness

- Fatigue

- Difficulty concentrating or feeling as if your mind goes blank

- Irritability

- Difficulty sleeping

As with other mental health concerns, if you're struggling with clinical anxiety symptoms, seek help. You can—and deserve—to feel better.

BUSTED

Myth: Stress is causing my infertility.

We've all heard the stories: people struggling to conceive go on vacation, come back, and immediately get pregnant. Dr. Lobel says this perpetuates the idea that stress is a major cause of infertility. That's just not true.

"Sharing such stories and perpetuating the belief that a woman's distress is preventing her from conceiving can lead someone to blame herself. This only adds to the suffering that a woman may experience."

Alicia lets us in on how she coped. "Therapy, staying busy, self-care, and focusing on ourselves as a couple helped find positivity and lessen the feelings of anxiety."

Fear

Fear is probably one of the easiest to recognize—even at its lowest levels—because it's such a powerful emotion. Fear is also closely tied to anxiety, but the key difference is your body's *response* to fear. Our bodies naturally react to fear with a fight-or-flight response.

For Melanie from Ontario, Canada, fear was the hardest emotion during her infertility journey.

"It just seems to make everything more complicated. Sadness, grief, and anger are all manageable, but when fear is thrown into the mix with any of those emotions, it seems to escalate the primary negative emotion so much faster and farther."

One of my most memorable experiences of fear happened when I was hospitalized for internal bleeding. Earlier that day in April 2015, I'd had my second egg retrieval. As far as I knew, the procedure went as expected—certainly no one at my clinic indicated otherwise. But that afternoon, I suddenly felt sharp, shooting pains in my shoulders—particularly on my right side—and was having trouble and pain when breathing or talking. Although she didn't tell me what she suspected, the on-call nurse at my clinic advised I head to the emergency room at my nearest hospital.

We'd recently purchased and moved into a house in southern Maryland to get away from the hustle-and-bustle of the city. On a normal day, we relished in the slow pace of the county we now called home. However, on *that* day, we were astounded by the lack of urgency exhibited by doctors in the *emergency* room.

We arrived around 5 p.m. and didn't receive a diagnosis until shortly before midnight:

I was bleeding internally and might need emergency surgery. At some point during my egg retrieval, something was nicked that shouldn't have been—or didn't cauterize when it should have. And blood had filled my abdominal cavity and was now pooling around my diaphragm, hence the troubles breathing and speaking.

I immediately had a panic attack. I'd never had one before—at least, not to my knowledge. I must have jerked in response because I could feel the blood suddenly overwhelm my diaphragm and completely cut off my ability to breathe—or so I thought. I'd endured so much throughout my journey up to that point— infertility itself, four miscarriages, stillborn twins—and *I might die in this hospital tonight all because I wanted to have a baby.*

Meanwhile, the doctor just stood there, silently watching me. No visible reaction whatsoever.

I managed to gasp out, "What's happening to me?!?" I couldn't see my own face, of course, but I know I *felt* extremely afraid—felt like I hadn't drawn a breath in an inordinately long time. Surely my expression was communicating that fear.

She slowly and calmly—almost nonchalantly—replied, "You're having a panic attack. It will pass."

Again, in a barely audible voice, I asked her, "Will it pass before I die?"

"Yes," she said coolly, "before you die."

It did pass, and thankfully, I didn't even require surgery. By the time they figured out the source of the bleeding, it had stopped on its own—the situation already resolving itself. Given the late hour and continued symptoms, I was kept overnight for observation and released in the morning.

Like my internal bleeding experience, there will always be situations you cannot anticipate, but make a list of the known fears, as well as things that might come up that would scare you, why these things are scary to you, and how you plan to respond to those fears. If you can, talk them through with a loved one or a mental health professional.

Nune described fear throughout her infertility journey in a memorable way. "Infertility has been a monster chasing me around a dark forest. I don't know how to get out of the forest, and I'm scared that I'm going to die here. Every time I start a new protocol, I'm scared that it

---

WARRIOR ACTION STEPS
Facing Your Fears

Our fears are always with us. Most of the time, they are down below the surface and aren't really a threat to our mental state. But when fear and panic do take over, be prepared:

- **Voice your known fears.** No matter how small or silly it seems, fear is a powerful emotion. Talking about it when you are less emotionally stressed helps you work through your fear and take away its hold on you.

- **Find a way to focus your breath.** When you're extremely scared or panicking, focus on your breath. Some people do this by counting to 10, while others repeat phrases like "I'm safe" until the feelings pass.

- **Don't visit Dr. Google.** It will only feed your fear. While many people say that knowledge is power, that's only true if the information is credible and accurate. Otherwise, you'll just start worrying about completely different issues. I like to compare Dr. Google to an ex-boyfriend. You broke up with him for a reason, so stop going back to him! Go directly to a trusted source, such as the *Beat Infertility* podcast or an infertility coach.

won't work. It's as if the monster starts chasing me again, and I have to run as fast as I can to get hope to save me."

If you know in advance something is going to scare you, it's easier to control your response. However, you won't always know what's coming, so learn to expect the unexpected. Get comfortable with the uncomfortable feelings. And, as Nune suggests, talk them through with a loved one or even a mental health professional.

Positive Emotions

I'm happy to report that not all of your emotions throughout this journey will be negative. In fact, you'll have positive moments frequently—even if they are truly that, just small moments. It isn't all doom and gloom!

Let's discuss some of the more common ones. If you know what they are, you can recognize them in your own experiences and make the most of them.

Cautious Optimism

Cautious optimism can best be described as "hopeful, but . . ." or hope with a contingency. Something seemingly positive has just happened, but in an effort to protect yourself, you don't want to celebrate it just yet. This can be anything from finally seeing a positive pregnancy test to receiving a good embryo fertilization report—and many other scenarios in between.

You could approach cautious optimism in one of two ways. You might decide to control the situation by not feeling too much—still living in stress and anxiety. Or, the more productive route, you might say to yourself, *Whatever happens, I got this. If something good happens, I receive it. If something bad happens, I am going to embrace it in my flexibility. I am going to let go of the outcome.*

"I know how scary that is," says Dr. Rothenburger. "But set that intention, and do everything that comes your way in terms of

---

WARRIOR ACTION STEPS
Making the Most of Cautious Optimism

Unlike the negative emotions of infertility, cautious optimism isn't a hurdle to overcome—it's an opportunity. Take advantage of your cautious optimism with the following steps:

- **Practice opening up to joy.** Cautious optimism has an inherent asterisk. You're ready for good but not expecting it. When you're feeling emotionally safe, explore more positive emotions like happiness and pride. Even if things take a bad turn, you have a right to recognize what you've accomplished at this stage in your infertility journey.

- **Breakdown your cautious optimism.** It's completely natural to be cautiously optimistic about some aspects of your situation (like your beta tests doubling) but

still worried about other parts (like the possibility of a miscarriage). Examine where you still have reasonable concerns so you can truly enjoy what you've accepted as possible, and practice self-care when you're still resistant to optimism.

- **Don't tie hope to mile markers.** It can be tempting to say, "I'm halfway there. Once I reach this point, I can be hopeful." Hope will arrive on its own schedule. If you try to force the next step, it can lead to disappointment.

becoming a parent because you trust. If you're religious, you trust God. If you are like myself, very spiritual, you trust the universe. Even if you're not religious or spiritual at all, perhaps you just trust *yourself* because you know you are going to take every opportunity and follow through with it. This projects more ease externally, and it brings more ease internally to your body. It gets rid of your fight-or-flight response, it turns on your reproductive organs, and it's just a much easier way of being."

Sheri experienced cautious optimism with each step—doctor consultations, new treatments, different holistic approaches, etc. Especially in the beginning, she was optimistic that the next "thing" would work. However, as the years went on, her fight-or-flight mode kicked in. "There was still always a smidge of cautious optimism, but it was as if I was in survival mode and this was the only way to protect my heart."

This is completely understandable and expected. It's exhausting to keep up cautious optimism when your journey drags on for months or even years. But Alicia offers some great advice. "After being in the world of infertility, I felt that being cautiously optimistic was crucial. It was more helpful to live in this state than to be negative."

For Dr. Madeira, cautious optimism is great because it helps us creep toward that "we've got this" moment, confident that we have the tools and the determination to navigate this journey.

Hope

The most positive emotion is hope. Unlike cautious optimism, as I prefaced in the previous section, hope is the belief that the future will be better than the present *and* you have the power to make it so.

"I chose to see hope in a lot of places like driving by a school or a playground," says Sarah from Ontario, Canada. That decision helped her on her journey. "There are so many children in the world and I was hopeful that one day, in some capacity, I would be a parent."

It's like a weight has been lifted off your shoulders. You suddenly are feeling happier, seemingly out of nowhere. You find yourself smiling more and thinking about what the future might bring.

I ask every guest on the *Beat Infertility* podcast about hope, and most admit to a complicated relationship with this particular emotion. Different aspects of the journey make different people hopeful. You might not feel hopeful until you have a child in your arms.

On the other hand, Alicia shares that hope was the driving force for her and her husband to *reach* their child. "Hope helped us to keep moving forward. Hope is motivating and something needs to motivate you during the tough times of infertility."

Two distinct moments of hope happened for me. With the twins, I finally felt hopeful after coming out of my 18-week appointment with my high-risk ob-gyn—all pregnancy complications to date were resolved. I finally knew in my heart—my soul—that our lives were about to change dramatically. I felt hopeful for the first time in 2 years!

Unfortunately for my future hope, everything *did* change dramatically when I lost the twins—although obviously not for the better.

And so, feeling hopeful again was much more difficult in the future. I did develop a sense of cautious optimism during my pregnancy with Aurora, but not until we "graduated" from our fertility clinic to the ob-gyn. Even then, I wouldn't feel hope until we brought her home from the NICU.

"It was incredibly hopeful to reach a place in our journey where using a donor was an option we felt excited about," reminisces Alicia when asked about her most memorable hopeful moment. "It took a while to get there, but once we were, it was like a new door opened up and that was a good, hopeful feeling."

I've had many regrets throughout my infertility journey, and one of them is not allowing hope to play a bigger role. Similar to cautious optimism, know in your heart and mind that good things *will* happen along with the bad while you're battling infertility, so unlike me, be open to seeing them. Honor the hope that you feel. It's okay to let it run wild or rein yourself in. Trust yourself, even if you don't trust your body.

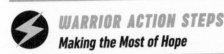

WARRIOR ACTION STEPS
Making the Most of Hope

Hope is something to be excited about—not something to fear losing. Revel in your newfound hope by trying to:

- **Separate hope from specifics.** It's one thing to be hopeful you'll become a parent—it's another thing to be hopeful you'll conceive naturally, have an uneventful pregnancy, and deliver in less than an hour on your due date. What's important is the outcome: a happy future. This will help you maintain hope if there are unexpected twists along the way.

- **Sharing your hope with those you trust.** Be open with your loved ones (and your partner if you have one) and let them know what you're hopeful about. This is a positive development, and they'll want to know you're excited about—not fearing—what comes next.

- **Record your hopes.** Often when we journal, we focus on the negative. Don't forget to document the positive. In the future, you're going to want to remember what it felt like to finally believe in a happy ending, no matter how that looks.

A big part of coping with your emotions is examining how your needs change because of your feelings. This will show you what types of support you need. Just remember that your needs can—and likely will—evolve over the course of your infertility journey. The key is to practice identifying your needs and then communicating your needs.

We've talked a lot about triggers in this chapter. They are what catalyze your emotions, but they are not the root cause of the issue. For example, you're not angry because your friend is pregnant. You are angry because you are struggling to become a parent.

When you begin to see the root causes of your feelings, the path to dealing with them becomes clearer. Sometimes you'll have to get creative. But you can take other steps to mitigate your pain. You can focus on other aspects of your identity so you feel more balanced during your journey.

Unsupported through her journey, Natascha looks back on how her needs were unconsidered. "I wish I had been more open about my grief and sadness. I also would have liked to be honest, strong, and sometimes mean to all the folks telling me to relax or adopt or do whatever they think I should do."

There are two parts to communicating your emotional needs during infertility. The first is just getting it all out, no matter how incomprehensible your words.

A couple of years into her journey, Sheri realized that it was important to communicate her emotional needs and be clear and direct with friends and family about how she wanted to be treated. "I knew they were sad with me and wanted to support me but didn't necessarily know how. I asked my friends who were at a similar stage in life to not treat me with 'kid gloves,' not treat me any differently, and just tell me—like they would anyone else—their news: announcing their pregnancies, their gender reveals, their labor stories, their kids' firsts, everything."

Speaking about her own journey, Dr. Rothenburger says, "I was not eloquent a lot of the time, and that's okay. Most of the time when people come to me for help, it's because they have reached the end of their rope. I remember seeking help for the first time and being absolutely appalled that I cried. It was just an absolute lack of control, and it was really embarrassing for me. And now, I laugh at myself because I'm much more capable of letting go and crying in front of people."

Once you've vented, restate your needs when your feelings are less intense. Be specific about ways people can help address your needs. For example, if you need an afternoon of self-care, ask your partner to run that day's errands. Or, if your emotions always get the best of you at appointments, Dr. Madeira suggests bringing an appointment buddy. They can support you by taking notes so you can review the information with a calmer mind.

→

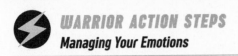

WARRIOR ACTION STEPS
Managing Your Emotions

There are things you can do every day to manage your emotions in a healthy way:

• **Meditate.** It helps you observe your emotions and not react to them. Instead, determine how they are affecting your body. This removes you from the subjective experience of the actual feeling and makes you more objective.

• **Talk.** The more you can get those emotions out, the more peaceful you will feel. Neuroscience research with MRI imaging now reveals that if you express your emotions, your brain activity shifts from the emotional parts of the brain to the prefrontal sections that are involved with rational thought and processing.

• **Journal.** It doesn't have to be written—you can speak it. It can be as long or short as you want. There are no rules!

• **Exercise.** Cardio, aerobics, strength training . . . There's something for everyone! Just don't overdo it (see chapter 8).

• **Connect.** As you already know or will soon find out, infertility is extremely isolating. Join the Beat Infertility community. Attend in-person RESOLVE support groups. Don't go through infertility alone.

WARRIOR WISDOM
Finding a Renewed Appreciation for Your Strength

"I spent a long time being unhappy and hating myself and my situation. I let my fertility failures define me. But after my miscarriage, I decided to put my mind, body, soul, and well-being at the forefront of my healing. It has made all the difference in the world. My struggles forced me to grow into a better person, mother, and wife."

—Krista, New Jersey

WARRIOR CHECKLIST
Navigating Infertility Emotions

❑ Recognize that your emotions are not wrong and you are not alone.

❑ Know and practice the five steps to working through your emotions in a healthy manner.

❑ Become familiar with the common infertility emotions and develop a self-care plan for how to deal with them when they pop up.

❑ Learn how to identify your emotional needs throughout your infertility journey and be willing to ask for what you need.

❑ Incorporate general coping mechanisms into your routine.

Add more items to your Warrior Checklist or jot down any notes here:

_____

_____

_____

Strategies for Becoming Stronger Than Infertility

CHAPTER 15

I STARTED THE *BEAT INFERTILITY* podcast for selfish reasons. I needed to feel hope again. If I helped just one other person out there feel hope again, too, great. But at the time, I was thinking mostly of myself.

I had intended to air episodes once a week featuring interviews with other infertility warriors to reassure myself—and potentially others—that it was possible to survive this journey. When I heard that iTunes would be featuring the podcast on their homepage, I reached out to Dr. Allison K. Rodgers, a reproductive endocrinologist with Fertility Centers of Illinois in Chicago who'd expressed interest in becoming my regular medical contributor and quickly put together two episodes for the official launch. To my surprise, both shows—the warrior stories and the guest expert—were equally popular, and I've continued airing the show twice a week ever since.

The other surprise was that my plan actually worked. I was feeling more hopeful—it helped me hear that success was possible while also learning about every imaginable aspect of infertility. And I was helping other people feel hopeful, too. My listeners are located in nearly every country around the world. I started to receive emails about how the show had changed the course of people's infertility journeys—that they wouldn't have their child if it wasn't for me. I had somehow turned the darkest moments of my life into a movement—one of hope, education, resiliency, and self-advocacy.

People often ask why I've kept up with the podcast—or became an infertility coach or committed to writing this book, for that matter—despite having my daughter, despite transitioning to "the other side." To me, there's no better way to honor where I've been than to give guidance to other warriors in any way I can. Infertility changed me in so many ways—negative *and* positive. And although I wouldn't wish my experience on anyone, I've learned to own my story rather than let it own me. I know deep in my soul that I've beaten infertility. Not in a medical sense, of course, but in a mental sense. I'm stronger than infertility.

Transitioning from Hopeless to Hopeful

Believe it or not, it is possible to feel and be better during your infertility journey. It means developing new skills and changing your perspectives, but you can be *stronger than infertility*.

I think this starts with changing how we approach hope. Infertility takes a lot of control out of your hands, leaving you with feelings of hopelessness. Cycles fail. Test results deliver bad news. Treatments leave you feeling stressed and exhausted. And there's absolutely *nothing* you can do about it, right?

That's not entirely true. I define hope as the belief that the future will be better than the present, and *you* have the power to make it so. That better future might not be exactly as you expected or wished, but it *is* possible if you do the work.

In this chapter, I'll give you a lot of tips and tricks to try, but know that not every method is right for everyone. What makes you stronger might not help your partner or your fellow infertility warriors. But you won't know what works unless you try.

Developing Resilience, Transitioning to Growth

Adrienne and her husband, Matthew, from New Jersey began their journey in 2017. They tried on their own before moving on to multiple IUI and IVF cycles, which all ended in miscarriages. It wasn't until August 2020 that they began their success story.

"I do feel like this journey has given me lots of opportunities to practice resiliency!" Adrienne shares. "After each miscarriage, I was left feeling so devastated. It took time to adapt, but somehow, I was able to find some additional will to keep going. For me, that meant being open to adjusting my course of treatment and even my doctors at multiple points during the journey."

BUSTED

Myth: I can't be stronger than infertility.

Infertility is a formidable beast. Even on your best days, it can loom over your life, threatening your happiness. Understandably, many infertility warriors struggle to see how they could ever win against such a foe. But people have done it before, and so can you.

As I write this, I'm gearing up for a frozen embryo transfer in the hope of giving Aurora a sibling. It's an odd feeling to be back in fertility treatment mode, but this time around is completely different. And not because I already have a child—I definitely don't feel my family is complete just yet. Instead, I feel in control. I am educated about all the options available to me, and I'm taking advantage of as many of them as possible. I understand the first transfer might not work, but I believe everything is going to be okay in the end—and that's empowering and liberating.

"Whatever the outcome, whatever happens along the journey, you're going to be okay," says Kara from North Dakota. "It's going to be really hard, and there are probably going to be times when you're not so sure that you're going to be okay, but in the end—whatever the end is—you will be."

Just remember: Your "okay" likely looks different from mine—and that's okay. Thinking back, I didn't truly reach my "okay" until about 2½ years after Aurora was born—once most of her medical issues cleared up and my body was no longer in constant fight-or-"flight" mode as I advocated for her care. But you might find your okay at *any* point during your journey—from before you visit a fertility clinic to when you first hear a heartbeat to graduating to an ob-gyn to bringing home a baby to reaching acceptance about living child-free.

Strength during infertility is made of two interconnected parts: becoming resilient and growing as a result of the stress and trauma. These skills will help you process and move through your pain. You have to decide how much power and control you give that pain over your life.

Resilience

In nature, plants and animals learn to adapt to environmental changes and other threats around them. We infertility warriors are no different. When the odds are set against us, we adapt and become stronger than before. *That* is resilience.

Some people are naturally resilient. It's part of their personality, or previous life events have forced them to develop adaptive behaviors. For others, resilience is tough. The way we experience and process the trauma of infertility is not one-size-fits-all—everyone brings their own prior baggage.

"Resilience is about healing from pain," explains Dr. Maria T. Rothenburger, a psychotherapist who specializes in infertility at Miracles Happen Fertility Center in Salem, Oregon. "Everyone has a baseline, and when a traumatic event happens, you are now below your baseline in terms of emotion. Resilience means you have healed enough to come back to baseline."

Before getting back to baseline, some people resist. They want their circumstances to be different so badly that they fight tooth and nail against what's happening. According to Dr. Rothenburger, this resistance leads to prolonged suffering.

Resistance is avoiding consulting a reproductive endocrinologist for fear of what they might say. Resistance is believing treatment will never work after a failed cycle. Resistance is refusing to ever be around pregnant people.

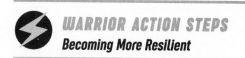

WARRIOR ACTION STEPS
Becoming More Resilient

Resiliency is a skill. You can learn how to process and recover from pain more effectively. Your infertility journey won't suddenly be a cakewalk, but the following steps may help you keep moving forward:

- **Face fears.** No matter what they are, be willing to deal with your fears. Maybe you're scared of another miscarriage or that your partner will leave you. Examining those fears will help you see ways you can adapt to alleviate stress surrounding those issues.

- **Focus on perspective.** Infertility is just one part of your life. Granted, it's an excruciating part, but it's not everything. Maintaining perspective helps you see opportunities to be grateful and learn. Acknowledge and celebrate what you already have—your partner, family, pets, great job, etc. This will lessen the power your pain has over you as a whole person.

- **Be forgiving.** We'll get into *self*-forgiveness later, but to become resilient, you need to forgive others. Holding on to grudges—such as against friends and family who've made insensitive comments or a boss who passed you over for a promotion—is a form of resistance that tethers you to your negative emotions. Forgiveness isn't about the other person—it's freeing yourself from the hurt you feel because of someone else.

- **Form cautiously optimistic plans.** Resilience prepares you to move forward. The next step is going back to working toward your goal. If that is still building a family or if it's now to live child-free, making plans restores your hope in a better future.

If you are too rigid, you may snap. But being resilient means accepting the challenges of your situation and finding healthy ways to adapt and move forward. It's okay to fall into darkness—just don't stay there.

Adrienne's advice: "Try and keep a degree of flexibility throughout the process because there are just so many variables at play."

Post-Traumatic Growth

Resilience is about bouncing back to where you were—dealing with stress and trauma so you can recover from that pain. Dr. Rothenburger, who wrote her doctoral dissertation on the topic, says post-traumatic growth is becoming *better* because of the trauma.

"I know it's really difficult to wrap one's brain around this because most people say, 'Why on earth would I ever say I'm better *because* of infertility?'"

But this is possible, and Dr. Rothenburger says she's experienced it herself. While it's a process for most people, she can point to a moment in her life when a switch turned on.

"I had a feeling like my life was purposeless and meaningless and terrible things were happening, all related to infertility," she shares. "But there came a point when I decided infertility wasn't going to take over anymore. I began to consciously make choices that matched that idea. Then I started noticing things in my life were way better than they were even before starting my infertility journey."

There are five pillars to post-traumatic growth. You can experience positive change in one or more of these areas. With Dr. Rothenburger's help, let's walk through these pillars:

• **Appreciation of life:** Before trauma, people tend to view life with certain expectations, and as a result, parts of our lives become mundane. We take having a home or friends and family for granted because that's what we're *supposed* to have. When trauma like infertility threatens one of our expectations (*it'll be easy for me to have kids when I'm ready for them*), it can help us gain a new appreciation for the positive parts of our life.

• **Relationships with others:** This goes beyond appreciating the people in your life. It's about identifying your true friends and building your community. After infertility, you begin to separate who is supportive and who isn't. Meaningful relationships strengthen and deepen, while the other relationships fall away or end (see chapter 16).

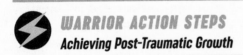

WARRIOR ACTION STEPS
Achieving Post-Traumatic Growth

Post-traumatic growth doesn't just happen. But you have the power to cultivate positive changes through your actions. Here are some steps to help you become stronger after the trauma of infertility:

• **Put yourself out there.** Even if you're introverted, find ways to develop meaningful connections. Whether this means offering support to other infertility warriors or sharing your story on a blog, open yourself up to enriching interactions.

• **Go through the window.** The saying goes when a door to an opportunity shuts, a window opens. In order to grow, you need to go through that window. Don't let your fears or past pain keep you from seizing the possibilities that present themselves.

• **Develop your new world view.** This is big-picture stuff, but as you learn and grow during your infertility

journey, acknowledge how those lessons play into your larger belief system. For example, after asking you a hurtful question about infertility, a friend might surprise you and ask you to educate them. Finding a friend who is willing to support you and walk through the journey alongside you shows the power of a solid friendship—and gives you the opportunity to serve your friend in return when she or he needs you.

• **Consciously foster growth.** Make it a habit to examine each of your decisions with a growth perspective. Ask yourself: Will this choice help me improve or keep me stuck in my pain?

• **New possibilities:** Simply put, this is when your eyes open to new opportunities or different life paths you'd never considered before. This could be extreme, like going skydiving, or small, like nightly bubble baths. Or it could be more meaningful. For me, that looked like starting the *Beat Infertility* podcast and changing careers and following my calling to become an infertility coach to support other people on this journey. Regardless of what makes sense for you, keep your eyes open and don't let life not going as planned keep you from other pursuits.

• **Personal strength:** This is when some part of you speaks up and says "infertility won't get me." It's when you recognize your pain and feel that pain but don't allow it to break you. Developing personal strength also can trickle into other areas of life, such as becoming a better advocate for yourself with doctors, at work, or even in your relationships.

• **Spiritual change:** Often, infertility challenges our belief system and spirituality. But with post-traumatic growth, that develops into a new sense of meaning in something greater than ourselves. It's not something that's tangible—sometimes it's just a thought, an intention, an awareness around the need to create meaning from your journey.

"There is no doubt this is a traumatic experience, but I think it's taught me a lot about myself," Adrienne shares about her growth. "I feel much more able to empathize with others—not just about fertility issues but in general. I have definitely learned that even with the best preparation and intention, things don't always go according to plan and sometimes even science can't explain why. At times like these, being open to new avenues or even new goals can be the best way forward."

Regaining Your Sense of Self

One day during your journey, you may look in the mirror and not even recognize yourself. This is not uncommon because it's nearly impossible to come out of infertility exactly the same. You do, however, have a *choice* in how infertility impacts your identity.

Regaining a sense of self and refining your identity is a process. But be aware of who you are and how infertility has changed you so you can be proud of who you end up being.

Dr. Rothenburger shares her analogy of bamboo, "You feel the pain, you acknowledge the pain, you accept the pain, and you slowly rise again. After a hurricane, a bamboo tree

BUSTED

Myth: Strength means being tough and unyielding.

Strength is often seen as being impervious or undefeatable—that you can't be strong if you cry or have negative emotions. But being vulnerable and admitting that things are tough is brave. Asking for help is courageous. There are many forms of strength that you need during your infertility journey.

"To me, strength lies in one's ability to be flexible rather than rigid around how they want things to go. That way when a catastrophe happens, the ability to move through it becomes much easier," says Dr. Rothenburger.

She advises infertility warriors that instead of trying to be giant, thick oak trees, be bamboo. A strong enough hurricane can snap a mighty oak tree in two. But bamboo, which is also strong, will bend and survive because of its flexibility.

is very flexible and comes up slowly from the ground. It says, 'This sucks. I don't want to be here. It's very painful. But I am accepting that I'm here.' And then, just like all emotions, it's transient. You begin to pop up slowly, slowly, slowly, slowly, slowly until you're your normal self again."

Accepting Change Is Inevitable

A lot of infertility warriors want to know how they can return to their former selves after experiencing infertility. Dr. Rothenburger argues that's not the best approach.

"The fact of the matter is you're *not* who you were before," she says. "You've experienced this very big thing. Maybe you don't even want to go back to who you used to be. The next step may not be who you were before but be a newer version of yourself."

It can be healthier to look at how you've changed and embrace positive improvements. For example, many infertility warriors become more compassionate and empathetic as a result of infertility. That's not something you want to give up so you can be your old self.

"I learned how to identify my role in the situation and understand what is out of my control," says Brianna from Pennsylvania, whose journey started in February 2019. "Before, when I would experience setbacks or failures, I would go down an emotional spiral. I now practice better skills to encounter these situations with a levelheaded mindset."

Integrating the Infertility Experience into Your Identity

We've said this before, but let me reiterate: You are *not* defined by your infertility. When you're working to regain a sense of who you are, remember that infertility is an experience, not an identity. Your task now is to find ways to integrate that experience into your identity.

Look at it this way: Maybe you fell off your bike and broke your arm when you were a kid. Despite the pain, maybe that moment gave you a taste for danger. Once you're an adult, when someone asks you to tell them about yourself, you don't say "I'm someone who fell off my bike when I was 11." Instead, you describe yourself as adventurous or a bit of a daredevil.

You can find ways to look at your experience with infertility and see the ways that it shaped your identity without being defined by it.

Choosing Your Reactions

One thing you have control over is your reaction to situations. Remember, reactions are different from feelings. After a failed cycle, whatever feelings pop up, pop up. But you get to decide what you do with those emotions.

"When you deal with any intense life issue, you get to decide how it shapes you. Will it destroy you or will it enhance who you already were?" says Dr. Rothenburger.

Throughout your infertility journey, ask yourself if your choices and behaviors align with your sense of self. This will help you stay connected to your core identity. For example, after a frozen embryo transfer, Elyse and her husband, Brad, from Minnesota decided not to take any home pregnancy tests. She knew that could bring out a less desirable version of herself.

"I heard too many stories from other people about [testing before the beta test] being stressful, and I just know my personality. I know I probably would've been pretty obsessive about it, so I really just tried to be at peace with whatever was going to happen."

Nurturing Other Aspects of Your Identity

It's easy to sacrifice other aspects of your identity because of infertility. The experience steals your attention, energy, and time. Still, it's essential to make an effort to maintain other factors that add to your identity.

"In order to become stronger than infertility, I highly recommend staying engaged in passions and hobbies that are not related to infertility," says Lisa Stack, a support coordinator at CNY Fertility in Syracuse, New York. "This serves as a constant reminder that you are so much more than whether you are fertile or not, and your worth is not intrinsically connected to conceiving."

You may not be able to keep up with all your interests at the same levels, but don't give up activities that give you joy. Meghan from Ohio has a farm with horses, cows, and a bull. While it involves hard work, caring for her animals helped her stay grounded during her infertility journey.

"My animals helped take my mind off of infertility. I would stay in the barn for hours with my horses," she shares. "I think our new filly could tell how I felt because she all of a sudden started giving hugs and wrapping her head and neck over my shoulder. Animals know how you feel, and mine would always make me happy or at least calm my soul."

Practicing Self-Love, Self-Forgiveness, and Self-Care

Taking into consideration that your sense of self can change throughout your infertility journey, remember that how you *treat* yourself should remain the same. You deserve care and respect during these tough times, and that starts with your own behavior toward yourself.

Self-Love

Self-love isn't always easy. It goes beyond self-esteem and self-respect—it's the foundation of how we view ourselves. The amount of self-love we have influences how we behave and think about ourselves. And with infertility, it can be difficult to extend ourselves the courtesy of love.

Dr. Rothenburger suggests a good way to start loving yourself is to imagine a vulnerable puppy on its back wanting a belly rub. The thought of kicking that puppy is obviously inhumane and gives many of us a queasy gut wrench.

During your infertility journey, you're in the same position as that puppy—vulnerable and desperate for affection. If you wouldn't kick the puppy, don't kick yourself, either. Don't deny yourself the kindness and love you desperately want, need, and deserve.

"Love yourself," advises Allison from New York. "You are already whole. Just like you don't need a partner to complete you, you don't need a child to complete you, either. These are added life bonuses and blessings. Don't feel like you are unworthy."

Self-Forgiveness

Dr. Rothenburger says it's important to feel your emotions but to do so without judgment.

"Stop beating yourself up!"

Punishing yourself is unproductive. You want to always move forward during your infertility journey, and blame will keep you from making progress.

"There's a quote I really love that says, 'What you think, you become,'" shares Suki from Florida. "The more that I kept thinking about my useless uterus, the more my uterus was useless."

It won't happen overnight, but piece by piece, you can free up your mental space for thoughts and actions that lead to strength and change rather than condemnation. Don't get me wrong: "Just stay positive" is incredibly unthoughtful advice and not what I'm saying here *at all*. But torturing yourself with self-blame is just that—torture. It serves no purpose and doesn't deserve a place in your life.

Self-Care

With every challenge life throws at us, we are better equipped to cope when our basic needs are met. But still, it's easy to forget about self-care.

"Basic behaviors like eating healthy meals, drinking plenty of water, sleeping enough each night, being physically active, having a good support network, and managing stress as much as possible are all important aspects of self-care," says Mia Joelsson, a licensed clinical social worker at Shady Grove Fertility in Harrisburg, Pennsylvania.

Self-care is about taking the time to check in with yourself and recognizing when you need to put yourself and your physical and mental health first. That looks different for everyone. Some people spend an evening watching a marathon of their guilty pleasure reality show. Others spend more time training at the gym. Pay attention to what activities give you a break from infertility so you can recharge and achieve better balance.

Brianna took wonderful care of herself—physically and mentally. "During cycles, I made sure to keep my workload as 'stress free' as possible. I got my nails done, took care of my appearance—small things that helped me feel more put together. I also went into each new cycle as if it were my first. Every IUI had a fresh new opportunity."

Going from Suffering to Surviving to Enjoying Life

Every infertility warrior knows there are certain events and triggers that cause them pain. You think your only option is to learn how to grin and bear it. But that's not true. While you won't be able to change all of your triggers into happy moments, there are ways to go from suffering to enjoying your life.

WARRIOR ACTION STEPS
Loving, Forgiving, and Caring for Yourself

Self-love, self-forgiveness, and self-care are unique to each individual. But there are some overarching steps you can take to help you find what works for you:

- **Be self-aware.** Paying attention to your emotions and their changes will show you where you're struggling and why. For example, maybe you notice you're particularly hard on yourself in the days leading up to a doctor appointment. Once you spot that trend, you can make the decision to practice more self-care in preparation for the anxiety-inducing event.

- **Try something new.** Yes, in the middle of your hectic infertility journey, I want you to make time for new activities. Why? Because even if you don't like it or suck at the activity, you'll learn something new about yourself. Spend time loving yourself for those new dimensions of your identity.

- **See yourself through a loved one's eyes.** While your sense of self-worth shouldn't be based on someone else's opinions, getting an outside perspective can help you fight negative feelings and behaviors about yourself. When you're at your lowest, hearing your partner loves how intelligent you are can give you a positive mantra to focus on and direct you away from darkness.

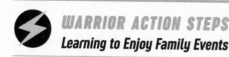

WARRIOR ACTION STEPS
Learning to Enjoy Family Events

This is a process, so don't expect to suddenly relish the idea of big family gatherings filled with children. Work on these steps over time to get to the point where you look forward to these formerly dreaded events:

• **Practice open and honest communication.** Many people assume if they see you happy on one occasion, you've moved past all your "hang-ups" about family events. But there are nuances to your pain. Share your progress with your loved ones, but remind them of areas where you're still struggling.

• **Give yourself an out.** If you feel like you cannot emotionally handle the event—or even take away from others' joy if you go—give yourself permission to back out. Trying to grin and bear it will hurt your progress and might take you a few steps backward. Be open and honest with people about why, and then forgive yourself for not going.

• **Create your own rituals.** For many of us, one reason family events are hard is we've envisioned how we'd pass traditions down to our children. Infertility is taking that away. Create your own child-free rituals that are focused on your relationships and love.

"This was a slow transition," Brianna admits. "I let negative thoughts and doubt take over much of my time. I realized through time and self-work that my goal was still *so* attainable. I just needed to keep my head high and appreciate life in between. So much of my life was passing by as I sat in despair. I learned to keep moving forward and find joy and hope in every day."

Family-Focused Events and Seasons

Infertility can turn the holidays and family events, once joyous times, into nightmares.

"Holidays are very hard for those going through infertility because just seeing all the babies and the families reminds you what you don't have right now, even though you're longing so much for it," explains Abbey from Wisconsin.

The key to participating in these events is establishing boundaries. Just as you don't want to feel isolated because you don't currently have children, you don't want your loved ones to feel excluded because they do.

If you feel safe doing so, explain your emotional triggers to your friends and family. Let them know if there are specific parts of celebrations that you can't be a part of and why. Especially during the early part of your infertility journey, talk about how you're going through the process. You don't want to avoid family events forever, but you need time and support to build up your strength.

Also, try to find ways to make your infertility journey part of the rituals. For example, let's say you've experienced a pregnancy loss. During gift-giving holidays, ask your loved ones to make donations to organizations like the March of Dimes in recognition of the possible child you lost or to RESOLVE in recognition of your and other infertility warriors' struggle.

Beth from Utah says attending family events where children will be present can be a chance to get more support from the people in your life.

"I was always very open and honest with my friends and family, and even coworkers, about our infertility struggle. Being able to be real about what I was going through strengthened my relationships because it allowed my friends and family the opportunity to support me."

Birthdays, Anniversaries, and Other Milestones

Birthdays, anniversaries, and infertility or pregnancy-related milestones can be particularly triggering. Dr. Rothenburger says it's important to weigh each of these occasions for how they make you feel and what they can signify about your journey.

- **Your birthday.** In most cases, birthdays are times of celebration. But when you're facing infertility, each year can represent a drop in your chance of conceiving or even just a reminder of how long you've been trying. Be aware of this and how it may change your feelings about your birthday.

- **Anniversaries.** Whether it's the date you were diagnosed, when you miscarried, or an anniversary in your relationship, certain days will weigh heavily on your heart. As time passes, it's essential to note which dates are harder for you so you can prepare ahead.

- **Other milestones.** Due dates and key doctor appointments will remind you that if you had had a successful pregnancy, this day would feel very different. To make it through these days, it's important to consider your needs. Do you need a day of self-care? Would a distraction be welcome? Decide what plan for these days will help you gain a sense of control so you can self-soothe.

It also helps to find ways to bring a sense of celebration—no matter how small—to bring positivity to hard days. Some people like to recount how far they've come during the year. Others like to create rituals that express their love for the child they don't yet have. Donate a toy to an organization that helps children in need, or write a letter to your future child. The key is finding a way to redirect your feelings toward something positive or hopeful.

"Birthdays were the most difficult thing for me during this process. I have felt enormous

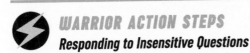

WARRIOR ACTION STEPS
Responding to Insensitive Questions

If you're ready to push back on ignorant questions and comments, it helps to have prepared ways to respond. This helps you react with compassion rather than anger. Here are some common situations infertility warriors find themselves in and ways to flip the script so you can walk away feeling empowered and proud instead of sad and ashamed:

- **"Doesn't it feel like something is missing from your life?"** There's no such thing as a perfect life. But there's also no such thing as one life that is less valuable than another. Explain that even though you'd like to be a parent, you are not defined by that role.

- **"Don't you wish you didn't wait so long to try?"** First, many causes of infertility are unrelated to age. Even if that's not your situation, explain that people of all ages struggle to build a family. Then talk about what it means to you to be ready to build a family now. You want to give your potential child the best life possible

and think they deserve for you to have all your ducks in a row before bringing them into this world.

- **"Have you tried just relaxing?"** Many fertile people have a fundamental misunderstanding of how babies come into the world and all the steps leading up to that point that have to go just right. Acknowledge that you know they're trying to help, but stress does not cause infertility—infertility causes stress. People have been having babies in stressful situations for as long as our species has been around.

pressure given my age. My third egg retrieval was the day before my 40th birthday, and I just had this irrational feeling that I had to get those eggs out before they all expired!" Adrienne recalls. "My advice is that families are built on all different timetables and in all different ways. Looking around in my life for examples of this was really helpful for me. Age is certainly a factor, but it doesn't have to be the deciding factor in your journey if you are open to multiple pathways [to parenthood]."

Confidently Talking About Infertility

It might seem weird, but many infertility warriors derive a sense of joy by working to overcome the stigmas surrounding infertility. Answering questions and sharing your story helps you find purpose and joy.

"It's so common to be going through infertility issues, and you feel so much better when you talk about them," says Mindi from Ohio. "Then you make discussion become the norm because it's really not something that you should be ashamed about."

We'll discuss more about advocacy and stepping up by talking about infertility in chapter 27.

Big Picture Ways to Cope and Get Support

Throughout this book, we've explored ways to cope in specific infertility situations. However, some skills and actions are so essential that they can help you through every stage of your journey and lead to you becoming stronger than infertility.

Finding and Building Your Support Team

Dr. Rothenburger believes that infertility will reveal your strongest and truest connections. These relationships will become your support

BUSTED

Myth: Being strong means doing it all alone.

Isolation can be overwhelming. You think no one else can understand what you're going through, and therefore, you need to do it all alone.

We are not alone. In the United States, one in eight couples are facing infertility. "If you live in an apartment building, there's somebody real close to you who has been through infertility or is going through infertility," says Dr. Alice Domar, an expert in mind/body health and infertility. "Every time you see a pregnant woman or a baby, you cannot assume that it was easy. You cannot assume that the baby is genetically connected to or carried by them."

team. They are the people who will stick by your side (and you by theirs) no matter what.

"Find others who understand," says Joelsson. "Going through infertility can be a very isolating experience, and having a couple of people who know what it feels like can be really helpful. Having a team behind you can make all the difference in feeling strong while going through infertility."

For many infertility warriors, like Elyse, the best part of infertility is the relationships that develop in the trenches.

"Easily the brightest spot was meeting all these other really strong, amazing, capable, hilarious, creative warriors—an immediate community—and really connecting with them in ways that I couldn't connect anymore with my friends who weren't experiencing it. We were in this sisterhood, there was a secret code, and we knew what to ask each other."

WARRIOR TIPS
Joining Online Infertility Communities

Whether you're not ready to share your infertility journey with those in your life or you haven't gotten the support you deserve, there are numerous online communities to help you find your allies. Check out:

- **Beat Infertility.** My podcast and the surrounding community is a safe place to get real about infertility. We strive to be honest as a way to empower ourselves and take back control during the infertility experience.

- **RESOLVE.** Aside from offering resources about infertility, RESOLVE also hosts infertility events and provides information about in-person support groups you can join.

- **FertileThoughts.** An online forum that covers all aspects of infertility. Think of FertileThoughts as a social media platform for the infertility world.

- **Peanut.** A social app where you can meet, chat, and learn from like-minded people across infertility and parenthood.

Sharing Your Story

To find your team, you're going to have to be vulnerable. You'll need to take a chance on people—sometimes complete strangers—and have faith they'll catch you when you fall. The first step in this process is sharing your story.

Stack says once you put your story out there, either publicly, privately one-on-one, or online, that's when your team will emerge. Your struggle will resonate with others (both in the infertility community and outside it), and a new connection will be formed.

While you'll have to put aside any feelings of shame or fear, it's almost always worth it. Plus, you might be surprised who understands what you're going through.

"When you share, you'll find you know other people in your family, or group of friends, or even at work who have also been through infertility or are also going through it now," says Joelsson. "Those people will have a special bond with you and be your tribe."

Even if it takes time to find your allies while you share your story, the process itself can be very cathartic. Angela from Missouri says talking about her infertility not only got her family and friends invested in being there for the highs and lows, but also helped her reconceptualize her situation.

"I let my narrative change," she says. "I think we all dream of a Beyoncé Instagram baby reveal in the beginning. That wasn't going to be my story. My narrative pivoted. I shared my story, openly and completely."

Creating a Community

Sometimes you have to start completely from scratch to find your team. While I had support from people in my life, a big part of my infertility journey was creating the *Beat Infertility* community. Beyond the podcast, at first, my listeners used Facebook as a platform to swap stories, ask and answer questions, and overall support each other. But through the generosity of networking platform Mighty Networks, we gained access to a free custom, branded app devoted to our community that relinquished us from the pain and triggers that Facebook often causes. The community has grown over time, and I'm frequently told it's the best online support network. It's a judgment-free safe space where warriors jump at the chance to help each other in any way they can, even after they become survivors on the other side. I'm so honored and humbled by the connections and true friendships that now exist because of this community I built.

Adrienne shared of her experience within our Mighty Networks community. "My husband has been incredibly supportive, but beyond that I really relied on the *Beat Infertility* community. Connecting with other women—especially after my miscarriages—was incredibly helpful as I was so isolated otherwise. What I found the most helpful of all was trying to support others through *their* challenges. It really gave me a sense of purpose during those darkest times."

Using Mind-Body Techniques

There's been a lot of chatter about mind-body health practices in recent years, and with good reason—these practices work. The idea is that your body already knows what it needs to cope and heal, and these strategies help you identify ways to address those needs. They provide a framework for you to explore all your feelings head-on in a safe way—there's no room for avoidance—and they help you reach a state of acceptance.

• **Meditation and mindfulness.** Being mindful means observing your current state without judgment. You take note of your emotions and situation so you can be present in the moment. Activities like meditation allow you to objectively examine your thoughts and emotions without making them feel too big. What's going on with you doesn't exist outside that moment.

• **Visualization.** During your infertility journey, your anxieties and negative emotions don't just impact your mind. They affect your *physiology*—a rapid heartbeat, inability to catch your breath, and other side effects. Visualization allows you to calm your body by focusing on images that help you feel safe and lead to positive emotions associated with those images.

• **Hypnosis.** Many people picture hypnosis as people clucking like chickens after hearing a trigger word. But in reality, hypnosis is about accessing parts of your subconscious associated with your brain's belief center. When you tap into that, you're open to suggestions that can help you better understand and process your emotions so you can be in a better state.

WARRIOR TIPS
Using Mind-Body Tools

When people say there's an app for everything, it's true. There are even multiple niche apps and tools to specifically walk infertility warriors through mind-body exercises. Check out:

• **Circle + Bloom.** This company offers a free meditation program, as well as many paid programs. As you might recall, I used its IVF program during my final cycle.

• **FeriCalm.** Because every infertility situation is different, this app has 500 ways to cope in 50 different distressful aspects of infertility.

• **Mindful IVF.** Create better mind-body habits by practicing 10 minutes a day each day of an IVF cycle.

• **Be Fertile.** Foster relaxation with these audio files customized to everything from trying to conceive to getting sleep once you have a child.

- **Emotional freedom technique.** While lesser known, the emotional freedom technique (EFT) is built on the acupuncture pressure points but doesn't involve needles. You tap on different parts of your body, like your hands or head, while making affirming statements. The combination helps calm your body and focus your thoughts.

Journaling

I can't say enough about the power of keeping a journal during your infertility journey. Physically writing things down will help you externalize your emotions in a positive and healthy way. There are countless ways to journal, each with its own benefits. Consider the following methods to determine what aligns with your situation:

- **Expressive writing.** The purpose of expressive writing is just getting your feelings out. For 20 minutes, you write every thought and feeling that enter your mind about a particular event or topic. Spelling, grammar, and to an extent comprehension don't matter. The point is to give yourself the freedom to get everything out.

- **Gratitude journals.** Sometimes negativity overtakes your life during infertility. Having a journal where you list what you're grateful for and what you've accomplished can help you gain perspective and remember everything that's still going well in your life.

- **Writing letters you'll never send.** After a breakup, someone might have advised you to write a letter to your ex and then throw it away. It helps you voice your feelings and gain closure. You can do the same thing during infertility. Write letters to people in your life or to infertility itself so you can process your emotions and express how you've been hurt.

- **Day worth living evaluations.** For my infertility journal, I found it helpful to start taking stock of each day and determine what I'd done to make those 24 hours worthwhile. It let me see how my actions have meaning beyond infertility.

Brianna found a different way to record her journey. "I did not journal, but I did photograph small moments from different cycles. I documented our IVF from egg retrieval to transfer through photos of the process. I fondly look back on these photos, and see such strength in the girl looking back at me."

WARRIOR WISDOM
Uncovering Your Strength

"You are not alone. You are stronger than you can imagine! It sounds cliché. But it's so true. So many people struggle to have a family. Infertility uncovered a strength that I never knew I had within me." —Rachel, Pennsylvania

WARRIOR CHECKLIST
Becoming Stronger Than Infertility

❏ Believe that you can be stronger than infertility.

❏ Revisit what it means to be strong in the face of infertility.

❏ Understand the differences between being resilient and growing after infertility trauma.

❏ Be prepared to regain your sense of self and redefine your identity.

❏ Practice self-love, self-forgiveness, and self-care.

❏ Be open to finding and building your support network or community.

❏ Discover which coping mechanisms will help you throughout your infertility journey.

❏ Develop strategies to transition from suffering to enjoying life.

Add more items to your Warrior Checklist or jot down any notes here:

Maintaining and Strengthening Your Relationships

CHAPTER 16

U P UNTIL MY SECOND MISCAR-riage, my parents and I weren't particularly close. We've always loved each other, of course, but they also would readily admit that I've always been independent—and we struggled in our relationship during my teenage and college years.

Before that second miscarriage, my parents and I rarely called each other—and even more rarely visited in person. I lived with my husband in the Washington, DC, area, and they lived near Chicago. We'd see each other for most Thanksgivings and Christmases, but that was it. We talked by phone maybe once a month at most. But that miscarriage was a turning point for not only my infertility journey, but also my relationship with my parents. They desperately wanted a grandchild, and when they finally realized what we were going through, they were all in. Phone calls increased to every weekend. Visits increased to more than just the holidays. We actually knew what was happening in each other's lives and offered support where we could from a distance.

Eventually my parents retired and moved from Chicago to Virginia to be near us. Although they still live 90 minutes away, making that drive is much better than getting on a plane! Ever since that first IVF cycle—and even more so since Aurora was born—they have become the two most important people in my life outside my daughter and husband. We talk daily. They've supported me in ways I cannot even put into words. We have our spats, sure, but overall, our relationship is the one I always dreamed I'd have with my parents.

And strangely enough, I owe all of this to infertility.

Finding Space for Other People

Infertility can turn your world upside down. Relationships that were once simple and easy now may require effort to maintain. But don't let infertility take away the love and support systems. You don't have to abandon your relationships and community while you work to build your family. You may actually *strengthen* your relationships while on your journey.

Maintaining Your Relationship with Your Partner

If you have a partner while navigating infertility, prepare to have your relationship tested. There will be fights. Some days—or perhaps even some weeks or months—you'll feel out of sync. But with the right tools and coping mechanisms, you and your partner will come out *together* on the other side.

Accept that infertility introduces a new variable into your relationship, and that how you or your partner react may surprise you. Your experiences may change the dynamic of your relationship, but it does *not* mean that the quality of your relationship has to suffer. In fact, facing a challenge together, head-on, can lead to growth and deeper connection. The key is cultivating open, honest, and nonjudgmental communication.

Dr. Angela Palmer-Wackerly, assistant professor of health communication at the University of Nebraska in Lincoln, says it's important to recognize that everyone—you and your partner included—deals with the ups and downs of infertility in unique ways. She stresses the importance of open communication when working to maintain your relationship with your partner.

"Ask for whatever you need to process, whether that be physical and emotional space, distraction, emotionally venting, or all of these," she says. "Just make sure you're moving closer to each other—by supporting and listening to each other—and not further apart when communicating."

Laura and her wife, both from New York, kept each other strong throughout the journey. At just 28 years old, Laura was diagnosed with severe diminished ovarian reserve and told that if she wanted to use her own eggs, she needed to move forward immediately.

"I think that my wife was really good at keeping my hopes up. And I was good at keeping hers up," Laura shared on the *Beat Infertility* podcast. "If one of us was feeling down, the other was being optimistic, and vice versa. And I think we also knew, hey, we've been warned, this could be a long road."

Possible Pitfalls

By knowing what to look out for, you can prepare to deal with—and perhaps even avoid—complicated situations involving your partner.

Letting Infertility Define You

It's easy to become obsessed with your infertility. You might spend hours upon hours researching or preparing for treatment. Plus, the process is so emotionally draining that it may leave you without the energy to focus on anything else. But this can throw your relationship out of balance.

"At one point, my husband looked at me and said that we no longer had a marriage. We only had infertility," explains Jannette from Ontario, Canada. She was hurt by her husband Michael's words, yet she knew they were true. "Infertility had infiltrated every aspect of our lives. Work was purely to get money to pay for IVF. Sex was no longer spontaneous.

WARRIOR TIPS
Hiring an Infertility Coach

Imagine being able to put your infertility journey into a box and then handing it over to someone else to manage. The only time you would have to open the box would be when you had a question for the person in charge of the box. How awesome would that be?

That's what an infertility coach does. Essentially, they're your guide through the process so infertility doesn't consume your relationship or your life. My career as an infertility coach has been so incredibly rewarding and fulfilling, and you can find plenty of options in RESOLVE's Professional Services Directory.

WARRIOR ACTION STEPS
Regaining a Healthy and Fun Sex Life

It may seem strange to offer a set of guidelines for maintaining or regaining the fun and enjoyment of a healthy sex life. But that's what many couples need to get infertility out of their bed. If you're worried that your work to conceive has hurt your sex life, try the following:

Talk to each other. Yes, it can be awkward, but broach the subject. Tell your partner about what you like, your insecurities, or the ways your needs are or aren't being met. No matter how long you've been together, your partner isn't a mind reader, so you'll have to ask for what you need.

Break the routine. When you're focused on conception, sex can get vanilla. You have a schedule to stick to, after all. Make an effort to try something new or to enjoy being intimate outside of your most fertile times.

Don't limit yourself. There are many forms of intimacy and pleasure. Take bubble baths together. Make out in the backseat of your car. Find ways to show you're attracted to each other regardless of your ability to conceive.

Relationships with people with children and especially pregnant friends were strained."

Infertility can become not only the focus of your relationship with your partner, but also a constant catalyst for arguments. Ariane from Minnesota says that after her second miscarriage, she and her husband, Ben, struggled to connect. They used to be able to talk about anything, but infertility consumed Ariane.

"I couldn't think of anything else," she admits. "I wanted to talk about it all the time, and everything was a trigger for me. I would get mad at him because I couldn't imagine how he wasn't thinking about it all the time."

Dr. Alice Domar, an expert in mind/body health and infertility, advises couples to have a life outside of infertility. "Limit the time you spend talking about that," she says. "Do things that you love that don't involve children." This will give you time to nurture other aspects of your relationship while recharging mentally and emotionally.

Ultimatums

Early in your infertility journey, you may feel that you already know how far you're willing to go, such as stopping after two IUI cycles. But as your journey continues, I encourage you to open your mind and heart to other possibilities.

Take Elyse and her husband, Brad, from Minnesota: He was not a fan of IVF initially. Not knowing much about the process, he thought of it as "weird, science-fictiony, and creepy." When Elyse wanted to consider IVF, she was worried that he'd flat-out refuse.

"It's so funny how, throughout the journey, every time you get to that next step, you can change your mind," she says. "It was really important for Brad and me to stay aligned throughout the process and make sure that we were checking in with one another."

Over the course of their journey, Brad and Elyse had a lot of tough conversations about what they were willing to try. She says the key was to never give an ultimatum or make the other person scared of suggesting an option. "We tried to keep everything on the table, which was really helpful to us further down the path, so that is something I recommend a lot to other people who are struggling with their partners early on."

Replacing Lovemaking with Baby-Making

Sex and intimacy are important parts of any partner relationship. But with infertility, sex becomes clinical. It's scheduled, and sometimes there are medications to be taken in preparation. As Sharon N. Covington, director of psychological support services at Shady Grove Fertility in Rockville, Maryland, says, "Something that was once fun becomes a tedious job."

A 2018 study in the *International Journal of Reproduction, Contraception, Obstetrics, and Gynecology* found that 64.5 percent of couples dealing with infertility have sex only in an attempt to conceive. For 16.4 percent of the couples, sex was no longer fulfilling or enjoyable.

Covington suggests that couples make a point to find time for intimacy outside of ovulation windows. Focus on romance, and remember that there are many forms of sexuality that don't involve intercourse.

"We have had many more arguments during our infertility journey than ever before," confides Cvetelina from Georgia. "Our sex life has suffered as that has become more focused on baby-making. For a while, my husband felt unappreciated—that I was only interested in sex for the sake of becoming pregnant and not because of him."

She continues, "Initially, I had to go through a lot of medical interventions, and I felt that I was more invested in the process than he was. We process things differently and at a different pace, but it is hard to remember that. I tend to blame him for not caring because he does not obsess over things the way I do."

Not Being on the Same Page About What to Share

Talking about infertility can put you in an uncomfortable position. Sometimes you want to protect your own privacy; other times you may shy away from breaking social norms and taboos. But you don't want to close yourself off. So, how much do you share and with whom?

Many couples struggle with this issue. For example, you might want to talk with a friend about your fertility struggle, but your partner may want to keep it quiet.

Lisa Stack, a support coordinator at CNY Fertility in New York, encourages couples to focus not on *what* you want to share, but rather *with whom* you're sharing it. "Infertility patients often feel like they need to share every detail of their cycles with friends and family. This can cause an extra burden of stress, frustration, and grief. You can maintain relationships while also maintaining privacy with regard to your fertility by only sharing your journey with those who will be truly supportive and understanding."

Come to a compromise by discussing which friends, family members, and coworkers are most likely to receive information without judgment or nosy questions.

WARRIOR TIPS
Sharing Your Story

It can be nerve-wracking to tell others about your infertility journey, but sharing your story can be empowering. Here are some things to consider so you can decide whether it's time to go public.

• **Understand that getting real goes both ways.** When you "get real" about what you're facing, people will respond in a way that's true for them. And sometimes that can mean their reaction is negative. Acknowledge this as a possibility so you can prepare yourself emotionally.

• **Weigh the fear of telling against the pain of not.** Not being out about your infertility struggle closes yourself off to support from your friends and family. That can make your journey harder. When you reach the point where the fear of telling people is less than the pain you're feeling from having to keep it a secret, it's probably time to share your story with someone else.

• **Be excited about taking off the infertility mask.** When you're going through treatments in secret, you have to hide your emotions and struggle. This means being a less honest version of yourself, which in itself can be painful. Celebrate how good it will feel to take off that mask and open yourself up to support.

Playing the Blame Game

Blame is a dangerous element in any relationship. In the case of infertility, if you blame yourself or your partner for not being able to conceive, blame can damage your relationship.

A 2018 study found that when men self-blame, they experience lower relationship satisfaction. When women self-blame, their partner experiences higher levels of anxiety and depression. Women who blame their partner to some degree are also more likely to be depressed. (The study didn't look at men who blame their partner, but we can guess that it's not great for the relationship, either.) Again, the blame game is lose-lose.

Patricia Sachs, a clinical social worker at Shady Grove Fertility in Rockville, Maryland, says a better approach is learning to see infertility as a "couple's problem." This allows you and your partner to feel like equal partners in supporting each other. "Most couples do not want to play a blame game," Sachs explains. "Mostly they want to work together, with the person they love and chose, toward some resolution."

Sometimes blame comes from outside the couple. Same-sex couples, for example, may experience judgment from people in their lives—or society in general—who are not accepting of their decision to have children. "On top of feeling the shame that hetero couples might feel about not being able to conceive, [same-sex couples] oftentimes receive some rude comments about being gay and not being able to build a family. Basically, it's just shame and blame on a whole different level," says Dr. Maria T. Rothenburger, a psychotherapist at Miracles Happen Fertility Center in Salem, Oregon.

Dealing with Finances

Finances are a big part of the infertility journey, and for people who are part of couples, it can be a point of contention. It's not uncommon for one partner to be willing to spend whatever they can to build their family, while the other partner feels extremely worried about future stability. And anyone who worries about the cost of fertility treatments may be reluctant to speak up because that conversation could mean putting a finite monetary value on becoming a parent.

After a long journey to finally having a son, Laura says, "It was all worth it. I think that's the number one thing. You look back on how hard it was on your body and how hard it was on your marriage and how hard it was financially. And you just feel like, 'I would do it again a million times to get him.'"

The lowest point during the journey for Katie and her wife, Linda, from Wisconsin was when their first embryo transfer didn't work. They were doing reciprocal IVF—Katie's eggs and Linda's uterus—and had only two embryos. With one gone, their minds immediately turned to finances. "Frankly, if [the second embryo] didn't work, I don't know if we could have done it again financially at that point because of where we were in life. It was just Linda and me together, because we weren't telling any of our family we were going through this," she shares.

Try to separate what you *would* pay versus what you *can* pay. Of course you'd pay a million dollars if it meant guaranteed success building your family. But if you don't have a million dollars, that doesn't matter.

Throughout your journey, check in with your partner about your financial situation. Establish a baseline standard of living you won't fall below. Remain open to suggestions about ways to save money or pay for treatment (see chapter 20), but discuss your options with an understanding that you won't let your situation get worse than you're willing to endure.

Identifying Needs

Again, you and your partner will experience infertility differently and benefit from different forms of support. But the first step is figuring out what works for each of you as individuals. Remember that your needs will change and evolve throughout your infertility journey. Knowing how to check in with yourself will ensure you're able to be there for each other.

Get to the root of your worries so you can better express what you need. If you're struggling with self-blame, how can your partner assuage your fear? Would you like the two of you to attend more doctor appointments together so you feel like you're in treatment together? Or do you need assurances that your partner loves you whether or not you become parents? Working it out in your head or in a journal can be a good way for you to sort through complicated feelings. Later, you can review your thoughts and concerns and determine how each of you can support the other.

Communicating Needs

"Communication is so important!" says Cvetelina. "It is crucial to talk about where each person is in the process mentally, emotionally, and physically. It is important to listen to the other person without judgment, but this is so hard because we can easily become defensive or blame the other person for the way they feel."

It can be just as hard to *express* your needs as it is to identify them. But it is important to communicate clearly with your partner, in a way they can understand. Again, one of the keys to success throughout your infertility journey is having open, honest, nonjudgmental conversations.

BUSTED

Myth: You and your partner will feel the same way about the infertility experience.

You and your partner are two separate individuals. No matter how much you have in common, you will both have—and are entitled to—your own reactions and feelings. You'll process problems and losses differently and at your own pace.

Sachs says it's essential to accept that partners won't always be in the same place emotionally. "It may take one longer than the other to come to a decision about a new treatment path, and this should be not only allowed but respected," she advises.

Remember that there's no right or wrong way to deal with infertility. Even if you don't understand what your partner is feeling or why, hear them out and acknowledge their emotions as valid.

⚡ Sometimes it's hard to communicate what you need when you're in the middle of an emotional breakdown. Dr. Domar recalls a solution to this problem she heard from a patient. "Each person should make a list of twenty things that the other person can do for them when they're having a bad day," she explains.

Some people share feelings in order to be heard—but not necessarily because they're in need of solution. Listening actively can be just as helpful as trying to "fix" a problem. If you want your partner to simply listen to you, and not to try to fix the situation, tell them this directly. If you are a "fixer," try to remember that your help may not always be wanted, and tamp down on that urge to act.

It's also important to talk about how your body impacts your emotional needs. If you're the one with an infertility diagnosis, your experience is not only emotional but also physical. And this can be difficult for your partner to understand.

⚡ WARRIOR ACTION STEPS
Maintaining Your Relationship with Your Partner

Relationships are built on more than communication. You and your partner's behavior and actions (and reactions) will play a big part in maintaining the quality of your relationship. Individually, you both will have to make an effort.

Here are some additional actions steps for you and your partner to take to maintain your relationship:

Give each other space. When infertility becomes overwhelming, give your partner space and permission to focus on something else. Encourage each other to take time off, spend time with friends, or do something you love—whatever you're into—so you can have a break from the emotional stress.

Share positives. Make it a habit to share the good highlights of each day with your partner. This will remind both of you that not everything is terrible. It will also help a partner see they don't need to fix every aspect of your life to make you feel better.

Practice self-care. If you don't take the time to care for yourself, you can't be who your partner needs and deserves.

Be present. This process is a team effort. Go to as many appointments as possible, be well versed in the procedures and steps, help your partner with any treatments, and be there for each other.

Avoid unhealthy coping mechanisms. It's okay to want to escape from infertility and to seek activities that distract you from the situation. But be sure to avoid unhealthy behaviors, like heavy drinking or spending, that signal you're unwilling to deal with issues.

Accept that sometimes things can't be fixed. It can be difficult to do nothing. But when you're constantly throwing yourself at a problem with no solution, it wears on you.

"If you are undergoing the majority of testing and procedures, explain to your partner that you may have constant reminders of infertility throughout the entire bodily experience," says Dr. Palmer-Wackerly. "In other words, when infertility treatments are happening to your body, you may feel each cycle's failure more intensely, which can increase grief."

If you're part of a same-sex couple, the conversations around fertility treatments look different from the beginning. You may need to decide the source of sperm, eggs, *and* uterus. You may think that the process will be fast and straightforward once those decisions are made, but it can be frustrating—to say the least—when you find that there are further barriers to your fertility.

"When you're dealing with all of that hard stuff, emotions start to head in the upward, intense direction. You might find some anger coming out—some frustration coming

out—and misdirect it at your partner," explains Dr. Rothenburger. "I encourage you to keep living your life to keep doing the things that make you happy. Find time for yourself and your partner, just as you would had you not been going through this process."

It can be hard for some people to communicate their emotional needs. Nune from California reflects on how she supported her husband: "I gave him space to deal with his emotions even though he didn't show them to me. If I was able to, I would suggest things to do so that we weren't sitting on the couch sinking into our depressions."

When your partner talks about their worries, impressions, opinions, and ideas about the future, it communicates a lot of information that can transition into emotional needs. Get in the habit of waiting to have a conversation until any high-level feelings of anger and frustration have subsided. According to

BUSTED

Myth: Your fertile partner would be better off without you.

It's common for the partner with the infertility diagnosis to feel like they're depriving their partner of the opportunity to be a parent. This is the thought process: You both want to build a family, but *your* medical condition is preventing it. Therefore, it's best for your partner to leave you for someone else in order to get that desired family.

Jahsmyn from Queensland, Australia, admits that at first, such thoughts led her to push her husband, Drew, away. "I told him to leave, and that if he was with any other woman he'd have his family by now," she says. "Luckily, he didn't listen and continued to tell me that if I was his only family, then he was the luckiest man alive."

Stack reminds infertility warriors that their partner didn't choose them for their fertility. "It is good to remember that you two chose each other for many reasons beyond your ability to conceive," she says. "Remind each other of the many reasons you chose and continue to choose them, and you'll continue to grow in the security of your relationship."

Dr. Rothenburger, the best time to have conversations about emotions and needs is when you can say that, on a scale of one to ten, your feelings register at a four or lower.

She also points out that "I don't know how I feel" is a valid and valuable way to express yourself. "Sometimes there aren't words," she says. But at least in saying "I don't know," you

are participating in the conversation. And that's a step in the right direction.

Strengthening Your Relationship with Your Partner

The only upside to infertility is that it forces you to grow stronger. Throughout your infertility journey, you'll need support from your loved ones. Learning how to open up, ask for help, and be appreciative of the love in your life will help you strengthen a number of relationships.

Sachs says it's a common misconception that infertility drives couples apart. "In fact, it often makes them stronger," she says. "This may be the first real challenge they face as a couple, and they can seize the opportunity to develop new coping tools for future challenges."

Annie from Kansas had always wanted a baby, but she wanted to build up her career before starting a family, so didn't get started until she was 36 years old. Her wife was not interested in carrying a child, so they decided to start IUI treatments with Annie. Unfortunately, IUI didn't work. It turned out that Annie's egg quality was not good.

"For some reason, I hadn't anticipated that this would be possible. I was getting older,

WARRIOR TIPS

Don't Wait Until Problems Are Insurmountable

••

Infertility challenges even the strongest relationships. Admitting that you and your partner need help is not declaring defeat or the end of your relationship. For many infertility warriors, couples counseling can help them tackle problems that are too big to process alone.

"If you find that you are at an impasse or your usual coping strategies aren't working in the relationship, counseling may help," says Dr. Rothenburger. "Don't wait until things get critical."

Check out the following resources to find a mental health professional who specializes in infertility:

• American Society for Reproductive Medicine

• RESOLVE's Professional Services Directory

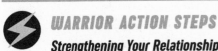

There's a difference between maintaining and strengthening. Even if infertility hadn't affected your life, you and your partner would, ideally, have worked continually toward building a deeper connection. Don't let your journey stop that process. Instead, use infertility as a way to tackle challenges together and build a stronger partnership.

Value your partner's contributions. Whether it's a second set of ears at a doctor appointment or a foot rub after a hard day, recognize your partner's actions. Say thank you. Let them know you appreciate what they're doing and that it's helping you deal with infertility.

Give each other permission to be vulnerable. Find strength in sharing fears and pain.

Don't take things personally. If your partner is expressing anger or frustration, try to remember that the situation is created by infertility, *not* you. If your immediate reaction is to take things personally, your partner is more likely to shut down so they don't feel like they're hurting you.

Open up. You may feel like you're protecting your partner by hiding your feelings, but in reality, it can make them feel isolated and alone.

Acknowledge new things you learn about each other. During infertility, you will see new sides of your partner. Share what new things you are discovering and loving.

Step up. Many couples develop a dynamic about who does what. Maybe you track the budget and your partner cooks the meals. If your partner is going through treatments, there are going to be days when they can't physically or emotionally fill their old role. Before that happens, show them you can pick up the slack.

sure, but I thought plenty of women that age become pregnant," she shares. "So it was disappointing that I didn't produce enough good eggs. But it was really clear from the blood tests and the ultrasound. There was no doubt that it was going to be much easier for us to get pregnant with my wife's eggs. She's 8 years younger than me. But it was difficult."

No matter who's been diagnosed with infertility, you and your partner are a team. You won't always be in agreement about treatment or other decisions, but how you learn to work together can bring you closer—strong enough to face anything else life decides to throw at you.

Maintaining Your Relationship with Family and Friends

I'll say it again: *Do not try to make it through infertility alone.* Please, for your own sake, lean on your loved ones during this heartbreaking journey. But also be aware that your friends and family will make mistakes. Though your emotions may be fried, you'll have to be patient and forgiving as they learn to support you.

Laura shares how she and her wife maintained their relationships with friends and family by agreeing on how they wanted to communicate about their journey. "We are open to friends and family asking us questions about our relationship. It gets a little more touchy when you're talking about having children. It's one thing to talk about your relationship when it's the two of you. But then you think about bringing a child into the world, and suddenly you get incredibly sensitive about how you want people to communicate with them and treat them. You really want to protect them."

She remembers, "Early on, people would ask, 'Who's the father?' and 'Did you choose a dad?' We became very clear very quickly. That's not the language we're going to use. You can ask us about the donor. We're going to talk openly about the donor in our family as our children grow up. But there's no father, there's no dad—these are not words we're using."

You need to balance your need for space and support. At the same time, loved ones need to navigate the treacherous waters of infertility as outsiders. As the one going through the emotional distress, learn how to set boundaries and guidelines surrounding your needs and the types of support family and friends should offer.

BUSTED

Myth: Infertility leads to divorce.

It's a fact of life: Relationships don't always survive difficult situations. However, while some marriages do break up during an infertility journey, it's not as common as you think. In fact, a 2017 study published in the *European Society of Human Reproduction and Embryology* found that infertility does *not* increase the risk of divorce. It might even make your relationship stronger.

Elyse says she saw her husband, Brad, make a big improvement in how he communicated with her. "Brad learned how to be more empathetic, and he learned how to acknowledge my reality and how to say, 'I see you're anxious, and I get it. How can I help you?' rather than 'You really shouldn't be anxious because there's no reason to be,'" she explains. "He's changed and grown so much throughout the journey, and it's made him such a great partner. I'm so appreciative of that."

Possible Pitfalls

Imagine you meet a good friend for coffee. You hug her when you arrive, but as soon as you sit down, she starts speaking another language. You have no idea what she's saying and don't know how to react when she gets frustrated that you don't understand her.

This may be what it's like for your friends and family when you first open up to them about your infertility. Unless they have experienced infertility themselves, they likely know little to nothing about the topic. They'll say the wrong thing or misunderstand your emotional responses. But by knowing the typical minefields, you can better prepare to protect your relationships—and your own heart.

Fertile Myrtles

When you're unable to conceive, it can be painful to be around pregnant friends or celebrate new births in the family. However, your loved ones may also feel hurt when you start crying after they give you fabulous news.

Krista from New Jersey describes her sisters-in-law as "the most fertile bunch an infertile can hope to be blessed with." She says: "It took work for me to celebrate their baby showers and stuff, but they never pushed or questioned my need for space or boundaries. But I had to figure out the boundaries. That was the most important part."

⚡ If you know that you have friends and family members who are trying to become pregnant, then, if possible, have the "I'm happy for you but sad for me" conversation. Explain that you will be excited for them and don't want to take anything away from their experience once they're pregnant. But at the same time, being reminded of your own infertility will stir up less positive emotions.

Dr. Palmer-Wackerly suggests asking your loved ones to give you time to process their announcement privately first. Before they publicly share the news, ask if they can send you an email or text. Promise to keep their secret, but explain that having space initially will help you celebrate after the public announcement.

Unsolicited Advice

Well-meaning family and friends *will* offer you advice. Without understanding your medical history or even how infertility works, they'll say things like "Just relax!" or "Why don't you just adopt?"

Part of the infertility process will be educating your loved ones. (Perhaps hand them a copy of this book? Wink wink.) But as Dr. Domar says, unless your family and friends have been through infertility themselves, they have no business doling out advice.

Let people know that you have a professional team to walk you through your options. What you need from friends and family is support. Tell them that if they'd like to help, the best thing they can do is ask what you need or how to best offer support.

The Hope-Grief Cycle

As we talked about in chapter 14, grief ebbs and flows during your infertility journey. Some days you'll feel great and be able to have lunch with your pregnant sister. Other days, hearing her voice will make you burst into tears.

It's hard for your family and friends to understand and accept that your reactions and feelings may shift—unpredictably. They might feel frustrated if you have to change plans at the last minute because your grief popped up. But as Dr. Rothenburger says, it's important to give yourself permission to cancel; you can explain to your loved ones ahead of time that you're prioritizing your mental health and sometimes they'll just need to be flexible.

"I encourage honoring wherever [you are] in the moment," Dr. Rothenburger says. "Please do *not* be afraid to politely decline. You'll be surprised how much anxiety melts away at this permission—and how much easier it is for you to navigate difficult waters."

Creating "Eggshells"

When you bring your family and friends into your infertility journey, it's important to set boundaries and explain your triggers. But Dr. Rothenburger says there's one caveat: Don't encourage your loved ones to walk on eggshells.

If your family and friends are scared to bring up your infertility, they can't be there to offer support. Once again, the answer is open, honest, and nonjudgmental communication.

In Dr. Rothenburger's own battle with infertility, she remembers she asked her mom to stop bringing up other family members' pregnancies. "She didn't realize it was so painful, so I had to communicate that. Then I asked for what I needed," she shares. "Be open about what is going on and say what is helpful and what is not. This will give family clear guidelines for how you need to be treated during this process."

Borrowing Money

It's not uncommon for infertility warriors to borrow money from friends or family to help pay for their treatments. If your loved ones are able to help out, that's great, but it can complicate your relationship.

Elyse and Brad borrowed money from his parents for their second cycle of IVF, and while they were appreciative, it did create a sense of pressure. "If it doesn't work, is my mother-in-law going to be mad at me? I don't want to throw their money away, but on the other hand, I felt pretty hopeful and confident going into the second round," she says.

Consider how borrowing money from friends or family might impact your relationship with them. If the pros outweigh the cons, broach the conversation with them and detail how much you're seeking and what the money would go toward. Then, as unfriendly and untrusting as it may sound, regardless of whether the money is a gift or a loan, write out the terms. If the money is a loan, detail how and when it will be paid back—including any interest, if charged. This will give everyone peace of mind. (For more on this, see chapter 20).

Identifying Your Needs

Just like you'll have to work to identify what support you need from your partner, you'll also have to figure out what you need from family and friends. Because you can't reliably predict anyone else's reactions and behavior, this can be a process.

To begin, pay attention to your emotional triggers. For example, some people who struggle with infertility might find it is hard to attend baby showers. Others might find their emotions are too raw to attend any event that falls close to the anniversary of a pregnancy loss.

"The holidays and family events were so very hard. There was a time when I was at my lowest right around Christmas. I avoided people. I shut those close to me out," confesses Brianna from Pennsylvania. "I look back on this person, and I wish I could tell her to somehow continue to find joy during the holiday season. To appreciate loved ones more, and not let the pain come through as anger. I wish

I would have talked about my struggle more, and let people in."

It's important to figure out what's really causing your pain—your triggers—so you can engage with your family and friends as much as possible. Know, too, that your triggers might change over time, with old ones no longer as painful but new ones popping up.

Communicating Your Needs

Remember two things when communicating your needs to family and friends. First, they likely *want* to help. Their hearts are in the right place. Second, they're likely blissfully ignorant about infertility. You'll have to give more in-depth explanations so they can better understand your situation.

"To garner support, always, always, always ask for what you need," says Dr. Rothenburger. "Even if you don't know what you might need, say that, and ask if you can have a voucher for future support. Good friends [and family] are likely to welcome you asking with open arms."

Introverted people might prefer to write emails, send texts, or have conversations one-on-one. Others feel more supported when they talk to their loved ones as a group. Figuring out *how* you want to communicate your needs is just as important as identifying them.

WARRIOR ACTION STEPS
Maintaining Your Relationships with Family and Friends

Infertility can strain relationships because it introduces a new dynamic. To maintain the quality of your relationships, you'll have to work together to find a new sense of normal. This creates a new framework that allows you and your family and friends to remain close during your infertility journey. To begin, try the following:

Explain what won't change. After you communicate all your needs to loved ones, they can feel disoriented. Give them some stability by discussing what's staying the same. No, you won't be going to your new baby cousin's christening, but, yes, you'll still be at Sunday family dinners.

Don't make it all about you. Infertility is difficult. But so are a lot of things in life. While it's okay to take time and space, you still need to be there for your family and friends when they're struggling. Relationships go two ways.

WARRIOR ACTIONS STEPS
Strengthening Your Relationships with Family and Friends

Use your infertility journey as an opportunity to *strengthen* your relationships with family and friends. Stack suggests taking inventory of your relationships to see where there are opportunities to do just that.

For example, if you could benefit from more one-on-one time with your sister, take an art class together. A creative outlet can help you better express your emotions while giving you a new connection with your sister. Here are a few other ways to strengthen your relationships:

Be grateful. It's hard to show genuine appreciation when you're emotionally strained. Whenever you're feeling up to it, take the time to thank your friends and family members. Small but meaningful gestures can help them see how glad you are that they're in your life.

Take risks. Your friends and family members can't step up if you don't give them a chance. Give them the benefit of the doubt, and let your walls down enough to share your experience and feelings.

Strengthening Your Relationships with Family and Friends

Leaning on loved ones during your infertility journey can lead to a stronger relationship with them. It gives your family and friends a chance to step up in ways you never imagined. Along the course of your journey, you can have meaningful experiences with others that deepen your love and trust in them.

Jahsmyn found her friends instrumental in keeping her optimistic and cheerful while she struggled to start a family. "Through it all, they were willing to listen or to distract me when I needed it. They gave me space without me having to ask and came to pick me up when I got so down I didn't recognize myself," she shares.

When a Relationship Cannot Be Saved

Sometimes relationships with friends don't survive infertility. If you've communicated your needs to a friend, but they continue to behave in a way that hurts you, it's time to cut ties.

"It helps to ask [friends] their perspective and what they might be struggling with in understanding your situation," says Dr. Palmer-Wackerly. "But if certain friends are unable to understand your situation and offer support, then you may need a break from those friendships, perhaps even permanently."

Elyse says infertility taught her the meaning of true friendships. "It's really easy to be friends with somebody when things are going well," she explains. "It's harder to be friends with someone when someone's going through a divorce, depression, or some other trauma happens."

Infertility can force you to examine who you really want and need in your life. If you find certain relationships have become toxic or one-sided, have the strength to move on and focus on getting the support you need and deserve.

Sadly, I lost friends on my journey, but these broken relationships were outliers. For the most part, my friends and family have rallied around me and my husband. But be sure to stand up for your own needs in every relationship—again, they go two ways—and recognize when you need a temporary break or permanent separation. You deserve to have only nontoxic people in your life!

WARRIOR TIPS
Finding Your Rock

"My friends were my rock because my family didn't get it. But my friends came through. They went on the long drives to my reproductive endocrinologist. They injected my medication when I needed them to until I was comfortable. They let me cry on them. My baby is here because of them." —Angela, Missouri

WARRIOR CHECKLIST
Maintaining and Strengthening Your Relationships

❑ Understand how to avoid the typical relationship pitfalls that occur with infertility.

❑ Know how to identify and communicate your needs in every relationship.

❑ See infertility as a chance to strengthen your connections with the important people in your life.

❑ Be prepared to pause or end relationships that continually cause you pain and deny you support.

Add more items to your Warrior Checklist or jot down any notes here:

Miscarriage and Recurrent Pregnancy Loss

CHAPTER 17

I DIDN'T TELL MY PARENTS—NOR did my husband tell his—about my first miscarriage until the second one happened.

No one knew we were trying to build our family. We'd kept it a secret. If I'm being completely honest, I wanted that big reveal of "We're having a baby!" However, keeping our baby-making efforts to ourselves came at a cost. It meant suffering in silence when complications arose, rather than receiving the support we desperately needed.

That changed after my second miscarriage, which was devastating *and* frightening. I just needed my mom. When I called her, I asked her to go into a room where my dad couldn't hear the conversation. I wasn't ready for him— or anyone else—to know. I was deeply sad, but also ashamed. *This is my fault. I own these losses.* But I knew she'd been through several miscarriages herself—although I didn't know the exact details—and needed to hear that everything would be okay.

Although I strongly suspect she told my dad about at least some of that conversation afterward, I'll always be grateful for the call. It was a turning point in my infertility journey— and in my relationship with my mom.

Dealing with the Unthinkable

Pregnancy loss. It's one of the most difficult parts of infertility to talk about. After trying for so long, there's the elation when you discover you've *finally* conceived. To have that hope and joy yanked away shortly thereafter is devastating. But it's a reality many have to face.

Because getting pregnant is already complicated, pregnancy loss can be particularly difficult to understand and process for infertility warriors. And, as Jamie Kreiter, a maternal mental health therapist, explains, "It is important for both patients and clinicians to understand that grief after any reproductive loss is not based on the duration of the pregnancy, but rather many other factors influencing the pregnancy and the success of future pregnancies. This includes, but is not limited to, the patient's age, financial means, previous losses, attachment to the pregnancy, and remaining viable embryos."

"In our society, miscarriages are so taboo," says Dr. Alice Domar, an expert in mind/body health and infertility. "No one talks about miscarriages and they become this big secret— something to be ashamed of."

Because people are hesitant to discuss miscarriages and recurrent pregnancy loss,

Myth: Miscarriages and pregnancy loss are rare.

The American Pregnancy Association estimates that between 10 and 25 percent of pregnancies result in a miscarriage. You are *not* alone. In fact, chances are someone you know has experienced a pregnancy loss. Even more likely, they experienced a pregnancy loss and didn't even know it.

"The statistics are that it happens often—and often before the fertile population even knows they were pregnant," says family therapist Penny Joss Fletcher. "But people in treatment test very early, so they, unfortunately, have the knowledge that they were pregnant and have now miscarried, rather than just thinking they're experiencing a late period."

When you're going through the pain of pregnancy loss, it can be helpful to find a support network of people facing the same situation. "You are not alone in the process," says ob-gyn Katherine Green. "There are many couples who are going through a similar experience, and talking through one's experience may be healing. [Not talking] can result in feelings of isolation."

Elizabeth and her husband, James, from Alberta, Canada, always knew they wanted to be parents. However, they faced several issues building a family. During their second cycle of IUI with donor sperm, Elizabeth had a chemical pregnancy. It was difficult, and she and James mourned their loss. But for Elizabeth, opening up about her experience with her mom helped a lot.

"My mom had experienced a miscarriage as well when they were building their family. Hearing her experience gave me a lot of strength, and I think drew me closer to her," she says.

---

it's difficult to get a sense of how to handle the situation. Knowing more about miscarriages and other forms of pregnancy loss won't make experiencing them any easier. However, it will help you understand your options and where to find support and resources.

Trigger warning: This chapter is going to be tough.

Types of Pregnancy Loss

Medically speaking, there are many ways to lose a pregnancy. It's important to know the symptoms and effects on your body to avoid major health risks.

Biochemical Pregnancy

Home pregnancy tests have become incredibly accurate. They identify signs of hCG—human chorionic gonadotropin, the pregnancy hormone—very early in the pregnancy. With a biochemical pregnancy (also known as a chemical

pregnancy among infertility warriors), the fertilization of an egg followed by implantation of an embryo creates hCG, leading to a positive pregnancy test. However, the embryo loses viability shortly after and never develops enough to be seen via ultrasound.

Before I go any further, let me say that I *loathe* this term: biochemical pregnancy. I realize it's the official medical terminology used by reproductive endocrinologists and other physicians, but somehow it diminishes the loss. My dear friend, loss is loss. If you are mourning the loss of a pregnancy, don't get wrapped up in the terminology. You and I both know your loss is real—and felt deeply.

Because this is a very early form of miscarriage, many people who aren't going through fertility treatment experience it without ever even having known they were pregnant. They often experience the miscarriage as normal menstruation. But because infertility warriors take pregnancy tests just days or weeks after treatments, they are more likely to be aware that a chemical pregnancy is occurring.

The symptoms of a chemical pregnancy include:

- Cramps that feel similar to menstrual cramps

- Vaginal bleeding

Miscarriage

Miscarriages are generally defined as the loss of a pregnancy after it's been clinically confirmed via ultrasound but before 20 weeks of gestation. Most happen during the first trimester, but they can occur later in the pregnancy. Types of miscarriage include:

- **Blighted ovum.** A fertilized egg implants in the uterine wall, but an embryo never develops, or it stops developing. The woman may still feel typical pregnancy symptoms like nausea, but at the first ultrasound, a doctor will discover an empty gestational sac.

- **Missed miscarriage.** Early in the pregnancy, the fetus stops developing. However, the body does not expel the tissue. The woman may continue to have pregnancy symptoms. There may be some cramping or vaginal discharge.

- **Molar pregnancy.** A chromosomal issue with the fertilized egg leads to overdeveloped pregnancy tissue. This prevents a viable fetus from developing. After ending a molar pregnancy, patients need to have their health closely monitored. Molar pregnancies can lead to invasive moles or choriocarcinoma, a type of cancer that develops at the placental site.

Each miscarriage is different, but common warning signs include cramping, back pain, vaginal bleeding, or the passing of tissue. Unfortunately, light bleeding and cramping can be side effects of many fertility treatments. These symptoms even occur in successful pregnancies. (I bled *heavily* with Aurora for 10 weeks!) Reach out to your doctor immediately if you're concerned your symptoms are the signs of a miscarriage.

Dr. Mark Perloe, an ob-gyn, estimates that about 70 percent of pregnancy losses are due to chromosomal issues. This is why many fertility specialists recommend IVF with preimplantation genetic testing (PGT; see chapter 4).

However, even embryos shown to be chromosomally normal with PGT can still result in a miscarriage. Other causes include:

- Uterine polyps

- Fibroids

- Adhesions

- Poor uterus receptivity

- Inflammation

- Infection

- Cervical insufficiency

- Hydrosalpinx (a buildup of fluid in the fallopian tube)

- Undetectable genetic issues with the embryo (PGT isn't perfect)

If you've miscarried, reproductive endocrinologist Dr. Allison K. Rodgers with Fertility Centers of Illinois in Chicago recommends getting a saline sonogram, preferably with 3D imaging, or another uterine cavity evaluation at a minimum to rule out any issues with the uterus. This will help you and your doctors develop treatments that will lower the chance of another miscarriage.

Ectopic pregnancy

An ectopic pregnancy is when the fertilized egg implants somewhere other than the uterus, like the fallopian tubes. Ectopic pregnancies can cause pelvic discomfort, feeling like you

BUSTED

Myth: Miscarriage is your fault.

It's the first thought many people have after a miscarriage: "I did something wrong." Maybe your diet wasn't as healthy as it should've been. Maybe you exercised too much—or too little. Maybe you should've been sleeping on your right side instead of your left.

Miscarriage is not your fault.

Unfortunately, not every embryo that implants is genetically capable of gestating to viability. Other times, there is no identifiable cause behind a miscarriage. Dr. Rodgers—who's had miscarriages herself—estimates this is the case with 50 to 70 percent of miscarriages. And yet, many people still blame themselves. But I repeat: Miscarriage is not your fault.

Mary and her husband, Charles, from Illinois miscarried their one and only pregnancy. Her doctor tested the products of conception and determined the fetus had a chromosomal abnormality. Mary wants other people in similar situations to know they are not alone—and most important, that there was nothing they could have done to change the outcome.

---

need to go to the bathroom, lightheadedness, gastrointestinal distress, nausea, severe abdominal pain, abnormal vaginal bleeding, and dizziness. If an ectopic pregnancy ruptures, blood will fill the abdomen, making symptoms more intense and even spreading pain to the back and shoulders. Surgery will be required to stop any internal bleeding and repair any damage, potentially leading to the loss of a fallopian tube.

Stillbirth

After 20 weeks of gestation, the loss of a fetus in the womb or upon delivery is classified as a stillbirth. The CDC reports that about 1 percent of pregnancies, or 24,000 a year, end in a stillbirth.

Most stillbirths happen for unknown reasons, but sometimes the causes are identifiable. They include:

• **Chromosomal defects.** Some birth defects allow the fetus to develop past 20 weeks but then cause loss of viability.

• **Umbilical cord incidents.** Having the umbilical cord knotted or wrapped around the baby's neck can lead to a stillbirth. Prolapse of the umbilical cord—when the cord enters the vagina before the baby and becomes compressed—can also cause a stillbirth.

• **Placental abruptions.** Trauma or infection can cause part or all of the placenta to separate from the uterus prematurely. If the separation is too severe, it can lead to a stillbirth.

• **Cervical insufficiency (aka incompetent cervix).** The cervix dilates too early in the pregnancy, leading to stillbirth. Cervical insufficiency itself is asymptomatic but is diagnosed by evidence of cervical dilation without full contractions, vaginal bleeding, infection, or water breaking. (This is what happened with my twins, Eric and Alexis.)

• **Infection.** Both bacterial and viral infections—like bacterial vaginosis, listeria, syphilis, and fifth disease—can cause complications that lead to stillbirth.

There are also several factors that can increase your risk for stillbirth:

• Carrying multiples

• Pregnancy that lasts longer than 42 weeks

- Physical injuries

- Carrier's age (women younger than 20 or older than 35 are more likely to have unexplained stillbirth)

- Poor maternal health (preeclampsia, uncontrolled diabetes, obesity, infection, lupus)

- Having previous difficult pregnancies, preterm labor, miscarriages, or stillbirths

- Abdominal trauma

Black women are more than twice as likely to have stillborn pregnancies than white women, according to data from the CDC. Researchers suspect that the many facets of systemic racism—such as reduced access to health care for Black communities, resulting in a greater likelihood of underlying health problems—have a role to play in this discrepancy.

WARRIOR TIPS
Count the Kicks

Once you are able to feel movement, determine a baseline for how often your baby moves and track it during your pregnancy—especially after 28 weeks.

If you notice a significant decrease in your baby's movements, contact your doctor.

Advocate for an Answer, but Accept When There Isn't One

While pregnancy loss is extremely difficult, it's important to talk to your doctor about what happened. The cause(s) behind your loss may give insight into your treatment plan and the path forward. If you experience recurrent pregnancy loss, encourage your doctors to approach each loss independently, as well as together as a whole. There's no guarantee that each loss was caused by the same factor.

Neonatal Death

A child who does not survive the first 28 days of life is classified as a neonatal death. Because the causes are typically related to the pregnancy or birth, many consider neonatal death a form of pregnancy loss.

Premature birth is one common cause of neonatal death. According to the March of Dimes, babies born prematurely are at greater risk for respiratory issues, brain bleeds, heart problems, infections, and other life-threatening conditions.

Another common cause is congenital birth defects. Babies with severe chromosomal issues may live for a few days, but often the defects cause a low quality of life and death.

Recurrent Pregnancy Loss

The American Society of Reproductive Medicine (ASRM) defines recurrent pregnancy loss as two or more unsuccessful pregnancies, whether those losses are caused by different factors, the same underlying medical issue, or unknown reasons.

Possible Causes of Recurrent Pregnancy Loss

It's not always possible to identify the cause of recurrent pregnancy loss, but some common issues include the following:

Genetics. A genetic abnormality in a parent can impact viability. Also, as the embryo cells divide, random mutations to chromosomes or individual genes can prevent the embryo from continuing to develop, leading to miscarriage. You and your partner (if you have one) can take genetic tests and/or start using PGT to determine whether genetics are leading to your pregnancy losses. If an issue is discovered, you may want to consider consulting a genetic counselor to determine your options moving forward.

Immunology. When it's working properly, your immune system fights and destroys foreign or harmful cells and organisms. However, there are certain autoimmune diseases that can cause your body to reject and attack an embryo. It's possible that an undiagnosed autoimmune condition—like Addison's disease, celiac disease, Crohn's disease, lupus, or multiple sclerosis—is leading to recurrent pregnancy loss. Your doctor can run blood tests, such as Pregmune, to see if this is the underlying issue. If an issue is discovered, you may want to consider consulting a reproductive immunologist to develop a treatment plan.

Infection. Certain infections lead to inflammation in the uterus that, left untreated, can cause recurrent pregnancy loss. These infections include listeriosis, toxoplasmosis, rubella, and herpes, but the most common is chronic endometritis, which can be diagnosed with a hysteroscopy and endometrial biopsy (see chapter 3). Once diagnosed, most of these infections can be treated with antibiotics or other inflammation-reducing medications.

Hematologic disorders. An undiagnosed or untreated blood clotting disorder, such as factor V Leiden thrombophilia, protein deficiencies, and the MTHFR gene mutation, can lead to recurrent pregnancy loss. Most of these disorders are diagnosed with blood tests and treated with blood thinners and supplements. Once diagnosed, you may want to consider consulting a hematologist to develop a treatment plan for future pregnancies.

Endocrine disorders. When they are not treated properly or uncontrolled, thyroid conditions and diabetes can lead to recurrent pregnancy loss. Thyroid conditions can cause hormone imbalances that lead to miscarriages. With diabetes, uncontrolled blood sugar impacts how the embryo is fueled and therefore develops, which can lead to miscarriage.

If an issue is discovered, you may want to consider consulting an endocrinologist, and possibly also a functional medicine practitioner, to develop a treatment plan.

Structural uterine anomalies. Polyps, fibroids, scarring, adhesions, and uterine deformities can impact everything from implantation to how the placenta develops and attaches. If you haven't had any tests that examine your uterus, like saline infusion sonography (SIS), hysterosalpingogram (HSG), or hysteroscopy (see chapter 3), consider asking your doctor to perform one to determine whether any anomalies are causing your pregnancy losses.

BUSTED

Myth: Stress is the cause.

Many people believe that stress directly impacts your ability to carry to term—that if you're excessively worried or stressed, your body will "reject" the pregnancy. But as Dr. Laura Covington, a social worker who specializes in infertility, grief, and loss, says, this just isn't true. "There is no consistent relationship between recurrent pregnancy loss and stress," she emphasizes. "Even people in really stressful situations get pregnant and stay pregnant."

However, don't let your stress go unchecked. Your mental health is *extremely* important. If you're feeling stressed, anxious, or depressed, seek help.

One potential cause not on this list? Your lifestyle choices. Dr. Green says recurrent pregnancy loss is rarely—if ever—caused by a woman's lifestyle. In other words, *it is not your fault*.

As Dr. Perloe notes, after a miscarriage, many couples want to try again immediately. Without an evaluation for possible causes, they leave themselves open to the possibility of another miscarriage. So, again, it's important to attempt to identify the cause behind each miscarriage. While it isn't always possible to pinpoint an issue, the more information you have, the better.

Know, too, that even if you've had multiple pregnancy losses, it is still possible to have a successful pregnancy. "After a first, second, third, or even more miscarriages, the odds are usually in the woman's favor that she will one day have a live birth," points out reproductive endocrinologist Michael Grossman. "A successful pregnancy is just as inexplicable as a miscarried pregnancy," he admits. "But we typically don't dwell on how much had to go correctly for that child to be born. And trust me—it's a lot. Persistence is the key."

Your Medical Options

Depending on the type of miscarriage, you'll have different medical options for passing or removing the fetal tissue. Some

---

WARRIOR TIPS
Getting to the Bottom of the Problem

After each pregnancy loss, it's important to discuss with your doctor what happened. Diagnostic tests can help refine your treatment options to avoid another future loss. While you won't always get an answer, it's important to try. Ask your doctor about:

Saline infusion sonogram (SIS). This is often one of the first diagnostic tests you receive to determine the cause of infertility, but many doctors like to perform an SIS after a miscarriage to check the uterus and fallopian tubes for new or previously undetected abnormalities. Your doctor will perform a transvaginal ultrasound and inflate your uterus with saline to check for polyps, scar tissue, and fibroids and evaluate the quality of your uterine lining.

Hysterosalpingogram (HSG). This uterine cavity evaluation test involves injecting dye into your uterus and fallopian tubes. Then your doctor will take X-rays to see if there are any blockages.

Hysteroscopy. With this test, your doctor will inflate your uterus and use a light and a camera to check for abnormalities in the uterus and fallopian tubes. If you are under anesthesia for the procedure, the doctor will most likely go ahead and correct any issues at this time.

Endometrial biopsy. Typically performed while you are already under anesthesia for a hysteroscopy, this small biopsy of your uterus is taken to check for conditions like chronic endometritis.

Endometrial receptivity analysis (ERA). This test, too, can be performed at the same time as a hysteroscopy—it's another small biopsy of your uterine lining, following a mock cycle with estrogen and progesterone. This test allows your doctor to understand *your* best implantation window—when your uterus is most receptive to implantation. It's most often recommended when patients have recurrent implantation failure, but it can also provide useful information following repeated chemical pregnancies. If you've been using IVF, it's possible you're transferring slightly outside your ideal window and thus the implantation is also not ideal.

Chromosome karyotyping. If you or your partner haven't had a chromosome karyotyping test before, consider one after experiencing recurrent pregnancy loss. The test is a simple blood draw and then the chromosomes in the sample are assessed. Remember that our chromosomes are passed on to the embryo, so if you or your partner show evidence of chromosome abnormalities, this can cause recurrent pregnancy loss.

Carrier test. This is also a blood test, but instead of looking just at your chromosomes, it checks for genes known to cause conditions that impede embryo viability.

Genetic testing of the products of conception (if possible). If you or your doctor are able to collect the products of conception (see page 305), they can be tested for any genetic abnormalities that may have led to the miscarriage.

people naturally pass all the tissue. Other times, a medical procedure might be necessary. Know that your choices and your doctor's recommendations will depend on a number of factors, including:

- How far along you are

- What procedures your doctor can perform in their office

- Your medical risk for complications like hemorrhaging

Wait and See

This is just what it sounds like—you wait and hope the products of conception will pass on their own. Ideally this will happen within a few days, but Dr. Rodgers says, "Instead of waiting to see if things don't happen in a timely manner, you can always then choose one of the other options."

It's rare, but if your body takes too long to pass the pregnancy naturally, a clotting complication called disseminated intravascular coagulation (DIC) can lead to hemorrhaging.

Medication

Your doctor might recommend that you take misoprostol, the same drug used to induce labor, to help the miscarriage process along. The pills can be taken orally or inserted as a vaginal suppository. The medication causes cramps and uterine contractions, and side effects may include diarrhea or fever, so taking it on a weekend with some support around is advised.

This is typically not an option for patients beyond 9 weeks.

Only a small percentage of carriers who use misoprostol for their miscarriage will need further surgical intervention.

Dilation & Curettage (D&C)

During a D&C, the woman is given anesthesia and her doctor removes the tissue from her uterus vaginally. As a result, the woman never has to see the products of conception.

Typically, it takes a couple of days to recover, with light vaginal bleeding and cramping being common side effects. A D&C has to be performed in a fertility clinic's surgery center or a hospital. According to ASRM, 10 percent of D&C patients get an infection, usually within a week of the procedure.

If you have *any* concerns following your procedure, always call your doctor immediately—but don't be surprised if you have more than the "light vaginal bleeding" they tell you to expect.

Collecting the Products of Conception

Whether you have your miscarriage at home or in a surgery center or hospital, or have a D&C, you can collect the products of conception to have them genetically tested. This may shed light on why the miscarriage occurred and even fill in some blanks about your infertility diagnosis.

Ask your doctors if they can, how much it costs, whether it may be covered by insurance, and when you can expect to receive results.

⚡ If you believe having your miscarriage at home is the best option for you, consult with your doctor about whether this is feasible and whether you want to have the products of conception tested.

Losing a pregnancy is an emotional minefield. It's not uncommon to feel guilt, anger, intense sadness, and inescapable hopelessness. Don't attempt to push these feelings down. It's not easy, but finding support and giving yourself room to cope is an important part of the grieving process. Given the complex emotions involved with pregnancy loss, this section is going to go into a lot more detail than in other chapters. First, let's revisit some general points about grief:

People grieve differently. Neither way is right or wrong, but you and your partner need to work to understand how the other is coping. See chapter 14 for general tips on how to support each other.

Grief isn't linear. Some days will be bad—even horrific. When negative emotions resurface after periods of positive emotions, don't think of it as a step backward but as a natural part of the process.

There's no shame in asking for help. Ignoring your mental health is dangerous. Failing to address grief and other negative emotions can lead to serious conditions like clinical depression.

Finding Out What You Need to Mourn

Many couples don't feel that they have "permission" to mourn their loss. But Dr. Covington stresses that openly mourning can be essential to many couples' healing process. "Find a way to connect with this much-wanted baby by doing something to ritualize the loss," she suggests. "This can be naming the baby, making a donation in honor of this baby, having a memorial service or funeral, buying a piece of jewelry or a memento for each loss, or even planting a tree in the baby's memory."

And don't confine your grief to a certain time period. When your due date passes or on the anniversary of the loss, feelings will resurface. Dr. Covington advises making a plan to help you deal on these days.

Every year, Rachel and Kit remember their stillborn daughter, Vivian. Their family and friends send cards and gifts. "Just remembering she exists is all the support we need," Rachel says.

Similarly, each year on Eric and Alexis's birthday, my husband and I light candles for our twins. We post photos on Facebook and ask our friends and family to do the same. Without a doubt,

it's a painful day, but the sense of community helps. It's a recognition of our children. Even though the pain doesn't cut as deep anymore, we will never stop mourning our loss.

Don't forget self-care. Dr. Rodgers says it's not uncommon for people to ignore their own needs when they're grieving. "It's hard to focus on ourselves when the list keeps getting longer—work, bills, cleaning the house, getting the oil changed—but it is important to take time to take care of you," she says. "Give yourself some time every day to do something that makes you happy."

Finding Out What You Need from Others

Immediately after your loss, it might feel like there's nothing in the world another person can do to make you feel better. In a way that's true; there are no magic words to soothe the pain. However, there are actions your support system can perform to make your life easier.

Find ways in which your loved ones can take responsibilities off your plate while you heal, physically and emotionally. For example, they could cook dinner for you, clean your house, walk your dog. And please, if you have a partner, one who didn't physically go through the pregnancy loss, don't assume that they will take care of all these tasks. They're hurting, too.

Because cooking and eating—keeping myself nourished—was the first thing I let go after each of our losses, whenever I hear about a loss in the infertility community, I send at least a week's worth of prepared meals. I've only ever received positive feedback about how much this helped! You can suggest that loved ones support you in this way.

Also, think of how you can ease yourself into opening up to support. Some infertility warriors need to spend several days alone. While that's okay, you can't isolate yourself forever. Maybe what you need next is to just sit with someone else for a few hours. You don't have to talk; you just need the presence of someone who loves you. From there, you can try talking about what happened and how you're feeling about it.

Keep in mind that the nonpregnant partner's experience and grief around a miscarriage may look and feel very different from that of the partner who was pregnant. Pay attention to your partner's language after a miscarriage and consider it from the perspective of how they're trying to make sense of the event and their place in it. This will help you understand what they're feeling and what forms of support they need.

WARRIOR WISDOM
Finding a New Strength from the Pain

During her 8-year battle with infertility, Krista from New Jersey had six miscarriages. She admits it never gets easier. But after each loss, she had a chance to rebuild and become stronger.

"Each baby I have to give back to heaven takes a piece of my soul with them," she says. "I am never the same after a loss."

Krista encourages other infertility warriors to continue pushing forward. "Don't ever give up on yourself because you are the only one who's going to get this done. No one else can do this for you. So, you have to find the energy to fight. Find a way to turn your pain into motivation."

Communicating Your Needs

Even the most loving and empathetic people have a hard time figuring out what to do when a loved one loses a pregnancy. Dr. Domar says that without meaning to, friends and family members will make mistakes.

"Be prepared for people to say stupid things to you," she warns. "People don't mean to be insensitive. They don't mean to be cruel. People in our society today just don't know what to say."

It's important to set ground rules. You have a right to grieve in your own way. Letting others know your boundaries or what you need will help friends and family support you in a productive way.

"Explain how you felt about this miscarriage," says Dr. Angela Palmer-Wackerly, assistant professor of health communication at the University of Nebraska in Lincoln. "You may need to take time to heal emotionally, physically, and mentally."

When communicating your needs to others, Dr. Palmer-Wackerly suggests you:

Politely decline to answer questions. It's stressful to answer questions, especially if you don't have any idea what caused your miscarriage. Let your friends and family members know that being asked questions and having to say "I don't know" adds to your stress and grief.

Set boundaries about how far information travels. A miscarriage not only is painful but also involves information about your private medical health. While you may want to share your story with your immediate family, you might not want every cousin or your parent's neighbors to know. Your support group needs to respect what details you want kept private.

Talk with a mental health professional. Mental health professionals and members of infertility support groups also help with the grieving process. These people either have experienced loss themselves or are trained to support people who are hurting. Sharing your feelings and concerns will help you process and move forward.

→

WARRIOR TIPS
Responding to Insensitive Comments

They're going to come your way, so you might as well prepare. Here are several common less-than-sensitive comments you might get after a pregnancy loss and tips on how to respond.

Don't worry, you can try again soon. Depending on how much this individual knows about your infertility journey, you might just want to say you're taking time to mourn and will try again if and when you're ready. If they are more informed about the time, energy, pain, and money you've spent trying to get pregnant, remind them of everything you've been through and that, for you, it's not as simple as just trying again.

It just wasn't meant to be. I find this statement ridiculous. It invalidates your feelings—like grief is somehow wrong in this situation. Even if you believe in fate, that doesn't lessen the pain of the loss. When you hear this comment, redirect the conversation to emotions, not what was or wasn't meant to be.

Next time don't . . . or next time try to . . . *Next time try to relax more. Next time don't exercise as much. Next time try to have more faith.* Again, you are not to blame for a miscarriage. These types of suggestions imply that you can control whether you carry to term. When people offer this advice, politely (or not so politely, depending on your mindset) let them know you prefer to follow the advice of your medical team.

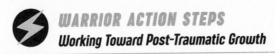

WARRIOR ACTION STEPS
Working Toward Post-Traumatic Growth

The general idea behind post-traumatic growth, which we discussed in chapter 15, is that you improve as a person *because of* your trauma and loss. But it's not easy. You have to lay down the groundwork with the following steps:

Honor your feelings. You can't move forward until you've dealt with what you are currently feeling or what you've felt in the past. After a miscarriage, let the feelings come. Acknowledge them and identify them, but do not give them permission to control you.

Take a step, any step. Whether you try another round of treatment or learn a new skill not related to reproduction, make a positive change in your life. It's not about being distracted or ignoring your loss—it's showing that you have the power to make choices that keep you from stagnating.

Check in with yourself. Losses are hard. Sometimes you experience so much pain that, while you know you'll eventually feel better, you feel unprepared to continue treatment. There's no shame in stopping or delaying your plan to build a family. You know how difficult fertility treatments can be, and if you're not emotionally ready, take a break and practice self-care.

WARRIOR WISDOM
This, Too, Shall Pass

"The pain you are experiencing won't last forever. You'll never forget the loss, but it won't consume you forever. Grief is normal, and it's okay to not be okay for a bit." —Sarah, Ontario, Canada

WARRIOR CHECKLIST
Understanding and Working Through Miscarriage and Recurrent Pregnancy Loss

- ❑ Know the warning signs of a miscarriage and understand your options after it happens.
- ❑ Remember that miscarriages are not your fault.
- ❑ Allow yourself to mourn and grieve.
- ❑ Ask for help and support. Miscarriages are not as uncommon as you might think, and there are others who understand your struggle.

Add more items to your Warrior Checklist or jot down any notes here:

_____

_____

_____

_____

_____

_____

_____

_____

_____

_____

_____

_____

_____

_____

_____

_____

_____

_____

_____

_____

Religion and Ethics in Infertility

LINDSAY AND HER HUSBAND, Jordan, from Louisiana started trying to conceive in late 2010. Lindsay's cycles were regular and there was no apparent reason why they wouldn't get pregnant quickly—but she was still worried.

"As a young teen, I had always feared that I would have trouble getting pregnant," she explains. "At the time, I had no real reason to think this, but it stayed in the back of my mind when we started trying to get pregnant."

After almost a year of trying, Lindsay went to her ob-gyn and asked for advice. They tried Clomid and IUI, and then did a hysterosalpingogram to check if her tubes were open. Nothing appeared to be wrong, but she still didn't get pregnant. They eventually started seeing a reproductive endocrinologist.

"We did two IUIs back-to-back with the [reproductive endocrinologist]," says Lindsay. "Each time, more and more aggressive with medicine. I responded great, but still no baby. We took a break from treatment—I desperately needed it."

During this difficult time, Lindsay relied heavily on her Christian faith. She connected with God through worship and praise. But she admits it wasn't always easy. When she failed to get pregnant month after month, she says

she wondered if her heart was aligned with God's. "Maybe not right at first, but eventually, I always ended up back before the Lord. I have seen faith do the same for my infertility sisters. Infertility is so uncertain. You have zero control over it, yet you can trust and rely on Jesus, who is always certain and is in control."

Eventually, she went back to the reproductive endocrinologist for another round of IUI, but without success. They decided to move on to IVF, and Lindsay admits she did face comments from people who thought they were "playing God."

"First, I do not think quite so highly of myself (or a doctor) to assume that I could begin to assume the role of God. I'm great and doctors are great, but not as great as God," she explains. "Others look at IUI and IVF as forcing a square peg in a round hole—that you are making something happen that is not happening naturally. This is a flimsy argument to me. If that is the case, then no one should ever seek medical help of any kind, not even Advil for a headache. Most would agree that is ludicrous."

After two rounds of IVF, Lindsay finally became pregnant and gave birth to a daughter. She and Jordan had planned to do a frozen embryo transfer when their daughter was a year old, but when she was 6 months, Lindsay discovered she'd gotten pregnant sponta-neously. Now that she has a daughter and son, she and Jordan are waiting to transfer their remaining embryos.

Lindsay says, "I had to continually remind myself that the Lord was in control and every single thing I was experiencing was going to ultimately work together for my good. It was hard to hold on to faith, but honestly, it was either hold on to that last shred of faith or completely fall apart. Falling apart could not happen, so faith it was!"

Faith, Religion, and Infertility

In this chapter, we're going to look at the ways in which religion intersects with infertility. The purpose isn't to espouse a certain set of beliefs, but rather to help you frame your own religion or spirituality throughout infertility.

This chapter isn't just for religious people. Even if you don't practice a particular religion or espouse a certain belief system, you might have people in your life who do. This will help you understand their perspectives and offer ways to navigate your discussions about infertility with them.

Every place of worship is different. Within religions, there are differences between congregations and communities. Some places of worship are more progressive, whereas others are traditional and adhere strictly to the tenets of the religion or denomination. Don't assume your specific religious community will follow all the guidelines of the overarching religious institution.

While everyone has their own idea of what it means to be faithful and religious, spirituality plays a big part in many infertility warriors' lives. A 2016 study from Yale University found that 72.5 percent of people facing infertility pray for support and guidance. That's significantly higher than the number of people who seek medical assistance for infertility, which is 52.6 percent.

The same study found that women with infertility issues are more likely to consult a religious leader (18.7 percent) than a support group (12.0 percent) or a therapist (8.6 percent). So if you are struggling with your faith during your infertility journey, you are not alone.

BUSTED

Myth: I will have to choose between being a parent and my religion.

When your religion doesn't agree with certain aspects of fertility treatments and then you find out you're struggling with infertility, it can be scary. You think you'll have to back a choice: your religion or being a parent. That's incredibly distressing!

However, according to Dr. Maria T. Rothenburger, a psychotherapist who specializes in infertility at Miracles Happen Fertility Center in Salem, Oregon, most people are able to find a way to stay true to their beliefs while on their infertility journey. "What I generally see is that people choose some kind of hybrid," she explains. "Most people choose to stay within their church or religion. Some will change churches within the same religion, but most people choose some kind of 'I understand the church's stance on [assisted reproductive technology]. I believe in most of the dogma of the church, but I don't believe in this part.'"

From there, most people find a way to integrate their faith with their feelings about assisted reproductive technology. Dr. Rothenburger does say, however, that it takes a lot of soul-searching. You'll need to really dig into what you believe and determine how that plays into your infertility journey.

Ethical Concerns

Even outside the religious world, there are debates involving the ethics of fertility treatments. For many people, the issues come down to the age-old morality question: It's not a matter of whether we *can* do something, it's whether we *should*.

Part of your infertility journey may involve navigating religious and ethical concerns as they apply to the paths to parenthood at your disposal. Having in-depth information about each will help you make choices that don't compromise your beliefs.

When and How Life Begins

If you believe that life begins at conception, certain fertility treatment options are problematic. With IVF, for instance, you must decide whether it's moral to fertilize more embryos than you need, to create embryos that won't develop into healthy babies, and/or what to do with extra embryos that aren't transferred.

For some individuals, a fertilized embryo is the moral equivalent of a fully developed person. As Michael Grossman, a reproductive endocrinologist, explains, "Biologically, an embryo only has a 5 to 25 percent chance of surviving to live birth, but the notion of 'people' wasting away or being discarded can be distressing to some." (Your state might also have laws that prohibit the discarding of embryos.)

Another issue for some infertility warriors is *how* eggs are fertilized. Most fertility clinics use intracytoplasmic sperm injection (ICSI; see chapter 7), a process that directly injects sperm into the egg. While there's still no guarantee that eggs fertilized through ICSI will develop into viable embryos, many feel the process gives too much control to human intervention. Normally the sperm has to work to fertilize the egg, and ICSI seems like humans "playing God."

If you believe that life begins at conception or ICSI is too "unnatural," you do still have options:

Limiting the number of eggs fertilized. If your egg retrieval yield is high, you can ask your doctor to fertilize only a few and then freeze the rest of the eggs.

Non-ICSI IVF. While it's not as successful, you can have your eggs fertilized by mixing the sperm and the egg, without ICSI.

Other forms of artificial insemination. IUI (see chapter 6) is always an option for women who ovulate and produce healthy eggs.

Leftover Embryos

Sometimes people end up with unused embryos. For many, it feels wrong to leave those embryos frozen indefinitely or even to discard embryos that have no chance of developing into healthy babies.

If you're done building your family and have leftover embryos, there are options:

Embryo adoption. There are organizations, most of which have religious affiliations, that will match you with another couple struggling with infertility who can adopt your unused embryos.

Compassionate transfer. Your doctor can transfer a leftover embryo or an embryo with a low chance of developing at a time that is less optimal for implantation. There's a low chance of getting pregnant, but at least the embryo is given a chance at life.

Preimplantation Genetic Testing

With preimplantation genetic testing (PGT; see chapter 4), your doctor checks for chromosomal anomalies that will lead to medical conditions like Down syndrome or cystic fibrosis. For some people, this creates a few ethical dilemmas.

First, there's the issue of whether it is morally right not to transfer an embryo because it has a genetic disorder. And if you decide not to use an embryo with abnormal PGT results, what do you do with it?

On the other hand, if you do not use PGT and discover during pregnancy that the baby has a condition that would lead to a low quality of life or early death, is it morally acceptable to end the pregnancy? Or, if the baby survives, is it worse to have a child who will be in pain every day?

For reproductive endocrinologist Allison Rodgers with Fertility Centers of Illinois in Chicago, another issue is the possibility of false PGT positives. "There is a small chance that the embryo is called abnormal, [and it is later found that] the trophectoderm (which becomes the placenta and the membrane) where the biopsy was done was abnormal but the inner cell mass (that becomes the baby) was normal," she explains. "Typically, the benefits [of doing PGT] greatly outweigh the risks, but again, this needs to be discussed between the physician and patient."

And then there's the ethical slippery slope. Currently, PGT looks at only the chromosomal makeup of the embryo and is intended to look for physiological disorders. But because sex is determined by chromosomes, you can also find out the sex of the baby. Is it ethical to choose to transfer embryos of only a certain sex?

There are other implications that follow. "At the moment, we can simply detect irregularities and avoid them," says Dr. Grossman. "But what will happen when we find the genetic peculiarities that allow for greater cerebellar coordination (natural athleticism), or easier memory retention (better grades in school), or neuronal connectivity (higher intellect and creativity)?"

With regard to PGT, here are your options:

Genetic testing of embryos. This allows you to avoid the development of embryos with genetic conditions that may lead to terminating the pregnancy or babies with a low quality of life.

Not testing your embryos. This gives every embryo a chance at a life, regardless of whether or not it's genetically "normal."

Choose a middle ground. Some clinics will tell patients the sex of embryos before transfer. If that's a step too far, ask the clinic and/or genetic testing company to keep that information hidden from your records until you are ready to know it.

The Role of Faith

Infertility causes many people to reexamine their faith in new—and sometimes scary—ways. It's a process. And while you absolutely do not have to give up what you believe, being open to exploration and change will help you make sense of your infertility journey.

For Those Who Already Have Faith

In many cases, infertility deepens faith. People struggling with infertility may find support not only in their relationship with a higher power but also at their place of worship. Praying, going to services, or studying religious texts provides guidance and comfort. Or they use their faith to help shape their next steps. Playwright Lisa Grunberger, in doing research for a play about infertility, spoke with many Catholics who took their diagnosis as a sign from God that they were destined for another path, making it easier for them to pursue options like adoption.

Infertility warrior Allison from California says she approached her faith with infertility in the same way she did other aspects of her life.

"Infertility is one trial. We all have trials, even if we aren't going through infertility," she says. "The question we are faced with is whether we will turn toward God or away from Him as we figure out how to get through the trial. In my experience, the path is always easier when you lean on God."

For Those Who Find Faith

Let's take a minute to talk about the difference between having a religion and having faith. Elizabeth Hagan, senior minister of Palisades Community Church in Washington, DC, and author of *Birthed: Finding Grace Through Infertility*, defines the difference like this: "Faith is the belief in a power greater than you. Religion is an organized path that folks follow in search of a relationship with that power greater than themselves."

Following this definition, you can be part of a religion without having true faith—and vice versa. Even people who participate in the rituals of their religion don't necessarily have faith. For some infertility warriors, their journey is what brings them to faith.

"People who have never been heavily involved in areas of faith will turn to faith for comfort or guidance when infertility makes its unwelcome appearance in our lives," says Beth Forbus, founder of a Christian infertility support ministry. "Faith gives us something to hold on to when science runs out of answers."

Hagan says it's also possible for people to find faith but not religion during their infertility journey. "Faith is the belief in what we can't see. Faith is giving up control."

For Those Whose Faith Is Shaken

Neither infertility nor having faith is easy. Many people struggle to maintain their faith and religious beliefs on their journey. "For those struggling with infertility, I imagine there is much wrestling—as Jacob wrestled with the angel—to find a way to make peace

with this condition," says Grunberger. "I have seen this deepen one's faith, and I have seen it have the opposite effect."

Hagan admits to struggling with her faith during her infertility journey. She says the process challenged her basic beliefs about God. "I'd always believed as a Christian that God was with me. I never faced any of my troubles alone. But to live in a very fertile world and to have the desire to parent (which I believe can be a natural God-given desire) and then not be able to is difficult. It is very easy to feel like God has abandoned you or forgotten you," she says.

Know that it's not uncommon to doubt during infertility. Hagan says she explored a lot about her idea of God and the answer to the question "Is God good?" Asking these questions can help you better understand your beliefs. Hagan tells us, "The answer that I found my way to, that I wrote about in my book, is that I did believe that God was good. Even if my circumstances didn't feel good or weren't what I'd chosen, I could trust the character of God to bring goodness to my life even if the journey to get there was long or difficult. This one fact gave me much comfort during my infertility journey."

BUSTED

Myth: Infertility is a punishment for not being religious enough.

No matter your religious beliefs, infertility is *not* your fault. And along the same line of logic, a baby is not a reward for being pious. Yet Larissa from Ontario, Canada, who belongs to the Bahá'í faith, says she's met many infertility warriors who have this mindset.

"That kind of thinking fails to acknowledge that infertility is a medical problem," she explains. "If these same people had a burst appendix or a heart attack, would they feel like it was because they didn't have enough faith? Probably not."

BUSTED

Myth: My faith will be enough.

After an initial diagnosis, many infertility warriors believe that, as people of faith, if they pray, they'll get the family they want. Yes, prayer can be helpful when dealing with infertility, but know that it's just part of the process.

During her journey, Allison, a member of the Church of Jesus Christ of Latter-Day Saints, says she grew tired of people telling her that everything would work out if she just had faith.

"That's a great start, but faith without work is dead," she explains. "A friend of mine who struggles with infertility stopped by after a hard day. She has been praying for years to get direction. But she hasn't done anything yet. I boldly told her that faith and prayer are necessary. But until she acts and takes a step into the darkness, the light will never be shined in front of her."

Use the advice you've read in this book. Get a fertility workup. Research the best clinic and doctor for you. Then, take one step at a time down whatever path your journey leads you on.

Integrating Faith and Science

Science and faith have an interesting relationship. We tend to compartmentalize the two, which makes it difficult to understand different aspects of infertility as a whole. For example, infertility is a medical condition. Doctors develop treatments on the foundation of science. They use biology to explain our situation. Given that, how does a belief in a higher power fit in with scientific evidence and facts?

"Science and faith are actually not natural enemies!" argues Forbus. However, thinking the two are mutually exclusive creates issues for religious infertility warriors. Religious leaders may have trouble understanding the intricacies of fertility treatments and how they benefit people. Meanwhile, fertility treatment teams don't consider a patient's faith when recommending next steps.

Tailoring Fertility Treatments to Your Religious Beliefs

Doctors won't always take your beliefs into consideration when recommending certain fertility treatments and interventions. Some don't even feel comfortable asking about your spiritual beliefs because religion and faith are such personal topics. You're going to have to be proactive by asking questions and voicing your concerns. And remember, if your fertility team isn't willing to listen, you have a right to find another doctor or fertility clinic.

"Treatment teams must realize the importance that faith plays in a believer's life, even if that belief is different from their own," says Forbus. "When a patient makes a decision based on their faith, the impact will be felt far beyond what happens in the clinic treatment room. These decisions must be treated with respect and carried out as much as is medically possible."

After Jamie and her husband, Mike, from Ohio struggled for a year to get pregnant with their third child, she had a fertility workup and discovered she had low anti-Müllerian hormone (AMH) and a blocked left fallopian tube. Her doctor was very reassuring and told her neither should be a problem. He recommended doing an IUI during a cycle when her right ovary developed at least one follicle, because that tube was open. If she was still not pregnant after 6 months, he suggested discussing IVF. However, Mike, who had been raised Catholic, did not feel comfortable going down that path.

"It's not that he's against it," Jamie explains. "We are both amazed by science and everything that they can do to help almost everyone now, but it just wasn't for him. It wasn't in his heart. It wasn't something he wanted to pursue."

In the end, Jamie had a tuboplasty to open her blocked tube. She and Mike now have four children, two of whom were born after the procedure. She became pregnant with their third child during an IUI cycle with Clomid and gonadotropins and with their fourth child using only Clomid—no IVF needed.

Discussing Your Options with Your Fertility Team

When talking with your doctor about your options, it's important to be open and honest about your beliefs as well as your gaps of knowledge. Don't just dismiss a treatment because you assume it violates your faith. After learning more about it, you might see that the option is still on the table.

Dr. Rothenburger says it's not uncommon for people to not fully understand fertility treatments because no one expects to need them. "A lot of times, people have preconceived notions like, 'IVF is not okay. It's like you're playing God. I don't believe in that,'" she explains. "But then once they are diagnosed with infertility, they're able to dig deep and look at the topic, the actual issue, and their beliefs."

Once you've got a handle on your stance about different fertility treatments, talk with your doctor in order to tailor your treatment. During this conversation, remember:

Speak up. If your doctor recommends a treatment you're not comfortable with, ask for alternatives.

Explain your objection. Even people who hold the same belief might do so for different reasons. During discussions, you don't want your doctor to assume the reasons for your hesitancy about certain options. Clearly explain where your belief comes from and why it's important to you.

Ask questions. It's imperative that you understand all your options. As your doctor suggests various treatments, gather information so you can be confident you're morally okay with them.

Find out success rates. Often, alternative treatments are less successful than the one the doctor would recommend. Compare the success rates for the recommended treatment against the alternative so you can weigh whether changing course is worth it to you.

Demand respect. Again, you have a right to your beliefs. While your doctor does not have to agree with them, they do have to honor and respect your decision. If a doctor tries to push a treatment on you or scoffs at your decision to go a different route, consider finding a new care provider.

When Objection Comes from Family

Dr. Rothenburger advises that you be honest with yourself about who your family really is so you can anticipate what their reaction might be. You know your family better than anyone else, so you likely know what to expect.

"It's generally not a surprise. But before something happens, plan for a reaction," she says. "My advice is to react with love. You have your feelings. You might be angry and reject what they have to say. You might feel guilty. You might feel hurt. It's fine to have all the feelings. All you need to do is say to them, 'It hurts me when you say things like that' or 'I'm feeling really angry that this has come up.'

"From there," she continues, "the discussion depends on with whom you're communicating because some people might not receive things well. But the general idea is to have your feelings without needing to fire back. Learn how to react to people, particularly with your close family, by cultivating some sense of peace within yourself—any kind of feeling that comes out in a positive light."

You may not believe it's a higher power's will for you to suffer. Or that a higher power enabled the invention of the many different types of assisted reproductive technologies. Or that you're on your own spiritual journey that's no one else's business. Or perhaps you'd like to keep religion out of your conversations and decisions altogether. Only you can come to terms with your relationship with religion. Determine what that looks like, and know that you don't have to explain yourself to others—not even family.

When Objection Comes from Your Religious Community

Infertility can come with a societal stigma—and religious communities often multiply this stigma many times over by adding their own values-based judgments to the situation.

"For example," explains Rabbi Elchanan Poupko of the American-Israeli Jewish Network, "in many Middle Eastern cultures, there is readiness to address the issue of female fertility. And yet, when it comes to any issue that the male has, the man may be made to feel more ashamed to address the issue. When a man has a baby boy, his last name changes to the name of the boy. This is a central value in that society. And so, men in those societies who deal with infertility will often be stigmatized."

Ask yourself: What does my religion say about infertility, fertility treatments, and other paths to parenthood? If other people in my religious community have been diagnosed with infertility, how did others react? Would telling others in my religious community about my situation cause unnecessary pressure to make specific decisions?

"For every group, you have not only a religious setting but also a sociological setting," says Poupko. "Understanding sociology is key—just as much as understanding the religion itself—when speaking about infertility in religious communities."

There may come a time when you have to choose between violating your own right to privacy and being judged for something that isn't true. Again, only you can decide what makes you most comfortable.

When You Want to Keep It to Yourself

Eleanor* from Tennessee is Catholic and wanted to pursue fertility treatments in a way that would not conflict with her religion. She learned that her fallopian tubes had been damaged during her teenage years following a ruptured appendix, and it was clear she needed IVF. She was referred to a Catholic reproductive endocrinologist.

"[Our doctor] believes embryos contain life and we shouldn't be discarding them," Eleanor says. "So, if you're going to work with him, his policy is that you need a legal plan of what's going to happen to your embryos in a variety of different scenarios, such as a divorce—and all of those plans must include [giving them a chance of] life."

Eleanor and her husband decided that the embryos they created would go to the donation center only if she died. Because their doctor understandably did not want to create too many embryos at a time, they ended up with only four from her retrieval. The first transfer resulted in a miscarriage, but her second gave them their daughter. However, Eleanor remains uncomfortable with having two frozen embryos and plans to transfer both eventually (one at a time).

*Name has been changed

BUSTED

Myth: My faith will make my infertility journey easier.

Faith and religion can be a great comfort for people facing infertility. But it helps if you think of faith as something that can help you through—not prevent—the painful or difficult things.

Kelli, a Christian from Wisconsin, chooses to look at faith's part in her journey as a sign that God knows her strength. "God already knows exactly where each path is going to lead before you even start," she explains. "I'd argue that *because of my faith* in God, my journey and what followed with the traumatic birth of my son was tough. I know in my heart that I was given this path—the birth and postpartum journey—because I was strong enough to handle it."

Your view might be different from Kelli's, but it is essential that you figure out what faith means to you and how it will help you during your infertility journey.

They have not told their religious community about the IVF part of their journey. "I went to confession and confessed our sins [against the Catholic Church] there, but otherwise, it's not something we're broadcasting," she explains. "I wish I could tell more Catholic women that there is a Catholic option through a Catholic doctor. Even though we're respecting life, we're taking God out of the picture, according to the church doctrine. And unless you can get someone's attention [for a long time] to explain it, the fact that we did IVF as Catholics makes people think we're hypocritical."

You own your story. You determine who—if anyone—will hear it. If you want to form a support network, pick only the people who will be in your corner every step of the way, even if they do not share your religious views.

Faith and support go hand-in-hand. For many people, faith itself is a type of support. Additionally, religious communities rally behind one another in difficult times. However, because a lot of people don't understand or have experience with infertility, they won't always know the best way to offer their support.

Identifying Your Needs

During your infertility journey, you're going to explore your faith in ways you never imagined. You'll ask tough questions and have to be honest with yourself about your beliefs. Dr. Rothenburger points out that most religions have a built-in guide to help you figure out your needs.

"The one commonality that I find with most religions is this idea of what Christians call the Holy Spirit, but other religions call it different things. But it's that still, small voice that when you get quiet, and you listen to it, it's a guide and it's a way to gauge your truth," she explains. "So one thing that I would recommend regardless of what the church is saying—regardless of what your family and friends are saying, or even your spouse—is to really get quiet and pay attention to what is inside *you*. Pay attention to what your own truth is."

Once you understand your truth, you can look at your situation and see where there's discord between your truth and your life. Then, think of what you need to change—or simply accept that disconnect.

Communicating Your Needs

People can get very passionate about faith and religion, so it's important to ask for help in a way that doesn't make your loved ones think you're challenging their beliefs. The first step is to share your feelings in a clear way. Dr. Rothenburger says that if you're mad or hurt, let people know. But also tell them how they can better support you.

For example, many infertility warriors get angry when they constantly hear statements like "Everything happens for a reason" or "God will answer your prayers in His own time." These phrases are meant to be comforting, but for someone in pain, they minimize the complexity of their situation.

If this happens to you, explain why such statements hurt, but also explain that you understand the individual is trying to help. Then give them specific actions they can take to support you better. Whether you'd like them to pray for you or listen to your frustrations without judgment, most people will be willing to acquiesce.

→

WARRIOR ACTION STEPS
Making Faith Part of Your Infertility Journey

Thought, prayer, and self-reflection are big parts of keeping your faith when you're facing infertility, but there are additional action steps you can complete:

Educate yourself. When it comes to both your religion and fertility treatments, it's common to have preconceived notions about what's right and wrong. Before dismissing an option, research it and your religion's stance on it. This will help you refine your beliefs and make decisions that work for you.

Have prepared responses. It's likely you know the common religious and ethical objections to fertility treatments. Don't try to come up with responses in the heat of the moment. Think of how you can explain your positions *before* friends or family voice their opinions so you can address the topic clearly and calmly.

Remember, it's your relationship with your higher power. When push comes to shove, it's your faith and beliefs. While your religion offers guidelines and suggestions about moral issues, you're the one who has to be able to accept your decisions.

WARRIOR WISDOM
Finding Comfort in the Face of Uncertainty

"Questioning why things happen the way they do is part of our humanness, and God is big enough and personally cares about our questions, disappointment, loss, and pain. He is approachable, loving, and patient with us. Knowing this creates a safe haven to express our deepest hopes, fears, and hurts. In other words, the first place I turned in my infertility journey was God." —Kelli, Oregon

WARRIOR CHECKLIST
Faith, Religion, and Ethics

❏ Know that while faith can be an important part of your infertility journey, your faith—or lack thereof—is not the reason you do or do not end up with a child.

❏ Consider the different ways your faith impacts your infertility journey.

❏ Consider the different ways your faith can change during your infertility journey.

❏ Research your religion's stance on different fertility treatments. Think about whether those beliefs align with your own.

❏ Examine different ethical debates surrounding fertility treatments and determine where you fall given your personal morals.

❏ Start a conversation with your fertility treatment team about the possible treatment methods and their success rates so you can have a plan that doesn't compromise your beliefs.

❏ Determine what type of support you need and how you can effectively ask for it.

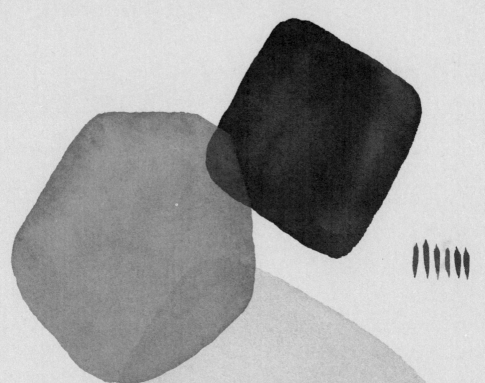

PART FOUR

The Practical Stuff

Understanding Your Insurance

(and Convincing Your Employer to Cover Infertility)

CHAPTER 19

ATIE LELITO AND HER HUSBAND always knew they wanted a big family. Four—that was the magic number of kids. However, they couldn't always agree on *when* to start building this family. They went back and forth until, finally, when Lelito was almost done with her PhD program, they decided they both were ready. She went off birth control, and they tried and waited.

"We're both biologists. We're both scientists," she explains. "And I'd like to say that we knew what we were doing."

After trying for 9 months with no success, Lelito was frustrated and went to consult with the ob-gyn at her university. That doctor told her not to worry because they hadn't been trying for a full year yet. Lelito persisted and convinced the ob-gyn to refer her to the campus reproductive endocrinologist.

The RE diagnosed Lelito with diminished ovarian reserve based on her follicle count and blood work. But Lelito admits that she didn't find her results foreboding. "I didn't really think it was that serious. I had a friend who just had some Clomid, and she got pregnant," she says. "I was really shocked when I went to my appointment, where my doctor gave me this diagnosis, and she told me that we needed to go straight into IVF."

This realization was terrifying, but another hit came soon after: Her RE informed her that IVF probably wasn't covered by her university insurance. The doctor gave Lelito the cost codes for the recommended procedures, and Lelito called her insurance company.

"I found out that nothing was covered," she says. "And I started to get really frustrated with the poor woman who was on the phone with me. But then she told me that [the insurance company] doesn't decide what is covered and what is not covered. And they had plenty of plans that covered IVF."

Lelito learned that her employer, the University of Michigan, needed to make a change to its insurance plan in order to add coverage for fertility treatments. She decided to write a letter and ask the university to update its coverage so it would be more inclusive. The only problem was she had no idea where to start; given the size of the university, it was unclear whom she needed to contact.

"I contacted the president of the university, the academic university, the CEO of the University of Michigan hospital," Lelito says. "I contacted Association for Women in Science groups. And honestly, when I would meet with these university admins and community members, they had no idea that we didn't have [infertility] coverage."

While most of these people agreed that fertility treatments *should* be covered, many didn't think any updates would be coming soon because the university was going through budget issues. But Lelito kept up her advocacy, and eventually the university expanded its health insurance coverage to include $20,000 toward IVF for people who were diagnosed with infertility and $5,000 toward medications.

Insurance Isn't Unbeatable

Insurance is not as black-and-white as many people think. It's not as simple as whether or not a treatment or medication is covered. You will have opportunities to self-advocate, so you don't have to limit your treatment options from the start based on insurance and financial constraints. Unfortunately, you won't win every battle, but know that you *do* have a right to fight.

In this chapter, we'll look at an overview of the insurance process, how it works, the current laws surrounding infertility and insurance coverage, and the appeal avenues available to you if your claims are denied. We'll also discuss how to advocate for improved coverage with your employer. While it might seem overwhelming, know that you have the power to work through all the red tape. Infertility warriors have done it before and *so can you.* It just takes knowledge, patience, and the willingness to try.

BUSTED ═══════════════════════════

Myth: Fertility treatments are luxuries.

It has always bothered me—and likely you, too—that society views fertility treatments as luxuries. Because most people can conceive without help, the general population doesn't understand why options like surrogacy or IVF should be seen as "normal" routes to building a family.

But infertility is a *medical problem*. And insurance companies exist to help individuals pay for their *medical* costs. Every time infertility warriors stand up and ask for coverage, they change how others view fertility treatments. It shows the world that these are not luxuries but treatments required to address medical conditions. No one goes to a reproductive endocrinologist—whether to plan timed intercourse or IVF—because it's the fashionable thing to do. We do it because, for many of us, it's the only way to build our families—something everyone else takes for granted that they can achieve on their own.

Insurance Coverage Basics

Insurance is one of those boring but vital topics, especially within the infertility community. Unfortunately, many decisions we make about building our families come down to cost. Having a solid grasp of what your insurance covers today—and the ways in which you might influence that coverage—will benefit you immensely. Let's start with the basics.

A health insurance policy is an agreement between you and your insurance company. You and/or your employer pay the cost of that policy—the fixed premium—to the insurance company. In turn, the insurance company pays for various health-related expenses on your behalf. Your policy details which health services are *covered* and *uncovered*. The insurance company agrees to pay for all or a portion of covered services, and you agree to pay for uncovered services. When a health-care provider accepts your insurance, they are considered *in network*. If they do not, they are considered *out-of-network*. Some policies will pay for a portion of out-of-network services, so check the fine print. Most health insurance policies call for an annual deductible—an amount that you pay for covered services before the insurance company starts to pay for them. Some policies have separate medical and drug deductibles, so read your policy carefully.

A *medical necessity* is a test, drug, treatment, or other service that your doctor has decided is necessary. A *medical benefit* is a test, drug, treatment, or other service that your health insurance policy covers. For the most part, insurance companies decide what tests, drugs, treatments, and other services they will cover with each plan. However, employers sometimes have a say in determining coverage based on what group plan (see page 326) they choose.

A *preexisting condition* is exactly what it sounds like—a condition you had prior to applying for a health insurance policy. Before the Affordable Care Act (ACA) went into effect in 2014, many people were denied health insurance coverage for costs related to a preexisting condition, including infertility. Under current law, however, insurers can no longer exclude coverage to people with a preexisting infertility diagnosis.

Types of Plans

Health insurance policies vary even within the same insurance company. In other words, just because you and your friend both have a policy with Aetna does not mean you have the same coverage.

Group Insurance

To help keep premiums low, group health insurance plans spread the cost over all members of the group. Group health insurance policies are purchased by an employer and offered to eligible employees and their eligible dependents. You will also see these policies referred to as employer-sponsored health insurance and job-based health insurance.

	TYPICAL GROUP HEALTH INSURANCE PLAN TYPES			
TYPE OF GROUP PLAN	REQUIRED TO HAVE A PRIMARY CARE PHYSICIAN (PCP)?	REQUIRED TO HAVE A REFERRAL TO SEE SPECIALISTS?	IN-NETWORK COSTS COVERED?	OUT-OF-NETWORK COSTS COVERED?
Health maintenance organization (HMO)	Yes	Yes	Yes	No
Preferred provider organization (PPO)	No	No	Yes	Yes (at least partially)
Exclusive provider organization (EPO)	No	No	Yes	No

	TYPICAL GROUP HEALTH INSURANCE PLAN LEVELS		
LEVEL	PROJECTED HEALTH-RELATED EXPENSES COVERED BY INSURANCE	PREMIUM	OUT-OF-POCKET EXPENSES AND DEDUCTIBLES
Platinum	90%	Highest	Lowest
Gold	80%	High	Low
Silver	70%	Low	High
Bronze	60%	Lowest	Highest

Individual Insurance

If you do not have a group health insurance policy, you must purchase individual insurance. You will have to pay the entire premium yourself—but you will also get to select the plan that's right for you, rather than having an employer, for example, choose a policy on your behalf.

Jon Belinkie, an insurance broker with Health Insurance Specialists, Inc., from Derwood, Maryland, recommends working with an insurance broker licensed in your state. (Agents work for a specific insurer, whereas brokers work directly with consumer clients.) "You want to understand what your state

mandates require the insurance companies to provide, and a good independent insurance broker can help you do that," he explains. "You wouldn't go to the IRS without your accountant. You wouldn't go to court without your attorney. And you don't want to deal with a billion-dollar insurance company without somebody who knows the system. Going directly to the insurance company is a prescription for not asking questions the right way and getting an answer that's not entirely accurate."

Belinkie advises selecting someone who not only knows and understands the local market but also has a vested interest in you. "Those people [at national insurance companies] want to make sales. That's their job. They are faceless people on the phone. Your local person gets to know and care about you, which I think is a better approach."

I wish I had known that individual insurance was an option! My home state of Maryland requires—with some exceptions— that individual insurance policies must cover the cost of three IVF cycles per live birth. Having that coverage would have changed our decision-making process—and, of course, not put us in such a risky financial position.

"You don't have to accept your [insurance] situation as the status quo," Belinkie says. "I used to have a mug that said, 'My work starts when they say no.' And it really is that way. There are ways to get around stuff. There are ways to structure [policies] to try and derive the maximum benefit."

Public Insurance

Public insurance programs are run by the federal, state, or local government, and premiums are paid in part or in full by the government. Two examples include Medicaid, which is a federal–state partnership that provides health care for low-income families, and TRICARE, which insures active and retired military members and their families (see chapter 22).

Private Insurance

Private insurance is any health insurance plan not offered by the federal, state, or local government. It includes plans offered by commercial insurance companies (Aetna), nonprofit insurance companies (Blue Cross/Blue Shield), and self-insured employers (explained later in this chapter). Even though the Health Insurance Marketplace—sometimes called the health insurance exchange—is managed by the federal government under the ACA, the plans themselves are offered by commercial and nonprofit insurance companies.

Fully Insured

When the insurance company—not the employer sponsoring the plan—takes on all the risk of the plan, the plan is considered to be fully insured. Because the insurance company is taking on the risk, it also gets to dictate which services are and are not covered within the plan. However, this does not mean your employer cannot choose to offer a new plan that has more inclusive coverage like fertility treatments.

Self-Insured

When the employer, not the insurance company, takes on all the risk of the plan, it is considered self-insured. Because the employer is taking on the risk, it gets to dictate which services are and are not covered.

Mandates, Laws, and Exceptions

The differences between group, individual, public, private, fully insured, and self-insured plans become important when determining what laws apply to your plan.

Mandates

No federal law requires infertility-related health insurance coverage. At the state level, you may (depending on your state) find one of two types of mandates:

Mandate to cover. Health insurance companies must cover fertility treatments as a benefit in every policy.

Mandate to offer. Health insurance companies must make policies that cover fertility treatments available for purchase, but employers are not required to select these plans as options for employees.

Currently only twenty states have infertility insurance mandates, and only twelve have fertility preservation laws (mandated coverage for medically necessary egg and sperm freezing, such as prior to cancer treatments). There are too many nuances to list here, such as unique definitions of infertility and exclusions of specific fertility treatments, so I encourage you to visit the RESOLVE website for complete details.

Exceptions

Barbara Collura, president and CEO of RESOLVE, warns, "Even in states with mandates, there are fine-print rules that affect your coverage." If your insurance is employer-provided, here's what you need to know to understand which exceptions apply to you:

Whether the plan is fully insured or self-insured. The Employee Retirement Income

INFERTILITY COVERAGE BY STATE*		
STATE	MANDATE	FERTILITY PRESERVATION
Arkansas	Cover	No
California	Offer	Yes
Colorado	Cover	Yes
Connecticut	Cover	Yes
Delaware	Cover	Yes
Hawaii	Cover	No
Illinois	Cover	Yes
Louisiana	Cover	No
Maine	Cover	Yes
Maryland	Cover	Yes
Massachusetts	Cover	No
Montana	Cover	No
New Hampshire	Cover	Yes
New Jersey	Cover	Yes
New York	Cover	Yes
Ohio	Cover	No
Rhode Island	Cover	Yes
Texas	Offer	No
Utah	Cover (only for public employees and Medicaid recipients)	Yes
West Virginia	Cover	No

*As of February 2023

Security Act of 1974 (ERISA) is a federal law that sets minimum standards for most private health insurance plans. For example, ERISA requires plans to establish a grievance and appeals process. However, ERISA applies only to fully insured plans, mandating that they follow state law (unless the employer falls under one of the other exceptions below). Self-insured plans, on the other hand, are exempt from state law and instead follow federal law. And remember, no federal law currently mandates infertility coverage.

The total number of people employed at your company. In many states, companies with fewer than twenty-five or even sometimes fifty employees do not have to offer infertility coverage.

The state in which the policy was *written*. If the policy was not written in a state that mandates infertility coverage, your employer is not required to offer it. Tricky, right?

Whether your employer is considered a religious institution. Often, religious organizations are not required to offer certain types of—or any—infertility coverage.

Whether your employer is considered a governmental organization. Public insurance programs run by the federal, state, or local government are not covered by ERISA. The Access to Infertility Treatment and Care Act, first proposed in 2018 but still under consideration by Congress, would require the Federal Employees Health Benefits Program, TRICARE, and the Department of Veterans Affairs to offer infertility and fertility preservation coverage. Reach out to your legislators to advocate for this type of legislation (see chapter 27).

In my case, although my family resides in Maryland, my husband works for the government in Washington, DC, and so we are covered under the Federal Employees Health Benefits Program. Our plan covered the costs of diagnostic testing, but we had no coverage for anything else.

Nicole had health insurance through her Maryland-based employer, but because of several exceptions, her insurance plan did not cover infertility. So, she contacted an insurance broker and told him about her goals and what she might need coverage for. "We didn't know how hard or easy [getting pregnant] was going to be at that point, but I wanted to find out the best plan as far as pregnancy and fertility treatments, in case we needed them," she explains.

If you want to go the independent insurance route, Nicole advises planning ahead. Enrollment is open only once a year for a few months, starting in November. "Select the best option for what you *might* need, because you cannot change your mind in 3 months or 6 months. You have to wait until the next open enrollment, and people don't always have that much time."

Keep in mind, though, that *all* insurance policies—regardless of whether or not they are employer-provided—have exceptions. Read carefully and weigh your options before making a decision.

BUSTED

Myth: You can't win arguments with insurance companies.

Davina Fankhauser, cofounder of the advocacy group Fertility Within Reach in Newton Highlands, Massachusetts, has helped many infertility warriors going through the insurance appeals process— and she's seen a high rate of success. "Approximately 70 percent of the appeals I've personally witnessed have won," she shares. "I would point out, from my experience, that people win. People win because they have science on their side. They have logic on their side."

Verifying Benefits with Your Insurance Company

Before initiating any fertility treatment, it's in your best interest to receive written verification from your insurance company of what is and is not covered by your health-care policy—your fertility clinic might even require it. However, no one likes dealing with insurance companies, and most people find these conversations confusing. But when you know exactly what questions to ask, you can pick up the phone feeling empowered and confident.

Step 1: Gather all available information.

Before you call the member services department of your insurance company (the phone number will be on the back of your insurance card), make sure you have the following sitting in front of you:

- Name, date of birth, and Social Security number of the policy subscriber

- Employer name (if applicable)

- Insurance plan name

- Member ID

- Group or enrollment code/number

- Plan effective date

- Summary plan description and certificate of coverage (if you have access to it online or through your employer)

Step 2: Document, document, document.

Every time you are on the phone with a representative of the insurance company, document the individual's name, the date and time, and the details of your discussion. After all, you may need this information down the road in the event that one of your claims is denied and you need to submit an appeal. Every time you have a conversation with or receive a communication from your insurance company, record and save the details. Also, after any personal conversation with a representative, ask whether that person can send you a follow-up email summarizing your conversation.

Step 3: Ask questions.

When it comes to deciphering their insurance benefits, most people don't know where to begin. Here is a list of questions to get you started so you can determine what your insurance policy covers.

Summary Plan Description and Certificate of Coverage

The summary plan description, in compliance with ERISA, helps you understand your benefits. The certificate of coverage—also referred to as a service plan benefit brochure or booklet—describes what is and is not covered in more detail. If you have not yet purchased insurance and are evaluating your options, many insurance companies readily provide these documents online. You may also obtain them through your employer.

Although the certificate of coverage looks thick and intimidating, draw your attention to four sections in particular (the exact names may vary):

Family planning. This is likely a subsection under "Medical services and supplies provided by physicians and other health-care professionals."

Reproductive services. Again, this is likely a subsection under "Medical services and supplies provided by physicians and other health-care professionals."

Covered medications and supplies. This will likely be a subsection under "Prescription drug benefits."

General exclusions. This section should detail what is *not* included in your infertility-related coverage.

Are infertility diagnostic tests covered?

- Which specific diagnostic tests are covered?

- Is there a limit on how many diagnostic tests can be run?

- Will there be any out-of-pocket expenses for these diagnostic tests?

Are fertility medications covered?

- Which specific medications are covered?

- Are they covered only for certain types of treatment, such as IUI?

- Is there a dollar maximum for these medications, either in a year or over a lifetime?

- Will there be any out-of-pocket expenses for these medications?

Which fertility treatments are covered?

- Is my doctor or clinic considered in-network?

- Are there limits on how many cycles of treatment are covered, either in a year or over a lifetime?

- Is there a dollar maximum for fertility treatments? If so, is it for all treatments or is it different for each form of treatment?

- Must I wait a certain amount of time before beginning treatment or moving on to the next type of treatment?

- If I stay on the same policy, are the same treatments and medications covered every year?

- Will there be any out-of-pocket expenses for these treatments?

Are there eligibility requirements?

- Do I need certain tests to "prove" infertility? If so, what are they and are they covered?

- What factors are considered in determining eligibility for fertility treatment? (These can be both biological or situational. Some policies, for example, cover procedures like IVF for heterosexual couples only if the male partner's sperm is used.)

Is fertility preservation (or egg, sperm, or embryo cryopreservation) covered?

- How long will insurance pay for storage?

- Do I have a choice in which facility stores my egg, sperm, and/or embryos?

BUSTED

Myth: It's the insurance company's fault that I can't get infertility treatment.

It's easy to point the finger at your insurance company and say, "This is who's keeping me from building my family!" But this isn't always the case. If you get health insurance through your employer, the employer has a huge say in what is covered through the group policy.

"They don't call them medical benefits for no reason," says Lelito. "They are something that your employer offers you to say, 'We will take care of you in these ways if you work for us.' They're *benefits*, and that's why your employer has the ability to cover whatever they want. They can cover pet health insurance. They can cover any benefit that they think is going to retain and attract employees."

We'll get into more details about talking to and educating your employer below, but remember to consider your employer's perspective when you approach them about expanding health benefits. Show them how fertility treatment coverage will keep you happy. After all, they don't want employees changing jobs just so they can build a family.

Step 4: Obtain preauthorization and written verification of benefits.

Your plan may require that you receive preauthorization (authorization by your insurance company based on proof of medical necessity provided by your doctor) for certain services. Angela from Missouri advises, "Get as much prior authorization for any and all procedures as possible. My insurance had pretty good coverage, but I had to call and activate the benefit before any treatment would be covered. Check your spouse's insurance coverage as well."

Unfortunately, even though it may be a necessary step, preauthorization alone does not guarantee coverage. So, whether or not your fertility clinic requires it, ask your insurance company for a written verification of benefits. I know I feel more assured when an agreement is in writing! Having this information can help you plan for—and perhaps save up for—future treatments.

Step 5: Learn about the appeals process.

Although you will hopefully never need it, ask your insurance company for a written description of their appeals process (we'll talk more about appeals later in this chapter). Each insurance company handles appeals differently, and some have a very quick timeline, so if your claim gets denied, you don't want to waste a moment having to learn about the process itself.

Working with Your Employer/Organization to Expand Infertility Coverage

Believe it or not, *you* have the power to bring significant change to your employer or organization's health insurance plan options. Although you can draft an external appeal letter (more on that later) requesting that an exception be made for your particular needs, advocating for a different plan altogether might be the better option.

Collura emphasizes, "Understand that it's not a big, bad insurance company that's calling all the shots. If you want to blame someone, then blame your employer. People need to speak up and let their HR department know what benefits are most important to them."

RESOLVE has some amazing resources for how to do this, but I'll walk you through the basics here. Also, please note that despite the use of the word "employer" throughout, this advice can also be used for other organizations, such as labor unions and trade associations. If you've been following the recommendations in this chapter, you should have already completed the first two steps.

BUSTED

Myth: One person can't make a difference.

We'll talk more about advocacy in chapter 27, but know now that one person *can* make a difference. In the case of getting more inclusive insurance coverage, sometimes just making your employer aware that one employee is struggling is enough.

Believe it or not, Lelito has advocated for insurance changes—and won—with not one, but two employers. With her second employer, it only took one letter. She had just started a new job and was worried about bringing up that she was trying to build a family and needed better insurance coverage. Still, one day she attended an "Ask Human Resources" event where she sat down with a member of her new HR team and asked if it was possible to get infertility coverage.

"She said, 'Oh, I didn't know we didn't have it. Okay, I'll ask,'" says Lelito. Later, she wrote a letter with her personal story and sent it to the HR employee she'd spoken with at the event. Within a few months, her employer extended the company's health care coverage to include fertility treatment.

"That's all I had to do: send this letter. I was honestly floored that they changed things so quickly and painlessly," she remembers.

Step 1: Determine what type of health insurance plan you have.

Is it a group or individual plan? Public or private? Fully insured or self-insured? In what state was the plan written?

Step 2: Confirm fertility-related state mandates, laws, and exceptions.

Does the state in which the plan was written have a mandate regarding fertility treatments? If so, what does it entail? What are the exceptions?

Now on to step three.

Step 3: Identify the decision-maker(s).

Who makes decisions regarding benefits? What is the best way to contact them? Do they have a gatekeeper, such as an administrative assistant or deputy, whom you might have to speak with first, prior to speaking to the decision-maker themselves?

Because you are asking something of this person, perhaps during your first ever interaction with them, it's important to understand as much as you can about their role within the organization, how they prefer to communicate, and even their personality and approach to these types of conversations. Ask around to find out if anyone you know has ever worked with them before to gain some insight.

Step 4: Find and leverage your allies.

Lelito wrote a detailed guide on her website— League of Extraordinary Uteri—with tips for crafting a winning argument and uploaded the actual documents she submitted.

Lelito suggests that you find allies in your community to campaign on your behalf. Examples include local reproductive endocrinologists (not just your own, but also any others in your area), infertility support groups, women's groups, and more. The idea behind this strategy is that you are not the only one struggling with infertility, and convincing your employer to offer infertility coverage as part of their health insurance plan would impact other employees—and might inspire other companies in the area to follow suit.

Your communication with these individuals and groups is twofold. First, ask how infertility coverage would impact them and others in the community. Second, suggest ways they can help your effort, such as signing a petition, writing letters of support to your employer's benefit plan decision-maker (always offer to write a draft they can edit), and reaching out to other people who might be willing to join your cause.

In addition to people and organizations in your area, identify allies within your company. Are there people who would be willing to join your quest for infertility coverage, whether it would help them personally or not? The more the merrier, but even better if one or more of these individuals has sway with the decision-maker.

Step 5: Pinpoint coverage areas that don't offer a "cure."

One of the biggest arguments against covering fertility treatments and medications is that they offer no guarantee. But many other health conditions that are commonly covered by insurance plans also offer no "cure." Lelito cites bariatric (weight loss) surgery and autism intervention as examples—these services are not guaranteed to work but are often covered by health insurance plans.

Go back through your certificate of coverage (i.e., the service plan benefit brochure) to look for these precedents. What treatments and medications that aren't always effective does the plan already cover?

Another common rationale given for not offering infertility coverage is that fertility treatments are considered "experimental" with low success rates. That's an out-of-date understanding. The oldest IVF baby is now more than 40 years old and has a child of her own, so it's time to do away with this notion! Find up-to-date research that shows the good chances of success with fertility treatments.

Step 6: Find out what competitors offer.

Many companies use their employee benefits, including health insurance, as a way to attract potential employees and set themselves apart from competitors. As a former employer myself for more than a decade, I kept up on not only the services and pricing of my competitors, but also the benefits they offered employees.

Make a list of your employer's competitors, and try to determine what health insurance plans they offer. You may need to befriend their employees to get the details, but the companies also might have this information directly on their websites. If any of them offer infertility coverage, you can make the argument that your employer should match or beat it to attract and retain employees. If these competitors do not offer infertility coverage, expand your search to indirect competitors—companies in similar industries.

Step 7: Align infertility coverage with the company culture.

Most companies have a mission and values statement. Read it. What kind of employees is your employer attempting to attract? Is the company trying be more inclusive? When you write your letter, use your findings to enhance your case.

"We framed our argument for fertility treatment coverage as an issue that spanned gender, race, class, and sexual preference. More and more women delay their childbearing years to be competitive with their male counterparts and find out they need reproductive assistance when they finally want to start their family," says Lelito.

Step 8: Prepare to address possible concerns.

For your employer, the main concern about expanding health-care coverage is likely to be cost, but your allies might help you come up with a larger list. For each concern, develop an evidence-backed response. Two good starting points are *The Policymaker's Guide to Fertility Health Benefits* by Fertility Within Reach and *Employers and Evidence-Based Infertility Benefits* by EMD Serono (both are available online). However, be sure to include the most recent references possible. Some commonly cited studies are a decade or more old and therefore are no longer representative of today's insurance landscape. You don't want that to be held against you!

Step 9: Research possible coverage options.

Familiarize yourself with the various coverage options, and develop suggestions for what gets covered, limitations, and exclusions. Be sure to think beyond just your own needs. What would best serve all employees who are struggling with infertility while keeping costs to your employer reasonable? Again, you can refer to *The Policymaker's Guide to Fertility Health Benefits* for some examples and inspiration.

Step 10: Understand the timeline.

Open enrollment for benefits at most organizations starts in October or November, and decisions about coverage options must be made well in advance. Although insurance companies can turn around quotes relatively quickly—just a few days in most cases—give your employer plenty of time to investigate and consider your request prior to the open enrollment period.

Step 11: Customize the RESOLVE letter template.

It's finally time to approach your employer's employee benefits decision-maker! RESOLVE was kind enough to draft a letter template as part of its Employee Toolkit you can customize for your use. However, I'd like to emphasize the word *customize*—it should be considered just a starting point. Combining Lelito's advice with my own, be sure to include:

Your journey. Unlike any letters you might write to your state or insurance company, this one should evoke emotion. Facts, research, and data still matter, but your employer is also interested in how benefits impact its employees personally.

Current coverage areas that don't offer a cure. Using your investigation from step 5, list examples of health-care interventions that are not guaranteed to work but still covered by your insurance policy.

Competing companies that offer infertility coverage. According to a 2017 survey by Reproductive Medicine Associates of New Jersey, 57 percent of respondents would be willing to switch jobs if a new employer offered infertility treatments. Another survey by RESOLVE found that people needing IVF who had employer-provided infertility coverage were more satisfied with their employer. If you can provide evidence of direct and/or indirect competitors offering infertility coverage, you'll definitely have the decision-maker's attention.

How offering infertility coverage would align with the company culture. Leaders at every company are concerned with developing and maintaining a strong, positive company culture. Present a case for how adding infertility coverage would do just that.

The reality about common infertility treatment misconceptions. Here's where the facts, research, and data come into play. For every myth you want to bust, back up the reality with evidence.

Coverage options. Outline coverage must-haves and nice-to-haves. Lelito adds, "The most important thing is to ask to be part of the conversation on deciding what gets covered and the details like limitations and exclusions." In other words, this letter will not be a one-and-done scenario. Expect it to be a process—one you want to be a part of.

Step 12: Submit and track your request.

Your request should contain more than just your customized letter. Use your best judgment about submitting everything electronically and/or by hard copy, but after making a copy of everything for yourself, include:

- A cover letter that lists every document the decision-maker will find inside

- Your letter

- Copies of every study you reference in your letter, if possible (your fertility clinic likely can obtain these for you)

- Any letters or other documentation provided by your allies

Especially if you submit your request electronically, confirm that the person you send it to receives it.

Step 13: Be patient.

Now it's time to wait—again. (Isn't this whole journey just a bunch of waiting?!?) Once you've asked for the decision-making timeline and the opportunity to participate in discussions, you'll have done all you can to make infertility coverage a reality at your workplace. Feel good about that! I truly hope you're successful.

"Adding benefits is a process," says Fankhauser. "Human resources will consider your request. They research the cost to add benefits. They present their information and recommendation to the executives. And if they are approved, the benefits will likely be added into the following open enrollment period."

The Appeals Process

In an ideal world, you'll have insurance coverage for infertility treatments, and you'll avoid having any claims denied by obtaining written verification of your benefits and preauthorization for any services you use. However, we live in an imperfect world. Let's say the insurance company has denied your claim. Now what?

As Collura says, "Don't be afraid to appeal a denial for an insurance claim."

WARRIOR TIPS
Types of Appeals

There are several types of appeals:

Internal appeal. A letter written to the insurance company that asks it to reconsider its decision about a claim.

External appeal. A letter written to the office of patient protection within your state's department of health and human services (the exact name of these offices varies by state) after an internal appeal has been denied. If an external appeal is approved and the insurance company doesn't fight the appeal, your claim is approved.

(However, if your policy is self-insured, it isn't regulated by state insurance laws and your appeal will have to go through the US Department of Labor.)

External complaint. If you feel your insurance company has violated a state law or regulation by denying you coverage, you can submit a complaint to your state insurance department.

In this chapter, I focus on the most common types of appeals: internal and external.

Internal Appeals

Step 1: Abide by the timeline and process.

Remember, you might have to submit your appeal quickly. Be sure not to miss the deadline! But you've worked ahead by arming yourself with the details on when and where to send an appeal and the information to include. You're already ahead of the game.

Step 2: Determine what was denied.

Call your insurance company. Again, always document the name of the representative you speak to, the time and date of the call, and the details of your discussion. Request written verification—preferably by electronic means rather than snail mail—of the specific reasons why your claim was denied. The more detailed, the better.

Step 3: Develop a strategy.

Upon receiving the denial letter, compare it to your certificate of coverage (the service plan benefit brochure). Your strategy will depend upon why your claim was denied.

For a service that was supposed to be covered under your plan, you'll use language from the brochure to counter the denial.

For a service deemed not medically necessary, you'll ask your reproductive endocrinologist (and any other doctor who might bolster your argument) to write a letter on your behalf explaining why the service was, in fact, medically necessary in your particular case.

For a service that was not covered under your plan, you'll request an explanation of how the insurance company developed the relevant guidelines. Conduct your own research and ask your reproductive endocrinologist—and again, any other doctor who might strengthen your argument—for any additional documentation that might prove helpful in your counter to the denial.

Step 4: Write your internal appeal letter.

Start with an overview of the claim in question, including:

- The claim and policy number

- The date(s) of service

- Your reproductive endocrinologist's (or other doctor's) name, organization, address, phone number, and email address

- Any other relevant background information to help the insurance company understand which denial is in question

Using your copy of the denial letter and your service plan benefit brochure, make note of the insurance company's terminology and use it throughout your appeal. While you can include a brief—and I do mean *brief*—personal story to make your letter stand out, for the most part, leave emotion out of it. Instead, the overall tone of your letter should be that the insurance company made a mistake in denying your claim because it did not have all the information. In other words, the decision to overturn the denial ultimately will be based on facts, research, and data—so provide plenty.

Be clear and specific about the resolution you're seeking (for example, that you want one IVF cycle covered). Follow with the steps you're planning to take should the denial be upheld. (For example, if you have to pay for the IVF cycle yourself, your financial situation will

---

WARRIOR TIPS

Should I Hire an Attorney?

In short, no. This type of work is not profitable for most attorneys. Plus, including an attorney in the process may come off as confrontational rather than cooperative. You've got this all on your own!

result in medical decisions not recommended by the American Society for Reproductive Medicine—you will transfer two embryos, which could result in twins and ultimately cost the insurance company more down the road.) The insurance company will ask doctors to review your letter—it won't be just some bureaucrat—so, again, it cannot be overstated that you must support your statements with facts, research, and data.

If a letter from your reproductive endocrinologist or another doctor might add weight to your appeal, draft a letter on their behalf to make it easy for them to participate. They'll likely edit it, but at least you've given them a head start.

Finally, if you're available, tell the insurance company that you want to attend the review hearing. Denying a living, breathing person standing in front of you is a whole lot harder than denying words on a sheet of paper! Just remember that you'll have to keep your emotions in check.

Step 5: Send and track your appeal.

After making a copy of everything for yourself, in a *single package*, include:

- A cover letter that lists every document the reviewer will find inside

- Your appeal letter

- Copies of every study you reference in your letter, if possible (your fertility clinic likely can obtain these for you)

- All relevant medical records

- Any letters or other documentation provided by your doctor(s)

Send the package via certified mail. *This is important!* You want to be able to track its every move and for a real person to sign for it upon arrival. Approximately 10 business days later, call the insurance company to ensure that the entire package—*every* document listed in your cover letter—ended up in the right hands.

Step 6: Keep your employer in the loop.

Regardless of whether the denial is upheld or overturned, if you get your insurance through your employer you should explain what happened to your employer's benefit plan decision-maker. In my experience, where there is one dissatisfied employee, there are others. Your employer selects the plan(s) available to employees, so this individual has the power to make future changes. Often, the problem lies in a lack of knowledge about employees' needs.

External Appeals and Complaints

If your internal appeal to the insurance company is denied, you can request an external review from your state's department of health and human services, often through its office of patient protection (the exact name varies). An external review is conducted by an independent doctor or other health-care professional working in the area of medicine in question. You cannot be charged more than $25 for an external review, and sometimes it is completely free. If an external appeal is approved, the insurance company can appeal again, but they rarely do.

The process varies from state to state, so determine what you need to submit and by when. You'll need all of the documents that you sent to the insurance company, plus the final adverse determination letter (the letter from the insurance company denying your internal appeal), but your state might require you to complete additional forms. As far as the external appeal letter itself, you can start with your internal appeal letter. Just update it to be addressed to the appropriate agency, tweak the language for this new audience (if necessary—you be the judge), and add in details about the internal appeal denial.

"If in your original appeal you provided all your information—letters from doctors, research supporting you—I have never had anyone lose an external appeal case. But most people are too tired or beaten down, [and they] give up by then," says Fankhauser.

In other words, if you believe your test, treatment, or medication was medically necessary and should be covered, don't be afraid to fight for it.

An external *complaint* is slightly different from an appeal. Here, the basis of your argument is that by denying coverage for certain treatments or medications, your insurance company is violating state law. You'll need to thoroughly research the details of your state's laws and explain how the law was violated. It's still important to have letters from your doctor and research backing your claim, just as with an external appeal. Instead of going through the department of health and human services, complaints are submitted to your state's department of insurance.

COPING AND GETTING SUPPORT

Advocating for better infertility insurance coverage can be a long and tiring process. Make sure you're taking time to destress and renew yourself during the fight so you don't further deplete your energy reserves. Following the steps and plans laid out in this chapter will make the process easier, but always take time to care for yourself.

One of the best things you can do is get help from your partner (if you have one), your family and friends, and other members of the infertility community. Wherever possible, ask them to take on part of your burden. While they won't be able to make the phone calls or do all of the legwork, here are some small but impactful ways others can support you:

Editing your letters. It never hurts to have another set of eyes read your letters and appeals before sending them off. Especially if you know people who are proficient writers, see if they can check your letters for everything from typos to flow to effective word choices.

Sharing research. Knowing the latest research is essential. Chances are others in the infertility community also keep up with new studies and reports that can bolster your argument. Ask them for suggestions on what sources to read and use.

Giving you an escape. It's easy to get lost in hours of phone calls and research, but that's not sustainable in the long run. Plan times to see your friends and family members when you do not discuss your insurance issues. This will help you maintain balance in your life.

→

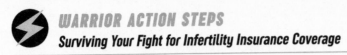

WARRIOR ACTION STEPS
Surviving Your Fight for Infertility Insurance Coverage

Unfortunately, your emotions aren't always your friend when you're trying to get better health insurance coverage. Take the following steps to maintain your sanity:

Don't lose your temper. Whether you're talking to an HR employee at your company or an insurance company representative, don't allow yourself to get angry or raise your voice. Losing your temper will only hurt your argument.

Give yourself time for a breather. While it's important to follow the timeline and deadlines of these processes, knowing what they are beforehand allows you to build in a breather— a time to step back and gather your thoughts

so you can approach your advocacy and appeals with a cool head.

Understand that trying is a victory. Even if your requests and appeals are denied, know that *trying* helps move the conversation about infertility forward. Every time someone outside the community learns about the reality of infertility, they become more sympathetic to the cause. Even if the answer you get is a no, you're laying the groundwork for the next infertility warrior, who might get a yes, to step up.

WARRIOR WISDOM
Assume the Best Is Possible

"Assume that your employer has good intent. Assume that they just didn't know that they don't have the coverage. Assume that they don't know that it is a huge benefit for attracting and retaining employees. And I think all of us will be pleasantly surprised at the number of employers who feel 'you know what, this is a good decision for our company.' So, assume that they might say yes." —Katie Lelito

WARRIOR CHECKLIST
Dealing with Health Insurance

❏ Understand the different types of health insurance policies, the terminology associated with them, and how they impact your options for coverage of infertility treatment.

❏ Know what your state's mandates, laws, and exceptions are so you can advocate for better coverage.

❏ Learn the ins and outs of what your policy covers and what it doesn't.

❏ Form a plan to ask your employer for better coverage using your story, research, and other arguments to make your point.

❏ Know your appeal options in case you are denied coverage.

❏ Be willing to ask others for support during your quest for better infertility insurance coverage.

Affording Family-Building

BOTH MY HUSBAND AND I grew up in middle-class families. My mother was a teacher and my dad a scientist. His mom was a school administrative assistant and his father an agricultural engineer. Like most people, we wanted our children to have at least as much as we did, and hopefully more. So, although we married young, we spent the first 6 years building our careers rather than our family. After all, we wanted to be "financially stable"—a nebulous phrase if ever there was one. Little did we know we'd use nearly every penny we'd saved *creating* a child rather than raising her.

Once it became clear that IVF was our path, and given that our health insurance policy wouldn't cover it, we thought we had only one shot. *Better make it count.* Two transferred embryos, two stillbirths, and a transabdominal cerclage later, we were no closer to our goal of building a family—and out of money.

There were two turning points in our financial situation: our fertility clinic grandfathering us into a package and my parents giving us money.

When we explained our financial situation to our reproductive endocrinologist, he took our case to the clinic's internal review board. They decided we were good candidates for the three-cycle package, which included three retrieval and fresh transfer cycles and unlimited frozen transfers. All we had to do was pay the difference between what we'd already paid and the cost of that package.

If only we could afford to pay what they were asking! We are people who need a certain amount in the bank in order to sleep at night. What if something happened to our house or car? What if one of us lost our job? Our bank account was the emptiest it had ever been.

When my parents—without us asking—said they would give us the money we needed, a variety of emotions overwhelmed me: gratitude, shock, guilt. We would still end up paying more because the package did not cover medications, but with my parents' help, we could make it work. But how would that gift change the nature of our relationship? None of us knew for sure, of course, but we ultimately took them up on their offer and told the clinic we'd accept their offer too.

Years later, I don't regret a thing. None of us do.

Financial Infertility

Infertility is a medical condition. Your genes and biology are the only things that impact the success of your treatment, right? Unfortunately, no. A person may have a high chance of success with certain fertility treatments but be forced to forgo them because they can't afford the cost. Pamela Hirsch, cofounder of the Baby Quest Foundation in Los Angeles, has two daughters who went through fertility treatments. Luckily, Pamela and her husband were able to help them pay for treatments, but it got her curious about what financial support other infertility warriors could use.

"I found that the existing resources were very slim to none," she says.

Hirsch's organization, which provides need-based financial assistance through fertility grants, and others like it are making great impacts, but it's important that we acknowledge the existence of financial infertility. The fact that money is a limiting factor for many people needs to be a part of the advocacy conversation.

Let's Get Real About Treatment Costs

Research conducted in 2020 by Jake and Deborah Anderson-Bialis, cofounders of FertilityIQ in San Francisco, in coordination with NerdWallet, confirmed what we all know: IVF is expensive. The survey also revealed that most respondents had *no* infertility health insurance coverage.

The same study also found that family-building is a wealthy person's pursuit—again, depressing but not surprising.

In a perfect world, we would have full health insurance coverage for all people and all treatments. But even in this imperfect world, regardless of the way you build your family—timed intercourse, a gestational carrier, or anything in between—there are many ways to finance it.

In this chapter, we'll go through all the different ways you can make the costs of family-building more affordable. As with all the other topics in this book, no one route works for everyone. Depending on the avenues you're pursuing and your current financial situation, some options will work better than others.

Before we dive in, the following has to be said: Do *not* bankrupt yourself during your infertility journey. Even if you end up with a child, you need to be able to provide for them. We'll talk about the available resources and options, but always consider how these decisions will impact you over the long term, especially when you're taking out loans or opening credit card accounts.

Grants and Scholarships

I wish I'd known about grants when I was paying for treatments! There are too many state- and patient-specific opportunities to list here, but you can find comprehensive lists posted online by FertilityIQ, CoFertility, and RESOLVE. Below are some of the larger national organizations giving grants for fertility treatment and family building. Details are subject to change; visit the organizations websites for the most up to date information.

Baby Quest Foundation

The organization aims to award grants, which may be used to cover any expenses related to IUI, IVF, egg and sperm donation, egg freezing, and surrogacy. Unlike many other grant organizations, Baby Quest does not have a maximum income requirement but does require applicants to prove they have health insurance, even if they do not have infertility coverage.

Hirsch explains why she started the Baby Quest Foundation: "I distinctly remember sitting up in bed and wondering who was going to help these people who needed surrogacy, because the costs are astronomical." Listen to the Bonus 128 episode of the *Beat Infertility* podcast for insider tips about winning a grant from Baby Quest.

Hope for Fertility Foundation

This organization typically awards grants, which may be used toward adoption and in-clinic expenses associated with fertility treatments but not medication. Single people are not eligible and couples must be legally married.

Journey to Parenthood

This organization awards grants to couples and/or individuals building their families through IUI, IVF, egg donation, surrogacy, and adoption (private, foster care, domestic, or international). Unlike many other grant organizations, Journey to Parenthood does not have a maximum income requirement but does require applicants to prove they will provide financially stable homes for their children.

Tinina Q. Cade Foundation

This organization in Owings Mills, Maryland, awards grants to assist with fertility treatments and domestic adoption costs. Grant applications are accepted twice a year. Dr. Camille Hammond, cofounder of the Cade Foundation, says, "You're not alone. Even though it feels scary and like things will never work out, they will—if you don't give up. You will overcome." Listen to the Bonus 120 episode of the *Beat Infertility* podcast for insider tips about winning a grant from this organization.

Financing Programs and Loans

When you're considering a loan, your credit history will play an important role in determining the interest rate for which you are eligible. Generally, a score of 720 or more is considered excellent, 660 to 719 is fair, 620 to 659 is poor, and lower than 620 is bad. Historically, credit scores tend to increase with age.

Don't know your credit score? The federal Fair Credit Reporting Act requires the nation's three major credit reporting agencies—Equifax, Experian, and TransUnion—each to provide you with a free copy of your credit report once every 12 months. You can request your report at AnnualCreditReport.com.

Third-Party Treatment Packages and Fertility Lenders

I'm lumping third-party treatment package providers and fertility lenders into one section because many companies offer both services. Treatment packages can be either financed or self-pay—hence the overlap in some cases. Fertility-specific lenders tend to offer higher-than-average interest rates, so explore this option with your eyes wide open.

If you want to explore this route, here are some considerations:

Type of lender. Does the provider specialize in fertility loans? If so, do they offer bonus services like direct payments to your clinic, pharmacy, or infertility coach? General personal loan lenders, such as a bank, typically do not offer much beyond the loan itself.

Credit score requirements. What is your credit score, and does it meet the lender's requirements? As I'm sure you know, borrowers with excellent credit have more options than those with poor credit.

Annual percentage rate (APR). What is the loan's APR? The APR calculation factors in the loan, the origination fee (payment made to establish an account with the lender), and the interest rate. The lower the APR, the less you'll pay in interest through the time period of the loan.

Fees. Does the lender charge any additional fees, such as an application fee or late payment or prepayment penalties?

Loan amount. How much money do you really need, and does the lender offer a loan that high (or low—some lenders have minimums)?

For more information about the current best fertility treatment loans, check out Investopedia, a financial media website that analyzes the options each year. It offers the pros and cons of each lender and can help you identify the best one for different circumstances (bad credit, quick funding, etc.).

WARRIOR TIPS

Third-Party Treatment Packages and Lenders
••

Although this is not a complete list, it will get you started (and remember details are always subject to change). It's important to note that each provider requires your clinic to be a member of its network, so if your clinic isn't, encourage your doctor to reach out about joining.

ARC Fertility. Packages are available for IUI, IVF, egg freezing, genetic testing, donor egg cycles, and more.

CapexMD. Offers loans to cover medications, fertility treatments, and preimplantation genetic testing.

LendingClub Patient Solutions. Offers financing toward fertility treatments, medications, genetic testing, egg freezing, and more. The short application does not impact your credit score, and there is an online calculator to help estimate your payments.

LightStream. Provides unsecured loans to be used for fertility treatments, medication, and/or surrogacy. There are no application fees, down payments, or prepayment penalties.

Univfy. Based on a variety of factors—your age, diagnoses, ovarian reserve, semen analysis, and body mass index—Univfy will generate a report of your IVF success probability. The results will determine if you qualify for a Univfy-backed IVF refund program.

WINFertility. Offers a treatment package for patients with no infertility insurance coverage that could include diagnostic tests, fertility treatments, medications, and/ or genetic testing. The bundle options vary by clinic but could cover IUI, IVF, FET, and donor egg cycles. If you purchase a bundle, WINFertility also offers a variety of financing programs.

Credit Unions

As a credit union member for more than a decade, I can personally attest to the low interest rates they offer compared to most commercial banks. To see for yourself, go to the website of the National Credit Union Administration (NCUA), where a comparison chart is updated each quarter.

Currently the Federal Credit Union Act prevents federal credit unions from charging more than 18 percent in interest—which is lower than the interest rate offered by many of the fertility-specific lenders discussed in the previous section—but this figure is subject to change. And again, the specific rate approved for you will depend on a variety of factors. Some downsides to credit unions include a "hard check" of your credit history that temporarily lowers your score, application fees, and a lengthy application and approval process.

To find a credit union in your area, use NCUA's online locator tool.

Credit Cards

I don't recommend credit cards for financing fertility treatments, but it's really common, so here's what you need to know.

If you have good credit and need to borrow only a small amount, you might qualify for a zero-interest card. If your credit isn't great, your credit limit likely will be low and your interest rate high, but this is still an option. Just keep in mind that carrying a balance will negatively impact your credit score.

After determining your credit score, a good place to start is NerdWallet's list of best credit cards with zero or low introductory interest rates. And if you have or open a credit union account, don't forget to check their credit card options.

BUSTED

Myth: I'll know all the fertility treatment costs up front.

When you go into a store to buy, say, a sweater, it's clearly labeled with a price. When you go to check out, there aren't surprise additional costs that take the sweater out of your price range—it costs just what the store said it would when it was hanging on the rack. However, that's not always the case with fertility treatments.

Mary Beth Storjohann is a certified financial planner in San Diego, author of *Work Your Wealth*, and host of the *Work Your Wealth* podcast, and even she was caught off-guard by certain costs during her infertility journey. During a round of IVF, her doctor recommended freezing all the retrieved eggs instead of going straight into a transfer. She agreed, not realizing there was an additional $5,000 fee for freezing the eggs.

"That was a surprise to me," she shares. "So I call [the clinic] crying and really upset because there was a lack of communication."

While your clinic will give you a breakdown of the costs for your course of treatment, always ask what additional costs might pop up. This way, even if there are changes to your treatment plan, you're prepared to handle them financially.

Fertility Clinic Discounts

Thankfully, most fertility clinics have at least one discount program. I know talking about money can be uncomfortable for some people, but put on your self-advocacy hat and speak up. Ask for what you need.

Treatment Packages and Refund Programs

Many fertility clinics—especially the ones within large clinic networks like IVIRMA—offer treatment packages and refund programs for IVF. Jake Anderson-Bialis of FertilityIQ surveyed more than three hundred fertility patients in 2017 and interviewed representatives of clinics and clinic networks that administer these programs. Key takeaways include:

• The price of refund programs and treatment packages is 25 to 50 percent less than what you'd spend on the same number of cycles individually.

• Because not everyone qualifies for a refund program, the majority (two-thirds) of those accepted into these programs succeed on their first fresh transfer, and more than half succeed on the first frozen transfer.

• Even though they are successful quickly and thus spend more money up front than would be otherwise necessary, most patients see refund programs and treatment packages as a good deal.

Let's unpack this. Although every clinic is different, you'll see the same overall approach: Only the patients who are most likely to be successful—and just as important, successful before the package is completely used up—are eligible. I've said this before, but fertility clinics are businesses. They offer these programs with the hope of maintaining their success rate and making more money than they would have otherwise.

However, the end result doesn't always work out in the clinic's favor. I'm a prime example. On paper at the time, I was a great candidate: We got pregnant with twins on our first transfer and only lost them because of a problem with my cervix—which we surgically

		SAMPLE COMPARISON OF PAYING FOR INDIVIDUAL CYCLES VS. TREATMENT PACKAGES		
TYPE	**POSSIBLE COST**	**POSSIBLE DETAILS**
Pay-as-you-go	$18,000	One retrieval, one fresh transfer ($15,000), and one frozen transfer ($3,000)
One-cycle bundle	$20,000	One retrieval, one fresh transfer, and unlimited frozen transfers
Two-cycle bundle	$25,000	Two retrievals, two fresh transfers, and unlimited frozen transfers
Three-cycle bundle	$35,000	Three retrievals, three fresh transfers, and unlimited frozen transfers
Three-cycle bundle with 100% refund	$45,000	Three retrievals, three fresh transfers, unlimited frozen transfers, and all money back if not successful after using all embryos

Source: FertilityIQ, https://www.fertilityiq.com/topics/cost/ivf-refund-and-package-programs. Date accessed: September 3, 2022.

corrected—and had four remaining embryos. I don't think any of us could have predicted that our seventh transfer—two retrieval cycles later—would be the successful one.

WARRIOR TIPS

Deciding If a Treatment Package or Refund Program Is Right for You

Ask yourself—and potentially your reproductive endocrinologist—the following questions:

- If I am eligible, why am I such a good candidate? Could I possibly spend less by paying for individual cycles?

- What is included in—and excluded from— the cost?

- After how many retrievals and transfers do patients with diagnoses and prognoses similar to mine typically succeed?

- How does the treatment package or refund program define success?

Eligibility

Multicycle treatment packages typically have no eligibility requirements and instead are designed for any patient without infertility insurance coverage. Refund programs, however, are a different story.

Each clinic has its own rules, so read the fine print. Here's an example from my clinic: Its Shared Risk 100% Refund Program, which included six retrievals (your eggs or donor eggs) and unlimited frozen transfers of the resulting embryos. To qualify for this program:

- The patient's physician will need to medically indicate the proposed treatment.

- Patients must be younger than 40 upon completion of the IVF cycles.

- Patients 41 and older can participate in the Shared Risk 100% Refund Program if they are using donor eggs. The clinic encourages the use of donor eggs for candidates older than 41 only if the prognosis with your own eggs is poor.

- Patients who need intracytoplasmic sperm injection (ICSI) or a gestational carrier, or who are having an embryo biopsy, are eligible.

- Patients who have no insurance benefits (or choose not to use benefits) are eligible.

I ultimately ended up in a customized version of this refund program, but determining my eligibility was not straightforward. I met all the requirements, but as I mentioned earlier, my doctor was not the decision-maker. Instead, my patient case was taken before an internal medical review board, and my reproductive endocrinologist had to present an argument in my favor. Because I had already become pregnant during my first transfer—with twins, no less—the board probably figured I'd get pregnant again quickly and I was therefore low-risk. Boy, were they wrong!

The lesson here is to find out who makes these decisions. Determine who administers your clinic's refund program, whether that's an internal medical review board or an external third-party like ARC Fertility. And ask your reproductive endocrinologist for help making your case.

What's Included

You're probably picking up on a theme here: Financial support varies from clinic to clinic. Some treatment packages and refund programs include all cycle monitoring, cryopreservation, and the first year of embryo storage and exclude medications and "extra" services like ICSI and preimplantation genetic testing. Other clinics refund programs may only include ICSI and some extra services on a case-by-case basis. Understand what you're getting at what cost—and what you'll need to spend on top of that.

Defining Success

Although you want a live birth, fertility clinics and third-party administrators might measure success with different parameters. A fertility clinic uses relative success to get your attention and use their services, while you are looking for absolute success. Again, make sure you are clear on the details. Get the full scoop on what qualifies as success in writing.

TREATMENT PACKAGE AND REFUND PROGRAM DEFINITIONS OF SUCCESS		
	CLINIC	THIRD-PARTY
Pregnancy	27%	16%
Pregnancy through the first trimester	22%	7%
Live birth	22%	28%
Take-home baby	29%	49%

Source: FertilityIQ: https://www.fertilityiq.com/topics/cost/ivf-refund-and-package-programs. Date accessed: September 3, 2022.

Risk vs. Reward

IVF is more successful than IUI—that's just a fact. But in this case, high reward also means high cost. According to the New York State Task Force on Life and the Law, "When payment is linked to outcome, physicians may encourage patients to accept aggressive treatments that increase the chance of success without due regard for what those treatments may entail."

In other words, some reproductive endocrinologists are encouraging IVF—and in some cases, donor egg IVF—as the first step. On top of that, many clinics now do frozen transfers only for embryos that have been proved normal through genetic testing, which adds genetic testing to the patient's final bill.

WARRIOR TIPS
Consider Mini IVF

A meta-analysis published in *Human Reproduction Update* found no difference in pregnancy outcomes between minimal stimulation IVF and conventional IVF. As you might imagine, the major cost difference between mini and conventional IVF stems from the reduced amount of medication required by the former. Ask your reproductive endocrinologist if mini IVF is likely to be successful for you. (Just remember: Saving money won't mean too much if the cycle isn't a success!)

Thankfully, in my case, the medical review board and my reproductive endocrinologist took the opposite approach, requiring that we transfer no more than one embryo at a time to be accepted into the refund program. Despite what I'd been through, I admittedly objected at first. *I've transferred two before, I now have a transabdominal cerclage to keep my cervix closed, and everyone else gets to transfer two,* I thought. However, after a little more time had passed and my emotional healing continued to progress, I realized they were right. Don't allow costs to force you away from what are considered the best practices for fertility treatments. I know it will be difficult, but I say this as someone who spent tens of thousands of dollars during my infertility journey. The risks—ovarian hyperstimulation syndrome, preterm delivery, and so on—are just too great.

Self-Pay Discounts

Let's say that your health insurance policy covers $5,000 annually for infertility treatment. That's a good chunk of change but not nearly enough to cover an entire IVF cycle. However, fertility clinics (and all medical offices) charge insurance companies more than they will charge you if you're paying out of pocket. For example, if the insurance company is charged

$25,000 for your cycle and your policy covers $5,000, that leaves you owing $20,000. However, in this scenario, if you were to self-pay, your total cost for the cycle might be $18,000—a savings of $2,000 over using your insurance benefits. Ask about self-pay discounts, and calculate whether or not to submit all of your claims—or only certain ones—to your insurance company. Your clinic's financial department should be a great resource here.

Need-Based Discounts

Some clinics offer discounts based on a patient's financial circumstances. If you're approved, the discount may be applied toward precycle screening, treatment cycles (timed intercourse, IUI, and IVF), other discount programs, medications, and more. Eligibility rules and inclusions will vary by clinic.

Discounts for Active Military, Reservists, and Veterans

I'll devote an entire chapter to navigating infertility in the military (see chapter 22), but briefly, your clinic may offer military discounts.

Nicole lives in Georgia with her husband, Jeremy. He is a member of the US military, and so they had a choice between a military treatment facility and a civilian clinic. "We found that different clinics offered different fees. Many of them had scholarship programs as well as generous refund packages. We chose a [civilian] clinic that offered military discounts, was highly successful, and had lower fees compared to many clinics."

Discounts for Clinical Trials

Pharmaceutical companies or other research groups conducting clinical trials for new medications or treatments for infertility typically recruit participants through clinics. Ask your reproductive endocrinologist if you qualify for any current trials. Before agreeing to participate, however, be aware of the potential benefits *and* risks.

Potential Benefits

• Access to new treatment protocols, techniques, technology, and/or medications

• Reduced-cost or free medications and/or treatments

• Guaranteed close monitoring and care, which you may or may not be receiving at your current clinic

Potential Risks

• Not being able to choose the treatment protocols, techniques, technology, and/or medications assigned to you

• The protocol, technique, technology, or medication you're assigned may not work for you

• Unanticipated—or more severe than expected—side effects

• Infertility health insurance (if you have any) may not cover any costs you owe as part of the trial

• More frequent testing and doctor visits

Tax Deductions

Here is some good news: Your infertility-related expenses may be tax-deductible!

Publication 502 produced by the Internal Revenue Service (IRS) explains the medical (and dental) expenses you can claim on Schedule A (Form 1040). Although that percentage and the expenses that qualify are, of course, subject to change depending on the latest tax code revisions, some medical expenses you can deduct may include:

- Acupuncture

- Annual physical exam

- Birth control pills

- Fertility enhancement procedures, like IVF, cryopreservation, and vasectomy reversal

- Home pregnancy tests

- Insurance premiums

- Laboratory fees

- Legal fees, such as those incurred when pursuing donor eggs/sperm/embryos, adoption, or surrogacy

- Lodging, such as when you have to travel for fertility treatments

- Mental health care provided by a psychologist

- Prescription medications

- Qualified adoption expenses (find details about this in IRS Form 8839)

- Smoking cessation programs

- Surgery

- Transportation to and from your fertility clinic

- Weight-loss programs

Always consult a certified public accountant (CPA) who specializes in tax preparation if you are unsure about any aspect of your filing—or simply to protect yourself against an audit.

Flexible Spending Accounts (FSAs) and Health Savings Accounts (HSAs)

If your employer offers them, you may benefit from enrolling in a flexible spending account (FSA) or health savings account (HSA). Both are types of savings accounts that, using pretax funds deducted from your paycheck, may be used to pay for qualified medical expenses not covered by your health insurance policy. Ask your HR department or check with the IRS for guidelines for setting up and using FSAs and HSAs.

Tara and her husband, Sean, from Minnesota have no insurance coverage and are paying for all medications and treatments out-of-pocket. They're using a two-part strategy to make their infertility journey as affordable as possible. "We maxed out our medical FSA contributions so we can use pre-tax dollars to pay for treatments," she explains. "We also have a 0 percent interest credit card. We put all of our medications and doctor appointments on that."

WARRIOR TIPS

Taking Advantage of Tax Deductions

· ·

Planning ahead is best, but if you did not itemize your qualified medical deductions from the previous tax year, you can file Form 1040-X to revise your return. Either way, here's what you need to do:

- Keep track of—or track down—all invoices and receipts.

- Maintain a log—including the date, cost, description, etc.—of all expenses. Don't forget to write down travel expenses, including mileage, tolls, parking, hotels, and meals.

- Save your log, invoices, and receipts for 7 years in case of a future audit.

FLEXIBLE SPENDING ACCOUNTS vs. HEALTH SAVINGS ACCOUNTS		
	FSAs	**HSAs**
Health insurance requirement	None; you are not required to have health insurance to have an FSA.	You must have a qualified high-deductible health plan (HDHP) with a minimum annual deductible and a cap on out-of-pocket costs.
Qualified expenses	See IRS Publication 502.	See IRS Publication 502.
Nonqualified expenses	Health insurance premiums and expenses covered under another health plan	Health insurance premiums, health coverage tax credits, and expenses incurred before you established your HSA
Interest and other earnings on the account balance	No interest or other earnings are tied to these accounts.	Interest and other earnings accumulate tax-free.
Contribution limits	See IRS Publication 969 for current contribution limits.	See IRS Publication 969 for current contribution limits.
Rollover of funds	Caps on how much you can roll over into the next year.	All funds can be rolled over to the next year.
Portable to other employers	No; if you leave your job, you lose your FSA unless you are eligible for continuation through COBRA.	Yes; you own the account, so if you leave your job, your funds go with you.

Source: Internal Revenue Service, *Health Savings Accounts and Other Tax-Favored Health Plans*, Publication 969 (for tax year 2021), IRS.gov/Pub969.

BUSTED

Myth: I can't ask family or friends for financial help.

It's not easy to ask your loved ones for help paying for treatment. Borrowing or accepting a gift of money from relatives or friends carries with it the risk of changing that relationship. Ultimately, it's your decision whether to tell your family and friends about your financial troubles and ask them to help. But there are some ways to ease the awkwardness of approaching the topic. We'll dive into exactly how to do this later, but consider how Chrissy and her husband, Lee, from Maryland included crowdfunding in their quest to pay for treatment.

"If you don't feel comfortable directly asking people for financial assistance, post a link to a crowdfunding page on social media that tells your story and asks for donations indirectly," she says. "We created a crowdfunding page and posted a link on our website. We regularly posted updates to it and would include the link in any blog posts or videos we created. We were fortunate that we raised $5,000 from friends and family to put toward our journey."

These types of approaches take away the pressure of asking for help point-blank. Your family and friends can contribute if they're able, and there's no awkwardness that comes from taking a large sum of money from one person (unless they choose to make the donation on their own, which does happen).

Other Creative Funding Strategies

When it comes to raising money for fertility treatments, people can get very creative. Here are a few that have worked for people I know or worked with.

Crowdfunding

Jacob and his wife, Sarah, used GoFundMe to raise nearly $15,000. Their son, Gabriel, is nothing short of an IVF miracle. "For us, ease of use was really important," Jacob says of choosing from among the different crowdfunding platforms. "I wanted to make it easy for my grandmother and grandfather to use."

He also looked at the fees—both the amount and how they are charged. "I liked GoFundMe because the fee is taken out after the donation is made. I didn't want the fee to be passed on to the donor. I'd rather it came out of us."

Finally, he evaluated how the platforms handled the donations. "Some sites won't let you withdraw the money until you've reached your goal. Some sites won't let you extend the goal to continue the campaign." GoFundMe allowed them to withdraw as they needed, as well as extend the campaign beyond the original goal.

Asking for Money in Lieu of Gifts

Have a birthday, wedding, holiday, or other gift-receiving event coming up? Open up about your journey, and request gifts of money to pay for medication and treatments.

Garage/Yard Sale

If asking for money in lieu of gifts and crowdfunding both make you a bit queasy, having a garage/yard sale might be more up your alley. Chrissy suggests, "You could do a 'donation only' sale where the customer pays what they can/feel comfortable paying, or [you can] tag everything with predetermined prices."

Consider asking friends, family, and members of your broader community to donate items for sale. Again, if you're up front about your journey, you'll almost certainly find people in your life who want to help.

Get a Part-Time Job

Starbucks famously offers infertility insurance coverage to both full- and part-time employees, but it is hardly the only company with great fertility benefits. Check out FertilityIQ's Workplace Index for a list of more than 250 employers and details on the fertility benefits they offer.

Sign Up for Airbnb

If you own your home and have family or friends you can stay with, Airbnb can be an easy way to supplement your income. In one year, Emily and her husband, Matthew, made $17,000 renting out their Indiana home via Airbnb. While it can be time-consuming to clean and set up the house between guests, and you'll have to lay out some money up front to get your home ready, Emily says it was nice to do things on their own timetable.

"You need a place to stay while renting your house," she explains. "We actually found a few people who rent their places and then stay at each other's houses while their place is occupied. We luckily stayed with family, which was less chaotic." (She recommends getting additional insurance to cover short-term rentals because it's likely your homeowner's insurance won't cover any damages that happen when you're renting your home.)

Personal Asset Loan

In a 2018 survey conducted by Student Loan Hero, approximately 14 percent of respondents said that they planned to pay for IVF using an early withdrawal from their 401(k), and 8 percent planned to take out a home equity loan. However, these types of personal asset loans come with plenty of risks and costs, so consult a certified financial planner before making any moves.

Create a Financial Plan

I would be remiss to wrap up this chapter without talking about budgeting. After all, if you discover your financial situation is not as dire as it seems, you might be able to avoid strategies that make you uncomfortable. Use the information in this chapter to scope your options, then work with a financial planner to make a plan that is best for you.

BUSTED

Myth: Less invasive treatments will be more affordable.

In most cases, technically this is true. On its own, a timed intercourse cycle is less expensive than an IUI cycle, which is less expensive than an IVF cycle. But when you're doing cycle after cycle, the costs add up quickly. Before you know it, you can go through several unsuccessful forms of less invasive treatment for the same price as one cycle of IVF.

This is why it's so important to talk with your doctor about each treatment option and its chance of success. If it's highly unlikely that you will get pregnant with IUI but you are a good candidate for IVF, you could end up *saving* money by going straight to IVF.

Step 1: Review your financial situation.

Storjohann says, "Coping with the treatments, terminology, and outflow of cash can be stressful." And she would know. Her husband, Brian, was diagnosed with male factor infertility, but they now have two children thanks to IVF.

Storjohann advises that you start by understanding exactly how much treatments and medications will cost—with and without insurance (even if you have some coverage). Then turn your attention to your available savings, your projected monthly income, your debt load, and areas in which you may be able to reduce spending.

"Determine where you currently stand in these areas," she says. "If you're not the kind of couple that has a budget in place, now is certainly the time to take action in that category. It's going to be incredibly important to understand where your money is going in the months ahead."

Step 2: Prioritize.

Of the funds you have available today *and* the money you were planning to set aside for savings in the future, how much of it are you willing to put toward building your family? This is a personal decision, says Storjohann. But thankfully, unlike so many aspects of this journey, in this arena *you* are in control.

"Each situation is unique, and you have to determine where each phase . . . falls on your list of priorities," Storjohann says. "If you are currently saving up for a down payment on a house or a big trip, is that money you'll reallocate toward the medical payments for treatment? Perhaps you'll cease making contributions and reallocate any future savings amounts toward your family planning goal."

Step 3: Create a plan.

For the financial plan itself, Storjohann advises that you determine:

- How much you can allocate *without depleting your emergency fund*

- The areas in which you will cut back in order to save more in the shortest amount of time

- Whether or not to open up a separate account to track your savings and expenses (this might be especially helpful come tax time!)

- At what point you're willing to finance treatments with a loan if you cannot save enough on your own

- Whether you would benefit from fertility clinic shopping to find more affordable—but obviously still quality—treatments

Krista from New Jersey recommends, "Look at it from every angle possible. We didn't take elaborate vacations or spend extravagantly. We took hand-me-down furniture so we could put the money [we would have spent] toward treatment. We got rid of extra monthly debt—besides bills—so if we needed to take out a loan, we could swing a monthly payment."

Step 4: Start saving and adjust as needed.

You and your partner have agreed upon a plan, so now it's time to put it into action and start saving! Set up automatic transfers to a savings account on a weekly, biweekly, or monthly basis—whatever works best for you.

Nicole and Jeremy shopped around for the best savings account options and planned ahead. "Figure out how much you can afford to save. The earlier you save, the more money you can have," she advises.

Additionally, putting fertility treatments and medications on a credit card doesn't have to be a risky proposition—and in fact can help you save money. Storjohann suggests finding a credit card with good cash-back rewards and paying off any purchases immediately rather than carrying a balance.

"We would put all of our medical bills on our credit card and then immediately transfer the money from our savings to make a payment," she says. "This allowed us to stock up on travel points that we've cashed in for trips over the past few months."

Step 5: Know your limit.

Financially (and physically and emotionally), what's your limit? Three IUIs? One round of IVF? Adoption? Three retrievals was the limit for me. I will never, ever go through another one, even if we cannot complete our family with the four frozen embryos we have left. But your threshold might be lower or higher.

Storjohann says, "We were flexible, but we had a limit, and one round of IVF was it for me—physically, emotionally, and financially. If it didn't work after one round, adoption was our route, and we were okay with that."

Keep in mind that breaks aren't just for physical and emotional recovery—taking a financial break to save enough to continue your family-building goal might be just what you need at some point.

"It's hard to keep the numbers in mind with such an emotional issue, but as it goes with many things with your finances, you shouldn't put all of your eggs in one basket. While you may want to throw everything you can at this goal (which could work for a period of time), you can't let it wreak financial havoc on your life," warns Storjohann.

A 2022 report from the American Psychological Association found that 66 percent of Americans named money as a top source of stress in their lives. If you don't take time to deal with and alleviate financial stress, it will negatively impact multiple aspects of your life and relationships.

One of the best ways to cope with stress is talking about it. Unfortunately, it's not easy to talk to others about money—or your lack thereof. While it might be uncomfortable at first, find someone you can talk to about your worries without making it seem like you're asking for charity or pity. Start with other warriors in your support system; they understand better than anyone how difficult it is to manage your finances during your journey. It can be helpful to preface these conversations by letting your listener know that you just need to vent—you're seeking an empathetic ear, not advice.

It's essential to not give up all your interests and hobbies to save for fertility treatments. Yes, you can find ways to cut costs, but you shouldn't sacrifice everything you love. This is an open invitation for infertility to take over every aspect of your life, which is neither healthy nor conducive to long-term happiness. Find room in your budget for affordable self-care activities.

WARRIOR ACTION STEPS
Don't Let the Finances Drive You Crazy

Don't let financial stress get the best of you. Take the following steps to maintain your emotional and mental health, despite the pressure of paying for treatments:

Get organized. We've touched on this throughout the chapter, but I can't overstate the importance of having a good organizational system for your finances. Set up spreadsheets, have a filing system for your receipts, and develop a way to track your applications for grants or loans. It's best to have all this in place *before* you start going through treatments so there's one less thing to worry about.

Don't skimp on mental health counseling. Depending on your insurance policy, regularly seeing a mental health counselor can be costly.

But if you need professional help, do not go without. Talk to different professionals to find out which is the most affordable option. If you chose to pay out of pocket, many therapists will work with you to find a fee you're comfortable with.

Never dip into your safety net. You never know when a big expense will pop up. Sure, you can afford IVF with the money you have now, but if your car breaks down the following week, you're in trouble. Have the discipline to maintain some cushion so you have peace of mind in case disaster strikes.

WARRIOR WISDOM
Getting the Most out of Your Financial Options

"My husband and I saved for several years, so we were able to pay out of our savings accounts. We also used a nice credit card with really good rewards, so we paid for everything on that credit card and then just paid it off right away. We have about $1,500 worth of travel that we get to use here soon, too. So, if you have to pay out of pocket, it's a really great way to at least get something out of the deal." —Mindi, Ohio

→

WARRIOR CHECKLIST
Affording to Build Your Family

❑ Know the truth about the costs of fertility treatments and ways to pay outside of insurance.

❑ Research fertility grants and apply for the ones you qualify for.

❑ Learn about different financing and loan options.

❑ Ask your clinic about treatment packages and discounts.

❑ Consider other creative ways to raise and save money.

❑ Create a financial plan and stick to it.

❑ Find ways to cope with stress that arises due to finances.

Add more items to your Warrior Checklist or jot down any notes here:

Navigating Infertility in the Workplace

FOR 4 YEARS, JAHSMYN FROM Queensland, Australia, went back and forth with general practitioners about why she couldn't get pregnant. None of the doctors believed there was anything wrong and never recommended running any diagnostic tests.

Finally, she saw a reproductive endocrinologist. And although she didn't have a choice in doctors, she liked him. "I lived in the middle of nowhere, and [he] was my only option," she explains. "He was great. He listened to me and ran tests and got me diagnosed after years of doctors not listening."

Her doctor performed a hysterosalpingogram (HSG), an X-ray to show whether the fallopian tubes are blocked (see page 45), and Jahsmyn admits that she hates reliving that day. It was extremely painful, and at the end of the test, her doctor simply said IVF was her only option and left the room. Weeks later, she was told she'd probably have to have her fallopian tubes removed.

"I wish that my doctor had told me all in one hit. I also wish I was told what IVF was, why it was my only option, and the rates of success. I left my HSG appointment having no idea what was wrong with me or any information about my future. I was gravely uninformed."

Thankfully, Jahsmyn's job was a refuge during this rough time. She says it's important for all infertility warriors to figure out what helps get them through their day-to-day lives. "The thing that helped me the most was helping others. I'm lucky enough to have a job [as a teacher] where I do that every day."

When it came time to prepare for her IVF cycle, her employer and coworkers were accommodating and supportive. She'd already told them about her infertility battles, and there had been no issue getting time off for appointments or procedures. "When I told my boss I had to do IVF, he made sure I was emotionally supported and continued to monitor me," she says. "When I had to leave at a moment's notice, he never complained. When I got too overwhelmed, he made sure I had help to get back to where I needed to be."

While Jahsmyn understands that not everyone will have a supportive workplace, she still advises opening up to those you can. "Before that, I would never talk about it. I battled for years in silence," she says. "When I opened up, the support and understanding I received was unlike any other. And by being open, I helped other colleagues battling infertility, as well. If they don't know, they can't help you, so tell everyone you feel comfortable with."

Untangling the Web of Work and Infertility

We've already talked about how you can advocate for better health coverage at work (see chapter 19). Now let's get into how you deal with infertility *and* your career on a daily basis. This is a difficult topic because every workplace is different and every individual has their own idea about what it means to be professional.

In this chapter, we'll review your legal rights as an employee with infertility issues and the potential benefits and drawbacks of

---

BUSTED

Myth: My employer won't care that I'm having trouble building a family.

Though this may be true for many employers, don't be so quick to assume that your employer is among them. More and more employers are becoming more sensitive to what employees are dealing with in their lives.

When it comes to infertility, however, it's likely that your boss and the people you work with know very little about what you're going through. "They don't understand the environment and the needs [of people facing infertility] unless it's communicated to them or they've had experience with it in some way," explains Davina Fankhauser, cofounder of the advocacy group Fertility Within Reach in Newton Highlands, Massachusetts. "The employee finding the courage to come forward and express how this is something very important is very eye-opening to the employer. And they will listen."

---

sharing your story with your employer and colleagues. And as I've said before, you should never let infertility overtake your life. So, you'll also find tips on how to maintain a successful career during your infertility journey. Basically (prepare for a bad pun), this chapter will show you how to work it all out.

Understand Your Workplace Rights

To begin, if you share your personal medical information with your employer, you have a right to privacy. Even if you volunteered information about your infertility to your employer, your employer cannot share that information without your permission (unless there is some legitimate business-related reason to do so).

The law is likely on your side here. You probably already know that employers cannot discriminate against employees based on race, sex, sexual orientation, religion, national origin, physical disability, or age. But did you know that you—an employee battling infertility—have *additional* rights? Use this section to understand the power you have in the workplace—and what your employer can and cannot do under the law. (As always, laws are subject to change!)

Americans with Disabilities Act (ADA)

Tom Spiggle, an attorney and principal of the Spiggle Law Firm in Arlington, Virginia, explains, "The Americans with Disabilities Act (ADA) of 1990 prohibits discrimination against a qualified individual based on disability and requires employers to provide reasonable accommodations to its employees with disabilities."

Let's break down this statement, as defined by the ADA:

Qualified individual. "A person who meets legitimate skill, experience, education, or other requirements of an employment position that he or she holds or seeks, and who can perform the 'essential functions' of the position with or without reasonable accommodation." Essentially, if you have what it takes to perform the core responsibilities of your job, you're a qualified individual.

Reasonable accommodation. "A modification or an adjustment to a job or the work environment that will enable a qualified applicant or employee with a disability to participate in the application process or to perform essential job functions. Reasonable accommodation also includes adjustments to assure that a qualified individual with a disability has rights and privileges in employment equal to those of nondisabled employees." Providing time off work for infertility-related appointments and procedures would be considered a reasonable accommodation, according to Spiggle.

Disability. "A physical or mental impairment that substantially limits one or more major life activities." A life activity includes the "operation of major bodily functions" such as reproductive systems.

Your employer cannot discriminate against you because of your "disability"—yes, the medical condition of infertility is legally recognized as a disability. This is a good thing! It means you have more legal avenues to protect your rights. As long as you continue to do your job, your employer must grant you time off for appointments, procedures, and treatments. It also cannot pass you up for that big promotion you earned!

Family and Medical Leave Act (FMLA)

The Family and Medical Leave Act (FMLA) of 1993 requires employers to provide eligible employees up to 12 weeks of unpaid, job-secured leave—as well as continuous health insurance coverage during that leave—each year. However, only certain conditions qualify for this leave, and here's where it gets complicated for those battling infertility. Employees may take FMLA leave only if they have a "serious health condition."

"Unfortunately, neither the FMLA nor case law has definitely declared whether leave for infertility treatments is covered by the FMLA," says Spiggle. "The crux of the issue depends on whether infertility is considered a 'serious health condition,' which depends on the facts of each situation."

For argument's sake, let's say infertility qualifies as a serious health condition. You almost certainly won't need to take off 12 weeks at once. Does that mean you cannot apply FMLA leave to infertility treatments? Nope. Intermittent leave—either reducing your usual schedule or taking leave in separate blocks of time—is permitted so long as you "make a reasonable effort to schedule treatment so as not to unduly disrupt the employer's operation."

"It's possible the more invasive and time-consuming fertility treatments (requiring more time away from work), such as in vitro

---

BUSTED

Myth: If I tell my boss or coworkers that I'm working through infertility, I'll have to tell them all the details.

How you tell your story is one of the only things you have control over during your infertility journey. Which details you choose to share are *completely up to you*. You can post a sign on your desk that says "Ask me about infertility!" or you can never mention your journey to another soul in your workplace.

"If you do not want to disclose specifics to your team, explain that you are experiencing an unexpected health issue that requires you to miss meetings or come in late because of very precise treatment schedules that [are] out of your control," says Dr. Angela Palmer-Wackerly, assistant professor of health communication at the University of Nebraska in Lincoln.

At the end of the day, all that really matters is whether you can do your job. So, when deciding how much to tell others, focus on what level of disclosure will make you your best version of an employee.

---

fertilization, may meet [the serious health condition] requirements, but no court has reached that conclusion," says Spiggle.

He's right, although the *Culpepper v. BlueCross BlueShield of Tennessee* decision suggests that you could be covered if your reproductive endocrinologist or other doctor presents written evidence of your time away from work being medically necessary (and adheres to the other FMLA guidelines).

Bottom line: document, document, document. If you need time off work for infertility-related appointments, procedures, and/or treatments, keep written records and get notes from your doctor(s). In an ideal world, your employer won't challenge you as long as your work gets done, but you just never know.

Pregnancy Discrimination Act (PDA)

Title VII of the Civil Rights Act of 1964 and the Pregnancy Discrimination Act (PDA) of 1978 (an amendment to Title VII) prevent employers from discriminating against current or potential employees on the basis of sex, which includes pregnancy and "related medical conditions."

Spiggle explains, "For example, if an employee is fired for taking time off for in vitro

fertilization treatment, that can be illegal discrimination in violation of the PDA and Title VII. Firing an employee based on child-bearing capacity can be discrimination based on sex, not infertility."

⚡ If you lose your job because you took time off for an infertility-related procedure or treatment, your employer likely violated the PDA, and you should consider filing a complaint with the US Equal Employment Opportunity Commission (EEOC).

Patient Protection and Affordable Care Act (ACA)

The Patient Protection and Affordable Care Act (ACA) of 2010 requires employers to offer health insurance to their employees—but only if the company has more than fifty full-time employees. It also mandates certain health benefits as essential, meaning that they must be covered by health insurance policies. Unfortunately, infertility-related care is not among them.

In other words, infertility health insurance coverage has been left to the discretion of individual states and employers. See chapter 19 for tips about how to get the coverage you need.

Impact of Infertility at Work

Infertility is physically, mentally, emotionally, and financially exhausting—and it only makes sense that this exhaustion isn't limited to the time when you're not at work. In fact, we've all heard—and probably felt—that infertility can become a *second* full-time job.

Maria T. Rothenburger, a psychotherapist at Miracles Happen Fertility Center in Salem, Oregon, explains, "Between appointments and emotional factors inherent in infertility treatment, one's physical attendance and mental capacity in the workplace is likely to suffer. If one is not receiving medical treatment, mental health is often a factor contributing to difficulties in the workplace. Focus, concentration, and motivation are all negatively impacted by difficult medical conditions."

I was consumed by infertility—constantly in research and worry mode. My work situation

BUSTED

Myth: People at work will think I'm lazy if I keep taking time off for fertility treatment.

This is a big one. Many infertility warriors feel they have to share their story—because if they don't, missing work will appear to be slacking off. Even if they do want to tell their coworkers, they worry that their coworkers won't understand all that fertility treatments entail and will think they're making up excuses to avoid work.

Kate from Illinois had a supportive boss, but she was concerned about what her coworkers thought. "It was stressful for me to know my absence may have had an impact on my coworkers," she admits. "I worried my coworkers may think less of me for having to take time off for appointments or that I couldn't do 100 percent of my job."

Remember that infertility is a *medical condition*, and trust that your coworkers won't judge you any more than they would a colleague who needed to miss work for cancer treatments. Again, you don't have to tell them your exact medical condition, but most people will understand the need to leave work to address health issues.

Dr. Palmer-Wackerly suggests maintaining open lines of communication. "You may want to also recommend to your team that if they feel your absences are negatively affecting the team's performance, [they should] come talk to you so you can brainstorm solutions that can work for all. This way, resentment can hopefully be avoided," she advises.

was unique in that I owned my own business and had remote employees, so I was physically by myself all day long. While the environment allowed me to process bad—and good—news in the comfort of my own home without any onlookers, my employees and I were very close and in constant contact over the phone, text, and group chat. In fact, we "talked" more than any other group of people I've ever worked with! In other words, I still had social triggers—and you likely will, too, regardless of your position or workplace environment.

Dr. Rothenburger elaborates, "The social aspect of the workplace [can be] difficult to navigate, since others are invariably announcing new life milestones (weddings, pregnancies, births, etc.), which may serve to heighten the sense of isolation and feeling 'stuck.'"

Angela from Missouri has a daughter thanks to IVF, but she hasn't forgotten what it's like to battle infertility. "Our department had a baby shower for someone not on my team and everyone had to attend. I saw my teammate across the room with red eyes and blinking. She had her own infertility struggles. Before it was socially acceptable, I went across the room and got her out. The rest of our team followed like ducklings, unaware. I let my manager know privately why we left, and he was completely supportive."

Sharing Your Journey . . . or Not

Only you can decide whether or not to bring anyone at your workplace in on your infertility journey. This is one aspect over which *you* have control.

Dr. Palmer-Wackerly suggests that you "identify if infertility grief or infertility treatments are affecting your work performance—difficulty concentrating, crying, needing to take more breaks, calling in sick more often, late to meetings, missing important work-related events. If so, you may need to confide in your supervisor or a colleague."

She goes on to say it's important to weigh the advantages of telling against the possible outcomes. If disclosing will create more negative effects than positive, it might not be time to open up completely.

To determine if you're in a place where you will benefit from sharing your story, we can break down the process into four steps.

Step 1: Assess your workplace culture.

Do your coworkers, subordinates, and/or boss openly share personal information on a fairly regular basis? Or is everyone pretty private? If your workplace tends toward being open (what I call an open culture), you'll likely find a warm, welcoming, and supportive environment when sharing your story. If your workplace is more reserved (what I call a closed culture), you still might find support, but it likely will be more bureaucratic—for example, approving time off without wanting to know the details.

Step 2: Research company policies.

This is a boring but necessary step. Most workplaces have a human resources handbook. You likely received a copy on your first day but never read it. Get your hands on one now, and look up how the company handles medical conditions. Do you have a specific amount of sick leave hours or days? Are you able to work longer hours on some days in order to get time off on other days without touching that sick leave? Can you work remotely some days? Do you need permission to take sick leave? If so, whom should you inform? Keep in mind all of these questions as you read. The answers might give you more insight about whether you work in an open or closed culture. If after your research you're still not sure about your

How to Spot an Open vs. Closed Culture
• •

To help decide whether you work in an open or closed culture, here are some characteristics of each:

Open culture. At least some of your colleagues feel like family. You know their partners' names, birthdays, and so on. There's a lot of "water cooler talk"—the good kind, where people share what's going on in their lives. You and your colleagues would help each other out and fill in for each other no matter the situation—you've got each other's backs. Your boss tells you when you're doing a great job, and you have an overall good relationship.

Closed culture. For the most part, everyone keeps to themselves. You know nothing or next to nothing about your coworkers' personal lives. Success, promotion, and efficiency are valued over connection. Any "water cooler talk" is all workplace politics. You may not have coworkers you can rely on to help you out in a jam. Your interactions with your boss are infrequent, chilly, or just formal.

employer's sick leave policies, talk to your HR department, which must keep any medical information you disclose confidential.

"If your workplace does not seem supportive, you may want to talk to HR to see what options are available to you in terms of asking for accommodations," says Dr. Palmer-Wackerly.

Step 3: Determine how infertility will impact—or already has impacted—your job performance.

Be honest with yourself. Do you anticipate being out of work frequently and/or for an extended period of time? If so, can you still handle your current workload at the performance level your coworkers and boss have come to expect? Or will you need a colleague to help you manage everything and perhaps even start declining new assignments? Even in a closed culture, if this latter situation is more

accurate, you likely want to bring in at least one person—probably your boss—on your journey.

Fankhauser says that even if you can't give an advance list of every appointment date, you need to give notice if treatment will disrupt your workflow. "And I know that's tricky because sometimes the blood work and the monitoring with ultrasounds are 'Come back tomorrow' or 'We need you to come back in 2 more days.' But if you let them know in advance, 'I'm going to be undergoing an IVF cycle. This will require me to either be late or miss a little time to have these medical tests done during this procedure timeline,' that's giving them notice," she says.

Step 4: Check in with yourself.

At the end of the day, regardless of the workplace culture, company policies, and potential impact on your workplace performance, you might be paralyzed with anxiety about telling anyone—and that's okay. *You* are the final decision-maker. If you decide not to let anyone in, I would advise you to come back to these steps in a couple of months. Everyone is private about their journey . . . until they aren't. Your comfort level might change with time or circumstance.

Staying Private About Your Infertility

I f you've decided to keep your infertility journey to yourself or are undecided, this section is for you.

Cassandra Pratt, senior vice president of the HR department at Progyny, Inc., in New York, says, "Support during this time is incredibly important, especially since it can be an extremely isolating experience. But don't feel pressured that you need to disclose your fertility journey to someone at work."

She's exactly right. The choice is *yours*. However, there will come a point when you need to communicate *something*. After all, people will notice if you're routinely late for work—or take off for several hours during the middle of the day.

Pratt continues, "Remember, you don't need to share the details to have arrangements be made. It's important to be proactive at work and let your boss, coworkers, and team know about potential scheduling challenges, meeting attendance, or any other conflicts that may arise from your treatment. This will help your team plan in advance, adjust as needed, and support you appropriately during this time."

And that's it. If you're uncomfortable even discussing infertility as a vague "medical condition," don't lie—but don't offer more information than is necessary to maintain your workplace performance. As I always told my employees, as long as the work gets done, I'm happy. Hopefully your boss, coworkers, and subordinates will feel the same way.

Consulting with HR

Whether you are keeping your infertility journey private or being open about it at work, your HR department might be a good source of support. Beyond helping you decipher your health insurance benefits, HR staff can point you toward other company resources, such as an Employee Assistance Program (EAP) or other mental health benefits. "These services are completely confidential and can help you with different issues, including stress," explains Pratt.

Although it was not related to infertility, I once used my employer's EAP to connect with a social worker. I ended up seeing him weekly for therapy for the next 3 years—long after I left the company for another position. Our first six sessions were covered by my employer, and the rest were covered under my health insurance

policy. After more than 10 years of working in the career management and human resources industries, I can say with certainty that most people are unaware of all of their employee benefits. Ask, then take advantage of any resource available to you.

Creating a Workplace Strategy Around Infertility

Yes, it *is* possible to manage your workload while also going through fertility treatments! Let's talk strategy.

Step 1: Identify your allies.

Wouldn't it be nice to brainstorm with someone about balancing work and fertility treatments, taking time off, ways to lighten your workload, and so on? Or perhaps just to reduce the burden of carrying around the weight of this secret struggle by sharing it with someone else?

You likely need to let your boss (or HR) in about what's going on—vaguely, at a minimum. However, if you can identify the right person or people in your workplace who can become your ally, you'll feel more confident and supported leading up to that big conversation.

Dr. Rothenburger suggests asking yourself the following questions:

- Do I trust this person?

- Could disclosing my condition to them impact our work relationship? If so, in what way?

- Could disclosure impact my future at this company? If so, in what way?

If the answer to any of these questions reveals too much risk—whether about your medical situation specifically or about your personal life in general—then this person is not your ally.

Dr. Rothenburger shares her experience: "When I told one or two people at work what I was going through, I trusted them wholeheartedly. I asked them to not disclose this to other people before I did, and they honored that."

Your group of allies can be as big or small as you desire. *You are in control.*

Step 2: Determine when and for how long you'll need their support.

Talk to your reproductive endocrinologist about the foreseeable future—the current treatment plan, as well as the plan (or two) that might come into play if the current one fails. Keep in mind what you're able to pursue—financially, physically, and emotionally. I won't pull any punches—this will be a difficult step. It's hard to picture the worst-case scenario, especially when you're prepping for a conversation you may have been dreading for a while. But you need to have a solid sense of what you're asking of both your coworkers and your boss.

Once you have an idea of what the next 3 to 6 months might possibly look like, determine how much time off you'll actually need or want. At first glance, a timed intercourse cycle might require less time away from work than an IVF cycle, but what about scheduled mental health days to give yourself time to grieve? Or a day off with your partner to actually enjoy the timed intercourse and make it as spontaneous as possible? (Sex gets a lot less fun once doctors are involved!) If your clinic offers early morning monitoring (not all of them do), you can likely get away with a shifted schedule on those days rather than taking time off, but there's a lot of variability here depending on your workplace culture, company policies, and so on.

Pratt reminds us that doctor visits are not always "in and out" scenarios. "Add a grace period to make sure you're not consistently running late or missing meetings," she advises.

I'm a hard-core planner, so I would prefer mapping everything out on a calendar—probably with color codes for every aspect—but your method is up to you. Regardless, make sure you give yourself some wiggle room—create best-, middle-, and worst-case scenarios.

Step 3: Develop a productivity and time management plan.

Now you know how much time you'll need away from work, but what about how your time will be spent when you're at work? As I always told my employees, never come to me (your boss) with a problem (for example, needing time off to deal with infertility) without also having at least one suggestion for a solution (for example, a plan to reduce the impact of your time off on the company). The final solution might be one you and your boss develop together rather than exactly what you first propose, but the extra effort is appreciated. The same goes for approaching any coworkers you plan to ask for help.

When you're on the clock, your mind and energy should be spent on work. I know, I know—easier said than done. But setting an intention is a crucial first step. Dr. Rothenburger suggests that being productive might help you too. "If you are completely immersed and focused on whatever you are doing in the moment, it's going to help you cope with the roller coaster of emotions caused by infertility," she says.

There are many ways to go about this, but my favorite is to create a to-do list every evening for the following day. Break it up into tasks that (1) must be completed, (2) would be nice to complete, and (3) could be started if everything else gets wrapped up earlier than expected. Then, when you arrive at work in the morning, tackle the easiest must-complete tasks first. Checking one or two items off your list quickly will give you a boost of energy *and* prove to others that you're serious about keeping your head in the game.

Keep in mind, too, that you might have to get creative with your time. For example, several of my infertility coaching clients have to travel more than 90 minutes each way for doctor's appointments. Regardless of how early their clinics open, they often spend their mornings in their car rather than at work. Sound familiar? If you're able to work remotely, consider clocking in at a coffee shop or library—anything with reliable Wi-Fi—near your clinic. You can either put in your full day there or stay until commuter traffic dies down. If your role doesn't lend itself to remote computer work, consider scheduling calls while you're in the car on your way back to work. Just be sure you're hands-free and safe!

Pratt adds, "If you know you're a morning person, aim to work from home early before appointments—or at night, if it's better for you. Know when your most productive time is, and focus on key projects during that time. Often, people are able to accomplish more in the off hours when there are fewer distractions."

Tara and her husband, Sean, from Minnesota are currently going through fertility treatments. "I try to make my appointments early in the morning or after work so it disrupts my day the least amount as possible," she says, "but things like IUI are on a specific timetable, so that's the main struggle. Our clinic is also open Saturday morning, so I'll try to schedule at that time if possible."

If you have a partner, they also will require at least some time away from work—more if they want to attend routine appointments to support you. Elizabeth from California says, "[My husband and I] have a shared Google calendar so we can keep track of each other's schedules, which made it much easier to plan appointments around our work responsibilities."

Step 4: Develop a communication strategy.

Remember how your workplace can be open or closed? You can feel the same way—either in general or about this issue in particular. Even when you choose to bring others in, that doesn't mean you have to disclose *everything*. You'll likely want a strategy for each individual you plan to tell about your struggle with infertility.

Step 1: Consider your workplace culture and your internal assessment.

If your workplace has a closed culture, you likely want to keep details to a minimum across the board. If it's open, you may feel more free to share details.

As for your internal assessment, this is a gauge of how open *you* are. It's perfectly acceptable to work in an open culture while feeling closed yourself. You can share as much or as little as you'd like with each individual.

Step 2: Determine the best timing and location for the initial conversation.

Regardless of whether you yourself feel open or closed, Dr. Rothenburger advises beginning from a place of hope. "Infertility is fraught with seemingly endless hope-disappointment cycles. One would do well to begin disclosing to others when they are in the 'hope' part of a cycle."

Depending on the individual and your workplace, you may have to schedule a one-on-one meeting or just grab them at their desk or in the hallway during your break. Or you may prefer a lunch date outside the office so you don't run the risk of being overheard. Perhaps one or both of you work remotely, and thanks to the wonder of video calls, only your pets could possibly listen in. Choose whatever makes you most comfortable.

Step 3: Outline what you'll say.

Regardless of the individual, you may want to begin simply by saying you have a medical condition, and then use your best judgment in terms of adding more details. Be genuine and authentic—even vulnerable, if the situation calls for it.

When disclosing to your boss, give details on how it may impact your work. Then emphasize how much you value your job and explain the plan you've developed to address those impacts. If possible, end on a positive work-related note, such as an important task you just completed. If, based on company policy, you'll need a letter from your doctor(s) confirming your diagnosis, acquire that ahead of time.

When disclosing to a coworker or subordinate, keep in mind what you will be asking of them. If you're simply informing them you will be missing certain days or meetings, the conversation can be just that. If you're looking for emotional support, the conversation will likely be more detailed and intimate. If you're seeking workload support, the conversation should be solution-oriented—suggest at least one way you can work together to accomplish the work at hand, but be open to other options.

Pratt says, "Be transparent. Even if you aren't ready to discuss fertility treatments, let your team know you will have doctor commitments for 'X' period of time and what you will be doing to address the extra time out of [work]. Discussing expectations can save a lot of frustration down the road."

Again, as a planner, I would prefer to bring a notecard or piece of paper with bullet points to these conversations so I don't forget to mention anything important. I may not use it, but it's there if I need it. You, on the other hand, may prefer to just wing it.

Step 4: Prepare for all possible responses.
People can surprise you—negatively *and* positively.

Remember how supportive Jahsmyn's boss was in the story at the beginning of the chapter? That's a best-case scenario. But you should brace yourself for whatever might come up and the emotions you might feel. Try to stay poised and professional, if possible. Plan an escape route ahead of time, as well as a safe location where you can recover afterward.

Dr. Rothenburger admits that it's not possible to have prepared answers to *all* potential questions. However, she suggests having an answer that sets limits on questions you're not ready to answer. For example, she says, you could respond with "I'm not ready to talk about that just yet" or "I'm sorry, I don't have the answer to that yet" or "I'm not sure, but I'm working on it." She notes, "One may also consider rounding back to the impact on job performance. For example, 'I don't have the answer to that yet, and I don't believe it's likely to impact my job performance.'"

⚡ Similar to limits, it's important to set boundaries. Pratt advises telling your boss and allies up front if you do not want others to know about your infertility. Additionally, if you prefer that they don't ask questions—or prefer that they do—tell them. "Be honest about what you need during this time and let them know in the beginning," she says.

Step 5: Develop a self-care plan.
I saw an unattributed quote on Facebook that applies here: "You are not required to set yourself on fire to keep others warm." In other words, your job and workplace relationships are important, but *you* matter in this situation too. It's unavoidable: You're going to be physically and emotionally uncomfortable at work. Maybe not all of the time, but at least occasionally. Considering everything you've learned and planned to this point, develop a separate plan to care for *yourself*. This can include anything from 5-minute breaks throughout the day to spa treatments on the weekends—whatever helps you feel like you're not setting yourself on fire, so to speak.

Remember your pre-infertility hobbies? It took me a while to recall mine, but once I did, I incorporated 30 minutes of reading every night before bed. This helped me turn off my brain to my own troubles for the evening. One of my coaching clients gets up 15 minutes early every morning to meditate before starting her day. Another client goes golfing once a week with her girlfriends. The specific activity and timing depends on your situation, but don't skip this step.

Step 6: Execute.

Okay, it's that time! You can do this! You are prepared, and I believe in you.

Keeping Your Career on Track

Pratt says, "Infertility and fertility treatments can feel like a roller coaster, and your job can actually be the perfect distraction. So much of the process involves waiting. Your job can be a good way to occupy the space during the waiting periods when you don't have control over timing."

I completely agree! But I bet you're thinking, *Is it possible to be an exceptional employee (and/or coworker and/or boss) **and** beat infertility?* I'm here to tell you the answer is yes.

Be Aware of Limitations

Fertility medications—and the journey in general—can take a toll on you physically. Work around your body's schedule. Do you get headaches in the morning? Perhaps start your workday a little later. Are you exhausted in the middle of the day? Extend your lunch break a bit and take a walk. Does your brain start to fog in the late afternoon? Shift your work schedule earlier. Discuss it with your boss, of course, but many workplaces will accommodate employees to allow them to work when they are most productive—regardless of the reason they might be unproductive at certain times. After all, getting the work done well and on time is what really matters.

Your doctor will let you know if you'll be limited by any physical restrictions or precautions at any point in your cycle. If they will impact your work in any way, ask your doctor for a note and your workplace must accommodate. Alternatively, if you have the option, it never hurts to take some days off every once in a while!

⚡ Everyone has limitations. Learn to recognize yours. Take breaks. Ask for help when you need it. Now is not the time to set yourself on fire.

Follow Your Productivity, Time Management, and Self-Care Plans

You've hopefully already created these plans, as discussed earlier. Now it's just a matter of following them.

Pratt adds, "It's important to remember that you need to be mindful of your emotional health during the process. You should consider taking a few personal days when feeling particularly stressed. Your EQ (emotional quotient) is a critical part of how you perform at work, including initiative, decision-making ability, productivity, and surrounding employee morale. Being able to decompress during treatments is as important for your career as it is for yourself."

Speak Up When You Need to Change the Plan

Things happen and even the best-laid plans must change. It can be hard enough to navigate a change of course as an individual—but it can feel especially insurmountable if flexibility and adaptability are not part of your workplace culture.

⚡ But remember—if you need something, you have to advocate for yourself. Don't be afraid to ask for what you need.

Learn the Art of Letting Go

So . . . about all that planning you've done? Plans are an excellent foundation, but they should be fluid rather than etched in stone. Dr. Rothenburger offers some pointers on learning how to be more flexible and accepting during your journey:

Keep your dream and move easily toward it—don't barrel through obstacles on your way. Imagine a river flowing toward the ocean. Along the way, the banks guide the river, nudging it in different directions. The river never stops to fight against the banks—it just moves around them. Like self-advocacy, learning to let go when something doesn't go according to plan is a skill that takes practice. You'll likely begin by thinking "This river must run absolutely straight because that is the shortest distance between two points," but setting those expectations is hard on you, mentally and emotionally. So, with time and practice, acknowledge the banks and move smoothly around them.

Trust yourself. So much of this journey erodes trust. But when you trust yourself, you can react to obstacles with a state of calm rather than fear. There are times when you will feel like a gazelle being chased by a lion, but eventually you have to trust you're safe and stop running.

Set broad goals and let go of little expectations along the way. Rather than specific expectations (timelines, deadlines, etc.), set goals that allow you to be open to possibilities. Dr. Rothenburger's example is "I want to live a fulfilling life." She explains that when you let go of the little stuff, you begin to see more and bigger opportunities in your life. One of my coaching clients had a professional opportunity that would enhance her career, but the required work trip would set her IVF cycle timeline back by 2 weeks. When I suggested that she live her life and IVF would be waiting for her upon her return, she thought I was nuts—but went on the work trip anyway. Upon her return, she was renewed—she received a bonus, felt more confident than ever in the workplace, and completed her most successful IVF cycle ever shortly thereafter. Had she not let go of a little expectation—the exact start date of her IVF cycle—she never would have reaped those benefits.

Be Honest with Yourself and Others

Routinely check in with yourself and ask:

- Is my work performance suffering because of my infertility journey?

- Is my infertility journey suffering because of my dedication to my work?

- Are both suffering?

If the answer to any of these questions is yes, first recognize that this is a temporary situation for most people. Believe it or not, your infertility journey will not last forever. I've heard of people quitting their jobs or switching to part-time positions to focus on family-building. Although these are certainly options—nothing is off the table—don't feel pressured to make an extreme change. You can't do it all, but this doesn't need to be an all-or-nothing situation. Instead, consult your allies, speak with your boss, and perhaps even brainstorm with your reproductive endocrinologist. I believe you can come up with a solution that works for everyone.

One last thought from Dr. Rothenburger: "Know that you are doing the best you can in every single moment, even if you are laying in the fetal position bawling your eyes out. Even if you are so angry you cannot see straight. Remind yourself that you are normal, and you deserve ultimate compassion. When you come from that place internally, your workplace will respond in kind."

In this chapter we've focused on ways to get support at work, but for the most part, we talked about support that allows you to move forward with both your job and your infertility journey. There's a larger well of support that many infertility warriors get from people at work: emotional support.

Again, this isn't the best option for everyone. If all you need from your coworkers is to understand why you will be late to weekly morning meetings, that's fine. But if you feel safe trusting and leaning on your coworkers, take advantage of those relationships.

Identifying Your Needs

The last thing you want is to become fodder for the workplace rumor mill, so a big part of identifying your needs is defining the boundaries of who you want in the know. You might be okay with your best work buddy knowing but would rather that Karen in accounting didn't hear all the details of how you're trying to build a family.

If you're unsure of which coworkers you want to be in the loop, do a mental experiment. Imagine sitting at a table with each individual in question and talking about infertility with them. Pay attention to how that makes you feel. Does it make you anxious? Terrify you? Make you feel more relaxed? Trying out these situations will give you an idea of how you feel about the details spreading. Of course, make sure that whomever you do tell will respect your boundaries and wishes.

Communicating Your Needs

A big part of communicating your needs to coworkers is sharing your triggers. Depending on how well you've kept your emotions in check while at work, they may have no clue what sends you over the edge. They probably have no idea what comments *(It'll happen when you relax!)* or questions *(Why don't you just adopt?)* sting. Make this part of your conversation when you first talk about your infertility.

If you haven't shared all the details of your journey, it's okay to speak in generalities. You don't have to say something as specific as "That stresses me out because it reminds me of my miscarriage." You can instead say something more general, like "Infertility is complicated, and many people in the community are hurt by comments others see as harmless."

WARRIOR WISDOM
Being Open to Another Layer of Support

"Be as honest as you're comfortable with. I find the support of coworkers and my manager to be beneficial, but I'm an open book in many aspects of my life. And as more people are sharing their struggles of infertility, it helps others understand how common this is—and can maybe change your employer's benefit package!"

—Tara, Minnesota

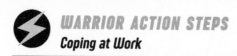

WARRIOR ACTION STEPS
Coping at Work

Be patient and forgiving with yourself when you're dealing with your career *and* infertility. This is a process, and no one figures it out overnight. To help you cope, be sure to:

Have a support code word. Emotions pop up, and sometimes you need a moment in the middle of the workday to deal. Have a code word you share with people to let them know you need to step away. Just be clear what your code word means. Is it a signal to your manager that you're not being disrespectful but need to step out of a meeting? Or is it a signal to your best work friend that they need to meet you in the bathroom with some tissues?

Celebrate your accomplishments. Many infertility warriors think that because they were able to get projects done on time or meet company goals before infertility, it shouldn't be a big deal when they continue to do it *after* being diagnosed. But it is. In a sense, you're relearning how to effectively do your job, so pat yourself on the back when you accomplish something, no matter how small.

Own up to your mistakes. If you mess up because you're distracted, don't try to sweep it under the rug. Remember that the goal is to be a great employee, not a perfect one. Avoiding your mistakes means denying a chance to learn and grow professionally. Be honest—you know that if you don't admit you made a mistake, it's going to create an extra layer of guilt you don't need. It might be tough in the moment, but addressing your work whoopsies now will allow you to move on more quickly.

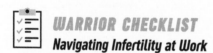

WARRIOR CHECKLIST
Navigating Infertility at Work

❑ As an employee battling infertility, understand your rights in the workplace.

❑ Understand how infertility might impact you in the workplace.

❑ Determine who in your workplace you want to know about your journey and to what degree you'll share details.

❑ Develop solutions for how you'll manage stress, time, and your workload—and when necessary, communicate the support you need from others.

❑ Recognize that you don't have to choose between building a family and building your career; there are ways to achieve balance.

❑ Find ways to cope with the emotional aspects of infertility in the workplace.

Add more items to your Warrior Checklist or jot down any notes here:

_____

_____

_____

_____

Navigating Infertility in the Military

CHAPTER 22

THE MILITARY COMMUNITY TELLS me that family-building in the face of infertility can be particularly isolating for service members. Your journey is distinct from that of other military members *and* from that of other infertility warriors, which is why I devote an entire chapter to your unique experience.

New Yorkers Jalina and Anthony got married in 2011. By 2013, they were ready to start building their family. Anthony, a sergeant in the US Marine Corps, was due to deploy in 6 months. They expected to get pregnant quickly, but when it was time for Anthony to deploy, Jalina still wasn't pregnant.

"We were surprised to not conceive before he left but were hopeful we would conceive shortly after his return," she says. "After his homecoming in April 2014, there was another 6 months of trying to conceive with no success."

During Jalina's annual visit to her ob-gyn, she mentioned they were having trouble getting pregnant. The doctor ran a basic fertility workup and diagnosed Anthony with male factor infertility. They decided the best plan for them was to focus on a natural approach of eating healthy whole foods, taking supplements, and eliminating toxins from their home. Jalina also used Softdisc menstrual cups after intercourse; she'd read success stories about how they could increase the odds of pregnancy. In May 2015, Jalina found out she was pregnant, but she miscarried at 7 weeks. Devastated, they decided to take a break.

The entire situation put a strain on their relationship. "Overall, navigating infertility while my husband was in the military was isolating and emotionally draining. I assumed my husband was young, fit, and fertile and was surprised when his fertility proved unrelated to his outward physical health," Jalina shares. "The pressure of infertility and Anthony unexpectedly not being allowed to reenlist at the end of his 6-year contract emasculated him and nearly destroyed our marriage."

Eventually they did get pregnant again, and their son was born in August 2016. Ten months later, they decided to try for a second child. Once again they conceived but miscarried, this time at 4 weeks.

They decided to try again immediately, and within a month, Jalina was pregnant. During this pregnancy, she was diagnosed with the MTHFR gene mutation and antiphospholipid syndrome, which can cause blood clots and miscarriage. Their second son was born in May 2018, and, in January 2019, they were surprised to learn they had conceived spontaneously.

Being an Infertility Warrior in the Military Community

First, thank you for your service and sacrifice. To add an infertility journey on top of that is truly heroic.

A 2018 report from Service Women's Action Network found that 37 percent of military women have difficulty conceiving. A 2018 study published in *Translational Andrology and Urology* reported that 43.5 percent of male veterans have infertility issues.

In this chapter, we're going to dig into the realities of being in the military community while dealing with infertility. And to be honest, it's not easy. Everything from deployed spouses to the impenetrable bureaucracy of

---

BUSTED

Myth: Soldiers are strong, virile, and fertile.

Servicemen and servicewomen are in peak physical condition. They go through grueling training. They fight wars, for Pete's sake. How could the best of the best not be fertile baby-making machines?

Jennifer, a military wife based out of California, says that thanks to a high dose of machismo, there's a misconception that men in the military "should be impregnating their spouses with just a look."

When servicemen and servicewomen struggle to conceive, it challenges this preconceived notion of super-strength. Many members of the military community don't feel comfortable disclosing their fertility struggles.

The truth is infertility *does* strike in the military community—just like in any other group. Fertility has nothing to do with strength.

---

the military health-care system complicates matters. But hopefully, with the stories of and guidance from your fellow service members, this chapter will help smooth your journey.

The Good, the Bad, and the Ugly

As with any journey, there are highs and lows when you're dealing with infertility. Knowing what those are for the military community will help you make the most of the good times while preparing for the tough times.

The Good

For all the challenges that come along with being part of the military community, there's a big benefit too: the bond that forms between servicemen and women and their families. The strength of those relationships can be invaluable during your infertility journey.

"The military really is a family you choose," says Jennifer. Her husband, Ryan, a lieutenant colonel in the US Air Force, was deployed while she was pregnant, but the members of her community stepped up. "When I had complications during the pregnancy, it was my military family that was in the doctor's office holding my hand. When our daughter was born, it was once again my military family that was there, holding my hand, supporting us, and even taking pictures of the moment our daughter entered the world via emergency C-section."

Even if those around you don't understand your struggle with infertility, they will get how difficult it can be to have your partner away during big life moments. Lean into that support, and you'll be surprised how powerful it is to feel that kind of love.

And while their absence is hard, their return can be one of the best ways to deal with the pressures of infertility. "Being in a cycle of my husband leaving for training and deployments and then coming home greatly enhanced our sex life," says Jalina. "It often took the pressure off trying to conceive. There's nothing that takes your mind off infertility like homecoming sex."

The Bad

Moving around as frequently as military families do can put a big snag in your infertility journey. Every time you're transferred to a new base, you have to find new doctors, get on new waitlists, and possibly start over with certain treatments. And because every doctor approaches infertility cases differently, you can end up with conflicting opinions and messages.

"Continuity of care is challenging. When working with medical providers, it is important that military families not only identify themselves as military families, but also point out exactly what that means: how long they think they will be in the area before the next permanent change of station and when the service member is likely to be gone for deployments, training, etc. This may impact the treatment plan," says Karen Ruedisueli, government relations deputy director of the National Military Family Association in Alexandria, Virginia.

Jane* was splitting her time between Oklahoma, where her husband was stationed, and her job in Michigan. Her doctor in Oklahoma wanted to perform diagnostic surgery, but that meant she would be in recovery—and unable to conceive—during the last few months before her husband's deployment.

Jane flew back to Michigan to see her former ob-gyn and ask his advice. "He suggested trying Clomid for a couple of months and, if it didn't work, we would have an entire year while my husband was deployed to run every diagnostic test imaginable." Opting for that route, she found out she was pregnant right before her husband deployed.

For some infertility warriors, one big hurdle is a lack of options when it comes to nearby

treatment centers. Many military bases are in secluded, rural areas and the top fertility doctors are rarely close by.

After waiting for months to see a doctor at a military treatment facility about her troubles conceiving, Jennifer was referred to the closest reproductive endocrinologist . . . who was 4 hours away. She and her husband both had to take a full day off work just for a simple consultation.

The endocrinologist then told them he was only willing to do IUI with fresh sperm and working around the female patient's natural cycle. "That meant that we would both have to drop everything when my body clock rang the alarm and take an entire day off work," explains Jennifer. The Air Force was not exactly understanding about that prospective schedule—or rather, the unpredictability of it—and so, as Jennifer puts it, "that spelled the end of the road for us."

The Ugly

Understandably, one of the hardest parts for couples facing infertility while in the military is the long separations. This often leaves couples with two not-so-desirable options: pausing the effort to conceive or having one of the partners carry on alone.

Jalina and her husband chose the first option. "For me, the worst part of going through infertility while being married to a military member was not even being able to try during certain months while he was gone for training or deployments," she says.

Mary and her husband, Wes, a Navy fighter pilot, went with the second option, which meant that Mary was forced to take on the burdens and stress of fertility treatments while Wes was thousands of miles away. "I often had to go through treatments on my own. Or I had to make arrangements to make sure things would work while Wes was gone. For example, freezing his sperm prior to his departure with

Name has been changed.

the military so we could complete a round of IVF while he was away."

Wendy from Virginia, who is married to a US Navy SEAL, points out another difficult consequence of long separations: If you *do* get pregnant via fertility treatments while your spouse is deployed, you either have to explain your struggles to conceive to everyone or let whispered rumors of whose baby you're carrying follow you around the base. As a result, many infertility warriors in the military community decide to do IUI and IVF cycles only when their spouses are on base.

"People don't always know that you're going through fertility treatments," says Wendy. "So there's the rumor mill and all that stuff. And I think that might be why people are uncomfortable [doing treatments] when a spouse is deployed."

And then there is the matter of the frequent moves. Military families are used to moving, but when you are an infertility warrior, there are extra complications to consider: transporting frozen eggs, sperm, and embryos. While this is safe in most cases, it's not a perfect system.

Kerry, a former member of the US Coast Guard and current volunteer for the Service Women's Action Network (SWAN) located in San Leandro, California, needed to ship her embryos from California to Virginia, and the embryologist failed to properly seal the container. During shipping, the glass straws holding the embryos vibrated so much they broke, and her embryos were lost.

"The package wasn't damaged, so the shipping company denied any responsibility and the clinic that packed them would not take any responsibility. Insurance wouldn't cover it for property damage and we were left with nothing but the prospects of having do to at least another treatment to replace what we lost," she says. In the end, she had to go through two more egg retrievals before she and her husband had any new embryos.

If you have to transport frozen eggs, sperm, or embryos, Kerry recommends the following:

• Ask beforehand if the clinic or storage facility uses glass or plastic straws for transport.

• Learn about their packing process and success rates.

• Find out if the clinic and the shipping company have insurance or accept liability in the event that your eggs, sperm, or embryos do not safely reach their destination.

Active Duty

Real talk time: It's not easy undergoing fertility treatments when you or a partner are active duty. First, there are inherent challenges that come with a military career. Deployments, frequent relocations, and the lack of treatment center choices make it hard to create and stick to a plan of action.

Then there's the health-care system in place for the military community. As with any large bureaucracy, there are waitlists, a lack of flexibility, and behind-the-times processes. Because infertility is different for every individual, the established military health-care systems don't fit every person's needs.

Let's try to make sense of the situation.

TRICARE

If members of the military community need medical care outside of the military health system, TRICARE provides insurance coverage. However, TRICARE doesn't currently cover assisted reproductive technology procedures like IUI or IVF. So, if you choose one of these treatment options through a civilian fertility doctor, you will have to pay out of pocket.

TRICARE does cover some testing and medication related to infertility, especially if your infertility is a result of an active-duty injury.

BUSTED

Myth: The military will cover everything.

The military takes care of its own. And many families are grateful, especially for the free health care extended to active-duty military and family members. Just one problem: TRICARE doesn't currently cover fertility treatments.

"TRICARE insurance is just like any other insurance in that certain things are excluded, and anything surrounding infertility falls into the excluded category," explains Jennifer.

Even if you are stationed in a state that mandates infertility coverage, TRICARE will not pay for most fertility treatments. "TRICARE is not subject to state laws," says Ruedisueli. "The only infertility treatment policy exception is related to service members who lost their natural reproductive ability due to a serious injury or illness while on active duty."

Ruedisueli says it's important to remember that coverage is often based on medical necessity. For example, Wendy was diagnosed with endometriosis before struggling with infertility. Her doctor performed ultrasounds and other procedures to treat her endometriosis, and TRICARE paid for them. But at the same time, those procedures provided information about and treatment for Wendy's infertility.

"There are many nuances to a TRICARE policy and what was true for your neighbor may not be true for you," explains Ruedisueli. "For most families, TRICARE coverage for infertility treatment is limited."

Find a complete list of what TRICARE does and doesn't cover at tricare.mil.

Military Treatment Facilities

Even though TRICARE does not cover many fertility-related procedures, there are military treatment facilities (MTFs) that perform those treatments.

However, Ruedisueli explains, "the [military health system] runs infertility treatment programs at select military hospitals to support the graduate medical education of uniformed medical personnel." In other words, the main purpose of these clinics is to provide practice for service members seeking medical degrees, and the treatment of infertility is just a by-product.

Even so, military families who live near these installations may be able to access IVF at significantly reduced costs. Ruedisueli also recommends members of the military community check with their MTF pharmacy to see if they can get free medications related to infertility that TRICARE won't cover.

Unfortunately, there isn't one resource that lays out the details of all MTF IVF programs, so let's go through some of the MTFs that currently perform assisted reproductive technology procedures. (Note that information about these medical centers and the services they provide are subject to change.)

Brooke Army Medical Center, Houston, Texas

Brooke Army Medical Center is a member of the Society for Assisted Reproductive Technology (SART). It is a full-service clinic through a partnership with the Fertility Center of San Antonio.

In 2020, according to SART, Brooke Army Medical Center performed 138 IVF retrieval cycles. Of the 138 cycles, for patients under 35, 26.7 percent resulted in live births. For patients between 35 and 37, 38.5 percent resulted in live births, and for patients between 38 and 40, 21.4 percent resulted in live births.

Madigan Army Medical Center, Tacoma, Washington

Madigan Army Medical Center's obstetrics and gynecology department addresses issues surrounding infertility and recurrent pregnancy loss. The urology department treats issues related to male factor infertility.

Some of the services this MFT provides include:

- Reproductive endocrinology testing and treatments for endometriosis, polyps, uterine scarring, and ovary and fallopian tube disorders

- IUI

- IVF with ICSI

- Hormonal evaluation

- Vasectomy reversal

- Varicocele repair

- Testicular biopsy

- Infertility-related counseling

SART data says that in 2020, Madigan Army Medical Center performed 129 rounds of IVF. For patients under 35, 29.6 percent resulted in live births. For patients between 35 and 37, 10.5 percent of cycles resulted in live births, and for patients between 38 and 40, 3.8 percent resulted in live births.

Tripler Army Medical Center, Honolulu, Hawaii

The Tripler Army Medical Center includes a SART fertility clinic that works out of the obstetrics and gynecology department, so it treats mainly female patients. Some of its services are:

- Fertility workups

- Genetic testing of embryos (PGT-A)

- IUI

- IVF with ICSI

According to SART, Tripler Army Medical Center performed 260 IVF cycles total in 2020. For patients under 35, 25 percent resulted in live births. For patients between 35 and 37, 17.6 percent resulted in live births, and for patients between 38 and 40, 8.3 percent resulted in live births.

WARRIOR TIPS
Protecting Your Fertility During a Deployment

At the risk of being called Captain Obvious, let me point out that being in the military can be dangerous. A service-related injury or exposure can negatively affect fertility.

Being on active duty can put you in contact with materials that could negatively impact your fertility. When possible, avoid or limit your exposure to:

- Benzene fuels

- Pesticides

- Asbestos

- Heavy metals like lead or arsenic

- Radioactive materials

You can guard against that possibility by having the following procedures *before a deployment:*

Sperm cryopreservation. Sperm can be frozen and stored by a fertility center or cryopreservation storage facility. Just check their policies on shipping samples in case you're reassigned to another base.

Egg cryopreservation. While it's a more involved and expensive process, eggs can be retrieved and frozen for later fertilization and transfer. Remember that younger eggs (typically) mean better embryo health. The age at which you retrieve your eggs is actually more influential than your age at transfer.

Walter Reed National Military Medical Center, Bethesda, Maryland

Walter Reed is affiliated with the ART Institute of Washington and works with that staff to provide the following services:

- Cryopreservation of eggs and embryos

- Genetic testing of embryos (PGT-A, PGT-M, PGT-SR)

- IUI

- IVF with ICSI

The fertility clinic affiliated with Walter Reed performs more procedures than other MTF facilities. In 2020, according to SART, the ART Institute of Washington completed 574 IVF cycles. For patients under 35, 42.5 percent resulted in live births. For ages 35 to 37, 20 percent of cycles were successful, and 10.4 percent for ages 38 to 40.

Private (Civilian) Clinics

While MTFs are certainly a more affordable way to get fertility treatments, many members of the military community choose to go to a private clinic because of their location or long waitlists at MTFs.

Mary and Wes decided to use a private clinic because there was a 3-year wait at their MTF.

"A 3-year wait would have been too long for my case, and we likely would've never had children at all," Mary explains. "My fertility was rapidly declining, and once diagnosed with diminished ovarian reserve, I needed IVF ASAP."

There's information on choosing a fertility clinic in chapter 2, but it is important to note an extra consideration for members of the military community: time and location. Private clinics aren't always familiar with the military lifestyle, so they may not consider that a patient or a partner might be deployed during a treatment. Not only does that take different planning, but also it requires being able to support a patient who's going through the process alone.

That said, private clinics welcome members of the military community and some may offer discounts.

WARRIOR WISDOM
Advocating for Better Options

We've talked a lot about how infertility takes away a sense of control over your own life. That loss can feel even more pronounced for members of the military community, who often have no say over where they are stationed and how that impacts their ability to receive timely, quality treatment.

"I felt I was stuck going to fertility clinics where I was stationed and not necessarily to the best clinics for me and in the end, I regretted using their services," says Kerry. "Your resources are finite, so don't waste them on a clinic, doctor, or fertility treatment that you are not 100 percent sure is on board with your goal of getting pregnant and having a healthy baby."

While it will take action and advocacy, it's important to start a conversation about improving servicemen and women's access to fertility treatment. As you can see in chapters 21 and 27, one of the best ways to achieve change is to share your story and ask for what you deserve.

Adoption

Sometimes adoption is the right choice for infertility warriors in the military community. In many ways, the process is the same as it is for non-military prospective parents (see chapter 12). But there are a few concerns specific to members of the military:

What if my partner is deployed? The adoption process will continue even if your partner is out of the country. However, it is important for them to sign a power of attorney document that gives you the authority to serve as their legal representative.

What if we move to another state? If there's any possibility of you or a partner being transferred, choose an adoption agency or attorney who can work in multiple states. Otherwise, you will have to start over completely when you move. Also, if you've already been through the home study in one state, it will have to be updated to ensure you still meet all the requirements for your new home state. Depending on differences in state laws, your attorney might have to update legal documents.

Are military families more likely to be turned down? When it comes to being evaluated as potential adoptive parents, being in the military shouldn't matter. Social workers and adoption agencies want only a safe and loving home for the child. Birth mothers do have more discretion, and some may not want their child to go to a military home. But many love the values and lifestyle you can provide for their child.

Benefits, Reimbursement, and Leave

The military tries to be as supportive as possible for adoptive parents. There are policies and benefits in place to accommodate your journey. Members of the military are eligible for the following:

Reimbursement for adoption expenses. As of this writing, the Department of Defense will reimburse up to $2,000 for qualifying adoptions. If both you and your spouse are in the service, only one can apply. You have up to a year after the adoption is finalized to apply.

Adoption tax benefits. Like civilian adoptive parents, members of the military community can receive over $14,000 in tax credit based on adoption fees, court costs, and travel expenses.

Deployment deferrals and extensions of assignments. If you adopt your child from a different state, it takes time for paperwork to go through. In most cases, commanders will approve deployment deferrals or extend assignments to ensure you can be with your child while the paperwork is processed.

Parental leave. All branches of the military offer some form of parental leave for adoptive parents. For the primary caretaker, it's up to 42 days. For a secondary caregiver, it's 14 days in the Navy and Marine Corps and 21 days in the Army and Air Force.

Health care for your child. Even after you bring your child home, the adoption won't be finalized immediately. The military will extend health-care benefits to your child from the moment the child is in your care, rather than after finalization of the adoption.

Veterans

Crystal from Colorado describes what it's like to deal with infertility as a veteran or partner of a veteran: "Navigating infertility related to my husband's service-connected injury has been anything but easy. We had so many questions when we first started and no one or nowhere to seek answers after his medical discharge."

She explains that she and her husband, Tyler, a medically retired corporal in the US Army, advocated for change because, until recently, there was little coverage for veterans. "Historically, you were only provided access to care when you are active duty, and once you were discharged, you were left to fend for yourself. Now, there is temporary coverage available for service-connected infertility post-discharge, but the system you have to work within is so broken."

So, what are your options for infertility treatment after military service?

If your infertility isn't due to a service injury, there aren't many. The Department of Veterans Affairs (VA) covers assisted reproductive technology and other infertility-related services, but not everyone qualifies. The requirements are:

- Having infertility because of a service-related injury

- Being in a legal marriage

- The veteran or partner can produce sperm

- The veteran or partner can produce eggs and has an intact uterus

If you don't meet those criteria, you will likely have to pay for the majority of any assisted reproductive technology treatments out of pocket. The VA offers reimbursement of costs for adoptions by veterans that were finalized after September 29, 2016, and were made necessary by a service-related injury that caused infertility.

WARRIOR TIPS
Becoming an Advocate for Change
....

In enormous organizations like the military, change comes slowly. But people being willing to speak up and shine a light on issues can get the ball rolling. Some organizations are working to better support members of the military in communicating about and overcoming infertility. Consider becoming an advocate in the following ways:

- Joining RESOLVE's #IVF4Vets campaign

- Joining Service Women's Action Network (SWAN)

- Writing to your representatives about current veteran infertility legislation (see chapter 27)

Affording Family-Building

You can review chapter 20 for a more in-depth review of infertility financing options, but there are a few additional opportunities for members of the military community. And as Mary explains, even small discounts add up: "My husband is a fighter pilot in the US Navy. We were sure to ask for military discounts anywhere and everywhere we could. Our surrogacy agency, attorney, and psychologist all gave us a military discounted price for their services. While it doesn't seem like much individually, we did end up saving about $2,500 with these discounts."

Financial Assistance for Members of the Military Community

Depending on your situation, there are many grants, scholarships, and fertility clinic or medication discounts available to both active-duty and veteran members of the military community. This is by no means a complete list, but a few current opportunities are:

Compassionate Corps. If you are a veteran with service-related infertility, or the spouse of one, and your insurance does not cover fertility medication, the Compassionate Corps program by prescription drugmaker EMD Serono may cover the costs of your medicine. Your doctor will need to verify your infertility and that IVF or other assisted reproductive technology procedures are right for you.

Heart for Heroes. This program, from MDR Fertility Pharmacy, provides certain fertility medications to class 2 or 3 veterans. You must have a service-related injury causing infertility, have no insurance coverage for IVF medication, and live in the United States.

Veterans In Vitro InitiAtive (VIVA). VIVA offers up to $5,000 to veterans with service-related infertility issues who do not qualify for VA assistance. IVF has to be an option for you, and your fertility clinic needs to be SART approved. Veterans who are excluded from VA assistance because they are not married, are in a marriage that is not legally recognized, or require egg or sperm donation are eligible through VIVA.

For more information, RESOLVE, CoFertility, and FertilityIQ keep a current list of grants, charities, and clinics that offer financial support for the military community.

BUSTED

Myth: I need to suffer in silence.

Many members of the military community believe they can't share their struggles. Infertility is particularly taboo, and as a result, it can be easy to believe no one else is going through anything similar. When you live on a military base, it can seem like there are children everywhere and everyone is pregnant.

In Marjorie's small Canadian military community, there were six pregnancies in 18 months. Still, those in her community were there for Marjorie when she finally talked about her struggles. "I had so much more support than I had ever expected," she says. "It also allowed a lot of other people to tell me their stories, and I was surprised I wasn't so alone."

Military and Infertility Dos and Don'ts

Given the uniqueness of the infertility experience for members of the military community, it's essential to get as much guidance as possible.

Do share your story.

Your first instinct might be to keep your struggle a secret, but Kate, a veteran of the US Army from Illinois, says that doing so cuts you off from much-needed support. Although Kate's infertility journey began after she left the military, she still reached out to her military family.

"I've shared my infertility struggles with some of them, and they're always willing to lend an ear," she says. "The bond of military personnel is a gift, especially through this season. You come to realize who you can really trust as a friend."

Kate also advises not hiding how infertility is impacting you physically. "Be open and honest. Your chain of command needs to know what your limits are. Have your doctor give you notes for light duty because the military always appreciates a paper trail."

Don't assume anything about other families.

It's tempting to be envious of how easy fertile families have it. Jalina says it's not uncommon to be surrounded by mothers and their young children, which can be triggering for those battling infertility.

"Do not compare yourself to these women," says Jalina. "As with any family, you can never know at a glance what these women have gone through or are still going through to build their family. We all have our own struggles no one else can see."

Some of these neighbors might have gone through similar situations you now find yourself in. Being envious or judgmental of them only causes you pain and prevents you from making a meaningful connection with others in your community.

Do ask for recommendations.

It's frustrating to put your fertility treatments on hold every time you move. You have to start researching your options all over again, leading to gaps in your efforts to conceive. Luckily, the military community is really good at word-of-mouth endorsements.

"Military families are great at providing advice and recommendations to each other," says Ruedisueli. "This is how many of us find the best schools, restaurants, and doctors at a new duty station."

After you arrive on base and get to know other members of the military community, reach out to fellow infertility warriors. However, Ruedisueli advises, don't rely on information your new neighbors have about TRICARE. Remember that TRICARE coverage is highly dependent on your unique medical situation.

Don't take no for an answer.

Unfortunately, there are a lot of hoops to jump through when it comes to the military and infertility treatment. But you're not completely at the mercy of military doctors and facilities. Don't be afraid to explore different avenues or push for the treatments that are right for you.

"Never give up hope or stop trying; You have provided an honorable service to our country; tell your story! Make sure not to let the VA tell you no," says Crystal.

Remember to advocate for yourself and continue your search for information about and access to the treatments right for you.

Kelly from California says says it's important to remember the only person who has your best interests at heart is you. "It is on you, the patient, to research the care you want to receive and then to actively request and advocate for those services," she explains. "Even though infertility is a time-sensitive condition, it is not treated with any kind of urgency. It will be on the member to stay on top of referrals, processing of paperwork, obtaining meds, and ensuring timely appointments are made with their medical provider."

As Crystal puts it, "It is a pain to navigate [the system] sometimes, but in the end, your family is worth the struggle."

Being a member of the military community is tough enough. Mix in infertility, and even the strongest and bravest need help. And you deserve support. But the first step to coping is being able to understand and address your needs.

Identifying Your Needs

I offer tips and tricks for identifying your needs in-depth in Part 3. As a member of the military community, you can absolutely use those every day. But if you are part of a couple, then you and your partner face one challenge unique to your situation: deployment. Whether it's you or your partner who's serving—or both of you—when you're apart from each other for months at a time, your needs may be neglected, so plan ahead.

Think about all the ways your partner makes your infertility journey more bearable. How do they calm your anxieties? What do they do to make sure you're not letting infertility define your life? How does your shared communication style help you work through your emotions? Use these answers to determine what you'll need to feel supported during deployments. After all, being alone while you or your partner is deployed may on its own make you feel isolated. Adding the extra stress of taking on infertility alone may intensify those feelings—and add new ones.

Communicating Your Needs

For people whose lives are built around sacrifice, it's not easy to ask for help. But as we established in the beginning of this chapter, you do *not* have to suffer in silence. Chances are when you ask others for support, they won't hesitate or ask questions before stepping up. Just be clear about your boundaries with regard to who you want knowing about your infertility journey. The military community is small, and it may be necessary to draw a line when it comes to your privacy.

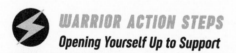

WARRIOR ACTION STEPS
Opening Yourself Up to Support

As a serviceman or woman or their partner, you have a lot on your plate. Adding more to that to-do list seems counterintuitive, but taking these small steps will help make your infertility journey more manageable:

Admit that you are not superheroes. Members of the military community are incredible. But you are not impervious to pain. When you're with loved ones, let down your guard and find ways to be vulnerable.

Establish communication plans. The people in your support network likely are all over the globe. During your infertility journey, reach out to those you need to lean on and agree on a check-in schedule. Even if they aren't dealing with the same issues, there's probably something in their lives they've been dying to vent to you about.

Speak up. Infertility may still be a taboo topic within your military community, making the journey that much harder. Find ways to share your story or educate others about the challenges infertility warriors face. This will open the door for a discussion about changes that can help you and others.

$\rightarrow$

WARRIOR WISDOM
Having Support Through Thick and Thin

"Being surrounded by military spouses within our community who often support one another through thick and thin was an advantage of walking the journey of infertility while in the military." —Mary, Rhode Island

 ## WARRIOR CHECKLIST
Navigating Infertility in the Military

❑ Let go of any preconceived notions about what it means to be a member of the military community *and* an infertility warrior.

❑ Be aware of the unique highs and lows of your infertility journey.

❑ Understand and explore the options available to you both within the military and outside it.

❑ Research the financial assistance programs that are available to active-duty and veteran servicemen and women.

❑ Learn from the wisdom of other infertility warriors in the military community.

❑ Lean on others in your support network during your fertility treatments and when your partner is far away.

Add more items to your Warrior Checklist or jot down any notes here:

_____

_____

_____

_____

_____

_____

_____

_____

_____

_____

_____

_____

_____

_____

_____

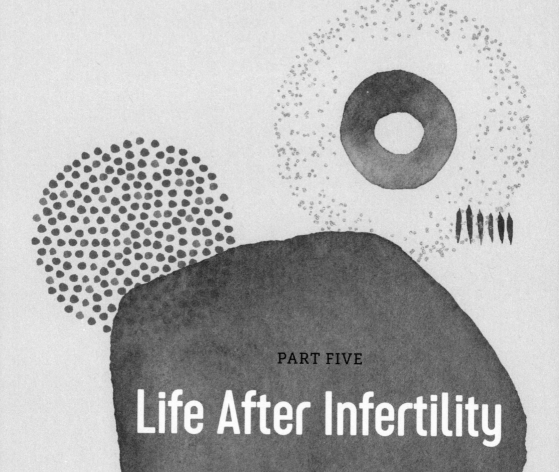

PART FIVE

Life After Infertility

Pregnancy After Infertility

I SWITCHED OB-GYN PRACTICES when I was pregnant with Aurora. Staying with the obstetrician who had delivered my stillborn twins stirred up too many painful memories. I found a practice that appeared to be a middle ground between standard and high-risk ob-gyns.

I was randomly assigned to a doctor, but as luck would (finally) have it, he was amazing. While I sat across the desk from him in his office, I voiced every concern I felt I'd have during the pregnancy—and he listened intently and took detailed notes. We had a quick peek at the fetus and the staff drew my blood for a noninvasive prenatal testing (NIPT), a genetic risk factor test.

Other than severe morning sickness (more like all-day sickness), everything went well for the next couple of weeks. At 12.5 weeks, I received an email from my doctor at around 8:30 a.m. "Genetics were normal. It's a girl." I'd somehow known it was a girl the entire time. We had referred to her as Aurora ever since our heartbeat confirmation ultrasound. But now it was official! Off to Facebook I went to share the good news.

Fast-forward to 3 hours later. I got up from my chair to make some lunch. As I entered the kitchen, I felt a rush of liquid streaming down my legs. I was covered in blood—and it just kept coming. I headed to the bathroom, leaving a trail of blood behind me. As I tried to sit on the toilet, I left a bloody handprint on the wall. To an outsider, it might have looked like a murder scene. I frantically called my husband and told him I was miscarrying—I needed him home NOW.

My next call was to my friend Dr. Allison K. Rodgers, a reproductive endocrinologist with Fertility Centers of Illinois in Chicago. She advised me to call my ob-gyn and head there as soon as possible. She was encouraged that I wasn't in any pain but also hedged that it was very possible I was miscarrying—and for the first time on our journey, she said surrogacy might be our next best step if that was the case.

The bleeding turned out to be a subchorionic hematoma—the second largest one anyone in my ob-gyn's office had ever seen—but the fetus was alive and well. I bled heavily for the next 10 weeks and finally got a break from the combined drama of the hematoma and morning sickness at around 22 weeks. It was a blissful 2 weeks until our next complication. At our 24-week appointment— viability!—we learned she was no longer growing as expected.

The rest of my pregnancy was fraught with worry. I began seeing both my ob-gyn and a maternal fetal medicine (MFM) practitioner once a week. They'd confer about whether Aurora was safer inside or outside my body. Although her growth continued to slow, all tests continued coming back normal—they could not determine a cause.

At my 33-week appointment, it was once again determined that in was better than out. However, that was the last time I felt Aurora move. After 36 hours of no movement, I called the emergency line at 3 a.m. and explained the situation. The ob-gyn on call told me not to come to the hospital. I told her, "Get ready, I'm coming in anyway."

We arrived at 6 a.m. (Our hospital was extremely far away from us in Washington, DC, and the city was recovering from the largest snowstorm it had seen in quite some time.) Within 5 minutes of being hooked up to the monitoring machines, I was in labor. Aurora wanted out. After 15 grueling hours of trying to stop the labor, she was delivered via emergency C-section at 12:33 a.m. on January 31, 2016. She weighed just 3 pounds 6 ounces. Moments after she cried for the first time, my ob-gyn—who wasn't even on call that day but came in because he heard I was in labor—stepped around the curtain and said something along the lines of "If we hadn't delivered the second we did, she would have been stillborn. Her cord disintegrated in my hands. She wasn't getting proper nutrients for . . . I don't know how long. You saved her life."

They allowed me to quickly kiss her forehead, then she was whisked off to the NICU. I wouldn't see her again for several days.

BUSTED

Myth: My anxiety will subside after . . .

Many infertility warriors experience anxiety throughout their pregnancy. After failed cycles or past miscarriages, you don't want to get your hopes up. There's a constant fear that, once again, infertility is going to snatch away your chance to be a parent. To deal with this anxiety, many women focus on pregnancy milestones.

We tell ourselves:

- I'll relax once I hear the heartbeat.
- Once I'm out of the first trimester, I will let my guard down.
- After the anatomy scan, it will finally feel real.
- Feeling the baby kick will finally allow me to enjoy being pregnant.
- When we reach viability, then I can sleep soundly.

Desirae Whittle, a birth doula at Harmony Births in Meriden, Connecticut, calls this "milestone chasing." She says, "Infertility makes you doubt everything, especially yourself and your body's ability to do something 'right.' The reality is the majority of women who are pregnant after infertility do not have a high level of joy during pregnancy without underlying intense bouts of fear."

Michelle from California is currently pregnant and admits dealing with anxiety has been incredibly hard. "After dealing with so much before getting pregnant, I had a hard time—still do—believing that this is actually happening. My anxiety still comes out before doctor appointments," she shares.

It is normal to feel anxiety and other negative emotions while you're pregnant. But it's also important that you find healthy ways to cope and share your (completely valid) feelings.

Finally Getting Pregnant

When infertility warriors finally get pregnant, they can ride a roller coaster of emotions. A lot of the experience of pregnancy will be influenced by the infertility journey.

In this chapter, we're going to look at the misconceptions of post-infertility pregnancy and prepare you for some of the challenges ahead, including new milestones and triggers that can be difficult for people dealing with infertility.

We'll talk about this in more detail, but however you feel during your pregnancy is *valid*. If you're in your third trimester and a stranger tries to congratulate you in the grocery store, it's okay to have an intense urge to throw produce at them. Don't do it, but know that having that internal reaction is understandable. There is no road map for pregnancy emotions, and trying to put up a facade of "everything is just fine" will only waste your energy.

To Test or Not to Test?

You'll hear time and time again throughout your journey not to test for pregnancy at home—and certainly not to test early. However, for those of us in the pee-on-a-stick (POAS) camp, who might (I'm not naming names) go as far as posting our early tests online for interpretation by others in the community, it's hard to resist the urge.

Unfortunately, there *can* be false positives, caused by the following:

- Waiting too long to look at the test (over time, the urine evaporates and can leave a faint line that looks like the desired "double line" positive)

- Expired pregnancy tests

- Fertility medications that contain hCG, the pregnancy hormone

- Pharmaceuticals like anti-anxiety medications, antipsychotics, anticonvulsants, diuretics, or antihistamines

- Residual hCG (after a miscarriage, hCG can remain in your body for weeks)

- Urinary tract infection

- Certain kidney diseases

- Ovarian cysts

- Ovarian cancer

In addition, as Dr. Rodgers points out, not all at-home tests are as accurate as a blood test. "You could have a very low level, get a negative, stop your medications, and cause your own miscarriage. And I've had patients do this," she says.

If you do have a positive at-home pregnancy test, the next step is scheduling an appointment with your reproductive endocrinologist for a beta-hCG blood test, referred to as a "beta." When you're undergoing fertility treatments, this test will be prescheduled for 9 to 14 days after ovulation, depending on the clinic. (Although you do not ovulate during some cycles, like a frozen embryo transfer, the test is dated from the day when you would have ovulated had it been a natural cycle.)

To confirm whether you're pregnant, your doctor will look at your hCG level. Although anything above 5 mIU/mL is technically positive, most doctors want hCG levels between 50 and 150, depending on the type of cycle and the number of days post-ovulation. The initial test will tell you only whether you are pregnant. It can't determine if the fetus is healthy or even if you're pregnant with multiples. Dr. Rodgers has seen an initial hCG level of just 11 lead to a healthy baby. In my own experience, I had an initial hCG level of around 530 and miscarried. This first number just doesn't mean too much.

More important than the initial hCG level is the pattern by which it rises. Early in pregnancy, hCG levels typically double every 48 to 72 hours. Your doctor will check that your levels are steadily increasing for the first week or 2, typically with a blood draw every 2 or 3 days. However, remember that many healthy pregnancies have hCG levels outside the normal range at first.

During these first blood draws, your doctor should also monitor other hormone levels like progesterone and estrogen to ensure the best likelihood of the pregnancy's success.

Between 1 and 5 weeks after a positive pregnancy test from your doctor—which is equal to 5 to 9 weeks of gestation—you'll receive multiple transvaginal ultrasounds to see if the embryo has indeed implanted in the uterus and is developing properly.

By around 5 weeks of gestation, your doctor should be able to see the gestational sac starting to form. By 6 weeks, the yolk sack (a little white ring) and fetal pole should be visible. By 7 weeks, the ultrasound should be able to detect the heartbeat, ideally at a rate higher than 90 beats per minute. During this time, the fetus should also be growing about a millimeter a day and be about the size of an unshelled pistachio.

If you were taking estrogen or progesterone during this cycle, it's likely your doctor will have you continue taking them during the early part of your pregnancy. While every doctor is different, you will likely taper off both between 8 and 10 weeks.

During this time, it's common to feel a wide range of emotions. You don't want to get your hopes up. Each test can trigger anxiety, and if you're not yet feeling any pregnancy symptoms (which is common), you might refuse to believe you're actually pregnant. Allow yourself to feel whatever comes up, whether it's joy or fear or even indifference.

First Trimester: Graduating from Your Fertility Clinic

Many post-infertility pregnant women spend most of their first trimester in the care of a reproductive endocrinologist. Unlike the general pregnant population, you'll likely be closely monitored, with ultrasounds and blood work to track the fetus's development, watch for early miscarriages, and taper you off any medications related to your fertility treatment, like estrogen and progesterone.

Once your doctor has confirmed the fetus is developing as it should, you will "graduate" to an ob-gyn—typically by 10 weeks at the latest.

Additional First-Trimester Tests

Aside from continued hormone monitoring and ultrasounds, you'll be introduced to a whole new group of tests to monitor your pregnancy. These may include:

Thyroid function test. During the first trimester, the fetus is relying on you for certain hormones to develop. Your doctor might check that your thyroid is producing enough—but not too much. For the first trimester, the Endocrine Society recommends your thyroid-stimulating hormone (TSH) be between 1.0 and 2.5 mU/L. Anything above 2.5 could put you at risk for an early miscarriage.

Noninvasive prenatal testing (NIPT). This screening, generally done at about 10 weeks, will check for common chromosomal disorders like Down syndrome, Edwards syndrome, and Patau syndrome. (This test can even confirm gender, if that's something you desire!)

Other genetic tests. Depending on your medical history, your doctor may want to screen the fetus for other genetic abnormalities that could prevent it from developing properly.

BUSTED

Myth: I can't complain while I'm pregnant.

Infertility warriors work hard to get pregnant, so they feel like complaining about their discomfort is a sign of being unappreciative of their journey. Dr. Alice Domar, an expert in mind/body health and infertility, says having conflicting feelings is common. "You think you can't complain when you get pregnant after infertility, even if you're nauseous, tired, swollen, and feel like crap," she explains. "You can't complain because everyone in your world thinks, 'Wait a minute; you fantasized so long about being pregnant.' You fantasize that it's going to be this perfect, amazing experience, and I think that's really hard to reconcile."

With infertility, it's also difficult because members of your support system are still in the middle of their fight. You remember how it felt when pregnant women lamented over how they were 'as big as a house' and don't want to face judgment or hurt others.

Heather from Missouri offers sage advice: Do you. "Do what you want to do, feel what you want to feel. Don't feel shame that you're pregnant or shame that you complain about pregnancy," she says. "Even though you prayed and begged for a child, that doesn't mean you can't complain about the process. Not all pregnancies are easy!"

First-Trimester Symptoms

Every pregnancy is different. I repeat: *Every pregnancy is different*. Even if you've been pregnant before, this time around you might experience completely different symptoms. I had only mild morning sickness when I was pregnant with twins, but I couldn't even stand upright on my own to take a shower with Aurora until I was at about 21 weeks.

Unfortunately, some early pregnancy symptoms can indicate a pending miscarriage (see chapter 17), so experiencing them can be very scary or trigger anxiety. When in doubt, call your doctor.

First-trimester symptoms can include:

- Extreme fatigue
- Tender or swollen breasts
- Vaginal bleeding
- Moodiness
- Headaches
- Nausea
- Constipation
- Frequent urination
- Heartburn
- Back pain
- Fluctuations in weight (gain or loss)
- Food cravings

Bleeding during the early part of your pregnancy can be terrifying for infertility warriors because they immediately think they are miscarrying. But as Dr. Rodgers says, bleeding is common and happens in about 50 percent of early pregnancies. Typically, as the placenta attaches to the uterus, a blood vessel bursts, causing a subchorionic hematoma and vaginal bleeding. In most cases, this does not threaten the pregnancy and will resolve itself. However, if you're feeling extreme cramping or pain (subchorionic hematomas are almost always painless), call your doctor. Also, if you're bleeding at a rate that saturates a sanitary pad an hour for more than 2 consecutive hours, call your doctor.

Announcing Your Pregnancy

First things first: You do not have to tell people about your pregnancy at any specific time. It's all about you and your needs.

"I was afraid to tell anyone well past the first trimester, and we didn't make a broader announcement until after the anatomy scan," shares Jamie from Wisconsin.

Dr. Rothenburger says this is not uncommon. Announcing your pregnancy makes it feel "real," and you can imagine what it'll feel like if you then have to tell everyone if something goes wrong. This is why you should be open and honest about your feelings when you do decide to tell people.

"A lot of times, infertility warriors find that [other] people are more excited for them than [the warriors] are for themselves. And that is because of the infertility experience," says Dr. Rothenburger. "My policy is absolute honesty and saying what's happening. It's okay to say 'I feel anxious' or 'I feel worried still.'"

There are also many different approaches to announcing your pregnancy, so here are some considerations:

Who do you want to know? You might want only a few people to know early in your pregnancy. If you want to keep from telling your entire family or everyone at work, that's fine. Just be sure you set those boundaries, telling your loved ones how far you want the news to spread and when.

Are you ready to answer questions? *How far along are you? Are you going to have a home birth? Do you know if it's a boy or a girl?* These are just some of the questions you'll get. Some post-infertility parents-to-be don't want an in-depth conversation. If that's how you feel, it might be better to make your announcement through email or social media so you avoid a barrage of in-person questions in that emotional moment.

How much of your journey do you want to share? Some infertility warriors include their entire story as part of their announcement. It makes them feel better and helps others understand why they may feel complicated emotions during the pregnancy. (With Aurora, I created a short video that chronicled our entire infertility timeline.)

WARRIOR TIPS
First-Trimester Triggers

Dr. Maria T. Rothenburger, a psychotherapist at Miracles Happen Fertility Center in Salem, Oregon, says that most of the emotions you feel during your pregnancy will be unexpected. The first trimester can be particularly anxiety-inducing because infertility warriors know what can go wrong.

For some warriors, the following can trigger anxiety, sadness, or other negative emotions:

Upcoming tests. Some people feel intense worry that each series of tests will reveal something is wrong. Some find it's worse when they don't fully understand a test—what it's looking for and why. Others find comfort in not knowing the worst possible result.

Pregnancy symptoms. Both the presence and absence of symptoms can cause worry. Spotting or even heavy bleeding, for example, can be completely normal. But for post-infertility pregnant women, it can cause an intense fear. Some women also worry when symptoms like morning sickness suddenly disappear. (I can tell you from experience that symptoms can come and go, both throughout the day and from day to day.)

Choosing an ob-gyn. If you don't already have one, I personally recommend making this selection as soon as you feel comfortable. Ob-gyn offices often book new patient appointments very far out, and having gone through fertility treatments, you're now used to seeing a doctor weekly. This change can be scary, as it's likely you'll see your ob-gyn much less frequently.

"Your emotions are going to be all over the place," says Dr. Rothenburger. "I encourage people to seek some reassurance. There's no harm in calling somebody to ask a medical professional a question."

How will you tell people in the infertility community? Becoming a parent doesn't mean you no longer have a place in the infertility community. But remember what it felt like when you were struggling. If your friends have previously talked to you about how they prefer to receive pregnancy announcements, honor their requests. Also, give them room to react and take space if need be.

Second Trimester: Transitioning to an Ob-Gyn

By the time you reach your second trimester, you'll have transitioned to your ob-gyn. This change in provider is not always easy, so it's important to find the right ob-gyn for you. Discuss with your doctor the different ways they can support you during your pregnancy.

Dr. Alice Domar, an expert in mind/body health and infertility, says it's important to know what will help reduce your anxiety and to be willing to ask your ob-gyn to accommodate your needs. "If you had a pregnancy loss, and your anxiety decreases with more ultrasounds, tell your obstetrician," she says. "Ask, 'Can I come in once a week just to hear the baby's heartbeat?' Most will accommodate that."

⚡ Always be willing to fire your ob-gyn if you aren't getting the support you need. Do not put the pressure to be polite over the fetus's health or your emotional well-being.

Second-Trimester Tests and Milestones

A lot happens during your second trimester. For many parents-to-be, now is when you'll first see your future child's face and (if you want) find out the sex. While your individual pregnancy will determine how often and what tests you undergo, here's a general overview of additional tests and milestones:

Anatomy scan. For many, this is a big one. It typically happens at around 20 weeks. The scan allows your doctor to make sure the fetus is developing properly, anatomically speaking, and to check for signs of heart or brain defects. Often, if you so choose, this is when you find out the gender.

Alpha-fetoprotein (AFP) blood test. This tests for genetic defects like spina bifida.

Switching to maternity clothes. While the exact point at which you move to maternity wear varies, most women become big enough to need it during the second trimester. At that point, you'll put on about a pound a week. By week 27, most pregnant women have gained between 12 and 15 pounds.

Movement. Most women begin to feel their baby move around week 20. However, if you don't, don't panic! I never felt the twins move, even at 21 weeks. How much you feel often depends on the position of the placenta. Ask your doctor whether the placenta is anterior or posterior. Often, posterior placentas allow the feeling of movement earlier, more often, and stronger than anterior placentas. Knowing the position of the placenta will help you set expectations.

Viability. This is the other big one. The fetus officially reaches viability at 24 weeks.

Second-Trimester Symptoms

Some first-trimester symptoms will continue well into the second trimester, but in general, symptoms like nausea ease up now. You'll possibly notice new feelings and experiences such as:

- Body aches extending through your back, abdomen, groin, and thighs

- Swelling of your feet, ankles, fingers, and face

- Numbness or tingling in your extremities

- Darkening of the nipples
- A dark vertical line running down your abdomen
- Itching on your palms, soles, and abdomen
- Low blood pressure
- Pain in the ligaments that attach your uterus to your pelvis

Your Baby Shower (If You Have One)

Baby showers are controversial within the infertility community. For the general population, they're a celebration of the miracle of life. But for people who struggle to build a family, it can feel like they could "jinx" your pregnancy. (Even attending other people's baby showers may continue to be painful.)

It is your decision whether or not you have a baby shower. This is *your* pregnancy, and it may be one of the few parts over which you have control.

Chrissy from British Columbia, Canada, admits that she was terrified to have a baby shower. "What if my baby never came home? I could not come home to baby things. I could not see it in my house. It's like you're living in a dream world."

However, Chrissy goes on to say, fear shouldn't be the reason you don't have a baby shower or enjoy other aspects of pregnancy. Take time to think about whether a baby shower is right for you. It's okay to change your mind.

Dr. Rothenburger suggests looking at a baby shower as an exercise in receiving. "So much is given away and so much is sacrificed through the infertility process. It's hard to feel those feelings of reception."

Try receiving on for size. Pay attention to what it feels like when people congratulate you or give you a gift for the baby. If you see and enjoy the actions as a display of love and support, a baby shower could enhance your pregnancy. I was personally too terrified to have a baby shower when I was pregnant with Aurora, but thankfully, my friends and family threw me a surprise shower—and I'm so glad they did. I had a great time and created many wonderful memories surrounded by the people who love me. (Although, I'll point out, the shower was held a little more than a week before I gave birth!)

Third Trimester: Counting the Kicks

By the start of the third trimester, the fetus is fully formed—just a smaller version of the child you ultimately deliver. It's important to remember that while 37 to 41 weeks is considered full-term, many women go into labor early. And if you're carrying multiples, anticipate going into labor even earlier. This means it's important to not put off preparations until the last minute.

Third-Trimester Milestones

As your body prepares to give birth, you'll pass the following milestones and changes:

Visible movement. The fetus will be large enough that you can see it move through your abdomen. If you have a posterior placenta, other people should be able to feel movement if they put a hand on your belly. It's a little harder to feel movement with an anterior placenta.

First stage of lactation. Around week 31, your breasts might start producing colostrum. Colostrum can be clear, yellow, or orange. If you produce colostrum before giving birth, it will be only a few drops at a time.

Production of relaxin. This hormone loosens the ligaments in the pelvis to prepare for your baby's passage through the birth canal. It will cause shifts in your bones, making movement feel strange or clumsy.

Cervical dilation. Toward the end of the third trimester, your estrogen level increases to get your cervix ready for birth. It causes your cervix to soften and dilate while thinning out the mucus plug. In the weeks before your due date, your doctor will check to see how far your cervix has dilated.

Third-Trimester Symptoms

As your baby continues to grow, your body has to make room. During your third trimester, your intestines and lungs actually shift their positions. This can lead to new or more intense symptoms, including:

- Frequent heartburn

- Hemorrhoids

- Full-body aches

- Shortness of breath

- Frequent and sudden need to urinate

- Trouble sleeping

- Braxton-Hicks contractions

Giving Birth

For post-infertility parents-to-be, uncertainty is scary. It's not uncommon for them to create elaborate birth plans to help themselves feel in control and comfortable that all the bases are covered. Your plan will change and develop throughout your pregnancy, but be sure to research and discuss your options concerning the following:

Who will deliver the baby. Many people have their ob-gyn deliver the child, but some prefer to use or include a midwife or doula. This decision can impact where you give birth and the level of medical care available if there are complications.

Where you give birth. Home births are becoming more popular, and most studies find they are as safe as hospital births for low-risk pregnancies. If you want to give birth in a hospital, also consider whether that hospital has a NICU (see chapter 24).

What drugs you want to take. If you're not having a planned C-section, decide whether you want an epidural or other pain medication. (You can always change your mind later! A decision you make before you go into labor isn't necessarily set in stone.)

Who will be at the delivery. Maybe you want only your partner or a particular family member in the delivery room. Maybe you want all your family and friends waiting at the hospital. Know who you're going to contact when you go into labor.

How to handle risks. While it's not a fun conversation, it's important to talk with your partner and doctor about what to do if there are complications. Discuss your preferences on C-sections and what to do if your life or your baby's life is in danger.

Remember, your baby is going to come on his or her own schedule. So, while it's important to have a birth plan, accept and expect that you'll have to adapt. This can be hard for infertility warriors.

As Dr. Rothenburger says, "to plan for perfection is to plan for frustration." While changing your birth plan is a difficult decision, Dr. Rothenburger's advice is to voice your emotions before they get overwhelming. "It's still okay to be upset about it. What I encourage people to do is to feel those feelings, and then watch them dissipate."

For Beth from New Hampshire, the idea of letting go of a strict birth plan made her birth easier. She had friends who planned out every detail of their birth and then ended up disappointed. "After having so many things go wrong in infertility, I was completely fine with whatever birth I had," she says. "I just wanted to get out of the hospital with a healthy baby. It was freeing to let go of all that."

When Complications Arise

Complications can happen at any point during a pregnancy, even during the delivery. For infertility warriors, these complications feed fears and anxiety, so it's important to give yourself room to feel your emotions before making decisions.

Whittle says complications will exponentially worsen negative emotions, and she recommends people talk to a therapist to help them cope. "I also suggest they stay off Dr. Google and listen to their doctors," she says. "Only look at evidence-based information."

This will provide perspective and allow you to say, *Yes, this is bad, or unexpected, but my worst fears aren't likely.*

Post-Infertility Pregnancy Dos and Don'ts

Again, every pregnancy is different. You have the right to experience pregnancy however works for you. However, you have to not only deal with the big events and decisions but also live through each individual day.

Do allow yourself to feel both grateful and upset.

"Not being happy, being anxious or scared, or complaining about having morning sickness have nothing to do with being grateful for your pregnancy," Whittle reminds us. As a birth doula, she says it's not uncommon for the women she works with to mention something difficult about their pregnancy and immediately follow up with "But I'm so grateful." Again, one thing has nothing to do with the other.

Think of it this way: Your gratitude extends to the entirety of your pregnancy. Your momentary negative feelings are tied to specific details or situations of the pregnancy. By linking your long-lasting gratitude to anger, frustration, or worry, you're giving the feelings permission to expand into *all* parts of your pregnancy. Do *not* give them that power. Allow yourself to feel negative emotions without qualifying them so you can begin to move on.

Do celebrate.

Celebrating doesn't have to be big, like a huge baby shower or gender reveal party. You can still find ways to acknowledge even the smallest moments. This will help you find joy more consistently during your pregnancy.

Tina from New Jersey used the mantra "Today, I am pregnant" to help remind herself to acknowledge the joy and stay focused on the present. "It can be scary to think ahead. Just take things day by day and appreciate the moment," she advises.

Your celebrations don't have to be tied to test results or developmental milestones. Identify times when you find yourself smiling about your pregnancy—perhaps when you are making lists of names, or when you can no longer see your feet—and live in and recognize those moments.

Don't compare your pregnancy to others.

Even if you've been pregnant before, this one might be different. Do not go down the path of comparing your pregnancy to others. Your friend might have felt her baby move at 19 weeks, but you might not until 24 weeks. Comparing the two experiences will fill you with worry. Then when your baby finally does move, it might not be as exciting because in your mind it was 5 weeks late and something must be wrong.

Comparing pregnancies will also send you down the Dr. Google rabbit hole, and that's never fun nor advised.

"Don't Google all your symptoms," warns Jalina from New York. "Just like with infertility, each pregnancy is different. Unfortunately, you will never, ever find a story exactly like yours, and trying to find one will drive you crazy."

Know, too, that you shouldn't compare your emotional experience to that of others or their expectations. Dr. Rothenburger says post-infertility pregnant women think they have to feel and act a certain way. They fear the judgment of others or judge themselves for their emotions. And that's not healthy.

If your sister felt worried before her 20-week appointment but you don't, that doesn't mean you don't care about your child. You have a right to your own feelings and experience.

Do see a mental health professional.

"Start working through your feelings *during* pregnancy—the sooner the better—with a professional who specializes in infertility. Having a therapist can be particularly helpful when you don't have a large support system. I have patients who are pregnant who just come in to complain because [here is] the only place they can do it," shares Dr. Domar.

Having a safe place to let your guard down will do wonders for your stress levels during your pregnancy. Even with your most irrational fears, saying them out loud will help you begin to process and move on. If you're unsure how to find a mental health professional who specializes in infertility, check out RESOLVE's Professional Services Directory, which you can find online.

For many infertility warriors, finally getting (and staying) pregnant is its own roller coaster of highs and lows. You've gone through a lot (physically, emotionally, mentally) to get to this place; it's completely normal that your feelings will be all over the map.

Identifying Your Needs

Find a way to balance your physical and emotional needs during your pregnancy, because both deserve attention. Some physical pains and annoyances of pregnancy are easy to identify. Your feet hurt, so you ask for a foot rub. You have a craving, so you ask for peanut butter ice cream and pickles.

But sometimes your physical state impacts your emotional needs, and this is where things can get tricky. Cramping in your first trimester can trigger anxieties. You may then debate whether or not to call your doctor because you're not sure if your symptoms are really "that bad" or if they're augmented by your emotions.

The truth is that either situation should be addressed. Whether your physical symptoms require the attention of your doctor or your emotional state requires reassurance from them, don't dismiss either need because you're worried about seeming irrational.

It's also important for you to think about your needs with regard to your support system and community. When you have struggled with infertility, perhaps spending years avoiding pregnant women because it's too triggering, it can be hard to find a place where you fit in. You don't want to hurt people in your infertility community, but people who haven't struggled with infertility don't really get it.

Take time to think about each of your relationships and what you may need from those individuals. For example, if you have a close friend who is still struggling to build her family, you may not need her at your baby shower, but you do need to be able to talk to her about your anxieties. If your sister has three children and every pregnancy was a breeze, think about whether you want her advice. This process will help you identify the specific ways the people in your life can be there for you.

Communicating Your Needs

Don't let the fear of seeming ungrateful or high-maintenance keep you from getting the support you need. In fact, by sharing your emotional state, you help people better understand what is going on with you, making them less likely to be judgmental. For example, if you tell your doctor that you'd like more frequent ultrasounds because it helps with your anxiety, then they see you're not wasting their time. Instead, you're in need of an additional level of care. Same with your family and friends. It's okay for you to say it hurts when they give you pregnancy advice because it reminds you how different your experience has been.

With regard to seeking support from those still struggling with infertility, remember that relationships are a two-way street. After asking for what you need, find out what *they* need from *you*. This will help you find a mutually beneficial way to support each other.

WARRIOR ACTION STEPS
Processing Your Post-Infertility Pregnancy Emotions

Remember, if there's one thing you can control during this journey, it's yourself. Here are some actions you can take to help you process everything you're feeling during your pregnancy.

Journal during the good and bad times.
Journaling helps you not only process your feelings but also track how far you've come. You can look back at low moments and see how you found the strength to work through those issues. On bad days, you can reread about the exciting moments and how they made you feel to help you remember that the anxiety and fear can and will subside.

Voice your feelings, whatever they are. You are allowed to be upset. You are allowed to not enjoy every moment. Anyone who does not support your right to feel shouldn't be involved in your pregnancy.

Have a conversation with your infertility community. It's common to feel like a ship without a port when you're a pregnant infertility warrior. But remember, by not maintaining your relationships with your friends who are still going through infertility, you're also taking away a source of *their* support. Have an honest and nonjudgmental conversation with them about how you'll navigate your pregnancy.

Identifying Your Needs as a Partner

Many people supporting their pregnant partners approach pregnancy as problem-solvers. If there's an issue or their partner is uncomfortable, they find a way to fix the situation. This keeps them focused and helps them manage their emotions. Addressing the problem gives *their* fears and anxieties less power.

But remember that doing isn't the same as feeling. You're allowed to have your own negative emotions, and you're allowed to ask for support. To do that, you need to be able to identify your emotional needs.

Before you jump into a new problem, take a moment to think about why you're acting. Are you researching hospitals because you want to take something off your partner's plate? Or are you doing it because you feel like a bystander in the pregnancy? Looking at your motives can help you pinpoint your emotional needs. And be sure to be open with your pregnant partner, who might not realize that you're struggling. ("I'm painting the nursery so early because I feel like it's the only thing I can control.")

BUSTED

Myth: My only job is to make sure my pregnant partner is happy.

While it is important to support your partner both emotionally and physically, you're not a bystander for this journey. You'll get anxious. You'll feel joy. Events will trigger *your* past infertility traumas, even if you have different triggers and feelings from your partner. Don't try to push your emotions to the side.

Let your partner know what you want out of the pregnancy experience so you feel included. Let your partner know what you're worried about and what parts of the journey you're excited about celebrating. Having this discussion will show you both that you're together and supported.

$\longrightarrow$

Communicating Your Needs as a Partner

If you are supporting a pregnant partner, it's important to communicate, especially if you are having complicated or hard feelings. Just be mindful to avoid language that may make your partner feel responsible for your emotions. Phrases like "I'm worried you'll have another miscarriage" or "I'm scared you'll go into labor too early" put the burden on your partner. Phrases like "the chances of miscarriage scare me" or "I'm worried the baby will come too early" keep you united. Choose your words carefully, and have these conversations when you're not overly stressed, anxious, or angry.

WARRIOR ACTION STEPS
Being Supportive and Feeling Included in a Post-Infertility Pregnancy

It can be hard to balance your emotions while supporting your pregnant partner during a pregnancy. Take the following steps so you can be there for her while honoring your own emotions.

Back up actions with words. Taking action—painting the nursery to gain a sense of control, for example, or going for a run to work out your stress—can help you deal with your emotions. But your partner may not see the intent behind your actions and may be left feeling alone or helpless. Communicate with your partner to bridge the gap and help you stay united.

Be the buffer. Once you and your partner establish the boundaries of the pregnancy, you might have to reinforce them with your family and friends. If you decide to not have a baby shower and people keep asking your partner why, step in and reestablish those boundaries.

Welcome the complaining. Why would anyone want to listen to complaints? Because talking to an attentive, supportive listener makes people feel safe and heard. And who wouldn't want to do that for someone they love?

WARRIOR WISDOM
Take It All In

"This is what you've been waiting for! This is your miracle and your story. Do what you can to enjoy this time and to celebrate this sweet life." —Jalina, New York

WARRIOR CHECKLIST
Being Pregnant After Infertility

❑ Know that every pregnancy is different. Everyone feels differently while pregnant, and there's nothing wrong with that.

❑ Familiarize yourself with the different stages of pregnancy. Understand the milestones, symptoms, and, most important, possible infertility-related triggers.

❑ Take the time to identify your needs during pregnancy, then communicate them in a clear and honest way.

❑ Give yourself permission to feel the lows, and celebrate the highs of pregnancy.

Facing the NICU

I WAS THE LAST PERSON IN MY family to hold Aurora because she was whisked away from the operating room where she'd been born to the neonatal intensive care unit (NICU). I became very sick, vomiting for the next 2 days. Because the NICU is a sterile place—you have to scrub up before you enter—they didn't want me in there until I stopped vomiting. To see her for the second time after the brief kiss on her forehead in the OR, the orderlies wheeled my bed up next to her incubator because I still couldn't get up.

I was released from the hospital 5 days after giving birth. Despite the fact that I was recovering from a C-section, we drove to the NICU every day, a journey of 60 to 90 minutes each way depending on traffic. We stayed by her bedside from 8 a.m. to 8 p.m., leaving only to grab quick meals. We were surprised to see that during Aurora's 18-day stay, we saw another parent only once or twice. I imagine that was because most people had to return to work—or chose to work during their child's NICU stay so they could use their parental leave once their baby was released from the hospital.

I was an emotional wreck the entire time. Between our poor relationship with the lead nurse, my grueling recovery from surgery, and Aurora's delicate condition, I was at my breaking point. I cried frequently. Thankfully, she was born able to breathe on her own. She was admitted because of low birth weight, feeding issues, an inability to maintain body temperature, and, for the first several days, jaundice.

It's hard to describe what it's like to sit in the NICU. There are alarms going off almost constantly—and each time you hope it's not your child's. Whenever an alarm sounds, a team of nurses rush in to help.

Looking back, I would have done many things differently. I would have left her bedside *more* often—I didn't practice enough self-care. Breastfeeding never did work out—at the risk of TMI, Aurora's mouth was just too tiny and my nipples were huge. She wasn't able to latch—and the volume I produced was very low. So I pumped around the clock at her bedside when we were there, in the car on our way to and from the hospital, and overnight when we were home. I cannot remember a single time when I addressed my own needs.

After those 18 agonizing days, she was discharged from the NICU. She weighed exactly 4 pounds—the lowest end of the safe limit on her car seat. The drive home was terrifying, especially since she was hooked up to a bradycardia monitor, which would sound an alarm if her oxygen level or heart rate dipped too low. If it went off—which thankfully it didn't—we would have had to pull over to perform resuscitation. She was on that monitor—which went off dozens of times most days—for 7 weeks after coming home. In other words, physically leaving the NICU doesn't mean your NICU experience ends.

The Shock of the NICU

When you ask parents to describe the NICU, most say the same thing: It's terrifying. There's no use beating around the bush. If your child spends any time in the NICU, it will be scary, emotional, and exhausting. Putting all that on top of your infertility journey can be incomprehensible. Many warriors struggle to process how *something else* could go wrong on their journey to becoming a parent.

But the truth is, it happens. In 2016, for example, according to the National Center for Health Statistics, 9.85 percent of babies were born prematurely. And it's not just extremely premature babies that end up in the NICU. Research published in the *Journal of Clinical Medicine* in 2022 found that between 53 and 65 percent of babies admitted to the NICU are 37 or more weeks of gestation. Further, a paper published in *Seminars in Perinatology* in 2021 found that as many as 80 percent were normal birth weight. Birth defects, conditions of the delivery, and the mother's health can all lead to a NICU stay.

In this chapter, we'll walk through what happens in the NICU and what it's like to have a child staying there so you can be prepared.

Why Your Baby Might Require a NICU Stay

If a baby isn't healthy or stable enough to leave the hospital, the NICU is there to get them where they need to be developmentally and medically. After your baby is born, a doctor or nurse will check their temperature, heart rate, breathing, and color. If any of these factors fall outside the normal range, the baby will be taken to the NICU for testing or treatment.

Here are some common reasons as to why newborns—both preterm and full-term—need to stay in the NICU:

BUSTED

Myth: I won't be able to hold my baby in the NICU.

Newborns in the NICU have some sort of complication, and many are fragile. They might be hooked up to machines or kept in incubators. But the point is *not* to separate you from your child. In fact, most NICUs want you to hold and touch your baby.

Kangaroo care, or skin-to-skin contact treatment, is popular in most NICUs. Experts know that being held helps a baby heal and grow. While it might not be as often as you'd like, and NICU staff might have to help you, you likely will be able to have your child in your arms during their stay.

Aurora was so tiny and fragile that we were limited in how many times per day and how long each time we could hold her. It actually wore her body out to the point of setting off the monitoring alarms. But we took advantage every time we could.

Heather Reimer, director of the NICU Initiatives team at March of Dimes, suggests getting involved in the baby's daily care, such as diaper changes, taking temperatures, and bathing.

I was terrified to hurt Aurora, even during diaper changes. Meanwhile, my husband was a champ. He got into a routine with her right away. Although I struggled at first, the hiccups were only temporary. Just keep trying! You're doing the best you can.

WARRIOR TIPS
The NICU Parents' Bill of Rights

In 2013, the Preemie Parent Alliance (now the NICU Parent Network) released the NICU Parents' Bill of Rights as a way to get parents and NICU care providers on the same page. While the document is not legally binding in any way, it does serve as a good guide to the treatment and respect you deserve during your child's NICU stay. Many hospitals use the NICU Parents' Bill of Rights to inform their policies and help train their NICU employees.
   Some points include:

• Parents need to truly understand the baby's diagnoses in order to offer the baby the best care once he or she is home.

• Parents should be allowed and encouraged to hold their child as much as possible.

• Parents should participate in daily care (feeding, changing, etc.) as much as possible to ensure a seamless transition to being the primary caregivers.

• Parents are experiencing a lot of overwhelming emotions, and NICU staff should be patient and supportive, as well as share resources like support group information.

Preterm delivery. Often, babies born before 37 weeks of gestation are not developmentally ready for the outside world. Many have trouble regulating their body temperature or gaining weight. Depending on how premature the child is, there might also be respiratory, intestinal, neurological, or cardiac concerns.

Respiratory distress syndrome (RDS). If the baby's lungs are underdeveloped, he or she will need help breathing with an oxygen mask or breathing tube.

Infection. Babies with compromised immune systems will be monitored or treated for infections or sepsis.

Hypoglycemia. Babies with low birth weight or whose mothers had gestational diabetes might experience hypoglycemia (low blood sugar).

Difficult delivery. Sometimes, difficult deliveries cause decreased blood or oxygen flow in a baby. Left untreated, this can lead to brain injuries.

Maternal infections. Maternal chorioamnionitis (infection in the placenta or umbilical cord), group B strep, and many STIs can be transmitted to babies before or during birth.

Low birth weight (less than 5 pounds 8 ounces) or difficulty with feeding. Babies that aren't gaining weight will be placed on a feeding regimen or feeding tube in the NICU to ensure they get enough nutrition.

Birth defects. Any number of defects can cause seizures, heart problems, or neurological issues.

A Tour of the NICU

While each NICU is different, they can all be disorienting. There are machines you've never seen before and people with unfamiliar job titles. Alarms will go off and make you fear the end of your world.

On top of it all, your newborn is on display, while possibly hooked up to monitor wires or treatment tubes. Although it's the last place in the world you want to be, you'll spend hours in the NICU, so it's best to get an idea of what you can expect.

BUSTED

Myth: Being separated from my child will prevent attachment.

Having a baby in the NICU does mean you'll have to spend more time away from your child than you'd like. Some NICUs have limits regarding how long parents can visit, and again, many infants are hooked up to some sort of machine or monitoring device that can make holding them challenging.

But that doesn't mean you and your baby can't bond.

"Parents worry about attachment and that their relationship with their baby suffers during this time of being apart," says Sharon Covington, director of the psychology team at Shady Grove Fertility in Rockville, Maryland. "What we know is that attachment and bonding are ongoing processes and are very much occurring in the NICU and will continue long after."

You have a long time to form a bond with your child. If just one difficulty could hurt the parent-child relationship, no parent—not even ones without babies in a NICU—could form a strong bond with their child. Spending time in the NICU might seem like a rough start, but it will not define your relationship with your child.

The People in the NICU

The staff in the NICU are a lifeline. They will be the ones who not only take care of your child but also walk you through this difficult time. For many new parents, the NICU staff are the only light in the situation.

"Some of those women and men are angels on earth," says Ashley from Georgia, whose son spent 69 agonizing days in the NICU. "I was so surprised and relieved that there are people like them who truly love these children and do their jobs because they want to."

Some of the people who could be on your child's team are:

A primary nurse. In some NICUs, you can request a specific nurse to be your child's advocate when you're not there. This nurse will learn all the ins and outs of what's going on with *your* baby. They also get to know who you are so they can make decisions aligned with your wishes.

Neonatologist. A neonatologist is a pediatrician who's received additional training to specialize in caring for newborns.

Neonatal nurses. Most of the day-to-day monitoring and administration of treatment will be done by a team of nurses. They will also feed, bathe, and change your baby when you aren't able—or allowed—to. In most cases, the nurses in the NICU specialize in treating newborns.

Respiratory therapist. If your child has underdeveloped or compromised lungs, it's the respiratory therapist who will decide the course of action. They monitor any respiratory equipment, provide breathing treatment, and will most likely be present if your baby needs to be transferred or moved.

Physical therapist. Your baby will grow and change during their stay in the NICU. A physical therapist makes sure the baby is positioned correctly to encourage healthy development. Some physical therapists provide infant massage or help your baby learn to eat.

Lactation consultant. These consultants are on hand to teach you the basics of breastfeeding and support you as you and your baby figure it out together. If you are struggling or unable to breastfeed but still want to provide milk for your child, a specialist can help you pump and transition to breastfeeding when you and your baby are ready.

Mental health professionals. Many NICUs have counselors available for parents. While they may not be located in the hospital, they can be an important part of your NICU experience.

You will also see other parents in the NICU. Over the course of your child's stay, you'll get to know them and bond over your similar experience. Lean on and support each other. When asked about the other parents in the NICU, Azizah from California says she formed strong relationships. "I have friends for life in some of these women. We have been to hell and back together."

WARRIOR TIPS
Surviving the NICU as a Single Parent

The NICU can be isolating, especially for single parents. Don't think you have to go through this experience by yourself. "It's helpful when single parents can identify a family member or friend to function in that partner role and be part of the NICU journey," says Reimer.

You can form a team of friends and family to bring you food and sit with your child when you need a break.

Also make a conscious effort to meet and get to know the other parents. Once you head home, these are the people who will understand what you've been through. As your child grows, they'll provide understanding and support.

Choosing a Delivery Hospital with a NICU

I like how Dr. Alice Domar describes the NICU: "The NICU is not what you planned for. It's not what you anticipated. It's terrifying. It feels unfair because if you've gone through infertility, you've already suffered enough. You shouldn't have to also go through the terror of having a baby in the NICU. But most babies who go into the NICU come out normal, healthy babies."

With that peace of mind, let's talk about the difference between planning and preparing. Your birth plan will not include a trip to the NICU. But if it does become necessary, it helps to be prepared. If you want to deliver in a hospital, find out whether it has a NICU, and do research about it. We'll discuss this more in a minute, but not every NICU is equipped for every medical situation.

For example, Kelli from Wisconsin had her son via C-section. But her son had fluid in his lungs and had to be transported to a hospital with a NICU that could treat him. For the first 48 hours of her son's life, Kelli was recovering in a different hospital. "I'm his mommy, and the whole experience of having him taken from me 6 hours post-birth was traumatic."

She says the staff at her son's NICU were phenomenal. But if she had to do it over again, she would've given birth in a hospital with a NICU. "I'll never get those 2 days back."

If a hospital birth is part of your plan, consider the following NICU factors:

How many babies they care for and their success rates. There are two ways to approach what size NICU is right for you. Some parents are comforted by the fact that a NICU is smaller because their child will get more personalized care. Others prefer bigger NICUs because the staff are more experienced and have dealt with a wider variety of medical conditions.

Availability of specialists. If your child has already been diagnosed with a birth defect, like a heart problem, make sure there's a specialist on staff who can treat the condition.

Visitation hours and sleeping arrangements. Some NICUs allow visitors 24/7 and some even have places for parents to get some sleep. Others limit when you can be with your baby and offer no parent accommodations. While it's not healthy to *always* be in the NICU, make sure their schedule and setup fit your needs.

BUSTED

Myth: I can't question the care my child is receiving.

Many new parents are scared to question the nurses and doctors. They want what's best for their baby, so they keep their mouths shut. But after their time in the NICU, many parents say they wish they'd spoken up more.

"I would have asked to hold my baby more," says Kelly from Michigan, whose son had to be flown to a NICU across the country for special treatment. "There were some days when he was hooked up to so many wires that I knew it would take a team of people to put him in my arms. But I shouldn't have been worried about that. I should have just asked to hold him whenever I wanted."

We've been talking about self-advocacy throughout this book. Don't forget that skill once your child is born. Ask questions, make suggestions, and be involved.

As Covington says, it's important to have confidence in your NICU staff, but parents should listen to their gut if they feel something isn't right. Yes, the NICU team is a group of experts; however, this is your child.

Nutrition protocol. If you want to breastfeed your child, research the hospital's policies. Some will allow you to pump and leave the milk for the baby. Others work with donated breast milk programs.

Support for parents. A NICU might offer parenting classes and breastfeeding support to help you prepare for bringing your baby home. Some NICUs even have nurses who specialize in educating parents on any medical treatments they'll have to continue after their child is discharged. Other NICUs have mental health professionals on staff to help parents cope.

When I selected my ob-gyn, I took into account the hospital at which they deliver. Because of my previous experience, I knew preterm labor was a strong possibility and wanted a NICU that could provide my daughter the best level of care possible. Although it was a good distance from our house, I do not regret our choice.

Understanding Levels of Care

Not every hospital or NICU is equipped to care for every possible complication. They receive different levels of designation depending on the level of care and treatments they can provide.

• Level I: Provides basic care for healthy, full-term babies.

• Level II: Provides care for babies born after 32 weeks or who are recovering from serious health problems. These NICUs are further divided into Level IIA units, which do not provide assisted ventilation, and Level IIB units, which can provide assisted ventilation for less than 24 hours.

• Level III: Provides care for extremely sick babies. These NICUs are subclassified into Level IIIA units, which can care for babies born after 28 weeks, and Level IIIB units, which have more advanced ventilation options, a wider range of specialists, and more in-house testing and imaging capabilities.

• Level IIIC or Level IV: Provides care for babies at viability or in need of advanced ventilation or complicated surgeries.

Our NICU was a forty-six-bed Level IIIC unit. The NICU didn't offer any parent accommodations, so we went home to sleep every night. But it did provide a secure video stream on which we could watch her incubator whenever we weren't physically together. (A huge thank-you to the Verizon Foundation for the grant that made this possible!)

WARRIOR TIPS
Prepare for the Fishbowl Feeling
....

Dr. Rothenburger says many of her patients who had children in the NICU say they constantly felt like they were being watched. No matter how a NICU is set up, there's an openness to the layout. Other parents can see nurses interacting with your child. You can overhear sensitive conversations.

"There's a feeling of complete vulnerability," she explains. "It can seem like you're on display and being watched a lot."

This is at complete odds with how many infertility warriors approach their journey. You try to hide your emotions or want to keep what's going on under wraps, but that's not possible in a NICU. It's another layer of stress and trauma that you need to be prepared to tackle.

During Your Baby's Stay

A lot of parents with a child in the NICU feel helpless, like the only thing they can do is wait. But this creates a feeling of powerlessness that worsens stress. Take back some semblance of control by being proactive.

Keep Records

You're going to process a lot of information—to the point of being overwhelmed—during your time in the NICU. Dr. Maria Rotherburger, a psychotherapist at Miracles Happen Fertility Center in Salem, Oregon, suggests taking detailed notes as a way to regain some control. These can be about everything from how much your baby ate to what a doctor said or something you felt grateful for that day.

Keeping records helps you process information and identify what you have power over. "You take control of the things that you know you can, and then send the other things on their way with a gentle knowing that there are other people who can take care of this for you," says Dr. Rothenburger.

⚡ Try to be at the NICU when your doctors do rounds so you can stay up to date. Ask questions or request resources so you can better educate yourself about what's going on. Every few days, look back at your records and check in with how you've processed the information. When you're given new information or insight, what helps you understand it? This sort of record keeping and analysis can help you overcome feelings of helplessness.

Some infertility warriors recommend also documenting your experience with photos and videos. Chelsea from Massachusetts, whose twin daughters spent 52 days in the NICU, says her biggest regret was not taking more photos. "You may think you won't want to look at pictures of your baby looking so small, so sick, or with so many wires, but you will regret not having these later," she says. "I wish we had more photographic evidence to document and celebrate all the milestones that our girls hit while in the NICU."

Get Experience

Parents of premature NICU babies often aren't prepared for their children to be born so soon. They thought they had the rest of the pregnancy to educate themselves and buy baby supplies. For example, I went into labor on the day I was supposed to attend my first parenting class. We didn't yet have a car seat. And even if your child was born at term, there's no such thing as too much preparation before taking your child home.

"It might not seem like much, but having any interaction with your child in the NICU helps so much toward actually feeling like their parent," admits Chelsea. "I honestly felt so prepared when we brought them home that I think of our 7-week NICU stay as a 7-week parenting class."

Don't be too proud to get tips from the nurses and doctors.

The most valuable experience I received during our NICU stay was the required CPR and resuscitation class. That sounds frightening—and it was—but we used what we learned within hours of Aurora coming home because she didn't properly swallow her milk, cutting off her oxygen supply and reducing her heart rate to dangerous levels. Thanks to the training, we handled the situation well, even though it severely rattled us.

Don't Compare

When asked what advice she had for other infertility warriors with children in the NICU, Kelly from Georgia simply says, "Comparison is the thief of joy."

Each baby has a different path out of the NICU. If you compare your newborn's progress to that of other babies, you'll drive yourself crazy. Azizah admits to falling into this trap. She saw newborns who were just a pound but could breathe on their own. Why was her 4-pound son struggling? Eventually, she had to accept that his journey was his own. "They are all survivors, and they are all miracles," she says. "Your baby will get healthy on his or her own timeline."

Take Care of Yourself

Even if your NICU is always open for visitation, do not spend all your time there. I repeat: *Do not live in the NICU.*

"My best advice is to be kind and gentle to yourself," says Sharon Covington, director of the psychology team at Shady Grove Fertility in Rockville, Maryland. "This is a time when self-care is very important so that you can heal, get strong, and be prepared for the future."

If you haven't taken the time to rest and deal with stress, it'll make caring for your newborn once they come home even harder. Find something you can do every day to practice self-care, whether it's journaling, going for a walk outside, or taking a bubble bath.

Balancing Work and the NICU

Depending on the amount of parental leave you have and the length of your child's stay in the NICU, you may have to spend less time with your baby in order to return to work. It's another ball you have to start juggling during a difficult time.

Chelsea says a NICU's phone policy can complicate matters. If phones aren't allowed in the NICU, people—especially your work colleagues—may not understand why you can't be reached. "It was a huge struggle to find a balance between spending time at the NICU while also going to work, taking care of ourselves, and meeting other obligations," she says.

If you feel comfortable, talk with your employer or human resources department about your situation. They could be open to extending your parental leave or temporarily changing your work schedule. For parents whose child is at a NICU far away, see if you can work remotely during their stay.

When you do have to leave the NICU for work, Dr. Rothenburger suggests creating a ritual. If the NICU will allow, she says many parents find comfort in leaving a blanket, an angel figurine, or some other symbolic form of protection with your child. "The ritual can be praying or letting go of your guilty feelings of leaving your baby," she explains. "But if you're able to do the same thing every single time, it sort of sets you up for a feeling of comfort in knowing that your baby's well taken care of and is going to be safe while you're away."

Although my husband had 10 weeks of leave saved up, his employer insisted he come back to work just a week after Aurora came home following her 18-day NICU stay. This created an unexpected burden on us and robbed him of time he expected to spend with her. My mom was staying with us, though, so I did have help at home. As a result, and thanks also to the fact that I ran my own business (if I didn't work, I didn't get paid), I, too, went back to work very quickly.

Getting Discharged and Coming Home

It's the date you've been waiting for: taking your newborn home. Many parents assume the only criteria for being discharged is weight. While it is important, it's not the only one. Your NICU team will consider the following factors for your child:

- Being able to maintain a normal body temperature on their own

- Being able to eat adequately with a bottle or breastfeeding

- Gaining weight after feedings

- Having no apnea spells (periods of not breathing)

Also, know that it's not always best to rush your child out of the NICU. A 2016 study published in the *Journal of Perinatology* found that extending NICU stays by just 3 days resulted in better outcomes and lower overall healthcare costs.

Once your newborn has hit all the appropriate milestones and is ready for discharge, the NICU team will create a care plan for you. If your child needs medication or a medical device, a staff member will educate you about it. Many parents will also receive infant CPR training.

While you'll be excited to go home, remember this will be your first time being the sole caretaker for your child. Make sure you understand the care plan and ask as many questions as it takes for you to feel confident. Ask for a list of people or resources you can use if you have additional concerns once you're home.

⚡ It's also important to find a pediatrician and any specialists needed for future care *before* leaving the hospital. Assuming your NICU is close to your home, ask the staff for recommendations if you're not sure of your best options.

Once you're home, there will be an adjustment period—for you and the baby. Kelly from Georgia suggests recording the noises and the sensor alarms in the NICU before leaving. They may be frightening reminders to you, but they're familiar to your baby. Hearing them in their new home can be calming and comforting to your baby.

Make the transition easier on yourself by continuing certain aspects of your NICU routine. Record the same daily updates you did in the hospital. Continue to make time for self-care. And most important, ask for help when you need it.

Long-Term Cost of a NICU Stay

Worldwide, an estimated fifteen million babies a year are born premature—and the number is rising, according to the World Health Organization. The United States accounts for about 380,000 of those premature babies, costing an estimated $25.2 billion each year. And don't forget—it's not only premature babies who end up in the NICU.

NICU costs will, of course, vary according to duration of the stay, treatments, and location. Premature babies incur the highest costs due to their typically prolonged stays. The average length of stay for a baby admitted to the NICU is 13.2 days, according to March of Dimes. The average cost of a NICU admission is $76,000, with charges exceeding $280,000 for infants born prior to 32 weeks of gestation.

Paying for your baby's NICU care is expensive, but the cost doesn't end when you come home. Additional expenses might include additional medical care, early intervention services (such as the feeding therapy Aurora needed until she was 3), special education services for NICU babies when they're older (from ages 3 to 21), and lost work and pay for parents.

Those costs add up *really* fast, especially if you're paying out of pocket.

We were undeniably lucky to have amazing insurance coverage during each of my pregnancies. In the end, we owed nothing—not for my in-hospital bed rest with my twins nor for my C-section and Aurora's NICU stay. But not everyone is so lucky.

Many families start saving early for pregnancy and delivery expenses. Even if your baby does not require a NICU stay, knowing your financial options ahead of time will help give you peace of mind.

Paying with Private Insurance

Amy from Alabama gave birth to a daughter who needed 2 weeks in the NICU. Amy's private insurance didn't cover *any* of the $178,389.47 in hospital bills. The family considered bankruptcy but thankfully was able to figure out how to pay the NICU costs through payment plans—and supportive friends and family.

This is a cautionary tale. Find out which NICU expenditures are covered by your private medical insurance plan (see chapter 19). Add your newborn to your insurance plan as soon as possible after the birth (most plans have a 30-day waiting period). Many policies cover hospitalization for mother and baby but not expert or specialty care. Early communication with your insurer about your baby's medical bills, copays, deductibles, excluded treatments, and coverage limits is crucial.

It's also important to remember that many insurance plans have maximum payouts, in- and out-of-network providers, and deductibles. So even if you have insurance, you might still end up owing thousands of dollars.

Checking Your Bill

This is a good practice in general, but if you have questions about your hospital or NICU costs, ask for an itemized bill. It will detail each service you and your baby received, so you'll be able to see exactly what you're paying for.

Call your insurance provider if you have questions about any charges. You can appeal denials of coverage and argue why the service should have been covered under your plan (again, see chapter 19).

Paying with Medicaid

If you have Medicaid, ask the hospital's financial staff or a NICU social worker which charges are covered by your plan. If you don't have insurance or Medicaid, apply now! Medicaid eligibility varies by state. At-risk populations include pregnant women (and children younger than 6), so you may qualify while pregnant even if you didn't previously.

Paying with Supplemental Security Income (SSI)

Preemie parents may be eligible for SSI benefits from the US Social Security Administration throughout their baby's hospitalization. This option depends on the baby's birth weight and gestational age, and specific benefits received are based on the parents' income.

Asking for Financial Help

Again, the hospital social worker is your best friend. Ask about your options. They can help you find out what help is available and how to apply for it.

A hospital financial department is also a good option. For those who earn less than a particular amount each year (which varies depending on the hospital), many hospitals provide payment plans. They may also offer a discount for uninsured patients.

In some ways, infertility warriors are better equipped than most parents to cope with the NICU because they've already learned unique skills. "Yet, at the same time, it's also harder, as it is just another emotional challenge on the road to parenthood," Covington explains. Whenever you can, use the coping mechanisms you've practiced in the past, but understand that you may need to make adjustments to account for the unique experience of the NICU.

Identifying Your Needs

The birth of a child is typically a time of celebration. We have cultural norms in place to show new parents we love and support them. Having a baby in the NICU can complicate our rituals. The first step is to make checking in with yourself a habit.

Your needs at the beginning of your child's stay in the NICU will not be the same as after. For example, if you've had a C-section, you might need help with your physical recovery at the beginning. Or if you've put countless miles on your car, you might need help taking it to your mechanic for an oil change. If your baby was premature, your actual due date might be a particularly emotional day. Be conscious of what you're feeling each day and the new challenges you are facing.

Reimer reminds us that every parent will have a different process, so don't think you need to do what the other parents are doing. "The NICU is often a place of crisis for parents, and each parent needs individualized support based on their preferred coping style. For example, some parents may want to take action and be enabled to do concrete things for their partner and baby or babies. Others may want their partner to do things for them, such as interface with the medical team and provide updates to family and friends."

Communicating Your Needs

Be specific with your partner, your friends and family, and your NICU staff. The people in your life want to be there for you, but unless they've also had a newborn in the NICU, it's unlikely they'll know where to start.

Start by setting boundaries about what you need from them. For some parents, after spending all day in the NICU, they can't handle answering questions from all of their family and friends. If this is your case, let them know you'll update them when you can but won't be fielding daily calls asking about the newborn.

If you have a partner, set aside a time when the two of you can talk about ways to support each other. But do it when you're both not emotionally overwhelmed. If you have a long ride home from the NICU, take that time to be quiet and decompress. Then, when you get home, have a nonjudgmental conversation about your needs.

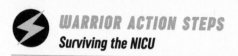

WARRIOR ACTION STEPS
Surviving the NICU

Aside from communicating your needs, there are other steps you can take to survive the NICU. Remember, the sooner you start preemptive measures, the less likely your stress and emotions will get out of control.

While you're in the NICU:

Ask the hospital for help finding resources. Sometimes, hunting down resources is exhausting. Chances are your hospital has information about therapists and/or support groups for NICU parents. If they don't provide these resources when you're admitted, ask.

Don't isolate. Typically, after giving birth, you'd be surrounded by family and friends. Don't let the NICU take that away from you. If your NICU will allow it, have family and friends come to celebrate when your newborn hits an important milestone. (Remember that NICU babies are very fragile. We required every visitor to have flu shots and any other vaccines our doctor recommended.) This will help them understand your situation and remind you that you're not alone. (Keep in mind that most NICUs limit the number of people per baby—including you—who can enter at one time.)

Once you and your child are home:

Give yourself permission to have bad days. Being a new parent is hard. Being the parent of a NICU warrior is even harder. There will be days when you're overly worried and nervously checking your baby's temperature every hour. Don't feel guilty for these feelings. Express your frustrations just like any other parent would.

Stay involved in the NICU community. Now that you're on the other side, try to continue to support other parents in the NICU. Stay connected with the parents you met. Consider getting involved with or starting a support group through your NICU so you can help future parents. You can be a valuable resource while getting reminders of how far your child has come.

WARRIOR WISDOM
Becoming Part of the NICU Community

"The biggest surprise was the bond I made with my fellow NICU moms. Imagine being in this strange routine all day long, sitting inside the NICU holding your sick baby, then taking breaks in the 'pumping' room. The conversations we had in that room were hilarious and moving. We laughed together, cried together, and shared our deepest fears. We were strangers thrown together in this horrible, unique situation, and it really created a deep connection."

—Azizah, California

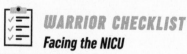

WARRIOR CHECKLIST
Facing the NICU

❏ Familiarize yourself with the different reasons your child might end up in the NICU.

❏ Research the NICUs in your area so you're prepared if your child needs to stay in one.

❏ Be as active in your newborn's care as possible.

❏ Take every opportunity to prepare yourself for your child coming home.

❏ Be aware of your needs and how they may change during and after the NICU.

❏ Ask for help whenever you need it.

Depression and Anxiety After Infertility

CHAPTER 25

AFTER **A**URORA WAS BORN, I struggled emotionally in many ways. Aurora developed a scary feeding disorder. In her first year, we had to attempt feedings every 90 minutes. Even once she moved on to solids, every new food we introduced began with a long period of complete refusal. She lost weight more often than she gained. We had to obtain a baby scale and weigh her every morning with her first diaper change of the day to keep track of her progress—or lack thereof. I think nearly any parent would struggle under these conditions, so I was not surprised when I was diagnosed with postpartum depression.

I was in constant fight-or-flight mode, functioning on sheer adrenaline. All I could think about day and night was keeping her alive. I felt like a failure on every level. *First my body couldn't get or stay pregnant, and now that our daughter is here, I can't get her to eat. I'm her mother. This is my responsibility—and mine alone. Why can't I do this?* These thoughts were heavy weights, and just when she made a little progress and I could take a breath, she'd regress and I'd be pulled back under.

I found a therapist who specialized in infertility and pregnancy loss—and had been

through both herself. She helped me realize that none of what was happening was my fault and that I was doing everything in my power to get the best care for Aurora. My biggest regret is not seeing someone sooner—for both my sake and my family's.

The Pain of Postpartum Mental Health Disorders

It's not fair, but sometimes the greatest joy in your life is followed by inexplicable sorrow. Postpartum depression and anxiety can make your first few months as a parent seem impossible. And after a long journey battling infertility, the situation can be even more complicated. But there is a light at the end of the tunnel when you have the tools and support you need to overcome postpartum depression, anxiety, and other mental health disorders.

Postpartum Depression

It's difficult to adjust to life with a new baby, especially when you've struggled with infertility. But left unchecked, negative emotions can develop into serious mental conditions that are harmful to you, your relationships, and your child. By educating yourself about possible postpartum depression, you can catch symptoms early and start your recovery.

Types of Postpartum Depression

Infertility, pregnancy, and having a new baby individually take a toll on your emotions and mental state. When you are dealing with *all* of these issues at once or in a relatively short period of time, feelings of sadness can manifest in different ways.

It's important to understand the differences between the types of postpartum mental disorders so you can be properly diagnosed and receive the help you deserve.

Baby Blues

After giving birth, your hormone levels change drastically. For many, these biological changes paired with the stress of adjusting to being a parent creates an unexpected sadness, or the "baby blues."

Believe it or not, having baby blues is quite common. While research on the prevalence of baby blues differs, the National Institute of Mental Health (NIMH) estimates up to 80 percent of mothers experience it.

The symptoms of baby blues are similar to those of clinical depression and postpartum depression but are milder and short-term. According to NIMH, in general, baby blues start presenting shortly after giving birth but last no more than 2 weeks. Typical symptoms include:

- Frequent crying

- Insomnia

- Fatigue

- Mood swings

- Sadness

- Feeling incapable of taking care of your baby

BUSTED

Myth: Anxiety and depression won't be an issue once you have built your family.

Most infertility warriors know postpartum anxiety and depression are real—for fertile myrtles, that is. After experiencing infertility, you can't imagine feeling anything but ecstasy when you're holding your baby.

"Some studies actually support the notion that those who have conceived via third-party reproduction are more likely to experience postpartum depression," says Dr. Maria Rothenburger, a psychotherapist at Miracles Happen Fertility Center in Salem, Oregon. She suspects the main reason is that infertility warriors don't recognize infertility as a trauma and believe having a baby will resolve all their difficult feelings. "The brain has, in fact, learned to behave from a traumatic place," she explains. "So, for example, the worry about whether a cycle will work translates to worry about whether the baby will continue to grow in utero, and then onto if anything will happen to the baby once born."

Also, remember that emotions originate from within. External factors cannot alleviate unresolved internal issues.

"Happiness comes from the 'inside,' from the cultivation of such qualities as trust, non-judgment, patience, compassion, non-striving, and acceptance," points out Janetti Marotta, a clinical psychologist and author of *A Fertile Path: Guiding the Journey with Mindfulness and Compassion*. "When these attributes are present, happiness arises. When actively engaged in the healing process, the inner resources you discover become the gift of a lifetime."

Postpartum Major Depression

The diagnosis requirements for postpartum major depression are the same as those for clinical depression (see chapter 14). The big difference, of course, is having an infant. The NIMH says that symptoms typically begin 3 weeks after giving birth but can start at any point during the first year of the baby's life.

Diagnosis of postpartum depression includes experiencing several of the following symptoms for a period of more than 2 weeks:

- Crying

- Difficulty concentrating

- Unexplained weight loss or gain

- Decreased appetite

- Insomnia or needing too much sleep

- Diminished interest in activities you previously enjoyed

- Unexplained aches or pains

- Feelings of worthlessness (especially with regard to your new role as a mother)

- Worry or anxiety

- Sadness

- Irritability

- Feeling disconnected from your child

- Suicidal thoughts or thoughts of hurting your baby

Postpartum Psychosis

Postpartum psychosis is rare (a 2017 report found that worldwide, fewer than 2.6 out of 1,000 new mothers have it), but it's particularly dangerous if left untreated. The *DSM-V* (the bible of psychiatric diagnosis) defines postpartum psychosis as a psychotic episode "with a postpartum onset." In most cases, symptoms start within the first 2 weeks after giving birth.

BUSTED

Myth: My feelings are wrong.

"There may be shame and guilt associated with feelings of 'I wanted this so much. How can anyone understand this when I can't?'" says Ellen Eule, a clinical social worker at Shady Grove Fertility in Rockville, Maryland. "So the inclination is to not tell, which in turn may lead to further feelings of being isolated and misunderstood."

But the truth is many people—both in and out of the infertility community—experience postpartum mental health disorders. They are not wrong or a sign that you are a bad or ungrateful parent. Denying your own feelings won't make them go away—in fact, it can make them worse.

Postpartum psychosis is often preceded by postpartum depression; however, the mother then develops delusions and/or hallucinations. These delusions and hallucinations can lead the mother to hurt herself, others, or even her baby.

Symptoms include:

- Confusion or disorientation

- Chattering nonsensically

- Unprompted feelings of rage

- Erratic behavior

- Rapidly shifting moods

- Seeing or hearing things that aren't real

- Believing things that aren't true

- Suicidal thoughts or attempts

- Intrusive and negative thoughts about your baby

Again, postpartum psychosis can be dangerous. Mothers who experience it can have periods of lucidity, but that doesn't mean the psychosis won't return. A 2016 study published in the *American Journal of Psychiatry* found that 31 percent of women who have had postpartum psychosis will experience it again after another pregnancy.

If you or your partner are showing signs of postpartum psychosis, get help from a mental health professional right away.

Risk Factors of Postpartum Depression

There is no one cause of postpartum depression or other mental health disorders. A combination of chemical and situational factors are at play. Still, it's important to know what risk factors could be present in *your* life. You can remove factors you have control over or make other preparations, depending on your degree of risk. However, know that there is a link between infertility and postpartum depression. A 2018 study published in the *Journal of Education and Health Promotion* found that new mothers who had struggled with infertility were more likely to have postpartum depression symptoms in the first 6 weeks after giving birth. A 2011 study in the *Journal of Midwifery and Women's Health* found that 25 percent of women who conceived via IVF had some degree of postpartum depression.

These correlations make sense to me. Infertility warriors have exhausted their time, energy, and possibly financial resources *before* becoming a parent. Emotional issues build up, and even after having a child, they can result in depression.

Dr. Alice Domar, an expert in mind/body health and infertility, says new parents who struggled with fertility issues are now struggling with a fundamental change to their identity. "They have identified as infertile for a long time and don't feel comfortable in the pregnancy [and parenting] world," she says. "They can't relate to [parents] who conceived easily, yet no longer fit in the infertile world. They can't complain to anyone since they feel guilty about feeling miserable."

Dr. Rothenburger argues that this sense of guilt can compound depression symptoms. People with fertility issues worked so hard and went through trauma to conceive a child. "Mothers think, 'This is what I asked for, this is what I strived to achieve. And now I'm having these feelings of sadness and despair. I don't get it,'" she explains. "So there's the self-judgment, this guilt, this shame associated with postpartum depression."

Let's break down some other risk factors for postpartum depression. According to the American Psychiatric Association and the American Psychological Association, contributors to postpartum depression include:

- Changes in hormone levels after giving birth

- Thyroid conditions

- Sleep deprivation

- Undiagnosed medical conditions

- Divorce or relationship problems

- Having a baby with health issues

- Stress surrounding your health

- Unplanned C-sections or other traumatic birth experiences

- Isolation

- Financial stress

- Lack of support both emotionally and in caring for your child

- Difficulty breastfeeding

- Previous mental health issues or a family history of mental health issues

Also, a 2022 study published in the *Journal of Affective Disorders* found that there is a higher prevalence of postpartum depression in first-time mothers, those younger than 25 years old, and mothers of twins (especially moms older than 40).

BUSTED

Myth: My feelings are my fault.

Just as infertility and any miscarriages were *not* your fault, neither is your depression and/or anxiety (yes, you can suffer from both). Infertility and parenthood have countless stressors, and it's not uncommon for emotions to become debilitating.

"Women are left to the task of monitoring our cycles, identifying fertility windows, and determining whether or not we conceived. Therefore, it follows that we feel a greater sense of responsibility, betrayal, and corresponding anxiety and depression when our bodies do not respond as we had hoped," says Debra S. Unger, a psychotherapist specializing in reproduction and infertility counseling in Bloomington, Indiana.

Your emotions are not your fault. And even if they were (*they're not*), that doesn't mean you have to endure them indefinitely. After everything you've been through, you deserve to be happy and enjoy being a parent, so please get professional help to begin on your road to healing.

Preventing Postpartum Depression

While there is no guaranteed way to avoid postpartum depression, you can take measures to lower your odds. Start by having a strong support system, which includes a mental health professional, in place *before* the situation reaches clinical depression levels. This person will not only help you shoulder your burdens but also catch early warning signs you may miss.

According to Dr. Rothenburger, this is especially important for women who have a family history of—or suffered previously from—depression, anxiety, bipolar disorder, or other mental disorders. She recommends that women with predispositions who are trying to have children start therapy as soon as possible.

This will help you gain the tools to deal with past traumas and the stress of finally becoming a parent.

It's also essential that you do *not* self-isolate, whether during your infertility journey or after becoming a parent. Separating yourself from your loved ones allows your negative emotions to grow and take over.

"[Isolating] can tend to exacerbate feelings of self-blame and shame," explains Unger. "When we share these emotions in either counseling with a therapist specializing in reproduction and infertility, support groups, or with close friends and family, research shows that it can help liberate us from these painful emotions and give women and couples some degree of relief, reducing their anxiety and depression."

Getting plenty of rest, avoiding alcohol consumption, and having a gentle exercise routine can also help minimize your risk of postpartum depression.

WARRIOR TIPS

Postpartum Depression Can Hit Anyone

We often forget that the infertility community includes celebrities. Kim Kardashian, Celine Dion, Brooke Shields, Emma Thompson, and many others have shared their struggle to build their families. It's a reminder that infertility doesn't discriminate.

Neither does postpartum depression. Chrissy Teigen, who conceived via IVF, opened up about her experience with postpartum depression in a 2017 essay in *Glamour* magazine.

When you see stories like this online or on social media, share your love and appreciation. After all, these people are part of our community and deserve our support.

Postpartum Anxiety

While there is high comorbidity with postpartum depression and postpartum anxiety, they are distinct disorders. And although postpartum depression gets more attention in the news, a 2013 study from Pennsylvania State University found that postpartum anxiety is more common. Of the study participants, 6 percent of mothers screened positive for postpartum depression, whereas 17 percent screened positive for postpartum anxiety.

It's normal for new mothers, especially those who battled infertility, to worry. But when that worry becomes excessive and debilitating, it's postpartum anxiety. According to Dr. Rothenburger, postpartum anxiety symptoms are the same as those of regular anxiety; there's just an additional focus on the baby. Symptoms include:

- Excessive worrying, despite how inconsequential the matter is

- Difficulty focusing

- Changes in appetite

- Insomnia

- Racing and repetitive thoughts

- Agitation

- Restlessness

- Being overprotective of your child

- Panic attacks

If you've never had a panic attack, they often present as an inability to catch your breath, pounding heart, chest pain or tightness, and sweating for no reason.

Looking back, even though my therapist never mentioned postpartum anxiety and instead focused on my postpartum depression, I definitely had anxiety. Not a moment went by when I wasn't excessively worrying or being overprotective of Aurora. I even frequently (wrongly) accused my mom and husband of making decisions related to her care that I thought would harm her in some way. I constantly thought she was going to die—and this lasted for months. I didn't get help nearly soon

---

BUSTED

Myth: It's just the sleep deprivation.

"I'm just tired." It's something we all tell ourselves when our mood starts to slip. Sometimes a good night's sleep will solve the problem, but understand how quickly things can go downhill.

After giving birth to twins, Adelle from Alberta, Canada, couldn't sleep because she was convinced that as soon as she shut her eyes, her children would die. "And I felt no one got it," she says. Feeling alone, she took on feedings by herself. Some nights, she would spend more than 5 hours trying to breastfeed, leading to a severe lack of sleep.

Eventually, Adelle was referred to a mental health specialist, whom she began seeing once a month. But when her children were about 5½ months old, she started thinking of ways she could rig her furnace to end it all. Thankfully, she arranged to meet with her psychologist more frequently and also sought out a sleep consultant. Soon, she was getting up to 4 consecutive hours of sleep each night and began to see the light at the end of the tunnel.

It's not just sleep deprivation. Recognize that your postpartum health needs attention. Getting more sleep helps, but you also need to cope with any negative emotions. And the sooner you seek support and treatment, the more likely you will recover quickly.

enough. Thankfully, my family was (mostly) patient with me, despite my emotional, terrible accusations against them.

Risk Factors of Postpartum Anxiety

Similar to postpartum depression, there's no clear cause of postpartum anxiety. However, most experts agree that changes to your hormone levels and sleep deprivation are big factors unique to postpartum women.

Dr. Rothenburger also says conditions surrounding you and your baby can lead to postpartum anxiety if they're not addressed. These include, but are not limited to:

- Health problems
- Previous pregnancy losses or infant deaths
- Lack of support
- Relationship issues

Women who have a family or personal history with mental disorders, especially anxiety disorders, are at higher risk for postpartum anxiety. The Pennsylvania State University study found that women who had C-sections or breastfed for a shorter period of time were more likely to have postpartum anxiety.

Preventing Postpartum Anxiety

One of the best ways to prevent postpartum anxiety is to remove as much pressure from yourself as possible. Dr. Rothenburger points out that many new moms, especially those who've struggled with infertility, want to be *perfect* moms. But setting unrealistic expectations and trying to be perfect is a recipe for anxiety. Perfection is not possible—for *anyone.*

She suggests that women who are at high risk for anxiety disorders start seeing a therapist while they're pregnant. Even if you aren't suffering from anxiety while pregnant, it helps you get ahead of your predisposition. You can learn and practice coping techniques when

you're not suffering. Then, after giving birth, use those tools to keep anxiety from getting out of hand.

⚡ It's also important to take time for yourself. Part of your anxiety stems from adjusting to becoming a parent. When you practice self-care, it connects you with other aspects of your identity that aren't tied to your worries and feelings of inadequacy as a parent. See chapter 23 for more on taking care of your mental health.

Finally, please take time to process your grief and emotions during your infertility journey. You're more likely to develop anxiety disorders if you don't learn how to cope with infertility's general fear of impending doom. Unger says it's understandable to want to hurry through treatments in hopes of succeeding sooner, but the pain piles up. "This can create a condition referred to as complicated grief, where the accumulation of loss can often heighten anxiety and make subsequent losses more painful," she explains. "In other words, the more we can stop and process our emotions along the way, the better able we are to cope with the impending feelings and consequences of our decisions."

Partners Experience Depression and Anxiety, Too

Yes, hormonal changes that occur after giving birth contribute to postpartum depression and anxiety. But any major life change can lead to the onset of mental disorders. This means new nonbirth parents are also vulnerable to depression and anxiety.

A 2019 meta-analysis of 47 studies published in the *Journal of Affective Disorders* found that new dads experienced both prenatal depression (14 percent in the first trimester, 11 percent in the second, 10 percent in the third, and 10 percent in all three) and paternal

BUSTED

Myth: You have to give birth to have postpartum depression.

After giving birth, hormonal changes can contribute to postpartum depression and anxiety. But life factors and changes are also in play. Becoming a parent means adapting to a lot of new situations in a short period of time. If you are unable to cope during your first few months as a parent, it is possible to develop postpartum depression or anxiety regardless of whether you gave birth.

Dr. Rothenburger, who is also an adoptive mother of two boys, says people who adopt, use surrogates, or are new non-carrying partners can develop these issues. She admits to feeling some level of depression after bringing her first son home. While she recognized how phenomenal it felt to finally be a mom, it was not easy to adjust to all the sudden life changes.

"My 18-month-old child was just ripped from all he knows. He was just ripped from his caretakers. He was just ripped from all familiarity," she explains. "You're watching your brand-new child go through a transition period, and there's nothing that you can do. There were even moments when he wanted nothing to do with me—did not want me to comfort him. I could not touch him and so it was really, really difficult."

All new parents are at risk for postpartum mental disorders. Learn the signs and take care of yourself.

---

postpartum depression (9 percent within 1 month of the child's birth, 8 percent within 1 to 3 months, 9 percent between 3 and 6 months, and 8 percent between 6 months and a year). Further, a meta-analysis of 23 studies published in 2021 in the *Journal of Psychosomatic Obstetrics & Gynecology* found that they also experience paternal prenatal anxiety and postpartum anxiety (both around 11 percent). For men who have unresolved issues stemming from their infertility journey, the risk can increase.

"What I see most often is that women take over the lion's share of the research and worrying while men tend to either avoid, minimize, or play a caretaker role in response to the woman's emotions," says Unger. "Most women present with both anxiety and depression while men appear to withdraw and internalize their despair—often to protect their partner—and experience some degree of depression."

Like new moms, it's common for new fathers to experience sadness, incessant worrying, or a tendency for isolation. However, with men, increased anger and frustration are also symptoms. If you are a new dad experiencing depression or anxiety symptoms (or if you suspect your male partner is), seek help.

A 2017 study published in *Perspective* found that the non-carrying partner in a lesbian relationship may feel insecure and uncertain about their new mothering role, leading to feelings of anxiety and depression. They may also feel envious of a breastfeeding birth partner. The researcher also pointed out that there is currently insufficient mental health support for LGBTQ+ partners both during and after pregnancy.

WARRIOR TIPS
Get Help

· ·

There is no shame in getting help for postpartum mental health disorders. These conditions are serious and can prevent you from achieving the happiness you deserve. If anything feels off after you have a child, check out the following resources to find support:

- Postpartum Education for Parents
- Postpartum Progress Support Groups
- Postpartum Support International

Please, do not ignore the signs of depression, anxiety, and other mental health issues. Address your emotions sooner rather than later. Reach out to a therapist at the first sign of trouble—or even before that—and practice the coping mechanisms you've learned throughout your infertility journey.

Identifying Your Needs

It's not easy to figure out what you need when you have postpartum depression or anxiety. Being overwhelmed and confused by your emotions is a by-product of these disorders. A big part of the recovery process involves avoiding isolation and being open to the observations of your loved ones.

After her daughter was born, Paula from Washington says she felt like a fish out of water. She wasn't able to produce enough breast milk for her daughter and felt like a failure. "I was overwhelmed," she shares. "I still didn't want to go out or have my husband touch me. Everything would either make me cry or piss me off."

Her husband, Konrad, was worried by the changes he saw in Paula and asked what he could do. Slowly, Paula was able to open up and heal.

"I was lucky that I have a great husband who talked with me and broached the subject," she says.

Even if you don't have a support system in place, find a way to make sense of your feelings and what may be causing them. Writing in a journal about what happened during the day and the accompanying emotions can help you start nailing down your triggers and fears so you can give a voice to your needs.

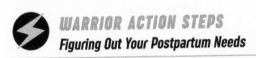

WARRIOR ACTION STEPS
Figuring Out Your Postpartum Needs

It's not easy, but sorting through your sadness and anxiety will help you figure out which of your needs aren't being addressed. Before your feelings get overwhelming, try the following:

Track changes. Some days will be better than others. Take note of what's different on days when you feel better or worse. Maybe you're facing new triggers and don't realize it.

Listen to your loved ones. Part of the issue with depression and anxiety is they become normalized for those experiencing them. You forget what you used to be like. Those around you will notice, however. When they voice their concerns, listen and try to see what they're seeing. This will help you address your emotions rather than just accepting them.

Don't neglect your nonemotional needs. It's not uncommon for people with depression and other mental health disorders to skip showers or meals or avoid cleaning their house. Even small tasks are too much some days. While this is completely okay, try to set small goals for yourself. Taking one shower a week, washing one dish in the sink, and cooking one healthy meal are all small ways you can tend to other needs.

Communicating Your Needs

It seems so easy in theory: Ask for what you need. But with infertility and postpartum depression and anxiety, there's a shame that often prevents parents from doing that.

"What we tend to do particularly with postpartum depression and anxiety is not only feel our emotions, but also judge ourselves because of them," says Dr. Rothenburger. As an extension, postpartum parents fear that voicing their needs will lead to judgment and rejection from *others*.

But the truth is your partner, friends, and family members want to see you happy. They want to offer support. Even if you can't clearly explain your specific needs, asking for help allows you to start down the road to feeling better.

Start small. Ask a friend to come over and help you put together a new baby toy or piece of furniture. You don't even have to bring up your emotions; this is about taking the small step of ending your self-isolation. Eventually, you can work up to talking about your depression and anxiety.

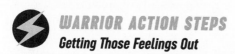

WARRIOR ACTION STEPS
Getting Those Feelings Out

Often, once you get talking about your feelings, it's like breaking through a dam. The words start flowing and they just don't stop. But how do you break through? When you're in a safe place, try:

Stream-of-consciousness writing. Sit down at your computer or with a pen and paper and just write. You don't have to worry about grammar or spelling, just start detailing what is going through your mind. Try to do this for at least 15 minutes, but you might find that once you get started, you don't want to stop.

Talk to "no one." Given the shame many postpartum infertility warriors feel, it's hard to admit how you're feeling to others. So talk to your dog, a photo of your mom, or an empty room. Saying how you feel out loud will take away some of the emotions' power and help you work up to talking to others.

Call a hotline. It may seem odd to open up to a stranger when you can't even talk to your partner. But many people find this easier. The volunteers at hotlines have no preconceived notions about who you are or how you *should* feel. They are trained and often available to talk to 24/7.

WARRIOR TIPS
Calling Postpartum Hotlines

There is *always* someone out there to listen to you. Whether you just need to talk or you're having thoughts of self-harm or suicide, reach out to one of the following resources:

Postpartum Support International:
1-800-944-4773 (phone) or 503-894-9453 (text)

Postpartum Education for Parents Warmline:
1-805-564-3888 (English) or 1-805-852-1595 (Spanish)

PPD Moms: 1-800-PPDMOMS (1-800-773-6667)

National Hopeline Network: 1-800-SUICIDE (1-800-784-2433)

→

Medical Treatment Options

Aside from therapy, some postpartum parents can benefit from medical treatment for their depression and anxiety. Depending on your diagnosis, you might be prescribed an antidepressant, mood stabilizers, antianxiety medications, or antipsychotics. With many of these medications, you will not be able to continue breastfeeding. In some cases of postpartum psychosis, electroconvulsive therapy might also be a recommendation. If you were already taking medications for a mental disorder, your dosage might need to be adjusted postpartum. Be open with your doctor about any new symptoms or changes in their intensity.

WARRIOR WISDOM
Finding Balance

"Brighter days outweigh the dark ones for sure, but out of nowhere a sadness will creep up out of my stomach and I will cry for my struggles and losses. But I have learned to honor those moments and them let them pass. It's all about balance and boundaries." —Krista, New Jersey

WARRIOR CHECKLIST
Understanding Postpartum Depression and Anxiety

- ❑ Understand the different types of postpartum depression and anxiety.
- ❑ Recognize the symptoms and potential risk factors for postpartum mental disorders.
- ❑ Build a support system that can help you deal with negative emotions after becoming a parent.
- ❑ Reach out to mental health professionals if you are having difficulty processing or adjusting to your new life as a parent.

Add more items to your Warrior Checklist or jot down any notes here:

_____

_____

_____

_____

_____

_____

_____

_____

_____

_____

_____

Parenting After Infertility

EVERYTHING I ENVISIONED ABOUT what it would be like to be a parent was wrong. Much of that has stemmed from my daughter Aurora's health issues, sure, but it's more than that. I've been more overprotective than I expected, I've been put in situations I never could have imagined, and my daughter is more like me than I care to admit most days.

Aurora has had some struggles including near-constant rejection of food, projectile vomiting what she managed to eat, severe asthma, and recurrent strep throat that led to her tonsils and adenoids being taken out at 16 months old. But there there has also been something unexpectedly amazing that's changed the way we approach parenting her.

At around 26 weeks gestation, I had an MRI of her entire body. There I was on Christmas Eve, barely fitting into an MRI machine, for 2 hours. Although they didn't tell us beforehand, our doctors were trying to determine if her brain was smaller than it should be at that point in pregnancy—in other words, if we should expect her to be developmentally delayed. Thankfully, her brain was perfectly fine. Still, we were told she should be monitored by a pediatric neurologist after birth as a precaution.

Although I had to advocate quite a bit until we found someone who would listen to our concerns, we eventually connected with an amazing neurologist. At one point, Aurora's overall growth was so behind due to her feeding disorder that her head growth also lagged. As our doctor explained, first goes the weight, then the height, then the head—and most often, once the head measurement is behind, it doesn't bounce back.

We turned our lives upside down to get food into her. With feedings every 90 minutes around the clock for her first year and then every 3 hours until she was 2½—and the fact that she would eat only certain things for certain people in certain places—we rarely left the house. But somehow we did it—her head measurement eventually got back on track. Our girl's still extremely tiny and thin, but she's lined up with her own growth chart now.

You're probably wondering, *Where's the amazing part?* The backstory is important, but here it is: Somehow, someway, after all she's been through, Aurora is off-the-charts smart. At 7 years old, she finished third grade math and fourth grade English—and was in third grade for everything else. And if I'm being honest, she often outsmarts us—in ways that are sometimes hilarious and sometimes maddening.

All in all, parenting is nothing like what I expected, and my infertility journey both created setbacks in my ability to adapt and uniquely trained me for situations that have arisen.

Being a Parent—Finally

Imagine it: You're a parent! All you feel is incredible joy, right? Yes . . . but also no. Parenting after infertility likely is not what you imagined. It's amazing, beautiful, and life-changing. But it's not perfect.

It's not uncommon for infertility warriors to idealize parenthood. While having a child is wonderful, it's important to acknowledge that being a parent isn't always easy. There are surprises and difficulties, and the infertility journey itself can leave lingering challenges.

Many parents who struggled with infertility think that once they have a child, they've finally put their infertility challenges in the rearview mirror. I hate to be the bearer of bad news, but that's not the case.

We're going to delve into the highs and lows of post-infertility parenthood. How is reality different from what you've imagined? How will past infertility trauma affect you as a parent? What can you and your partner do to be fantastic parents while balancing your relationship and happiness? Having all of these answers—and more—will prepare you for being the parent you want to be.

The Good, the Bad, and the Ugly

Real talk time: Parenting after infertility isn't all rainbows and unicorns. Yes, there are amazing highs in raising your child. But there are also things that flat-out suck. While knowing what to expect won't eliminate the low points, it can help temper the difficulty.

The Good

One thing that sets apart parenthood after infertility is your appreciation for having a child. Don't get me wrong: It's not that fertile myrtles are't grateful, but your journey gives you a different perspective. As Chrissy from British Columbia, Canada, puts it, you're

---

BUSTED

Myth: Every day of parenting will be a piece of cake compared to infertility.

After years of agonizing treatments and trauma, what could a baby or child possibly do that's worse than battling infertility? If you can survive all the obstacles you had to overcome to have a child, what are a few dirty diapers and sleepless nights?

First off, you're comparing apples and oranges. The difficulty of infertility doesn't make parenting easier. Though infertility can help you better understand how precious your child is, it doesn't mean there won't be days when you'll struggle.

Lisa Stack, a support coordinator at CNY Fertility in Syracuse, New York, says it's common for former infertility patients to assume that their journey gave them everything they need to be calm, patient, and grateful all the time once they become parents. "Remember that you are human!" she says. "You will be incredibly grateful, but you will also feel frustration, fatigue, and anger at times as well."

Beth from New Hampshire admits that when she was in the middle of her fertility treatments, she was sure gratitude for her child would make everything a breeze. "Baby up for the fourth time? Great, at least I have a baby! Diaper explosion? No problem, better than not getting to be the mom! Screaming toddler? I've got this, just like I had those PIO [progesterone in oil] shots!" she says. "Not so much. Parenting after infertility is just that: parenting. It's totally normal to be exhausted, grossed out, and frustrated."

always reminded of the miracle that is *your* child. "My son is and probably will always be my only," she says. "With him, I always know this will be the only time. The only time I give birth. The only time I throw a first birthday party. The only time I hear my child say 'mama' for the first time. Everything is to be celebrated and nothing is to be missed."

Bonding with your new baby is a powerful experience for most parents, no matter how the baby came into your life. It takes on a particular special quality if you are someone who dealt with infertility. But remember: The bonding process is different for every parent. For some parents it happens right away. For others it takes time—and that's okay.

Dr. Maria Rothenburger, a psychotherapist specializing in infertility, says it's important not to let worries about bonding build up.

BUSTED

Myth: All the other issues in my life will disappear once I have a baby.

Infertility directly and indirectly impacts many aspects of your life. It can create a web of issues that are difficult to unravel. But when your focus is honed like a laser on having a baby, you begin to think that once you achieve your goal, everything else will also get better.

Dr. Alice Domar, an expert in mind/body health and infertility, says it's important to know that's not the case. "You think, 'When I have a baby, I'm going to be happy. When I have a baby, I'm going to like my mother-in-law. When I have a baby, my husband and I aren't going to fight. My life is going to be complete and perfect,'" she explains. "But you can't pin all that on a 7-pound baby."

Getting your life to where you want it to be will take work, but it'll be worth it.

"Awareness is the key here," she says. "Know that you have the feelings, and simply let the feelings be what they are. Don't think they need to be any different. Some people's relationships grow a little bit slower."

Enjoy the process of bonding with your child. Getting to know who they are will be one of the best parts of parenting.

The Bad

Again, for all parents, there are bad times. But there are some common emotional hurdles specific to parents who battled infertility. A big one is guilt. Carol Toll, a clinical social worker, says many infertility survivors feel guilty about having negative—but totally natural—emotions. "After birth, parents are subject to all the rigors of caring for an infant while feeling they are never allowed to 'complain' about fatigue or doubt because they worked so hard to have this child."

Jay from New York says she didn't think it was possible to swing from gratitude to guilt as often as she did. And many other infertility warriors agree.

The guilt also plays into another difficult aspect of parenting after infertility: the pressure to be perfect. You've gone through hell to have a child, and now you must ensure their life—and your life—is perfect. You cannot drop the ball. Allison from California says the pressure she put on herself is her biggest parenting regret. "I worked so hard to get [my daughter] here and felt responsible that every minute be perfect because she and I both deserved that after the struggle. Especially since I couldn't have any more children," she shares. "But the truth is, I'm still an imperfect mom, and we are both going to have good days and bad days—and that's okay."

Maintaining their relationship is also a struggle for many couples. Becoming parents brings a completely new dynamic to a relationship. Taking care of the baby becomes time-consuming, and if you're not conscious about it, you might begin to drift apart. To avoid that, my husband and I spend Sundays together while Aurora is at my parents' house. That ritual has helped us stay connected to each other throughout the trials of parenthood.

The Ugly

No surprise, but some of the hardest parts of parenting directly relate to infertility. The triggers you experienced during your journey may not go away. In fact, new ones can crop up, especially if you had a difficult or high-risk delivery. Finally having a child will not erase the trauma.

"I spent a lot of time talking myself through my feelings when that trauma was triggered," says Beth. "I'd say out loud, 'This is my infertility scar making an appearance. It does not own the moment. It is a part of me, but it is not me.'"

We touched on this a little before, but wanting or trying to have another child can also bring up grief, sadness, and anxiety. Chrissy, for example, always feels torn about joining Mommy and Me–type classes. On the one hand, the classes are good for her son and her mental health. But on the other hand, seeing pregnant women or being asked if she and her husband are going to have more children triggers her pain.

If you do decide to try to have another child, returning to your old doctor and clinic will remind you of everything you endured last time. Dr. Rothenburger says that even if the treatments were free and conception was almost guaranteed, trying for another child would be very difficult emotionally. Getting your blood drawn, having an ultrasound, or seeing familiar faces could all become new triggers. As someone who has started a frozen embryo transfer cycle every year since 2019 in an effort to give Aurora a sibling, but never actually gone through with it, I can attest to this wholeheartedly.

Preparing for Reality

Once you know what you're facing, it's time to prepare to handle all that parenting can throw at you. Ideally, you'll be able to prep and plan before your child comes home with you, but if you can't, better late than never. Here are some good first steps:

Research parenthood. This sounds obvious, but a lot of people dealing with infertility avoid educating themselves about parenting in case something goes wrong—they fear they might jinx it. However, for many couples, it takes years to become parents, giving you plenty of opportunities when you're feeling strong to read or listen up on parenting.

BUSTED

Myth: I'll finally be "normal."

Part of the pain of infertility is the otherness of it. You can't conceive in a typical manner, instantly separating you from most of your friends and family. This leads many infertility warriors to believe that once they do have a child, they'll finally be "normal." They'll have a family, and the trauma they experienced during the process will no longer isolate them.

But as Toll points out, having a child isn't a "cure" for infertility. The resulting scars can make it difficult to feel comfortable becoming part of the parenting community. "Initially, [you] may even feel like an imposter during this transition into the fertile world of children and parents after the painful but familiar world of infertility," she says.

You'll love being a parent, but understand that the trauma of infertility *will* impact your experience. While you don't have to feel like an outsider, you won't suddenly feel like every other parent.

Talk out topics with your partner if you have one. It's incredibly difficult to make decisions when you're an exhausted and emotional new parent. Have conversations with your partner about how you'll handle common situations or choices. Discuss the rationale behind your preferences. This will get you on the same page about what to do once the sleepless nights come.

Have a relationship plan. Every relationship is different with regard to the amount of quality time and communication it requires. Some new parents maintain their relationship by having monthly date nights. Others set aside 20 minutes every day for adult conversation. Talk with your partner so you can identify your needs and come up with a plan that works for both of you—and be prepared to adapt it to fit your new circumstances and needs when a baby comes into the picture.

Post-Infertility Parenting Dos and Don'ts

There are no absolutes with parenting. But there are a few general tips that can help you navigate your new life with a child. More important, these dos and don'ts will help you work through challenges specific to post-infertility parents.

Do be aware of control issues.

Infertility often steals all sense of control over your life. It demands that you change your life plans and adapt to their rules. The struggle to take back control continues after you have a child. You might be tempted to cling to anything that gives you a greater sense of certainty.

For Katelyn from Ontario, Canada, it was stressful to let others hold her daughter, especially when the baby cried and the person holding her would try to calm her by themselves. "My stress level would go through the roof in those situations," she admits. But it wasn't easy for her to reassert control and ask for her daughter back. "My husband was good in that department. I would look at him and he would know to go grab our baby and give her back to me."

Dr. Rothenburger says it's very difficult to balance taking control over what you can—and should—with letting go and allowing your child to learn and experience life for themselves. She admits that after adopting her first son, she found herself going back and forth about control.

"As a therapist, I'm hyperaware of the inclination to be overprotective. I'm trying very consciously to allow my kid to do something on his own without me stepping in. But then there's a sense of guilt around that. 'Should I be giving him so much freedom? Should I be protecting him more?' It's this back and forth between 'Am I being overprotective?' and 'Am I doing the right thing by my child?'"

To say that I struggled with this same battle would be an understatement. At every stage of Aurora's life—whether it was when she came home with the apnea and bradycardia monitor or when we put baby gates on the stairs to keep her from climbing up them—my parents would joke that I'd be overprotecting her until college.

⚡ It's natural to have control issues after infertility. Be aware of your own feelings and weigh them against the well-being of your child. For example, if the thought of leaving your child with a babysitter causes anxiety, acknowledge those emotions, but also find ways that you can build up to becoming comfortable with leaving your child for a period of time because it's good for both you and your child to have some experience with separation. Don't let your desire for control in turn control you or prevent you from allowing your child the freedom to learn and grow.

BUSTED

Myth: I have to stick to "The Plan."

Every parent paints a picture in their head of the type of parent they'll be. They think about the holiday traditions they'll follow or how they'll approach disciplining their child. With infertility warriors, the journey to parenthood is longer and more difficult than normal, so there's a tendency to hold on to "The Plan" more tightly. *Gosh darn it, I finally have control over my life and I will make it as perfect as I imagined!*

But life is going to happen; you'll have to adapt and update your plan for being a parent. For me, I had to make changes regarding my work/life balance. Because my company at the time was made up of remote employees, for years I'd worked from home. I'd always imagined raising my children at home while I continued to work. It was important that I could be a role model for my future kids and have them *see* how hard I worked to provide for them. But when Aurora was born, that didn't turn out to be an option. By the time she was 8 months old, caring for her while I was also working was too much for me to handle, and we put her in someone else's care (we chose an early learning center for her, but there are many options).

I was devastated that I couldn't work *and* tend to all her needs. It wasn't the happy ending I imagined. But it was my reality, and it took time for me to accept that.

Remember our talk about being resilient in chapter 15? Building resiliency is key to the infertility journey, and you're going to have to continue to use that skill as a parent. Recognize when you need to make changes to your plan so you can be the best parent possible in your situation.

Don't isolate yourself from your new community.

Post-infertility parents often feel like outsiders in two communities. Now that they have children, they feel guilty being around people who are still struggling. But at the same time, they don't feel like they belong with "regular" parents. This feeling of isolation makes parenthood even harder.

Beth admits that she felt uncomfortable discussing kids and parenting when she first met other parents. "I wish I had put myself out there more to meet other moms with similar parenting attitudes and/or infertility experiences. I think it would have helped me transition to the parenting community from the infertility community."

⚡ Don't stop talking to your friends in the infertility community, as long as you can respect their boundaries about children. But it's also important to start building a support network of parents outside of that community. These new friends will help you adjust to your new identity as a parent and understand the daily struggles of having kids.

But as Kelli from Oregon found out, sometimes it's tough to find parenting peers your age. Many infertility warriors aren't able to have a child until their late 30s or well into their 40s. New moms tend to be younger.

"Most of my friends' kids are graduating from college, getting married, and having babies," Kelli explains. "While I can relate to young moms and to older friends preparing for retirement, there isn't anyone going through menopause at the same time they are raising little ones. But I laugh about it a lot and recognize that I'm uniquely positioned to connect with lots of people across the age spectrum."

If you take the same positive attitude, you'll build meaningful relationships in the parenting community.

Do use lessons from infertility.

One silver lining to infertility is the coping mechanisms you develop. The struggle makes you stronger, and Toll says the skills you learn can be a big help once you're a parent. "Perhaps you have strengthened partner relationships and learned how to ask for help. Or you know how to become an advocate while developing resilience from overcoming obstacles," she observes.

Take stock of everything you learned during your infertility journey and think of how that knowledge and perspective can come in handy as a parent. This will not only help you during difficult parenting times but also give some sense of purpose to the challenges you faced.

BUSTED ═══════════════════════

Myth: After having one baby, I won't be sad if I can't have another.

This is a tough one. After going through so much to have one child, it's difficult to accept both your gratitude *and* your desire to have more children. But many infertility warriors want to continue growing their family and struggle with their options.

Jay has two sons, one conceived through IVF and one spontaneously. But she admits she still wonders about how many kids she would have had if infertility hadn't been a limiting factor. "Fertile people ask, 'How many kids should we have?'" she says. "And infertile people ask, 'Can we afford the treatment to even try to have kids?'"

Dr. Rothenburger says it's natural to have trouble processing the happiness surrounding the children you have and your desire to have more. "There's absolutely zero wrong with wanting more children," she says. "But the idea that you'll successfully have one child and then never feel sad if it's a struggle to have a second is completely unfounded."

The self-advocacy skills I learned—albeit at the end of my journey—have served me well in advocating for Aurora's well-being. I've been her voice every step of the way, from getting her feeding disorder diagnosed and treated to ensuring she's receiving proper care and education.

Don't hide your story.

We've talked about the guilt you might feel being around people still struggling to build their family. You've been where they are, and you know how much seeing mothers and their children can hurt. And the guilt can be so heavy that you just want to keep your head down and stay under the radar.

Katelyn admits she used to see parents trying for a second child at her fertility clinic and think they were selfish and rude to rub their success in her face. "Fast-forward to today, and now I am one of those selfish, rude parents wanting a second child. It is so hard being at that clinic and having all the hopeful parents there watching me and my daughter. It's even

---

WARRIOR TIPS
Parenting a Child of a Different Race or Ethnicity
• •

It's not uncommon to end up being an adoptive parent of a child of a different race or ethnic background. As Dr. Rothenburger can attest, this presents its own challenges. She and her husband (who are both white) adopted their sons from Korea and acknowledge that you can't just ignore the fact that members of your family are of different races.

She and her husband make a conscious effort to expose their sons to both American and Korean culture. This allows them to embrace both aspects of their identity and normalizes their adoption stories.

EmbraceRace.org has a curated list of transracial adoption resources, and American Adoptions has a guide to transracial adoptions.

worse when some staff members squeal in delight when they see us and run up and hug us both."

She talked to her doctor about it, and he said to think of it as a way to show other infertility warriors that they, too, can succeed.

Instead of thinking of the harm you're unintentionally causing, focus on the good you can do. Talk to the women and men in those waiting rooms and swap war stories. Many other infertility warriors will walk away from your conversation with a renewed sense of hope.

COPING AND GETTING SUPPORT

It takes a long time to raise a child, and over that time, you're going to have different needs and varying support systems. It is important to know that you and your partner may not always be on the same page about what support you need or the best way to cope. Always pay attention to changes in yourself and your partner so you know when it's time to sit down and have a discussion.

Identifying Your Needs

At the beginning of your life as a parent, you're going to struggle with your new identity. For a long time, not having kids was a part of who you were. But now that you have a child to nurture and raise, you're going to discover new aspects of yourself.

Pay attention to areas where you're struggling to understand or embrace the new you. Ask yourself:

- What are my fears?
- What are my doubts?
- What do I think are my shortcomings?

Then identify what you would need to feel better about these aspects of your identity. Maybe you need more reassurance from your partner or to take a painting class once a week so you don't feel like you're losing your creativity.

After a few months with your child, you'll have gotten into a routine. Stop and consider how happy you are with your typical day. See if you can identify any challenging moments of the day when you could use more support or make changes to better address your needs.

Finally, think ahead to how you will talk to your child about their origin story. It will be a little different from the origin story of children whose parents didn't struggle with infertility, and you'll want to figure out how you plan to integrate that story into the narrative of your family. Other people—your own parents, other relatives, and friends—may have an opinion about what you tell your child and when, but none of that is their choice. This is your story to tell, and you should determine what you need to honor and respect it.

Think through and/or discuss the following questions with your partner:

- Are you comfortable with others talking to your child about how he or she came into your life if you're not present?

- What should your family and friends say if your child asks them questions about their origin story?

- Do you think it's important your child knows about their egg, sperm, or embryo donor? If so, how and when will you tell them?

Communicating Your Needs

When it comes to communicating your needs, if you have a partner, it's best to start with them. You two have been supporting each other throughout your infertility journey, and that doesn't stop after having a child. If you are a single parent, make sure you make space for these feelings— and be prepared to ask for help.

With Your Partner

Never assume that what you say will be interpreted in the way you meant it. Different people have different communication styles. One way to facilitate clear communication when you're talking about your needs is for you and your partner to get into the habit of restating what the other one just said to clarify that you heard and understood correctly. This ensures that you are on the same page about the best way to help each other.

With Your Family and Friends

It's okay to ask for parenting help and support. Angela from Missouri says that when she had trouble learning how to soothe her daughter, she turned to her mom. While it wasn't easy to admit, Angela knew she needed advice.

Whether you need a babysitter or someone to vent to, don't be scared to reach out. You'll find that the sooner you get help, the quicker things begin to get better.

However, know that not everyone will understand the enduring pain of infertility. Some people will incorrectly assume that now that you have a child, all your previous issues will be gone. You'll need to remind people about your triggers and how they can best approach topics surrounding infertility.

Despite having multiple miscarriages and going through several rounds of different treatments, Tina from New Jersey says it seemed like her friends and family "forgot" about her fertility issues once she had her son. "They'll make comments or jokes or blurt out pregnancy announcements that, although easier to hear than before I was a mom, sometimes still sting," she says. "I've needed friends and family to understand that my infertility is not 'over' and I'm not 'back to normal.' I'll never be 'normal' in that sense again."

If what your family and friends are saying or asking you hurts, tell them. Remind them that while you love your child, your child's existence does not erase your past trauma.

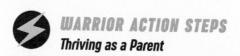

WARRIOR ACTION STEPS
Thriving as a Parent

Sometimes, honoring your feelings is the best way to get through the rough bits of parenthood. The following are ways you can cope with post-infertility parenting:

Allow for conflicting emotions. As a new parent who struggled with infertility, you might feel intense joy, gratitude, guilt, and depression—all within the space of 5 minutes. Instead of judging yourself, give yourself permission and room to feel whatever comes up. This enables you to accept your emotions instead of wasting energy trying to suppress them.

Be patient with yourself. Instead of spiraling into self-doubt and self-critique when you make a mistake, forgive yourself and focus on what you've learned, not what you did wrong.

Check in with your partner. Understand that while you may have worked through your grief, your partner might just be starting. Once infertility is no longer consuming you, it's not uncommon for negative emotions from that difficult time to finally surface.

→

Tackling Survivor's Guilt

If you're not familiar with the term, survivor's guilt involves the negative emotions someone feels when they've made it through a trauma while others haven't. With infertility warriors, it specifically applies to people who were able to build a family. You may feel bad because others in your community are still struggling.

"I felt so bad for the women still in waiting that I couldn't fully enjoy my pregnancy," shares Jalina from New York. "I couldn't shake the guilt that the sight of my baby bumps and then the sight of my children would be triggering for strangers in public who were in the same place I once was."

Becoming a parent—and feeling guilty about that—shouldn't separate you from the friends you've made in the infertility community. Discuss each other's triggers and how you can both support each other. It can also be extremely helpful to continue to advocate for other infertility warriors.

Jay, for instance, discovered she was stronger and in a better position to be an advocate and ally after becoming a parent. "It took me a bit to work out, but ultimately, you can walk that line between being a parent and being an infertility advocate," she explains. "I couldn't have been an effective infertility advocate when I was going through treatment, as I was dealing with both the emotional and financial strain of fertility treatment. Now I'm in a position where I can advocate for others who are where I was back then, unable to advocate for themselves."

WARRIOR WISDOM
Your Child Is Loved

"I think we put a lot of pressure on ourselves to be amazing parents because it is something we lost countless hours of sleep thinking about. We made plenty of pleas to the universe to just please give us a child. But having a real person that you are in charge of raising, one with their own personality and thoughts, is much harder than all the planning in the world. So don't be too hard on yourself. Your child is loved, and the only thing that matters is that they know that." —Erin, Ontario, Canada

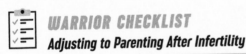

WARRIOR CHECKLIST
Adjusting to Parenting After Infertility

❑ Understand the reality of being a parent after infertility.

❑ Make preparations to deal with the highs and lows of parenthood.

❑ Find a balance between your two communities: parents and infertility warriors.

❑ Be able to identify your needs throughout your time raising your child. Be confident communicating them to others.

❑ Allow yourself to be imperfect as a parent and focus on the love you feel for your child.

Advocating for Fertility Benefits and Other Warriors

DAVINA FANKHAUSER, COFOUNDER of Fertility Within Reach in Newton Highlands, Massachusetts, is an expert on advocating for the infertility community, but she also has her own inspiring infertility story.

Fankhauser amassed valuable skills along her varied career path; she's been a teacher, a book buyer, a patient advocate at an egg donation bank, and the advocacy director for RESOLVE New England. In her capacity for that last one, she says, "I was at the Massachusetts State House every week lobbying to help pass legislation into a law. And we were successful, which is really exciting. From that experience, I decided to use that knowledge—and my teaching experience—to create Fertility Within Reach."

While balancing her work life, Fankhauser was also trying to build her family. She and her husband married young and immediately started trying to conceive. But at the age of 23, she was diagnosed with endometriosis. A year later, they still hadn't been successful, so

her husband also underwent fertility testing and was diagnosed with male factor infertility. After surgery to address the endometriosis, she finally became pregnant—but it ended in a miscarriage.

That pattern of pregnancy followed by miscarriage continued. "It seemed like we were getting pregnant once a year, but within 2 months, I would miscarry. And in total, we have had 10 pregnancies," she says.

When they moved to Massachusetts, they tried IVF, with genetic testing for the embryos. However, time passed and they remained unable to have a successful pregnancy. Further testing revealed that Fankhauser had a blood clotting disorder. Her doctors put her on blood thinners for her fourth cycle of IVF, which happily—finally—resulted in the birth of their daughter.

When they were ready to try for a second child, they miscarried another time. During the next IVF cycle, they transferred all of their available embryos to save money—and ended up with a triplet pregnancy. "That was a very difficult time because my body couldn't sustain a triplet pregnancy. And my cervix started to thin at 10 weeks," shares Fankhauser.

She saw three different specialists, and they all suggested reduction to a singleton, which caused tension between her and her husband. Ultimately, they agreed to proceed. Their son was born at 28 weeks. Despite the challenges that presented, Fankhauser didn't feel like her family was complete. "I was actually ready to try again," she says, "and my husband was like, no way, that is our last pregnancy. So, we did a lot of mental health support to help us end our journey. But we have two amazing kids because of it."

Now, as an advocacy expert, Fankhauser works to help others advocate for themselves and the infertility community through Fertility Within Reach. She doesn't want other infertility warriors to have to make detrimental decisions because of their financial status or lack of access to insurance. After she worked to help pass a law in Massachusetts that expanded infertility benefits, she was emboldened to do more. "After I experienced success changing the law in Massachusetts, I knew I could provide information and support to teach others how to experience the same success. But with less stress," Fankhauser says. "Really the motivation behind it was after experiencing what I did with my son's birth. It just felt it didn't need to be that way. And I wanted to see more safe pregnancies and healthy babies in the world."

Standing Up for Others

Whether you just started facing infertility, are in the middle of your struggle, or have finally reached post-infertility life, you've probably recognized two themes running through these chapters.

First, infertility is freaking hard. Plain and simple. It's exhausting, heartbreaking, and eternally challenging. Second, you have the power to speak up and own your journey. Self-advocacy is an indispensable part of becoming stronger than infertility.

In this chapter, we're going to talk about ways to advocate for other infertility warriors. As Dr. Alice Domar, an expert in mind/body health and infertility, reminds us, infertility is not uncommon. "In the US, it's one in eight couples. In the UK, it's one in seven. In Canada, it's one in six," she shares.

If you're still focused on acceptance and self-care, that's alright; you're still learning and growing on your journey. If you *are* ready to start advocating for the infertility community as a whole, it's time to step up and fight for those who can't.

Hopefully you're now a lot more comfortable with the concept of self-advocacy, even if you haven't yet mastered it. But advocating for others and the entire infertility community is a new adventure. If you're a little unsure of what the process entails or why you should

---

BUSTED

Myth: Advocacy isn't my responsibility.

You're just one person, and you've been through—or perhaps are still going through—a long fight to build your family. Why is it your job to continue fighting for someone else—someone you don't even know? Simply put, because someone has to speak up.

As Lee Rubin Collins, a member of the board of directors for RESOLVE, puts it:

"Our lawmakers aren't even going to think about infertility if we don't show up and tell our stories!"

Even if you play a small part, like writing a letter, it adds up. One voice might not seem powerful, but when infertility warriors speak up together, it becomes a roar.

---

even become a community advocate, you're not alone.

By better understanding the power of advocacy and why it's important, you can be more confident in your ability to create change.

The Current Landscape and Looking to the Future

No doubt you've encountered many logistical, financial, and legal issues on your infertility journey. You've faced a problem and thought, "There's got to be a better system for this." But you may not have considered how *legislation* can be part of the solution for these situations. So, let's take a look at some infertility issues, where they currently stand, and what the path forward looks like. (Note that all of this information was current at time of publication, but subject to change. And hopefully for the better! Visit the RESOLVE website for the most current information about legislation.)

Insurance Coverage

Most insurance companies—and by extension, employers and other organizations—do not willingly cover expensive but widely needed fertility treatments. Fertility preservation procedures, like egg or sperm freezing before chemotherapy, often aren't covered either. There's no federal mandate regarding infertility coverage. However, states can pass laws that require insurance companies to cover infertility-related diagnostics, medications, and treatments.

Current Legislation

As of February 2023, twenty states have laws related to insurance coverage and fertility treatments. These laws differ in terms of what they include, and some states are in the process of updating their laws to expand coverage to include treatments like IVF.

Where Things Are Heading

For infertility warriors who live in states where coverage isn't required by law, the next step is getting that ball rolling—drawing attention to the issue and asking legislators to write bills that will address it.

If you live in a state where coverage *is* required, don't assume the law is perfect. While it might have worked for your particular case, other warriors may be falling through the cracks. Educate yourself about possible loopholes in the law, and bring up these issues with your lawmakers.

BUSTED

Myth: You have to be an expert to be an advocate.

You're not a politician or legal expert, and no one is asking you to be. As Collins puts it, regular people make the best advocates. "It's your life experience—not your civics knowledge—that's persuasive to lawmakers. RESOLVE has been doing this for years and can guide advocates, bring people together, and make advocacy effective, gratifying, and even fun," she says.

Katie from North Carolina first attended Advocacy Day in Washington, DC, in 2015. She admits that even with RESOLVE's support, she was nervous about being an advocate. "I was still nervous that I hadn't memorized all the bills, and all the issues, and all the talking points. But it was so relieving to actually meet the staffers because it is not a script that you read to them. It's a conversation that you're having with people who influence changes in our policy."

Most likely you've had thousands of conversations about infertility throughout your journey. That's all advocacy is: telling your story. And you're *definitely* an expert on that topic.

Protection of Personhood

Are embryos morally equivalent to live people, and if so, what rights do they have? If states give embryos legal "personhood" (it's a legal term, but I'm not a fan), it would impact the availability of IVF. In some cases, it could also make the cryo-preservation of embryos illegal.

Current Legislation

According to RESOLVE, more than a hundred different bills surrounding embryo person-hood have been drafted. In the 2022 *Dobbs* decision overturning *Roe v. Wade*, the US Supreme Court declined to establish a base-line on fetal personhood; however, there's concern in the infertilty commumty about how fertility treatments may be impacted in a post-*Roe* world. These fights will likely play out at the state level going forward. A fed-eral bill introduced into committee in 2021 (H.R. 877–Sanctity of Human Life Act), states "each human life begins at fertilization, clon-ing, or its equivalent."

Where Things Are Heading

You can join a local advocacy group or a national group such as RESOLVE. If you join the RESOLVE Advocacy Network (it's free), it will send you information on your specific state. Information like how it impacts family planning options such as IVF, specific break-downs of the proposed bill, and how you can take action enables you to take charge and make your voice heard most effectively.

As of this writing, it is too soon to tell if or how fertility treatments will be impacted in a post–*Roe v. Wade* world. However, both RESOLVE and the American Society for Reproductive Medicine (ASRM) are keep-ing a close eye on state bills and laws. Visit their websites—RESOLVE.org and ASRM .org, respectively—for the most up-to-date information.

Infertility Insurance Coverage for Veterans

Until very recently, veterans with service-related injuries that led to loss of fertility did not have access to treatments like IVF through the US Department of Veterans Affairs (VA). For many veteran families, this put treatment out of their price range.

Current Legislation

Thankfully, Congress *finally* realized how unfair it is not to cover treatment for veter-ans who lost their fertility while serving their country. A bill passed in 2016 (and renewed in 2021) extended coverage to IVF procedures for qualifying veterans. However, this bill must be reauthorized each year and has not yet become a permanent benefit.

Where Things Are Heading

Since, as of this writing, those benefits expire after a year, it's important to continue to advo-cate for coverage for veterans. Many people are working to ensure *all* veterans and active-duty service members get coverage for *all* fertility treatments, whether or not their infer-tility relates to their service.

Adoption Accessibility

Adoption is expensive, and though the fed-eral government tries to help with the cost, it doesn't benefit everyone. This means many prospective adoptive parents are unable to afford to bring a child into their home.

Current Legislation

The adoption tax credit has been in place for years. However, in 2012, the law changed and "refundability" was removed. This means lower-income prospective adoptive parents receive a smaller tax credit or no credit at all—which can make adoption unaffordable for them. For adoptions finalized in 2022, there is

BUSTED

Myth: Legislators have better things to do than listen to me.

Politicians have a lot on their plate and are dealing with a lot of issues at once. Why would they be willing to listen to you and add another issue to their list? To put it simply: because it's their job.

"The fact is, legislators want to hear from you. If you think about it, they campaign, they go hungry for months, they are exhausted for months, they are raising money, and they are sacrificing a lot of family time—all so they can represent you," says Fankhauser. "And if they don't know what their people need, how can they really do the job that they worked so hard for?"

Honor the value of your opinions, and trust that your representatives value them as well. Unless people speak up, legislators are basically creating laws blindly, and that benefits no one.

"Know that your voice—your experience—is important," says Joyce Reinecke, executive director of the Alliance for Fertility Preservation in Lafayette, California. "Don't diminish your feelings or your needs. You are the one who went through this, and don't be afraid of expressing your opinion because you don't necessarily know the science or the technical aspects of insurance, etc."

---

a federal adoption tax credit of up to $14,890 per child. This sounds great, but then the non-refundable reality hits, and taxpayers can only use the credit if they have federal income tax liability.

As Collins explains, "Some families may not owe income taxes the year that they adopt, which leaves them without a tax bill from which their adoption costs are then subtracted. Or they may owe less in taxes than the value of the tax credit. They are allowed to spread the credit out over a few years but might not ever get the full value."

Where Things Are Heading

The Adoption Tax Credit Refundability Act of 2021 (S. 1156) is currently being considered by a Senate committee, but there has been no call to vote on the bill as of this writing. Because this is a federal bill, infertility warriors across the country should reach out to their senators to draw their attention to the issue.

LGBTQ+ Issues

In many states, the right to build a family is not protected for members of the LGBTQ+ community. Legal complications can make it harder or impossible for these infertility warriors, who need to use assisted reproductive technology or surrogacy, to become parents.

Current Legislation

There's a lot of variation between states, but, for example, multiple states don't allow gestational surrogacy. This automatically prevents many same-sex couples from having biological children and legally securing their parental rights to those children.

Where Things Are Heading

All allies should speak up for LGBTQ+ rights, including those related to infertility. The more legislators hear about these issues and *all* the people they impact, the more positive change we'll see. To keep track of the latest issues involving LGBTQ+ infertility warriors, check out the Family Equality Council's website.

How Legislation Becomes Law

While I love *Schoolhouse Rock!* as much as the next person, "I'm Just a Bill" does leave out a few key details about how laws are made. There are slight variations between states, so let's focus on the federal legislative process.

Writing and Presenting Legislation

Both senators and representatives can write new laws. Their ideas about legislation are influenced by what they hear from their constituents, which is why it's so important for you to contact your congressional representatives. In theory, they want to make you happy so you'll reelect them—and thus will pay attention to issues that matter to you.

The author of the legislation in the initial stage is called its sponsor. Once a bill is presented to either house, other congressional representatives can become co-sponsors of the bill to show their support. But at this point, the bill's sponsor gives it life.

Both the House of Representatives and the Senate set aside specific times when members can introduce legislation. (Fun fact: Bills introduced in the House of Representatives go in a box called the "hopper.") Typically, sponsors have 5 minutes to explain their bill and why it's important. After a bill has been introduced, the Speaker of the House or presiding Senate officer assigns it to the appropriate committee for review.

Congress convenes in sessions; unfortunately, if action isn't taken on a bill before the end of the congressional session in which it is introduced, the bill dies or needs to be rewritten and reproposed.

Committee Discussion

Governmental committees, like the Committee on Veterans' Affairs or the Budget Committee, discuss relevant legislation, among other things.

There are more than twenty committees in both the Senate and the House of Representatives, each with a different area of responsibility. After receiving a bill, they'll set a time to discuss it. If the committee decides to act on the bill, they'll take it through the following steps:

Discussion. Members consider the merits of the bill and whether it's worth moving forward.

Possible assignment to a subcommittee. Yes, there are *Inception* levels of hierarchy in Congress. When a bill is particularly niche, the appropriate subcommittee will take it over.

Hearings. In order to understand all the relevant intricacies, the committee may hold hearings to get information from experts. For example, with a bill related to infertility, the committee might call in doctors to learn more about it so they can decide what to include.

Subcommittee reports. If the bill went to a subcommittee, that's who will conduct the hearings. Once those are complete, the subcommittee reports its findings to the full committee.

Committee vote. The committee votes on the bill. If the vote passes, the bill continues on its journey. If it doesn't, the bill might be dead or further hearings and discussions will be called.

Mark-up sessions. At this time, committee members may make revisions or amendments to the original bill before taking it to the floor.

Taking Legislation to the Floor

After being approved by a committee, the bill is scheduled for discussion in front of the entire Senate or House of Representatives. When the bill reaches "the floor," it's up for debate. This is when things vary between the two houses of Congress.

In the House of Representatives, the debate is dictated by the guidelines of the Rules Committee. The sponsoring committee guides the debate, but both proponents and opponents of the bill are given equal time. Any proposed further amendments have to be germane—or relevant—to the bill. If there's a quorum present on that day, a vote will be called.

In the Senate, the debate is surprisingly a little like the Wild West. There are no limits on the amount of time a senator can hold the floor to debate a bill. What they say or add to the bill does not have to be germane. In fact, entire other bills can become riders—or amendments—to the bill on the floor. Senators opposed to a bill can filibuster, or essentially talk about whatever they want for hours to delay or prevent a vote.

In both houses, if the bill passes, it is sent to the other chamber, where the bill starts over with its respective committees. If it doesn't pass, the bill is dead.

Conference Committee

If a bill passes in both houses, it goes to the conference committee. These committees typically comprise senior members from both houses of Congress who iron out the final details. Remember, when the bill works its way through the second house, those members can make changes. It's the conference committee who works out a compromise between the two versions of the bill.

The conference committee writes a report about any changes it has made and sends it to both the House of Representatives and the Senate. If both houses approve the reported changes, the bill goes to the president.

Presidential Review

Once the president gets the bill, one of three things happens:

It's signed. The president has 10 days to review and sign the bill. Once he or she does, it becomes a law. Interesting twist: If the president *doesn't* sign the bill within those 10 days *and* Congress is in session, the bill becomes law anyway.

It's not signed and becomes a pocket veto. This is what happens if Congress adjourns before the end of the president's 10 days. While the president hasn't officially vetoed the bill, it's not a law and Congress will have to start the process *all over again* once it is back in session.

It's vetoed. The president vetoes the bill, and he or she can send the bill back to Congress with notes about why.

Overturning a Veto

The bill goes back to the branch of Congress in which it originated. The senators or representatives are then faced with a decision: scrap the bill and start over, or attempt to overturn the veto with a vote. If two-thirds of the originating chamber vote to override the veto, it goes to the other house. If the bill also achieves a two-thirds majority in the second house, the bill becomes a law. In the history of the United States, only 112 bills have become law after being vetoed by the president.

Communicating with Legislators

There are many ways you can communicate with your representatives to inform them about the issues that are important to you, like infertility. You can make suggestions for new laws or just let legislators know how you want them to vote on proposed bills.

As Fankhauser points out, there's one common factor behind all the current infertility-related insurance laws: the legislator who sponsored the bill was informed about the need. "Individuals like you and me educated the legislative leaders," she says. "Through lobbying, advocating, educating, whatever verb you prefer, it has been the desire to take action that evolves a vision into reality." Here are some steps inspired by advice from the ACLU (see pages 442–445). Their website is also a great resource for advocates.

Written Communication

While many of us have forgotten, there is power in a letter written on actual paper. Maybe it's the extra time and effort sending a letter requires. Or maybe it's seeing an actual person's signature. But letters to representatives hold weight. A letter is preferred, as email tends to be sent automatically to a system that responds with a form e-response and is not likely to be read by a real person. You can find good tips on writing your elected official on the American Civil Liberties Union (ACLU) website.

When Katie attended her first Advocacy Day, she brought with her stacks of letters from people in her infertility support network. "I gave these staffers piles of letters, and that indicated to them that this is not just an issue that I'm telling them about. It's an issue that's important to all these people represented in these letters," she recalls. "You just saw the look on their faces when I plopped this pile of papers on their desk. And it was representative of the voices that I carried there. It was just really powerful and the coolest thing I did on Advocacy Day."

However, there's an art to writing a moving and cohesive letter. By breaking down the process, you can ensure you balance both the elements of your story and the facts about infertility.

Step 1: Gather all available information. Legislation is written using complicated language, and there's a lot to dig through to ensure you understand the issue. While organizations like RESOLVE serve as a great starting point for your research, look for additional reliable information.

Be sure to compile the following:

The timeline for the bill. Has it just been proposed? Is a vote right around the corner? Has anyone even written a bill to address this issue yet? Where the bill is in the legislative process will determine what you're asking your representative to do.

BUSTED

Myth: I'll be judged for my choices.

All through your infertility journey, you're forced to make difficult decisions. It's understandable that you might be worried that when you share your story, your listener will judge your choices. But know that this is rarely the case.

"In my experience, advocates usually are received very warmly. Most legislators and policy makers are interested in their personal experiences, and many can empathize," says Reinecke.

And don't be afraid to reach out to a representative if they weren't supportive of infertility legislation in the past. Just because they didn't vote for a bill that would help the infertility community doesn't mean they aren't concerned about the issues. Legislation is complicated, and it's not uncommon for infertility to be a part of much more involved bills. Your representative might have been opposed to other aspects of the bill.

"But even if it was an infertility bill on its own, sometimes there's just a small portion of the bill they don't agree with. It prevents them from supporting the entire thing," explains Fankhauser. "So, they may support the cause. It just might be a problem with that particular bill."

Previous laws that set precedents. Because creating a law is a long, arduous process, representatives like to know that other similar laws have been effective in the past. This lets them know success is possible. It also informs how they write legislation and make their argument in Congress.

The latest research on the topic. This can include scientific research, articles that were recently published in peer-reviewed journals or respected mainstream media outlets, and data about the number of people the issue impacts. Focus on *credible* sources (and no, Wikipedia does not count).

How your story (or that of someone close to you) ties into the issue. Representatives love to hear about the human side of legislation. Telling a true story reminds them they represent real people. Fankhauser recommends gathering pictures or documentation that support your story.

Step 2: Select your key points.

Both infertility and legislation have many layers. It's impossible to cover all aspects of the issue in one letter. You need to focus on what's most important and relevant to *you*. Identify which points of your argument for or against a bill are most pertinent, urgent, and emotionally relatable.

Step 3: Identify and research your representatives.

This goes beyond looking up your state and federal officials. It's also important to look at your representatives' voting histories on past infertility-related and similar legislation.

If they've been an ally in the past, thank them and encourage them to continue fighting the good fight. If they haven't voted in a way that helps infertility warriors, think of ways you can change their mind. Many advocates

find that the best approach is sharing their story and explaining how the proposed legislation could have impacted their life—positively or negatively—if it had been passed during their infertility journey.

Step 4: Write your letter.

Actually, write multiple versions of your letter. It's not uncommon for emotions to surface during your first draft, making your words less cohesive.

Be sure it sounds like you. Yes, you are addressing an elected official. But that doesn't mean you need to fill your letter with legal and political jargon. When you write in a way that reflects your personality, representatives will be more likely to see the human aspect of the issue.

Be sure it makes sense. Unless they're trained writers, many people tend to write points and ideas as they come to them. However, this isn't how a reader processes information. To truly sink in, a letter needs to present information in a logical order and to flow in a way that connects the points and works toward the conclusion you want your reader to reach.

Take a break before sending the letter. Fresh eyes often spot mistakes you missed while writing a letter. Step away from your letter for at least 15 minutes—maybe even a day or 2—so your mind can reset for a final review. Additionally, consider asking one or more people to review it before sending it.

Fankhauser says it's also important to try to build a relationship through your letter. "In your opening paragraph, introduce yourself. If you are a constituent, indicate the town or precinct where you live. If you have heard your legislator speak on an issue or met them at an event, remind them of the meeting," she advises.

Step 5: Send and track your letter.

This one is simple: Send the letter via a method that allows you to track whether and when it arrives at your representative's office.

In-Person Communication

Meeting with your representative in person allows them to put a face to the issues. It forces them to realize that real people are being hurt because of the current legislation—or lack thereof. Yes, letters matter and make an impact, but as Fankhauser points out, in-person meetings take advocacy to another level.

"Legislators appreciate learning the stories of their constituents and find it easier to relate to them on a personal level, rather than a form letter," she says. "Legislators have told me over and over again, through our research and just through conversations, that one phone call or meeting from a constituent means more than two hundred written letters."

Having a real conversation allows your representatives to hear the emotion in your voice, making a deeper connection. They can also ask you questions so they can fill in their own gaps in knowledge.

Steps 1 and 2: Gather all available information and select your key points.

These are two separate steps, but I've combined them together here because, for the most part, the process is the same as when you're writing to your legislators. You're going to sift through credible sources to find the most salient information.

The main difference here is to consider how to commit relevant points to memory. If you're a nervous public speaker or have trouble keeping statistics straight in your mind, you might want to focus on simpler—but still important—points. Of course, you can bring printed notes with you. But for the most part, meeting in person is about having a natural conversation, not delivering a speech to your representative.

Also, think about which articles or studies you might want to bring to give to your representative. You don't want to overwhelm them with homework, but it helps keep them informed. "While it is important to get personal, you should always include evidence-based information to support your argument," says Fankhauser. "Provide results of studies, examples from other states, or even testimony from experts in the field."

Step 3: Identify your representatives and schedule the meeting.

It might seem unlikely that an elected official will have time to meet with you. But remember, you are one of their constituents. For all intents and purposes, you are their boss. That's not to say you should be pushy about demanding a meeting, but it should give you the confidence to schedule a meeting with your representative or a member of their staff.

Look up who your representatives are online. Then send an email or call to schedule a meeting using their official webpage and contact links. Some representatives have their own websites with a built-in scheduling tool.

Step 4: Make your pitch.

You and your representatives are likely strangers to each other. This can make sharing your story and making your pitch in person feel awkward and difficult. Try to start out with a simple way to get on a level playing field.

Collins recalls the trick of a longtime infertility advocate: "She used to walk into a lawmaker's office and look for a family photo on the wall or in a frame. She would point to it and say, 'This beautiful family that you love so much? That's all we want.'"

This quick connection to their own personal life changed the conversation for legislators. It reminded them that infertility advocates aren't asking for something exorbitant. They just want a chance to build a family.

Always remember to let your legislators know where you live so they know which area of their district you represent. And even though you're having a conversation, you need to have a clear "ask."

"Do you want them to sponsor a bill?" says Fankhauser. "And if you want them to write a bill, give them an example of a bill. That way they don't have to create one on their own. Do you want them to support a bill? Do you want them to protect their constituents by opposing a bill? Do you want them to get information for you?"

Be specific so they can be honest about whether they can do what you'd like.

Step 5: Follow up.

This is a step many forget. Etiquette suggests you send a thank-you note to your representative after your meeting. But this is also your chance to remind them of what you discussed. Don't rehash every point, but express gratitude for their time and repeat your overall request.

"Ask for a copy of their business card and ask if it is okay to follow up within 2 weeks," says Fankhauser. "Then do it. Legislators and staff can meet with hundreds of people each week on issues across the board. A friendly reminder will help keep your issue at the forefront."

Other Ways to Get Involved

Now that you know the overall process of creating legislation and advocating, what's next? Where do you start?

Everyone's advocacy path is different. To give you an idea of your options, we're going to use the issue of insurance coverage to see what you can do in addition to contacting your congressional representatives directly.

State Level

Collins says RESOLVE can always use help identifying new legislation to put on the organization's radar. Don't feel intimidated—you don't have to be a legal expert or thoroughly review the bill.

"Every year, we have to keep our eyes open for bills that could hurt or possibly help fertility treatment in the states. And we're always looking for volunteers who are there in the states that had issues to keep us up to date," she notes.

National or Federal Level

"The best way, hands down, to be an infertility warrior at the federal level is to participate in Advocacy Day in Washington, DC," says Collins. "On that day, RESOLVE and ASRM convene the infertility community—mainly patients but also doctors and business professionals—to go to Capitol Hill and advocate for the coverage we and our fellow infertility warriors need."

Advocacy Day occurs every year in May. RESOLVE can help you and will schedule times for you to meet with your representatives (in person or virtually). They'll also make sure you are set up for success by providing talking points and understandable descriptions of the bills and their consequences.

Each year the organization focuses on a different infertility-related issue. "Recently, we've advocated for the VA to provide IVF for wounded veterans; to keep and improve the adoption tax credit; to have the CDC issue a national action plan about infertility—and we've had a lot of success on these issues," says Collins.

Sue from Michigan started going to Advocacy Day in 2017 and says she'll never miss another one. "I was empowered beyond belief," she shares. "It was an incredible experience to lobby Congress and be a voice for the infertility community. It has altered my relationship with infertility."

Advocacy Outside of the Legislative Process

Not all advocacy is about creating or changing laws. Changing people's understanding of infertility and erasing the stigma that surrounds the topic is also necessary.

Share Your Story

For many infertility warriors, sharing their story is not easy. Infertility involves a lot of personal information and emotionally charged events. But when no one talks about it, those outside the community cannot become educated.

"I've really begun caring more about what people go through behind closed doors because we're all fighting a battle. Whatever it is, we're all fighting something, and I think that we need to be more open about that," says Abbey from Wisconsin.

Also, remember that there is strength in numbers. It's easy to sweep a topic under the rug when you think it doesn't impact that many people. "We are all in this together. The more we communicate to each other about our experiences, the stronger we can become," says Krista from New Jersey.

Here are a few ways you can share your story in a way that works for you:

Talk about your journey. Simply being open with others about your infertility can create moments for advocacy on an individual level.

Connect through social media. Use #infertility or #IFAdvocacy when telling your story or sharing information about infertility online. This will help others in the community find your posts.

Join a support group. Yes, a support group can help you work through your difficult times, but it can also help you become an advocate. When you tell your story, others feel less isolated.

Plus, you're teaching others about different aspects of infertility. They might become curious about a treatment you went through and feel empowered to ask their doctor about it.

Become a media spokesperson. If you enjoy public speaking, you can work with organizations like RESOLVE to become a resource to the media when they are looking for perspectives on infertility issues.

Start a blog. I'm sure you've spent hours reading other infertility warriors' stories online or listening to them on podcasts like *Beat Infertility*. Think about how much that helped you. Start your own blog and share your story. Or if you're short on time, offer to write a post for existing infertility blogs.

Volunteer

There are plenty of organizations that focus on advocacy outside of legislation. RESOLVE has volunteer opportunities that involve fundraising, building a support network, and running a helpline (866-NOT-ALONE) to provide caring listeners for those who are struggling.

Collins recommends emailing RESOLVE to find out what volunteer positions fit best with you. "Sending a note is a great way to introduce yourself. You can start a dialogue about what you're interested in doing, and RESOLVE can tell you what its needs are."

You can also always determine if your fellow infertility warriors need help making their lives easier. Ask if someone could use a homemade dinner after a failed cycle. Offer to role-play with a warrior so they can practice asking their boss for time off for treatment. Give recommendations about doctors, treatments, and other infertility support providers you've encountered.

Educate the Private Sector

Sometimes companies do the right thing not because the law requires them to but because they care. When it comes to issues like insurance coverage, employers can choose to support infertility warriors.

"More and more, private employers are voluntarily adding infertility coverage to the benefits they offer their employees," says Collins. "And do you know what makes them decide to offer it? Someone asks them. That's it."

If you want better benefits, talk to your employer or HR department. Explain why the current situation isn't working for you and what changes would offer the support you need (see chapter 19).

Advocacy Dos and Don'ts

Advocacy—for both yourself and others—is one of the hardest skills for infertility warriors to learn because, for the most part, we are people pleasers. We don't want to go against the norm. But the very idea that there is a "norm" is a huge factor in the difficulty of the infertility journey.

Most people expect that they'll have kids. Most people expect that *other* people will have kids. So not having children can make you feel like an outlier. Needing extra help or medical intervention to conceive can make you feel "less than" people who easily conceive on their own.

But it's through advocacy that we change the conversation about what is normal and how we approach infertility as a society. Knowing what works and what doesn't will help you seize advocacy opportunities.

Do show up.

This is the first step. Show up to advocacy events and be present for the infertility community. As Collins reminds us, there is power in numbers. "Just showing up is a big chunk of being a successful advocate," she says.

Sue points out that showing up when we're in a good place allows us to represent those who can't advocate for themselves on a large

stage. "Many people who are in the throes of infertility do not have the time, energy, or financial resources to go to Washington, DC, to lobby Congress," she explains. "If you have the opportunity to become an advocate, seize it. You will be the voice for the one in eight who are struggling with infertility. That's empowering!"

Don't let opportunities to educate go by.

When everyone you meet asks when you're going to have children, it can seem pointless to try to educate all of them about how hurtful that question can be. Does the level of energy you exert explaining infertility really lower the frequency of these hurtful—but common—inquiries? In the big scheme of things, yes.

"There isn't a societal norm for infertility," says Angela from Missouri. "People don't know when they've stepped in something. We have an opportunity as individuals to decide and craft what that norm is. You control the narrative and the dialogue, and I would encourage you to act with courage and act often when a situation or conversation doesn't feel right or allows misunderstandings to persist."

For me, every time a reporter contacts me to request an infertility-related interview, I jump at the chance. If the resulting article educates or changes the mind of just one person, it will have been worth my time.

Do use advocacy as a way to heal.

Hope and advocacy go hand in hand. In both cases, you believe in a better future *and* that your actions can impact that future. But with advocacy, you see an even bigger picture that can help you work through issues surrounding your individual infertility.

"Being an advocate for other people has been very healing. I think the best part for me has been helping other people on this journey," says Mindi from Ohio.

Even when you're still in the middle of your journey, advocating can give you that sense of success that has so often eluded you. As Katie explains, becoming an advocate helped nourish her hope and encouraged her to keep moving forward. "Part of advocating for others is having other kinds of success," she says. "If it is my hope to eventually have a family with children in it, then I'm going to make that happen anyway that I can." (Not too long after Katie provided this quote, she became pregnant and gave birth to her son.)

Advocating for others also helps you reclaim the control infertility stripped away. For many warriors, this is a huge and empowering step. "You're doing something other than feeling helpless," says Fankhauser. "You're no longer a victim of your infertility. You are taking action. You are doing something to make your life better and to help create this awareness."

Don't give up.

Take a moment to think back to our discussion of how legislation is passed. Did anything about that process seem speedy? Change takes time, and even when there are positive outcomes, we have to stay vigilant for threats that can lead us backward. But according to Crystal from Colorado, whose husband sustained injuries in the military that resulted in infertility, the fight is worth it. "Never give up," she says. "Because of advocacy work, there is now temporary partial coverage for service-connected infertility. This is a small victory, but if we stand together, there will continue to be bigger victories. Reach out to your local and national legislators to make your voice heard!"

However, remember to persevere with respect and politeness. As Fankhauser points out, you should never argue or lose your temper with a representative or their staff. This will just get you a bad reputation. "If they don't agree with your advocacy—and there are a lot of people who do not agree with infertility benefits—just learn from it and use that information to further your cause," she advises.

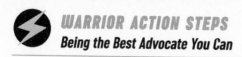

WARRIOR ACTION STEPS
Being the Best Advocate You Can

Every version of advocacy is awesome, but for you to get the most out of being an advocate, you need to find what form of advocacy might fit you best and be most fulfilling. You can do that in the following ways:

Take stock of your skills. Make a list of your skills and interests and assess how they can be of best use. If you're an artist, volunteer to design flyers for advocacy events. If you're a great listener, sign up with RESOLVE's hotline. You're aiming to find a way to get involved that makes you feel empowered and strong.

Continue to keep track of your journey and your feelings. Over time, you'll begin to view the history of your infertility journey differently, giving you new perspectives as an advocate. This will change how you tell your story and advocate for change. Don't assume what you do or say now will be the same in 5 years.

Celebrate your victories publicly. First off, you deserve this! Whenever your advocacy leads to positive change, go scream it from the rooftops. But also remember that the goal is to get everyone to step up and be an advocate. When you share your victories on social media or in your infertility support groups, you show others what's possible. This can help them on their journey and give them hope that they, too, will have the strength to advocate someday.

WARRIOR WISDOM
Changing the Conversation

"Advocacy, I think, can really make a material difference in a person's sense of hope. When I went from fighting for myself to fighting for everyone, it was an incredibly powerful change for my life." —Lee Rubin Collins, board member, RESOLVE

WARRIOR CHECKLIST
Advocating for Fertility Benefits and Other Warriors

❏ Understand why it's important to advocate for others in the infertility community and how you can do so effectively.

❏ Know how current legislation impacts the infertility community and what the issues are.

❏ Learn how laws are made or changed.

❏ Know the best ways to communicate with your representatives, both in writing and in person.

❏ Explore other ways to advocate outside of legislation.

❏ Use advocacy as a way to feel empowered and stronger than infertility.

Add more items to your Warrior Checklist or jot down any notes here:

_____

_____

_____

Diagnoses Appendix

What follows is an extensive list of conditions and diagnoses that can lead to infertility. I suggest reading through each one, even if your doctor hasn't mentioned it. If the listed symptoms of a particular condition are a potential fit with your experience, I hope you feel empowered to initiate a conversation with your doctor. Each entry includes a brief description of the condition, possible causes and symptoms, how it's diagnosed (some of these tests will have been covered in chapter 3), and how it might be treated and approached by your doctor. There won't be answers for everyone here, but I hope for some this appendix offers a missing puzzle piece.

Female-Factor Infertility Diagnoses

Female-factor diagnoses fall under one or more of the following broad categories:

Autoimmune Conditions

Antinuclear Antibodies (ANA)

Antibodies, which are supposed to attach to foreign or dangerous cells as a signal for the body to remove them, instead attach to a healthy cell's nucleus and may be markers for excessive or inappropriate immune responses.

CAUSE(S):
- Infection and inflammation
- Certain medications, like antibiotics used over a long period of time
- Aging
- Autoimmune conditions, such as lupus and rheumatoid arthritis

SYMPTOMS:
- Repeated fertility treatment failures or recurrent miscarriages due to inflammation around the embryo at the time of implantation or in the placenta after implantation
- Often there are no other signs of an autoimmune condition.

HOW IT'S DIAGNOSED:
A blood test

HOW IT'S TREATED AND APPROACHED:
Your doctor may prescribe prednisone, a corticosteroid, to suppress inflammation.

Antithyroid Antibodies

There are two types of antithyroid antibodies: antithyroglobulin and antimicrosomal. Both attack healthy cells in your thyroid gland. It is estimated that 10 to 15 percent of females have antithyroid antibodies regardless of their thyroid status.

CAUSE(S):
Autoimmune conditions, such as lupus, Graves' disease, Hashimoto's disease, hypothyroidism, Sjögren's syndrome, and rheumatoid arthritis

SYMPTOMS:
- Repeated fertility treatment failures
- Recurrent miscarriages

HOW IT'S DIAGNOSED:
A blood test after an 8-hour fast (you may have to refrain from taking certain medications before the test)

HOW IT'S TREATED AND APPROACHED:
- Your doctor may prescribe prednisone and/or dexamethasone to improve your chances of conceiving.
- High antithyroid antibodies levels could indicate an autoimmune condition and might lead to additional testing.

....

Lupus
A chronic autoimmune disease that impacts 1 out of every 185 Americans, 90 percent of whom are female. It causes inflammation in the skin, joints, blood, and kidneys.

CAUSE(S):
The exact cause is unknown but believed to be associated with a combination of genetics, hormones, immune system dysfunction, infections, and the environment.

SYMPTOMS:
- Joint and muscle pain
- Headaches
- Mouth or nose ulcers
- Persistent low-grade fevers
- Rash across the bridge of the nose and cheeks
- Extreme fatigue
- Weight loss

- Hair loss
- Sun or light sensitivity
- Pain in the chest when breathing deeply

HOW IT'S DIAGNOSED:
- A complete medical history, including any signs and symptoms of lupus
- Blood tests for complete blood count, antinuclear antibodies, and levels of proteins that are not antibodies
- A blood clotting time test
- Urine analysis
- Tissue biopsy

HOW IT'S TREATED AND APPROACHED:
Lupus itself does not cause infertility. Rather, the medications to treat lupus—such as Cytoxan and high doses of prednisone—can decrease fertility. Work with your doctor to determine a dose that keeps your lupus symptoms under control while maximizing your chances of conceiving.

....

Type 1 Diabetes
Your immune system attacks healthy insulin-producing cells in your pancreas. It's rare, accounting for only about 5 percent of diabetes cases.

CAUSE(S):
The exact cause is unknown but believed to be associated with a combination of genetics, immune system dysfunction, and infections.

SYMPTOMS:
- Increased thirst and hunger
- Dry mouth
- Nausea and vomiting
- Stomach pain
- Frequent urination
- Unexplained weight loss despite eating and feeling hungry
- Extreme fatigue

- Blurred vision
- Labored breathing
- Frequent infections of the skin, urinary tract, or vagina
- Hair loss
- Difficulty concentrating

HOW IT'S DIAGNOSED:
A blood test and urine analysis for sugar levels

HOW IT'S TREATED AND APPROACHED:
- Glucose monitoring and insulin administered via injections or an insulin pump
- Your doctor may also recommend IVF with preimplantation genetic testing because type 1 diabetes appears to impact DNA.

Blood Clotting Disorders

Antiphospholipid Syndrome (APS)
Antiphospholipid antibodies (APA) mistakenly attack healthy cells by binding to the cells' membrane. The syndrome is often described as "sticky blood." It causes improper blood flow and can contribute to blood clots. (Technically, this diagnosis could also fall under the autoimmune conditions category.)

CAUSE(S):
Beyond the presence of APA, the exact cause is unknown.

SYMPTOMS:
- Repeated fertility treatment failures
- Recurrent miscarriages due to blood clots forming in the veins or arteries prior to pregnancy or in the placenta after implantation

HOW IT'S DIAGNOSED:
A blood test to check for any of the three APA:
- Anticardiolipin
- Beta-2 glycoprotein I (β2GPI)
- Lupus anticoagulant

To be diagnosed, you need to have had either a previous blood clot or a pregnancy-related problem such as:
- Miscarriage prior to 10 weeks
- Recurrent miscarriages
- A stillbirth after 24 weeks
- Premature birth before 34 weeks due to preeclampsia

HOW IT'S TREATED AND APPROACHED:
- Your doctor may prescribe heparin and/or low-dose aspirin to reduce your blood's stickiness and prevent the likelihood of clots.
- Compression socks also are often recommended.

Factor V Leiden
A genetic mutation of factor V, one of the blood's clotting factors. Can increase your risk of developing blood clots in your veins, or thrombophilia.

CAUSE(S):
- **Genetic.** Inheriting only one copy of the gene mutation only slightly increases the risk of developing blood clots. However, inheriting two copies significantly increases the risk.
- High estrogen levels, both during fertility treatments and pregnancy, may also increase the likelihood of developing factor V Leiden thrombophilia.

SYMPTOMS:
- None, unless a blood clot develops
- Can lead to recurrent miscarriages due to blood clots forming in the blood vessels in the placenta during pregnancy
- In rare cases, individuals inherit both factor V Leiden and the prothrombin gene mutation, which may quicken the onset of blood clots and increase their severity.

HOW IT'S DIAGNOSED:

• Carrier test

• Activated protein C resistance test

HOW IT'S TREATED AND APPROACHED:

• Your doctor may prescribe heparin.

• Fertility treatments without added estrogen and progesterone might be considered, when possible, such as not prescribing hormone-based birth control pills and doing natural cycle IVF.

....

Methylenetetrahydrofolate Reductase (MTHFR) Gene Mutation

Extremely common condition in which the individual cannot convert folic acid or folate (vitamin B_9) into a usable form necessary for development

CAUSE(S):

• **Genetic.** There are two forms of mutations and three possible patterns:

• **C677T heterozygous (one copy of the mutation inherited from one parent):** Between 30 to 40 percent of the population has this particular gene mutation.

• **A1298C heterozygous:** Far less common and found in only 7 to 14 percent of the population.

• **C677T homozygous or one copy of C677T and A1298C (one copy inherited from each parent):** Rare but comes with a much higher risk of active symptoms.

SYMPTOMS:

None. Can increase the risk of:

• Cancer

• Cardiovascular disease

• Folate-related disorders, like spina bifida, in unborn children

HOW IT'S DIAGNOSED:

Carrier test

HOW IT'S TREATED AND APPROACHED:

• The MTHFR gene mutation is highly controversial in the infertility community. When folic acid builds up in the body, homocysteine levels also rise, possibly increasing your risk of a blood clot. Some believe the elevated homocysteine levels caused by the mutation lead to recurrent miscarriages and the risk of preeclampsia, Down syndrome, and other pregnancy-related concerns.

• Avoid folic acid, which is the synthetic form of folate that cannot be processed by individuals with the MTHFR gene mutation.

• Your doctor may prescribe a folate, vitamin B_6, and vitamin B_{12} compound to counteract any potential impacts of the mutation.

....

Protein C Deficiency

An individual who does not produce protein C, which regulates blood clotting, at necessary levels. Although many people have a mild form of protein C deficiency, the less their body makes, the greater their risk of forming a clot.

CAUSE(S):

• **Genetic.** There are 270 different gene mutations that can reduce or stop protein C production. The more mutations an individual has, the more serious their condition will be. The most severe cases occur when an individual has inherited two copies of the mutated genes, one from each parent.

• Blood thinners (warfarin)

• Liver failure

• Vitamin K deficiency

• Blood clots and other clotting disorders

• Removal of the small intestine

• Long-term use of antibiotics

• Certain tumors

• Childhood bacterial infections

SYMPTOMS:

- In the most severe cases, individuals experience blood clotting shortly after birth.

- In mild cases, individuals might not have a blood clot or blockage until puberty.

- Pregnant people are at increased risk of clotting, which can lead to recurrent miscarriages. If a person with protein C deficiency successfully delivers, their risk of clotting further increases after delivery.

HOW IT'S DIAGNOSED:

- A complete medical history

- A blood test for protein C levels

- Carrier test

- To determine if the cause is genetic, family members might also be tested.

HOW IT'S TREATED AND APPROACHED:

- Treatment might depend on whether or not you've previously had a blood clot. If you have or your case is more severe, your doctor might suggest long-term use of heparin.

- Fertility treatments without added estrogen and progesterone might be considered, when possible, such as not prescribing hormone-based birth control pills and doing natural cycle IVF.

Protein S Deficiency

An individual who does not produce protein S, which regulates blood clotting, at necessary levels. Although many people have a mild form of protein S deficiency, the less their body makes, the greater their risk of forming a clot.

CAUSE(S):

- **Genetic.** An individual needs to inherit only one copy of the gene mutation to increase their risk of developing blood clots. However, the most severe cases occur when an individual has inherited two copies.

- Although protein S deficiency is only rarely acquired, rather than being a genetic disorder,

it can develop as the result of another condition like liver failure or vitamin K deficiency.

SYMPTOMS:

- In the most severe cases, individuals experience blood clotting shortly after birth.

- In mild cases, individuals might not have a blood clot or blockage until puberty.

- Pregnant people are at increased risk of clotting, which can lead to recurrent miscarriages. If a person with protein S deficiency successfully delivers, their risk of clotting further increases after delivery.

HOW IT'S DIAGNOSED:

- A complete medical history

- Carrier test

- Protein S antigen test

- Coagulation test

- Factor V Leiden test

HOW IT'S TREATED AND APPROACHED:

- Treatment might depend on whether or not you've previously had a blood clot. If you have or your case is more severe, your doctor might suggest long-term use of heparin.

- Fertility treatments without added estrogen and progesterone might be considered, when possible, such as not prescribing hormone-based birth control pills and doing natural cycle IVF.

Prothrombin Gene Mutation (Factor II)

An individual who produces prothrombin, a blood clotting protein also known as factor II, at higher-than-normal levels. This is the second most common inherited blood clotting condition.

CAUSE(S):

- **Genetic.** An individual needs to inherit only one copy of the gene mutation (to increase their risk of developing blood clots. However, the most severe cases occur when an individual has inherited two copies.

SYMPTOMS:

- In the most severe cases, individuals experience blood clotting shortly after birth.

- In mild cases, individuals might not have a blood clot or blockage until puberty.

- Pregnant people are at increased risk of clotting, which can lead to recurrent miscarriages. If a person with the prothrombin gene mutation successfully delivers, their risk of clotting further increases after delivery.

- In rare cases, individuals inherit both the mutation and factor V Leiden, which may quicken the onset of blood clots and increase their severity.

HOW IT'S DIAGNOSED:

A carrier test

HOW IT'S TREATED AND APPROACHED:

- Treatment might depend on whether or not you've previously had a blood clot. If you have or your case is more severe, your doctor might suggest long-term use of heparin.

- Fertility treatments without added estrogen and progesterone might be considered, when possible, such as not prescribing hormone-based birth control pills and doing natural cycle IVF.

Hormonal Causes

Hyperprolactinemia

A disorder in which your pituitary gland produces excessive amounts of the hormone prolactin, which stimulates milk production. Although prolactin levels should be high during pregnancy and immediately after giving birth, they should remain low (5–40 ng/dL) if you are not pregnant.

CAUSE(S):

- A benign tumor on the pituitary gland (most common)

- Hypothyroidism (underactive thyroid)

- Medications you may be taking

- Recent orgasm or nipple stimulation

- Recent exercise

- Long-term consumption of high-protein meals

SYMPTOMS:

- Irregular periods

- Milk production when not pregnant

HOW IT'S DIAGNOSED:

- A blood test, typically after an 8-hour fast

- If your prolactin level is high, additional tests—including a blood test for thyroid levels, computerized tomography, and magnetic resonance imaging—may be performed to try to determine the cause.

HOW IT'S TREATED AND APPROACHED:

- Depends on the cause. If, for example, the cause is an underactive thyroid, a thyroid medication will be prescribed. If the cause is a pituitary gland tumor, a medication to shrink the tumor will be prescribed. If the medication doesn't work, surgery might be required.

- There is no cure, so once medication is stopped, surgery is unsuccessful, or if the tumor reappears in the future, high prolactin levels and corresponding symptoms will return.

Hyperthyroidism

Also known as an overactive thyroid, a condition in which your thyroid gland produces too much of the hormone that regulates how your body uses energy. Occurs in slightly more than 2 percent of people diagnosed with infertility.

CAUSE(S):

- Hyperfunctioning thyroid nodules

- Graves' disease

- Thyroiditis

SYMPTOMS:

- Sudden weight loss

- Sweating

- Rapid or irregular heartbeat
- Trouble sleeping
- Associated with an increased risk of miscarriage, preeclampsia, poor fetal growth, premature birth, and stillbirth
- Can reduce sperm count in men

HOW IT'S DIAGNOSED:
- A complete medical history
- Physical exam
- Blood tests that measure thyroxine and thyroid-stimulating hormone (TSH) levels. A high level of thyroxine and low level of TSH indicate an overactive thyroid.

HOW IT'S TREATED AND APPROACHED:
The specific approach depends on your age, weight, and underlying cause but can include oral radioactive iodine, antithyroid medications (propylthiouracil and methimazole/Tapazole), beta-blockers for the rapid heart rate, and occasionally thyroid surgery.

....

Hypothyroidism
Also known as an underactive thyroid, a condition in which your thyroid gland produces too little of the hormone that regulates how your body uses energy.

CAUSE(S):
- Autoimmune conditions like Hashimoto's disease
- Treatment for hyperthyroidism
- Radiation therapy
- Thyroid surgery
- Certain medications

SYMPTOMS:
- Fatigue
- Increased sensitivity to cold
- Weight gain
- Muscle weakness and aches

- Joint swelling and pain
- Heavier-than-normal or irregular menstrual periods
- Thinning hair
- Reduced heart rate
- Associated with an increased risk of miscarriage, preeclampsia, poor fetal growth, premature birth, and stillbirth

HOW IT'S DIAGNOSED:
- A complete medical history
- Physical exam
- Blood tests that measure thyroxine and thyroid-stimulating hormone (TSH) levels. A low level of thyroxine and high level of TSH indicate an underactive thyroid.

HOW IT'S TREATED AND APPROACHED:
Daily use of the oral synthetic thyroid hormone levothyroxine (Levothroid, Synthroid, others)

Ovulatory Disorders

Anovulation
When a person doesn't ovulate. It's not uncommon to occasionally experience an anovulatory cycle. However, chronic anovulation is understandably an issue.

CAUSE(S):
- Sudden hormone changes
- Body weight that is either too high or too low
- Extreme exercising
- High levels of stress

SYMPTOMS:
Heavy bleeding, similar to a period

HOW IT'S DIAGNOSED:
- Menstrual cycle history
- Blood test for progesterone levels
- Transvaginal ultrasound to examine the uterine lining and ovaries

HOW IT'S TREATED AND APPROACHED:
- If the cause is lifestyle-related, treatment may include regulating eating habits and moderating physical activities.
- If the cause is not lifestyle-related, your doctor may prescribe ovulation stimulation medication, such as Clomid or letrozole.

....

Diminished Ovarian Reserve (DOR)
Lower quantity and/or quality of a person's eggs than is typical. It impacts 10 to 30 percent of people with infertility.

CAUSE(S):
- Lifestyle factors (for example, cigarette smoking)
- Genetic abnormalities (such as fragile X and other X chromosome abnormalities)
- Aggressive medical treatments (such as radiation for cancer)
- Previous ovarian surgery
- Sometimes unknown

SYMPTOMS:
- Often, none
- As the condition worsens, you may notice shorter menstrual cycles.

HOW IT'S DIAGNOSED:
- A transvaginal ultrasound to perform an antral follicle count
- Blood draw on menstrual cycle day 2 or 3 to test follicle-stimulating hormone, estradiol, and anti-Müllerian hormone levels

HOW IT'S TREATED AND APPROACHED:
- Currently, no treatments increase egg quantity. Instead, patients are encouraged to hasten fertility treatments, freeze their eggs for later use, or, in late-stage cases, use donor eggs. Higher doses of ovarian stimulation medication will be needed to support fertility.

- There may be options to improve egg quality. See chapter 7.

....

Hypothalamic Amenorrhea
Menstrual periods and ovulation stop for several months or longer.

CAUSE(S):
A problem with the hypothalamus in the brain. When the hypothalamus reduces or stops the production of gonadotropin-releasing hormone (GnRH), the production of other hormones needed for successful ovulation also reduce or stop.

SYMPTOMS:
Lack of a menstrual period

HOW IT'S DIAGNOSED:
- A blood draw to test for follicle-stimulating hormone (FSH), luteinizing hormone (LH), estrogen, and thyroid hormone levels. Low levels of these four hormones indicate hypothalamic amenorrhea.
- **A "progesterone challenge":** If taking progesterone over a 7- to 10-day period does not induce menstrual bleeding shortly after discontinuing the medication, it indicates hypothalamic amenorrhea.

HOW IT'S TREATED AND APPROACHED:
Ovarian stimulation medications to induce ovulation and restart your menstrual period

....

Oligoovulation
Having infrequent or irregular menstrual periods.

CAUSE(S):
- Polycystic ovary syndrome (PCOS)

SYMPTOMS:
- Eight or fewer menstrual periods a year
- Menstrual cycles lasting 50 or more days

HOW IT'S DIAGNOSED:

- Menstrual cycle history
- Blood test for progesterone, follicle-stimulating hormone, and luteinizing hormone levels
- Transvaginal ultrasound to examine the uterine lining and ovaries

HOW IT'S TREATED AND APPROACHED:

To stimulate your ovaries, your doctor may prescribe Clomid or letrozole. Studies have shown the latter improves pregnancy rates.

....

Ovarian Cysts

Fluid-filled or solid sacs within or on the surface of the ovaries. Many people at some point in their lives develop harmless ovarian cysts without any symptoms. However, some cysts can impact fertility.

CAUSE(S):

- **Cystadenomas.** Cyst-like adenomas that develop on the surface of an ovary and can become very large.
- **Dermoid cysts.** Follicular cysts that have filled with different types of tissue, such as hair, fat, and bone or cartilage.
- **Endometriomas.** A cystic mass arising from a part of the uterine lining that traveled through the fallopian tube and attached to an ovary.
- **Follicular and corpus luteum cysts.** Cysts that occur as a result of the normal ovulation process.
- **Hemorrhagic cysts.** Follicular cysts that have filled with blood.
- **Polycystic ovary syndrome.** See the next section.
- Certain medications, such as Clomid and hormonal birth control, can increase the likelihood of developing ovarian cysts.

SYMPTOMS:

- Abdominal pain
- Irregular menstrual periods or midcycle bleeding
- Abdominal or pelvic swelling or bloating
- Breast tenderness
- Fatigue

HOW IT'S DIAGNOSED:

Transvaginal ultrasound to examine the ovaries

HOW IT'S TREATED AND APPROACHED:

- Endometriomas and polycystic ovaries are most likely to impact your fertility. When your uterine lining sheds each menstrual cycle, so too does the lining found in endometriomas. This can cause damage or scarring that blocks your tubes and interferes with other areas of your pelvic region.
- The other types of ovarian cysts impact your fertility only if they are too large to allow the proper production of a dominant follicle that will ultimately release an egg. Rarely, the ovary can twist if the cyst becomes too large.
- If your doctor determines they need to be removed, ovarian cysts can be drained via a hysteroscopy.
- If you've been taking Clomid to stimulate your ovaries, your doctor may recommend switching to letrozole (see chapter 5) because patients report fewer ovarian cysts—and overall side effects—from the latter.

....

Polycystic Ovary Syndrome (PCOS)

Accounts for 85 percent of diagnosed ovulatory disorders, making it the most common. People with PCOS do not properly metabolize insulin and produce inappropriate amounts of follicle-stimulating hormone, luteinizing hormone, and testosterone and other male hormones. The end result is irregular or complete lack of ovulation.

CAUSE(S):

Not well understood, although there is a genetic component. If your mother or sister have PCOS, you are more likely to develop it.

SYMPTOMS:

- Short or long menstrual cycles (outside the normal range of 25 to 35 days)
- Heavy, absent, or irregular periods
- Acne
- Excessive facial and/or body hair
- Being overweight or obese

HOW IT'S DIAGNOSED:

To be diagnosed with PCOS, you must have at least two of the following:

- Ovulatory dysfunction (irregular periods)
- Polycystic ovaries (fifteen or more cysts on either ovary)
- Excessive androgen levels

Multiple tests are needed, including:

- Complete physical
- Blood test for follicle-stimulating hormone, luteinizing hormone, and testosterone and other male hormones
- Transvaginal ultrasound to examine the ovaries

HOW IT'S TREATED AND APPROACHED:

- Depends on the criteria used to diagnose your PCOS. If you are overweight or obese, losing weight may improve a hormonal imbalance.
- To stimulate your ovaries, your doctor may prescribe Clomid or letrozole. Studies have shown the latter improves pregnancy rates.
- To improve your sensitivity to insulin, your doctor may prescribe metformin, a diabetes drug.
- If you have not conceived via timed intercourse after three cycles on these medications, you should consider IUI or IVF.

Premature Ovarian Failure (POF) or Primary Ovarian Insufficiency (POI)

A condition in which menopause occurs before the age of 40.

CAUSE(S):

- In some cases, unknown
- Exposure to chemicals or medical treatments that damage or destroy the ovaries
- Autoimmune diseases, such as rheumatoid arthritis, genetic disorders, thyroid disease, and diabetes

SYMPTOMS:

- Menstrual period irregularity
- Hot flashes
- Mood changes
- Decreased sex drive
- Vaginal dryness

HOW IT'S DIAGNOSED:

- Complete medical and menstrual period history
- Blood test for high levels of follicle-stimulating hormone
- Immunology testing to search for problems with the thyroid, parathyroid, and adrenal glands that may cause early menopause
- Carrier test
- Chromosome karyotyping
- Single gene test to look for genetic causes

HOW IT'S TREATED AND APPROACHED:

Currently, no treatments are available. Depending on your remaining ovarian reserve, your doctor may recommend IVF with either your own eggs or donor eggs. If using your own eggs, higher doses of ovarian stimulation medication will be needed.

Tubal Conditions

Distal Tubal Occlusion

A blockage of the distal fallopian tube, the section closest to the ovary, where fertilization normally occurs. Can range from mild adhesions to complete blockage that prevents egg pickup from the adjacent ovary.

CAUSE(S):
- Pelvic inflammatory disease
- Appendicitis
- Prior pelvic or lower abdominal surgery
- Presence of foreign bodies in the pelvis
- Endometriosis

SYMPTOMS:
None

HOW IT'S DIAGNOSED:
- Sonohysterogram or hysterosalpingogram
- Laparoscopy, if needed

HOW IT'S TREATED AND APPROACHED:
Tubal surgery, which increases the likelihood of an ectopic pregnancy, or IVF

Hydrosalpinx

A fallopian tube blockage occurring only at the distal end. The secretions do not drain out and instead build up and dilate the tube. Can be mistaken on an ultrasound for an ovarian cyst or tumor.

CAUSE(S):
- Adhesions
- Scar tissue
- Endometriosis irritating the fallopian tubes

SYMPTOMS:
None

HOW IT'S DIAGNOSED:
- Sonohysterogram or hysterosalpingogram
- Laparoscopy, if needed

HOW IT'S TREATED AND APPROACHED:
Because hydrosalpinges can adversely impact IVF pregnancy outcomes by as much as 30 to 50 percent, surgical removal of a fallopian tube (salpingectomy) or tubal ligation should be considered before undergoing IVF.

Proximal Tubal Occlusion

A blockage of the proximal section of the fallopian tube, where it connects to the uterus.

CAUSE(S):
- Mucus plugs
- Fibroids
- Endometriosis
- Scarring
- Pelvic inflammation

SYMPTOMS:
None

HOW IT'S DIAGNOSED:
- Sonohysterogram or hysterosalpingogram
- Laparoscopy, if needed

HOW IT'S TREATED AND APPROACHED:
- If only one tube is blocked, your doctor may recommend not treating it at all.
- If the blockage is mild, it can be removed in a doctor's office with a procedure similar to the hysterosalpingogram called proximal tubal catheterization, which is successful 60 to 80 percent of the time.
- If the blockage is a result of severe adhesions, scarring, or endometriosis, your doctor may recommend surgical removal.
- Regardless of the blockage treatment, IVF is the recommended approach.

Uterine Abnormalities

Adenomyosis

The inner lining of the uterus breaks through the muscle wall of the uterus, either in a single location or throughout. It's often initially misdiagnosed as uterine fibroids.

CAUSE(S):

The exact cause is unknown but believed to be associated with various hormones, including estrogen, progesterone, follicle-stimulating hormone, and prolactin.

SYMPTOMS:

- Heavy and prolonged menstrual periods
- Severe menstrual cramps
- Abdominal pressure and bloating
- Sometimes, no symptoms

HOW IT'S DIAGNOSED:

- A complete physical exam
- Transvaginal ultrasound
- Sonohysterogram
- Magnetic resonance imaging (in some cases)

HOW IT'S TREATED AND APPROACHED:

- Depends on your symptoms and how you wish to proceed on your infertility journey
- The only cure is a hysterectomy, which of course eliminates the option of carrying your own child.
- To relieve mild pain, your doctor may prescribe nonsteroidal anti-inflammatory drugs (NSAIDs) to take starting a couple days before your menstrual period begins.
- To temporarily reduce your symptoms in an effort to increase your chances of becoming pregnant, your doctor might recommend birth control pills, an intrauterine device (IUD), an endometrial ablation (minimally invasive procedure that destroys the lining of the uterus), or Lupron (gonadotropin-releasing hormone, or GnRH, agonist that lowers estrogen levels).

Arcuate Uterus

A Müllerian duct anomaly, or congenital abnormality that occurs when the Müllerian ducts do not develop correctly, that results in a mildly variant shape of the uterus. It is the most common Müllerian duct anomaly and the one least commonly associated with infertility.

CAUSE(S):

While in utero, female fetuses have two Müllerian ducts that merge to form one uterus. An arcuate uterus is caused by a failure in this process.

SYMPTOMS:

Often, none, although it is sometimes associated with recurrent miscarriage and premature birth

HOW IT'S DIAGNOSED:

- Transvaginal ultrasound
- Sonohysterogram or hysterosalpingogram
- Hysteroscopy

HOW IT'S TREATED AND APPROACHED:

If an arctuate uterus is diagnosed during a hysteroscopy, your doctor has the option to remove the extra tissue during the surgery since you are already under anesthesia. However, all surgeries have risks, and your doctor may recommend against treatment.

Asherman's Syndrome

Adhesions or scar tissue that form within the uterus and affect the endometrial lining.

CAUSE(S):

- Trauma to the uterine lining from a dilation and curettage (most common)
- Scarring after uterine surgery
- In some cases, unknown

SYMPTOMS:
- A lighter menstrual period or no menstrual period
- Pelvic pain
- Recurrent miscarriages or inability to conceive at all

HOW IT'S DIAGNOSED:
- Hysteroscopy (most common)
- Other diagnostic tests, such as transvaginal ultrasound, hysterosalpingogram, or sonohysterogram

HOW IT'S TREATED AND APPROACHED:
When this type of adhesion or scar tissue is diagnosed during a hysteroscopy, it is typically removed during the surgery since you are already under anesthesia. Afterward, a balloon catheter is typically placed inside the uterus to deliver estrogen therapy in an effort to decrease scar reformation. Unfortunately, recurrence is common.

Bicornuate Uterus
A Müllerian duct anomaly that results in two conjoined cavities and a uterus that appears to be heart-shaped.

CAUSE(S):
While in utero, female fetuses have two Müllerian ducts that merge to form one uterus. A bicornuate uterus is caused by a failure in this process.

SYMPTOMS:
- Second-trimester miscarriages and preterm delivery
- Possible cervical incompetence

HOW IT'S DIAGNOSED:
- Transvaginal ultrasound
- Sonohysterogram, hysterosalpingogram, or hysteroscopy
- Laparoscopy

HOW IT'S TREATED AND APPROACHED:
- It can be addressed via reconstructive laparoscopic surgery, but in most cases, doctors recommend against treatment.
- Instead, you may be advised about cervical cerclage options to keep your cervix closed during pregnancy.

Didelphys Uterus
A Müllerian duct anomaly that results in being born with two uteruses, two cervixes, and in some cases two vaginas. Each uterus has a single horn linked to one fallopian tube.

CAUSE(S):
While in utero, female fetuses have two Müllerian ducts that merge to form one uterus. A didelphys uterus is caused by a failure in this process.

SYMPTOMS:
- Pain during sexual intercourse
- Extremely painful and heavy menstrual periods
- Recurrent miscarriages and premature births

HOW IT'S DIAGNOSED:
- Transvaginal ultrasound
- Sonohysterogram, hysterosalpingogram, or hysteroscopy
- Magnetic resonance imaging

HOW IT'S TREATED AND APPROACHED:
Doctors rarely suggest corrective surgery, although it may help sustain a pregnancy if there is no other explanation for previous miscarriages.

Fibroids
Extremely common tumors of the uterine muscle. Almost always benign (noncancerous), though it is possible for them to be malignant (cancerous). Most are small and/or in areas that do not impact fertility, but their size and location are extremely important. There are three main uterine locations: on the outside surface, within the muscular wall,

and bulging into the cavity. The latter has the greatest impact on fertility.

CAUSE(S):
The exact cause is unknown but believed to be associated with a combination of hormones (estrogen and progesterone) and genetics.

SYMPTOMS:
- Often, none
- Heavy menstrual periods
- Irregular or more frequent menstrual periods
- Pain during sexual intercourse
- Painful bowel movements
- Miscarriages and other complications during pregnancy

HOW IT'S DIAGNOSED:
- Transvaginal ultrasound
- Sonohysterogram, hysterosalpingogram, or hysteroscopy
- Magnetic resonance imaging can be used to distinguish between fibroids and adenomyosis

HOW IT'S TREATED AND APPROACHED:
Large fibroids, or ones that bulge into the uterine cavity, can be removed via laparoscopic surgery. But like all surgeries, approach with caution. There is a risk of postsurgical adhesions and scarring. If your fibroids are small and asymptomatic, most doctors will recommend against treatment.

Mayer-Rokitansky-Küster-Hauser (MRKH) Syndrome

A condition that causes both the vagina and uterus to be underdeveloped or absent, though the patient still possesses a normal female chromosome pattern, ovaries, breasts, and external genitalia.

CAUSE(S):
The exact cause is unknown but believed to be genetic in nature, although most cases occur in patients with no family history.

SYMPTOMS:
- No menstrual period by sixteen years of age
- May have kidney dysfunction

HOW IT'S DIAGNOSED:
- Typically, if you fail to menstruate by the age of sixteen, you will first see a primary care physician, then be referred to a specialist.
- To make the official diagnosis, an abdominal ultrasound, magnetic resonance imaging, and/or laparoscopic surgery will be used.

HOW IT'S TREATED AND APPROACHED:
Although people with MRKH cannot carry a pregnancy, most can still produce biological children using IVF and a gestational carrier.

Polyps

Extremely common overgrowths of the uterine lining. Almost always benign, though it is possible for them to be malignant.

CAUSE(S):
The exact cause is unknown but believed to be associated with estrogen.

SYMPTOMS:
- Abnormal bleeding, such as between menstrual periods
- Repeated implantation failure or early miscarriages

HOW IT'S DIAGNOSED:
- Transvaginal ultrasound
- Sonohysterogram, hysterosalpingogram, or hysteroscopy
- Endometrial biopsy (to collect a specimen for lab testing)

HOW IT'S TREATED AND APPROACHED:
If the polyps are small and asymptomatic, your doctor might recommend a "wait and see" approach. However, most doctors will recommend surgical removal via a hysteroscopy.

Septate Uterus

The most common Müllerian duct anomaly that results in a thin membrane dividing the uterus, either partially or completely.

CAUSE(S):

While in utero, female fetuses have two Müllerian ducts that merge to form one uterus. A septate uterus is caused by a failure in this process.

SYMPTOMS:

- Often, none
- Recurrent miscarriages and premature births

HOW IT'S DIAGNOSED:

- Transvaginal ultrasound
- Sonohysterogram, hysterosalpingogram, or hysteroscopy

HOW IT'S TREATED AND APPROACHED:

When diagnosed during a hysteroscopy, the thin membrane that divides the uterus is typically removed during the surgery since you are already under anesthesia.

Unicornuate Uterus

The least common Müllerian duct anomaly that results in a uterus with a single horn and a banana shape. Many people with this condition also have a second smaller horn that either is solid or has a small cavity with a functioning uterine lining. Occasionally the smaller horn connects to the uterus and vagina.

CAUSE(S):

While in utero, female fetuses have two Müllerian ducts that merge to form one uterus. A unicornate uterus is caused by a failure in this process.

SYMPTOMS:

- People with a horn that contains a functioning uterine lining but does not connect to the uterus and vagina report painful menstrual periods because the fluid has nowhere to go.

- Recurrent miscarriages, premature birth, and stillbirth
- Cervical incompetence
- Overall difficulty becoming pregnant because often only one fallopian tube is functioning

HOW IT'S DIAGNOSED:

- Sonohysterogram, hysterosalpingogram, or hysteroscopy
- Magnetic resonance imaging

HOW IT'S TREATED AND APPROACHED:

- Most doctors will recommend laparoscopic surgery to remove a horn that contains a functioning uterine lining but does not connect to the uterus and vagina.
- Surgical correction of the unicornuate uterus itself is not possible. Instead, you may be advised about cervical cerclage options to keep your cervix closed during pregnancy.

Other Causes

Advanced Reproductive Age

Although not technically a medical condition, age does affect a person's ability to get pregnant, and that ability gradually declines from ages 30 to 35. After 40 years, there is a sharp decline. Miscarriages and chromosomal abnormalities also increase with age.

CAUSE(S):

As you age, you are less likely to ovulate regularly and more likely to have other medical problems, such as endometriosis.

SYMPTOMS:

Increasingly irregular menstrual cycles

HOW IT'S DIAGNOSED:

- A transvaginal ultrasound to perform an antral follicle count
- Blood test on menstrual cycle day 2 or 3 to check follicle-stimulating hormone, estradiol, and anti-Müllerian hormone levels

HOW IT'S TREATED AND APPROACHED:

- Currently, no treatments increase egg quantity. Instead, patients are encouraged to hasten fertility treatments, freeze their eggs for later use, or, in late-stage cases, use donor eggs. Higher doses of ovarian stimulation medication will be needed.

- However, there may be options to improve egg quality. See chapter 7.

Cervical Mucus Hostility

As ovulation approaches, cervical mucus becomes more like raw egg whites in consistency to create an ideal environment for sperm to move through the cervix. Hostile cervical mucus can be thick, dry, sticky, or acidic, or it may contain inflammatory cells or anti-sperm antibodies.

CAUSE(S):

- Hormonal imbalances
- Bacterial or yeast infections
- Previous infections where sperm was either present or involved
- Age and lifestyle factors (smoking, certain medications, etc.)

SYMPTOMS:

Around the time of ovulation, cervical mucus presents as anything other than raw egg whites in consistency.

HOW IT'S DIAGNOSED:

A pelvic exam and/or self-examination by checking the consistency around the time of ovulation

HOW IT'S TREATED AND APPROACHED:

- Depends on the cause. If you've been taking Clomid to stimulate your ovaries, your doctor may recommend switching to letrozole because patients report fewer cervical mucus—and overall—side effects from the latter.

- If your mucus is too thick, your doctor might recommend short-term use of cough medicine containing guaifenesin.

- If your mucus is too thin, your doctor might prescribe a synthetic estrogen and recommend reducing any antihistamine use.

- If you have a vaginal or cervical infection, your doctor might prescribe an antibiotic or antifungal medication.

- If you do not have an infection or anti-sperm antibodies and are trying timed intercourse, your doctor may recommend a sperm-friendly lubricant, such as Conceive Plus, Pre-Seed, or Astroglide TTC.

Endometriosis

A common painful, chronic disease where the uterine lining grows in areas other than the uterus, such as the ovaries, fallopian tubes, bladder, bowel, and other areas in the abdominal and pelvic regions. When your uterine lining sheds each menstrual cycle, so too does the lining found in these other areas. Because the excess lining has no way of leaving the body, the result is internal bleeding and inflammation.

CAUSE(S):

Unknown

SYMPTOMS:

- Pain before and during menstrual periods
- Pain with sexual intercourse
- Fatigue
- Painful urination and/or bowel movements during menstrual periods
- Gastrointestinal problems such as diarrhea or constipation
- In some cases, none

HOW IT'S DIAGNOSED:

- While a pelvic exam and transvaginal ultrasound might be helpful in some cases, the only true way to confirm endometriosis is via laparoscopy. ReceptivaDx, an endometrial biopsy test, may also help with a diagnosis (see chapter 46).

- In the past, physicians classified endometriosis—stages I through IV—based on pelvic adhesions, lesion appearance, and the anatomic location of the disease. More recently, they have begun using the Endometriosis Fertility Index (EFI) to better predict clinical outcomes following surgery.

The EFI rates endometriosis based on a combination of surgical observations and patient history. During surgery, doctors evaluate the patient's fallopian tubes, fimbria, and ovaries on a scale of mild, moderate, severe, or nonfunctional. They also assess factors such as the patient's age, years of infertility, and prior pregnancies. An EFI score of 0 represents the poorest prognosis, whereas 10 represents the best prognosis.

HOW IT'S TREATED AND APPROACHED:
- Depends on the doctor's personal knowledge of and experience with endometriosis. Treatment varies widely, ranging from over-the-counter pain medications like ibuprofen to hormonal therapy like Lupron Depot to stop ovulation to surgical removal via laparoscopy.
- Even when you do not currently have ovarian cysts as a result of endometriosis, the disease tends to degrade the quality—and sometimes the quantity—of your eggs.
- People with a high EFI score (9 to 10) may be advised to start with timed intercourse, whereas all others may be directed toward IVF.
- Although it is possible to conceive a healthy child without IVF, find a doctor who specializes in endometriosis cases to develop the right plan for your specific situation.

....

Luteal Phase Defect
Following ovulation, the uterine lining does not maintain thickness for a normal length of time.

CAUSE(S):
- Insufficient production of progesterone by the ovaries

- Another condition, such as anorexia, endometriosis, excessive exercise, obesity, or a thyroid disorder

SYMPTOMS:
- Frequent menstrual periods
- Recurrent miscarriages
- Spotting or bleeding in between menstrual periods

HOW IT'S DIAGNOSED:
- Transvaginal ultrasound to measure the uterine lining
- Blood test on menstrual cycle day 2 or 3 to check follicle-stimulating hormone, estradiol, luteinizing hormone, and progesterone levels

HOW IT'S TREATED AND APPROACHED:
- If you have an underlying condition causing the defect, treating that condition often resolves the defect.
- If your defect is not caused by another condition, your doctor might prescribe Clomid or letrozole to stimulate your ovaries, a human chorionic gonadotropin (hCG) to inject around the time of ovulation to trigger the release of one or more eggs, and progesterone injections, pills, and/or suppositories following ovulation to support your uterine lining.

....

Recurrent Pregnancy Loss
Two or more failed pregnancies, prior to 20 gestational weeks, that were confirmed by ultrasound.

CAUSE(S):
- A genetic or chromosomal problem with the embryo, anatomic abnormalities of the uterus, uterine fibroids, hormonal abnormalities, infection, antiphospholipid syndrome, and autoimmune conditions
- Untreated medical issues, such as diabetes and thyroid disorders
- Sometimes unknown

SYMPTOMS:
Symptoms will depend on the underlying condition or situation causing the recurrent miscarriages.

HOW IT'S DIAGNOSED:
- Ultrasound—transvaginal during the first trimester and abdominal during the second trimester—to confirm the pregnancy
- Two miscarriages prior to 20 gestational weeks
- To provide further information about the underlying cause, your doctor may order a recurrent miscarriage evaluation and coagulation blood panel.

HOW IT'S TREATED AND APPROACHED:
- Depends on the cause. If it's genetic or chromosomal, your doctor may recommend IVF with preimplantation genetic testing.
- If you have an underlying condition or infection, treating it may resolve the issue.
- If you have uterine fibroids or anatomic abnormality of the uterus, you may need corrective surgery.

Secondary Infertility
The inability to become pregnant or carry to term after previously giving birth, regardless of how you became pregnant in the past.

CAUSE(S):
- Any condition that can cause primary infertility—in other words, every condition discussed in this appendix—can also cause secondary infertility.
- Additionally, secondary fertility may be caused by risk factor changes for you or your partner, such as age, weight, use of certain medications, and complications from a prior pregnancy or surgery.

SYMPTOMS:
Depend on the cause

HOW IT'S DIAGNOSED:
Depends on the cause

HOW IT'S TREATED AND APPROACHED:
Although secondary infertility has too many variables to boil the condition down into a few bullet points, here are some general parameters:
- If you previously had a live birth and now—after a year of trying if you are younger than 35 and 6 months if you are 35 and older—cannot conceive or carry a pregnancy to term, it's time to head to a reproductive endocrinologist.
- If you are older than 30 and have irregular menstrual cycles, painful menstrual periods, or you or your partner have a known condition such as pelvic inflammatory disease or low sperm count, do not wait a year to see a specialist.

Unexplained Infertility
Infertility cases in which current medical science and technology cannot determine a cause of the inability to become pregnant or carry to term after a year of trying for people younger than 35 and 6 months for people 35 and older. Unfortunately, 10 to 20 percent of people struggling with infertility fall in this category after initial testing.

CAUSE(S):
Unknown

SYMPTOMS:
Varies

HOW IT'S DIAGNOSED:
Testing to eliminate other diagnoses

HOW IT'S TREATED AND APPROACHED:
- Educate yourself on the possible diagnoses that could explain your infertility, and seek a second opinion if necessary.
- If doctors truly cannot provide an explanation for your infertility, they will often start with medicated timed intercourse and progress to IUI after three failed cycles.

- If you have three failed IUI cycles, your doctor will likely recommend trying IVF. It's possible your doctor might determine a diagnosis during the IVF process once an embryologist can examine your eggs, sperm, and embryos in the lab.

WARRIOR TIPS

Dealing with Unexplained Infertility
. . . .

Sue recalls, "I suffered from unexplained infertility while my husband pursued his lifelong career aspiration of becoming the captain of a US Navy warship."

If you currently fall under the "unexplained" diagnosis like Sue, don't worry. Reproductive endocrinologist Dr. Edward Marut offers this reassurance: "There is rarely a true 'unexplained' infertility diagnosis. The reason may not be able to be determined or proven, but functional abnormalities are very common and often the easiest treated. Extensive testing has been replaced by logical treatments, during which answers may often show themselves."

Male-Factor Infertility Diagnoses

Male diagnoses fall under one or more of the following broad categories:

- Genetic disorders (page 468)
- Sperm abnormalities (page 470)
- Structural abnormalities (page 472)
- Other causes (page 474)

Genetic Disorders

Cystic Fibrosis

A genetic disorder that coats the lungs in thick, sticky mucus, resulting in chronic infections and decreased ability to breathe over time. Can also impact the pancreas, liver, kidneys, and intestines.

CAUSE(S):

Genetic. Individuals with cystic fibrosis (CF) inherit one copy of the gene mutation from each parent.

SYMPTOMS:

- Persistent cough
- Frequent lung infections
- Wheezing or shortness of breath
- Salty skin
- Poor growth or weight gain despite a healthy appetite
- Bowel issues
- No sperm in the semen due to a blockage or absence of the sperm canal

HOW IT'S DIAGNOSED:

- Carrier test
- Single gene test
- Most often diagnosed at birth, though your carrier status may not be discovered until later in life

HOW IT'S TREATED AND APPROACHED:

- Most males with CF still produce sperm, even though the sperm canal is blocked or missing. A reproductive urologist can surgically retrieve the sperm, which is then injected into eggs during IVF using a process called intracytoplasmic sperm injection (ICSI).
- To avoid passing on the condition, your doctor will likely recommend preimplantation genetic testing.

. . . .

Kartagener's Syndrome

A genetic condition that causes respiratory problems. It involves two main characteristics: primary ciliary dyskinesia (PCD) and situs inversus. PCD is when the hairlike structures (cilia) that line your lungs, nose, and sinuses don't move properly. Situs inversus is when your organs develop on the opposite side from what's normal in your body.

CAUSE(S):

Genetic. Individuals with Kartagener's syndrome inherit one copy of the gene mutation from each parent.

SYMPTOMS:

- Frequent respiratory, sinus, and ear infections and nasal congestion
- Sperm tails may be impacted, resulting in abnormal mobility

HOW IT'S DIAGNOSED:

- Semen analysis
- Carrier test
- Single gene test
- Most often diagnosed at birth, though your carrier status may not be discovered until later in life

HOW IT'S TREATED AND APPROACHED:

- Intracytoplasmic sperm injection (ICSI) during the IVF process eliminates the sperm mobility problem.
- To avoid passing on the condition, your doctor will likely recommend preimplantation genetic testing.

Klinefelter Syndrome

A chromosomal condition that impacts physical and cognitive development. A common cause of male factor infertility.

CAUSE(S):

Chromosome abnormality. The individual has an extra copy of the X chromosome. Some individuals have more than one extra copy of the X chromosome, which may result in more severe symptoms.

SYMPTOMS:

- Symptoms vary depending on the severity but can include lower testosterone levels, small testes, possible breast development, and more.
- Sperm count is very likely to be low or nonexistent.
- Individuals with more severe forms might also have intellectual disabilities, skeletal abnormalities, poor coordination, and severe speech problems.

HOW IT'S DIAGNOSED:

- Semen analysis
- Chromosome karyotyping
- Most often diagnosed later in life once fertility issues arise

HOW IT'S TREATED AND APPROACHED:

- About 20 percent of individuals with Klinefelter syndrome will have viable sperm. In this case, your doctor will likely recommend surgically removing sperm from the testicles and injecting it directly into eggs during IVF using ICSI.
- To avoid passing on the condition, your doctor will likely recommend preimplantation genetic testing.

Polycystic Kidney Disease (PKD)

A genetic disorder that causes noncancerous, fluid-filled cysts to form on the kidneys, enlarging the kidneys and causing them to reduce function over time. There are multiple types, including autosomal recessive PKD (or infantile PKD) and autosomal dominant PKD (or adult PKD).

CAUSE(S):

Genetic. Individuals with infantile PKD inherit one copy of the gene mutation from each parent. Individuals with adult PKD inherit one copy of the gene mutation from one parent.

SYMPTOMS:

- Varies depending on the severity
- Bloated abdomen due to enlarged kidneys
- Urinary tract or kidney infections
- Kidney stones

- Blood in the urine
- High blood pressure
- Kidney failure
- Very likely to have low or nonexistent sperm count due to obstruction of the ejaculatory ducts

HOW IT'S DIAGNOSED:
- Severe cases of infantile PKD are sometimes diagnosed in the womb. After 24 gestational weeks, it's possible to detect enlarged kidneys via ultrasound.
- In less severe cases, an ultrasound does not detect infantile PKD and cysts might not form until after birth.
- Despite the name, adult PKD is present in the womb but often goes undiscovered until later in life via ultrasound, computerized tomography, and/or magnetic resonance imaging once the individual becomes symptomatic.
- Carrier and single gene testing might also be beneficial.

HOW IT'S TREATED AND APPROACHED:
- If a testicular biopsy discovers viable sperm, your doctor will likely recommend surgically removing sperm from the testicles and injecting it directly into the eggs during IVF using ICSI.
- To avoid passing on the condition, your doctor will likely recommend preimplantation genetic testing.

Y Infertility
A chromosomal condition that impacts sperm production. The individual may have low or non-existent sperm count, low morphology, or low motility.

CAUSE(S):
Chromosome abnormality causing deletion of a piece of the Y sex chromosome in regions believed to provide instructions for making sperm.

SYMPTOMS:
- Often, none
- Occasionally, unusually small or undescended testes

HOW IT'S DIAGNOSED:
- Semen analysis
- Chromosome karyotyping

HOW IT'S TREATED AND APPROACHED:
- If a testicular biopsy discovers viable sperm, your doctor will likely recommend surgically removing sperm from the testicles and injecting it directly into the eggs during IVF using ICSI.
- To avoid passing on the condition, your doctor might recommend preimplantation genetic testing.

Sperm Abnormalities

Asthenospermia
Having sperm motility of less than 32 percent. In some cases, sperm motility is simply low. In other cases, sperm are completely immotile.

CAUSE(S):
The exact cause is unknown but believed to be associated with genetics, the man's age, and/or underlying health conditions or lifestyle factors.

SYMPTOMS:
None

HOW IT'S DIAGNOSED:
Semen analysis

HOW IT'S TREATED AND APPROACHED:
Depending on the percentage of motile sperm, your doctor may recommend up to three IUI cycles or immediately proceeding to IVF with ICSI.

Azoospermia

Semen that contains no sperm because of either problems delivering the sperm (obstructive azoospermia) or abnormal sperm production (nonobstructive azoospermia)

CAUSE(S):
Obstructive azoospermia:

- Missing or blocked ducts
- Absence of the tube (vas deferens) that transports sperm for ejaculation
- Ejaculation or emission problems, or others

Nonobstructive azoospermia:

- Genetics/chromosome abnormalities
- Hormonal problems
- Testicular failure
- Varicose veins in the testicles (varicocele)

SYMPTOMS:
Often, none, though that depends on the cause

HOW IT'S DIAGNOSED:

- A complete medical history
- Physical exam
- Blood test to check testosterone and follicle-stimulating hormone levels
- Semen analysis
- Possibly a testicular biopsy

HOW IT'S TREATED AND APPROACHED:

- For obstructive azoospermia, your doctor may recommend surgery. Afterward, many patients go on to achieve pregnancy without assisted reproductive technology. However, if that doesn't work, your doctor will likely recommend surgically removing sperm from the testicles and injecting it directly into the eggs during IVF using ICSI.
- For nonobstructive azoospermia, the treatment depends on the cause. Hormone deficiencies can be treated with medication, which can improve sperm concentration and motility. Varicoceles can be repaired surgically to tie off the impacted vein and reroute blood flow to healthy veins. Many cases will require surgical removal of the sperm from the testicles so it can be injected directly into the eggs during IVF using ICSI. If the cause of the nonobstructive azoospermia is a chromosome abnormality, your doctor will likely recommend preimplantation genetic testing.

Oligospermia

Semen with a low sperm count. Defined as mild (10–20 million sperm/mL), moderate (5–10 million sperm/mL), or severe (0–5 million sperm/mL).

CAUSE(S):

- Genetics/chromosome abnormalities
- Lifestyle factors (smoking, etc.)
- Underlying health conditions, such as varicocele, sexually transmitted diseases, hormone problems, ejaculation issues, and more

SYMPTOMS:
Often, none, though that depends on the cause

HOW IT'S DIAGNOSED:

- A complete medical history
- Physical exam
- Blood test to check testosterone and follicle-stimulating hormone levels
- Semen analysis
- Possibly a testicular biopsy

HOW IT'S TREATED AND APPROACHED:

- Depends on the cause. Varicoceles can be repaired surgically to tie off the impacted vein and reroute blood flow to healthy veins.
- Medications and antibiotics can treat infections and inflammation.

- Lifestyle changes, such as losing weight and stopping drug, alcohol, and tobacco use, may improve sperm count.

- Hormone deficiencies can be treated with medication, which can improve sperm concentration.

- If you're still unable to get pregnant on your own, your doctor might suggest surgically removing sperm from the testicles and injecting it directly into the eggs during IVF using ICSI.

- If the cause of the oligospermia was a chromosome abnormality, your doctor will likely recommend preimplantation genetic testing.

....

Teratozoospermia (or Teratospermia)

Semen that contains sperm with poor morphology, or a higher-than-expected rate of sperm with abnormal shape. Defined as mild (10 to 14 percent with good morphology), moderate (5 to 9 percent with good morphology), or severe (less than 5 percent with good morphology).

CAUSE(S):

The exact cause is unknown but believed to be associated with lifestyle factors, varicocele, and underlying health conditions, such as Hodgkin's disease, celiac disease, and Crohn's disease.

SYMPTOMS:

Often, none, though that depends on the cause

HOW IT'S DIAGNOSED:

Semen analysis

HOW IT'S TREATED AND APPROACHED:

- Your doctor might recommend taking antioxidants, like L-carnitine.

- Depending on the percentage of sperm with good morphology, your doctor may recommend up to three IUI cycles or immediately proceeding to IVF with ICSI.

Structural Abnormalities

Aspermia

Lack of semen, and therefore sperm, with ejaculation.

CAUSE(S):

- Retrograde ejaculation
- Ejaculatory duct obstruction
- Androgen deficiency

SYMPTOMS:

- Lack of semen with ejaculation
- Hazy urine following ejaculation
- Pelvic pain following ejaculation

HOW IT'S DIAGNOSED:

- A complete medical history
- Physical exam
- Blood test to check testosterone and follicle-stimulating hormone levels
- Semen analysis
- Postejaculate urine test
- Magnetic resonance imaging
- Transrectal ultrasound

HOW IT'S TREATED AND APPROACHED:

- Depends on the cause. If the cause is retrograde ejaculation, your doctor may first prescribe some medications focused on constricting the bladder neck during ejaculation, allowing semen to flow into the urethra.

- The next level of treatment might be a bladder sperm harvest, where semen collected in the urinary bladder is collected and then utilized during an IUI or IVF cycle.

- If neither of those methods work, your doctor might recommend a surgical approach: transurethral resection of the ejaculatory duct or recanalization of the ejaculatory ducts.

Cryptorchidism

A condition in which one or both of the testicles fail to descend from the abdomen into the scrotum. Also known as undescended testicles. Approximately two-thirds of cases impact only one testicle.

CAUSE(S):

The exact cause is unknown but believed to be associated with premature birth, low birth weight, genetics, lifestyle factors of the mother during pregnancy, and chromosome abnormality.

SYMPTOMS:

Not seeing or feeling a testicle where you would expect it to be

HOW IT'S DIAGNOSED:

• Usually detected by a doctor at birth. If the problem has not resolved by the time the baby is 4 months old, it will not resolve itself.

• It's also possible for previously descended testicles to retract through preadolescence (retractile or ascending testicle).

HOW IT'S TREATED AND APPROACHED:

• Most often treated surgically before the age of 1.

• If you're an adult with only one undescended testicle, fertility treatments may not be necessary. However, if you have two undescended testicles, chances are high you also have azoospermia and treatment would be approached similarly.

Ejaculatory Duct Obstruction (EDO)

A birth defect in which one or both ejaculatory ducts are blocked. If one duct is blocked, the result will be oligospermia or aspermia. If both ducts are blocked, the result will be azoospermia.

CAUSE(S):

• Müllerian or Wolffian duct cysts

• Inflammation caused by underlying health conditions, such as chlamydia, prostatitis, or cystic fibrosis

• Sometimes unknown

SYMPTOMS:

• Pelvic pain with ejaculation

• Blood in the semen

• Enlarged seminal vesicles

HOW IT'S DIAGNOSED:

• Complete medical history

• Physical exam

• Semen analysis

• Transrectal ultrasound

• Blood test to check testosterone and follicle-stimulating hormone levels

• Further evaluation, including a seminal vesicle sperm aspiration, TRUS-guided seminal vesiculography, and ejaculatory duct manometry, might be needed to make an accurate diagnosis.

HOW IT'S TREATED AND APPROACHED:

Depending on the severity, your doctor may recommend medication first. If that does not improve the blockage, your doctor might recommend a surgical approach: transurethral resection of the ejaculatory duct or recanalization of the ejaculatory ducts.

Epididymal Obstruction

One or both ducts that pass sperm to the vas deferens become blocked, preventing sperm from getting into the ejaculate. If one duct is blocked, the result will be oligospermia. If both ducts are blocked, the result will be azoospermia.

CAUSE(S):

• Birth defect

• Result of surgical error during a hernia or hydrocele repair

SYMPTOMS:

Unexplained pelvic pain

HOW IT'S DIAGNOSED:

- Complete medical history
- Physical exam
- Semen analysis
- Blood test to check testosterone and follicle-stimulating hormone levels

HOW IT'S TREATED AND APPROACHED:

- Your doctor will likely first recommend a testicular biopsy to look for viable sperm. If they are found, the issue is sperm delivery, not sperm production. At this point, your doctor may recommend a surgical bypass of the blockage.
- If you do not want this surgery or the obstruction cannot be bypassed, your doctor may recommend surgically removing sperm from the testicles and injecting it directly into the eggs during IVF using ICSI.

....

Hypospadias

A birth defect in which the opening of the urethra, which carries semen out of the body, is located on the underside of the penis rather than the tip.

CAUSE(S):

The exact cause is unknown but believed to be genetic in nature and is more common among twins and those born to mothers of advanced reproductive age.

SYMPTOMS:

In addition to the abnormal placement of the urethra opening, the penis often curves downward and has a "hooded" appearance because only the top is covered by foreskin, and the individual displays abnormal spraying during urination.

HOW IT'S DIAGNOSED:

- Usually detected by a doctor at birth
- More mild cases might be difficult to identify and thus persist into adulthood. These cases may be diagnosed with an X-ray of the urinary tract, kidneys, and bladder.

HOW IT'S TREATED AND APPROACHED:

- Most often treated surgically before the age of 1.
- If you're an adult with hypospadias, surgery will reposition the urethra, place the opening at the penis tip, and reconstruct the foreskin. Surgical complications are more likely in adults, so discuss the pros and cons with your doctor regarding your specific situation. However, surgical correction should resolve any fertility problems.

Other Causes

Androgen Deficiency (Hypoandrogenism)

When male sex hormones, such as testosterone, fall below levels expected for the individual's age.

CAUSE(S):

- Dysfunction or absence of the gonads (hypergonadotropic)
- Impairment of the pituitary gland or hypothalamus (hypogonadotropic)
- A number of underlying health conditions, such as Klinefelter syndrome and varicocele
- Lifestyle factors
- Certain medications
- Advanced reproductive age

SYMPTOMS:

- Symptoms caused by an underlying health condition
- Hot flashes
- Sweating
- Insomnia
- Decline or loss of sex drive

HOW IT'S DIAGNOSED:

- Complete medical history
- Physical exam
- Blood test to check testosterone, luteinizing hormone, and follicle-stimulating hormone levels

HOW IT'S TREATED AND APPROACHED:

- If the cause is not related to an underlying health condition, your doctor may recommend one of the many forms of testosterone replacement therapy. Typically, you will try this for 3 months, then recheck your hormone levels.

- If the cause is an underlying health condition, the approach will be to treat that specific condition.

Immune System Disorders (Anti-Sperm Antibodies)

When a person has developed antibodies that mistakenly attack their own healthy sperm. Often, anti-sperm antibodies attach to sperm and impact their motility or ability to fertilize an egg.

CAUSE(S):

Infection or physical or chemical injury that results in direct contact between blood and sperm. Once the blood/testis barrier is breached, sperm antigens escape their protected environment and launch an immunological attack.

SYMPTOMS:

Often, none

HOW IT'S DIAGNOSED:

- Semen analysis

- If semen analysis shows the sperm clumping together or other signs of an infection, your doctor may order additional tests, such as a semen culture, prostate fluid culture, urinalysis, and anti-sperm antibody test, which uses either a semen sample, a blood sample, or both.

HOW IT'S TREATED AND APPROACHED:

Your doctor may prescribe a steroid medication to destroy the antibodies. Additionally, the process of sperm washing that takes place during an IUI or IVF cycle can remove the antibodies.

Retrograde Ejaculation

A condition in which semen enters the bladder rather than leaving the body via the urethra during ejaculation.

CAUSE(S):

- Prior prostate or urethral surgery

- Diabetes

- Certain medications

SYMPTOMS:

- Little or no semen with ejaculation

- Hazy urine following ejaculation

HOW IT'S DIAGNOSED:

- Complete medical history

- Physical exam

- Semen analysis

- Postejaculate urine test

HOW IT'S TREATED AND APPROACHED:

- Your doctor may first prescribe some medications focused on constricting the bladder neck during ejaculation, allowing semen to flow into the urethra.

- If that doesn't work, your doctor might recommend a bladder sperm harvest, where semen collected in the urinary bladder is collected and then utilized during an IUI or IVF cycle.

Index

Acknowledgments

Writing a book is an incredible journey, and I am grateful to those who have walked beside me throughout the process. *Stronger Than Infertility* would not have been possible without the support, guidance, and love from those I am honored to acknowledge here.

First and foremost, I would like to express my heartfelt gratitude to my editor, Maisie Tivnan. Maisie, your passion, expertise, and patience have been invaluable in taking this book from a mere vision to a final product that fills me with immense pride. I am truly fortunate to have had the opportunity to work with you. To the entire team at Workman, especially Kate Karol, Barbara Peragine, Janet Vicario, and Analucia Zepeda: Thank you for your commitment to ensuring that *Stronger Than Infertility* shines in every aspect.

My incredible agent, JL Stermer, deserves a particularly special mention for her unyielding faith in this book over the past six years. JL, you have been part agent, part therapist, and part friend, and your guidance has been a beacon of light in this journey. Thank you for standing by me and for believing in the importance of *Stronger Than Infertility*.

To my loving family—my husband, Brett; my daughter, Aurora; and my parents, Bill and Terry—your unwavering support and strength have been the foundation upon which this book was built. Thank you for always being there for me, for providing the encouragement I needed, and for being a constant source of inspiration. Your love has carried me through the challenges and triumphs of writing *Stronger Than Infertility*, and I am eternally grateful.

Finally, I want to extend my gratitude to all those who have shared their expertise, personal experiences, and stories with me. Your knowledge, courage, and resilience have fueled my desire to create a resource that empowers and supports those navigating the complex and emotional journey of infertility. This book is dedicated to you and everyone who has ever felt alone in their struggle.